Patricia J

Low-Calorie
Foods
Handbook

FOOD SCIENCE AND TECHNOLOGY

A Series of Monographs, Textbooks, and Reference Books

Low-Calorie Foods Handbook

edited by

Aaron M. Altschul

Georgetown University School of Medicine
Washington, D.C.

Marcel Dekker, Inc.   New York•Basel•Hong Kong

Library of Congress Cataloging-in-Publication Date

Low-calorie foods handbook / edited by Aaron M. Altschul.
     p. cm. -- (Food science and technology ; 56)
    Includes bibliographical references and index.
    ISBN 0-8247-8812-5
    1. Low-calorie diet. I. Altschul, Aaron M. (Aaron Mayer).
    II. Series: Food science and technology (Marcel Dekker, Inc.) ;
56.
RM222.2.L655 1993
664'.63--dc20
                                                          92-44693
                                                           CIP

This book is printed on acid-free paper.

MARCEL DEKKER, INC.
270 Madison Avenue, New York, New York 10016

Current printing (last digit):
10 9 8 7 6 5 4 3 2 1

PRINTED IN THE UNITED STATES OF AMERICA

To
Sandra, Judy, and Frank
with affection

Foreword

Given today's food environment and sedentary lifestyle, one can confidently predict that, by the time they reach middle age, some 26% of the U.S. population will have become overweight. This outcome (including the adverse effects on health of the overweight condition) seems inevitable unless effective countermeasures are taken on a nationwide basis—a most unlikely contingency.

In the effort to combat overweight and obesity, two ingredients seem to be indispensable: first, a sustained desire to avoid being overweight (for whatever reason) and second, usable knowledge about the strategies that are needed to prevent or treat obesity. If people do not know *how* to control their weight, then even a strong motivation to become slender may be ineffective. On the other hand, it does not follow that, even if people know how to restrain energy intake and increase energy expenditure, they will automatically put this knowledge into practice. There is a sufficiency of overweight nutrition experts and other health professionals to bear witness to this fact.

Although we still have much to learn about how to help vulnerable individuals control self-damaging behaviors such as chronic overconsumption of food, there is no acceptable excuse for leaving people in ignorance about the adverse effects of obesity on health and longevity, or about the food choices that are appropriate if one wishes to consume a prudent diet, namely one that is both health-promoting and enjoyable.

In this *Low-Calorie Foods Handbook*, Dr. Aaron Altschul and a distinguished panel of contributors have assembled a wealth of authoritative information about the options that are now available to consumers who may wish to select low-calorie and low-fat food items in preference to their calorie-dense or high-fat counterparts. The goal of nutritionally tailored products (not necessarily realized in every instance) is to preserve the hedonic satisfaction of eating certain kinds of foods, but at a reduced cost in calories and fat (and often sugar and sodium as well). The *Handbook* examines the extensive repertoire of low-calorie foods and ingredients available (or soon to be available from the food industry) to use in the context of America's preoccupation with the problems of obesity, coronary heart disease, and cancer. Particular attention is given to the ingenious attempts of food scientists to solve the problem of reducing the fat and sugar content of high-calorie foods such as ice cream, cheese, spreads, and salad dressing with a minimum of sacrifice in palatability.

In theory, the systematic use of low-fat, low-calorie substitutes for "regular" foods whose energy density is high should help many people control their weight more effectively. But I suspect that, in some cases at least, these low-calorie analogs do not actually replace high-calorie foods but are consumed *de novo* because the reduced-calorie, reduced-fat label is interpreted as being almost a license to overeat. Paradoxically, this use of products reduced in fat and calories may simply add to the burden of dietary calories already being carried by the would-be dieter, but with a disproportionately small increment in the concomitant burden of guilt often experienced when one's eating control is thought to be compromised. In other words, the fat- and calorie-reduced products that are coming out of the food industry's R&D pipeline in increasing numbers need to be integrated appropriately into an eating policy carefully designed and administered to achieve the consumer's dietary goals, whatever they may be. Thus fat- and calorie-modified food products are not automatically beneficial—they can help or harm, depending on how they are used.

Whatever the case, the information available in this excellent *Handbook* can contribute greatly to the proper use by consumers of the calorie-modified foods appearing in ever-greater numbers in our markets. The members of the U.S. food industry responsible for these innovations are to be commended for their efforts to reduce the calorie and fat pollution that threatens our food environment. Dr. Altschul and those who have worked with him to prepare this valuable reference work deserve our gratitude for providing guidance to help us cope creatively with the long procession of low-calorie newcomers currently making their debuts on our supermarket shelves.

Theodore B. VanItallie, M.D.
Professor Emeritus of Medicine
Columbia University College of
    Physicians and Surgeons
New York, New York

Preface

The invention of new edible materials and new ways of processing existing edible materials to allow the formulation of low-calorie foods may in its totality be regarded as a milestone in the history of foods and food processing. We are witnessing the evolution of a new class of foods and a new purpose for foods: to control overconsumption. It is time to bring together the literature on this subject. But it is also time to stand back and review the rationale for these foods: to review how the public has taken to them, how the public has fared with them, and how health professionals react to them.

This is a book about processed foods that seek to mimic foods already in existence. These foods differ from their "normal" counterparts by containing fewer calories and less sugar and fat per portion. The idea is that consumers will like these foods and beverages enough to substitute them for the normal processed foods, thereby eating fewer calories and less sugar and fat. We describe the low-calorie foods—their history, technology, and prospects. We describe new edible products invented to make sugar and fat replacement possible and yet retain desirable flavor and texture. Meats are included because a serious effort is underway to reduce the fat in meat.

We also examine the social consequences of this very important development. The public considers low-calorie foods a tool to help change diet. Health professionals exhort the public to make changes in diet and lifestyle to lower the prevalence of obesity and to reduce the risk of diabetes and cardiovascular disease. Is the presence of low-calorie foods making a difference in calorie, sugar, and fat consumption? Are there fewer obese among us as a consequence? What action by the food and health communities might be taken to increase the effectiveness of low-calorie foods as engines of change?

The aim of this book, therefore, is twofold. First, we seek to provide a detailed exposition of the foods themselves, the strategies for replacing fat and sugar, and the problems of providing low-calorie foods equally as acceptable as the foods they seek to replace; in doing so, we describe the research underway to broaden yet further the types of foods that can be replaced with low-calorie versions. And, second, we examine the rationale for these foods. Is it sound, how well is it working, and what can be done to make this very successful new food development more useful to those who need it?

Food scientists and technologists seeking to design new fat or sugar replacements or who wish to use existing technology to formulate new low-calorie foods will find this *Handbook* indispensable to their needs. Those in the food industry who make policy should find useful the broadened approach to the low-calorie foods phenomenon as presented here as they seek strategies for the future. And teachers will find the handbook a basis for development of courses on low-calorie foods.

This book is also designed for health professionals of all kinds—those who advise the public about diet in a general way and those who, like primary-care physicians, nutritionists, dieticians, and counselors, make specific suggestions. They need to know about the composition of low-calorie foods and about the safety of their constituents. Those who serve the public in newspapers and periodicals need to know the low-calorie phenomenon from all its aspects as they seek to advise a public confused by the explosive character of this development. And, although this book is not designed for the general public, many may find it useful and interesting.

I acknowledge and thank the following, with whom I discussed this volume and who suggested potential authors: Mark A. Bieber, C. E. Butterworth, Jr., Sidney M. Cantor, Kenneth D. Fisher, Richard R. Hahn, Jules Hirsch, Lyn O'Brien Nabors, and Regina Ziegler.

Aaron M. Altschul

Contents

B. Low-Calorie Foods

C. Impact of Low-Calorie Foods

D. Impact of Diet Composition

E. Reflections

Contributors

Ramin Alemzadeh, M.D.   Department of Pediatrics, The University of Tennessee Medical Center at Knoxville, Knoxville, Tennessee

Aaron M. Altschul, Ph.D.   Departments of Medicine and Community and Family Medicine (Emeritus) and Diet Management and Eating Disorders Program (Emeritus), Georgetown University School of Medicine, Washington, D.C.

William M. Breene, Ph.D.   Department of Food Science and Nutrition, University of Minnesota, St. Paul, Minnesota

Elizabeth R. Burrows, M.S., R.D.   Cancer Prevention Research Program, Fred Hutchinson Cancer Research Center, Seattle, Washington

Floyd Michael Byers, Ph.D.   Department of Animal Science, Texas A&M University, College Station, Texas

Ellen Templeton Carroll, M.S., R.D.   *Cooking Light*, Birmingham, Alabama

Walter L. Clark, Ph.D.   Department of Food Science and Nutrition, Chapman University, Orange, California

H. Russell Cross, Ph.D.* Department of Animal Science, Texas A&M University, College Station, Texas

Adam Drewnowski, Ph.D.   Program in Human Nutrition, School of Public Health, University of Michigan, Ann Arbor, Michigan

Basant K. Dwivedi, Ph.D.   NuGen Foods, Ltd., Paterson, New Jersey

J. P. Flatt, Ph.D.   Department of Biochemistry and Molecular Biology, University of Massachusetts Medical School, Worcester, Massachusetts

Mary M. Flynn, M.S., R.D.   Nutrition Center, The Miriam Hospital at Brown University, Providence, Rhode Island

Amanda M. Frye, M.S., R.D., L.D.   Department of Foods and Nutrition, Kansas State University, Manhattan, Kansas

Robert C. Gatty   Gatty Communications, Inc., Columbia, Maryland

Janet K. Grommet, Ph.D., R.D., C.D.E.   Department of Health and Nutrition Education, Columbia University Teachers College, New York, New York

Kathleen A. Harrigan   Department of Food Science and Nutrition, University of Minnesota, St. Paul, Minnesota

Maureen M. Henderson, M.D., D.P.H.   Cancer Prevention Research Program, Fred Hutchinson Cancer Research Center, Seattle, Washington

Holly Henry, M.S., R.D.   Cancer Prevention Research Program, Fred Hutchinson Cancer Research Center, Seattle, Washington

Peter N. Herbert, M.D.   Yale University School of Medicine, and Department of Medicine, Hospital of Saint Raphael, New Haven, Connecticut

Janet Majewski Jemmott, M.S.   Cortlandt Group, Inc., Ossining, New York

Russell Lemieux   Calorie Control Council, Atlanta, Georgia

Fima Lifshitz, M.D.   Department of Pediatrics, Maimonidies Medical Center, Brooklyn, New York

Current affiliations:
*Food Safety and Inspection Service, U.S. Department of Agriculture, Washington, D.C.

Susan McCann, M.S., R.D.   Department of Social and Preventive Medicine, School of Medicine and Biological Sciences, State University of New York at Buffalo, Buffalo, New York

William T. Miller   The Beverage Research Center, Inc., Columbus, Georgia

Robert H. Moser, M.D.*   The NutraSweet Company, Mount Prospect, Illinois

Lyn O'Brien Nabors   Calorie Control Council, Atlanta, Georgia

Rosetta Newsome, Ph.D.   Office of Scientific Public Affairs, Institute of Food Technologists, Chicago, Illinois

F. Xavier Pi-Sunyer, M.D.   Department of Medicine and Obesity Research Center, Columbia University College of Physicians and Surgeons, and St. Luke's/Roosevelt Hospital Center, New York, New York

Lee Ann Quesada, M.S.   Department of Food Science and Nutrition, Chapman University, Orange, California

D. Elizabeth Randall, Ph.D., R.D.   School of Health Related Professions, State University of New York at Buffalo, Buffalo, New York

Paul Rozin, Ph.D.   Department of Psychology, University of Pennsylvania, Philadelphia, Pennsylvania

Marie Fasano Ruggles, M.S., R.D., C.D.E.   Division of Pediatric Endocrinology and Metabolism, North Shore University Hospital, Cornell University Medical Center, Manhasset, New York

Carole S. Setser, Ph.D.   Department of Foods and Nutrition, Kansas State University, Manhattan, Kansas

Norman S. Singer, Ph.D.   Department of Research and Development, The NutraSweet Company, Mount Prospect, Illinois

Nancy D. Turner, M.S.   Department of Animal Science, Texas A&M University, College Station, Texas

John E. Vanderveen, Ph.D.   Division of Nutrition, Food and Drug Administration, Washington, D.C.

_____

Current affilitation:
*School of Medicine, University of New Mexico, Albuquerque, New Mexico.

James L. Vetter, Ph.D.   Research Department, American Institute of Baking, Manhattan, Kansas

Charles H. White, Ph.D.   Department of Food Science and Technology, Mississippi State University, Mississippi State, Mississippi

Nedra P. Wilson, M.S., R.D.   Department of Nutrition Sciences, University of Alabama at Birmingham, Birmingham, Alabama

Low-Calorie
Foods
Handbook

1
Introduction

Aaron M. Altschul *Georgetown University School of Medicine, Washington, D.C.*

I. THE APPROACH

How do we present low-calorie foods? We surely should present them as examples of sophisticated food technology and of marketing of a new class of processed foods. Look at the record [1]. Alternate sweeteners replace sugar and other caloric sweeteners. New nonsugars provide functional characteristics formerly requiring sugar or other carbohydrates. Fat is no longer an essential ingredient of dairy foods. Fatty spreads and salad dressings "work" with much less fat or with no fat. "Fat feel" without fat is now possible. Indigestible oily materials are under serious consideration as replacements for cooking oil.

Food manufacturers developed marketing strategies for this special class of foods. They created names to differentiate these from their normal counterparts; among them are light, lite, low-cal, low-fat, and less. There is hardly a processed-food category that does not contain its subgroup of low-calorie items.

The pressure continues to improve and expand the list of low-calorie products: more artificial sweeteners to improve taste and safety; more bulking agents to replace sugar; more and better fat substitutes to reduce further the fat content of foods and to extend the low-calorie concept to more products. The pressure continues to reduce cost.

But that is not all there is to low-calorie foods. The public understands them as aids to problem solving, as tools to solve chronic health problems. Obesity and overweight are the most obvious, but cardiovascular disease, hypertension, and diabetes (and incidence of cancer) also respond to diet. Consumption of low-calorie (and low-fat) foods such as skim milk helps to lower fat intake as well as total energy intake. Food companies encourage the public in these expectations by the way that they present the low-calorie foods. This is why the public and the authorities scrutinize more carefully their labeling and presentation.

Do they work? Are the public and public health goals beneficiaries of these activities? This is a question being asked more often. The answer is not easy to come by.

It may help if we try to understand how this situation arose. Why have the fatness, sweetness, and saltiness of our diet increased so dramatically in this century? The answer must lie in a combination of human and environmental factors. Stripped of their great complexities, three factors can be identified: the preference by humans for the taste of foods that are salted, sweet, and fatty; the prosperity and technological advances that made it possible to satisfy such preferences at a reasonable cost; and aggressive marketing of the wide variety of available good-tasting foods. Our society encouraged lack of restraint in the choice of foods as long as they tasted good. It seemed that we achieved the goal of "having our cake and eating it."

Now, it seems that for many, if not most people, it becomes necessary to modify their hedonistic habits for reasons of appearance and health. A tension has been created between the need for restraint and the reluctance to give up the good eating life to which most of us had become accustomed. Some will be able to summon the degree of restraint needed to make the necessary adjustments in their diets (and lifestyles). But many are unable to do so at all or sufficiently well to meet their needs.

The same technology and prosperity that propelled this and other industrial societies into a situation that might be labeled "affluent malnutrition" has now created a new class of foods, low-calorie foods, for the purpose of reducing the restraint necessary to accommodate to the desires for better health and appearance. The new foods are being marketed aggressively, and consumers are responding positively.

It is no wonder that the question of "whether they work" is basic to the low-calorie foods phenomenon and illustrates the close relationship between food technology and public health concerns when dealing with low-calorie foods. Any serious treatment of the subject must include both aspects. This is our perspective.

We will describe the low-calorie foods—their history, marketing, technology, and prospects. We will deal with the targeted health problems, notice the secular changes in dietary habits, and try to assess what low-calorie foods may have contributed to any observed changes. We will describe the problems of utilizing low-calorie foods properly and opportunities yet untapped.

II. HOW THIS BOOK IS ORGANIZED

A. Introductory Section

Chapters 2 and 3 provide the background to the problem of obesity that provides the rationale for low-calorie foods. This is not a book about obesity, but obesity creeps in everywhere in the discussion, hence the need to provide the reader with the opportunity to acquire a background.

Chapter 4 provides a baseline of where we are and where we came from in our eating patterns. Several years hence a similar chapter would show where changes, if any, have taken place, and might suggest how successful low-calorie foods have been in changing eating patterns. Chapter 5 provides the reader with examples of the range of choices available to an individual who wishes to control the level of dietary fat.

These four chapters do not deal with low-calorie foods. But this is what one thinks about when deciding to become interested in low-calorie foods. Low-calorie foods are supposed to help the individual better manage weight and other problems considered under the rubric of overconsumption.

B. Low-Calorie Foods

Low-calorie foods are a subgroup of processed foods. They mimic in appearance, taste, and texture established and accepted processed foods with one difference: the food energy provided per portion or serving is substantially less. Some are truly low-calorie; others are reduced-calorie. Both are included.

These foods permeate the food supply. A catalog would include the following: artificially sweetened beverages with less or no added sugar; artificially sweetened foods and desserts; dairy products containing no fat or less fat than those derived from whole milk; spreads and salad dressings with less fat and no fat; low-calorie frozen dinners, canned foods, and soups; bakery products with less or no added fat; low-fat processed meats; and low-calorie snacks.

When we use the adjective low-calorie, we refer to processed low-calorie foods.

We introduce low-calorie foods with two chapters. Chapter 6 describes the tremendous, even spectacular, growth of this class of products and presents the results of surveys telling why individuals choose to use low-calorie foods. All low-calorie foods must be described on the label and in the marketing statements to provide maximum information to the consumer and avoid confusion. Chapter 7 describes the history of U.S. government regulations relating to these foods and brings the reader up to date on the latest published regulations.

Before it is possible to formulate a low-calorie food or beverage, it is necessary either to remove fat or sugar from the food and hope that it remains sufficiently attractive to the consumer (e.g., skim milk) or to replace sugar or fat or both in a food with new materials, lower in calories, that do the same for the food as expected from the original sugar and fat. The next four chapters deal with these ingredients. Chapter 8 deals with artificial sweeteners. Chapter 11 deals with materials that, in combination with the artificial sweeteners, make it possible to provide sweetness in foods without caloric sweeteners. Fat substitutes are described in Chapters 9 and 10. Some of the same materials described as bulking agents in Chapter 11 with some modification can also be used as fat substitutes.

The low-calorie foods themselves are described in Chapters 12 through 16. The field is changing rapidly, and new foods are announced almost daily. We present examples of the state of the development and some idea of the trends.

We have added meat and poultry products (Chapter 17) to the group of low-calorie foods. These are not considered low-calorie foods, but within this group there is a wide range of fat content and caloric density from bacon or steak to skinless white meat of poultry. Hence, an individual who chooses meat and poultry products with lower fat contents can, in fact, capture the effect of eating a low-calorie food. The trend, as described in this chapter, is to reduce fat content by breeding leaner animals, by feeding and management, and by removing more fat in the plant before the product reaches the consumer.

C. Impact of Low-Calorie Foods

We now turn to the impact of these new foods on aspects of our culture: food marketing, nutrition education, and recipe formulation.

A relatively new understanding in the food industry is that nutrition sells, and this has revolutionized the food-marketing industry, as described in Chapter 18. Nevertheless, taste remains the primary criterion in food selection. It is worth noting that stocking of "healthy" foods varies from store to store and area to area. In stores in the inner city, stocking of "healthy" foods is the exception rather than the rule.

Educators make dietary recommendations based on their knowledge of the prevailing consensus on the relationship between diet and health. They also must accommodate the changing choices presented by new food products. As described in Chapter 19, nutritionists have focused on increasing nutrition information on the theory that this alone would influence attitudes and dietary behavior. But new knowledge does not invariably result in changes in attitude and behavior.

People can consume low-calorie foods directly or incorporate them into recipes. Examples of how low-calorie foods can be incorporated into recipes are given in Chapter 20. A "wish list" of additional products that might make recipe making easier is provided for the attention of food manufacturers.

D. Impact of Diet Composition

The basic assumption of the marketing and presentation of low-calorie foods is that diet composition (i.e., the removal of all or some of the fat or sugar from a common food) by itself will cause a reduction in energy uptake. Is this true? What information bears on this point? The chapters in this section deal with this and related issues.

This specific question is the subject of Chapter 21, which summarizes the results of studies with human subjects. Data from extensive studies on experimental animals are documented in Chapter 22.

But reduction in intake of dietary fat is not always free of problems. Is there a minimum level of dietary fat intake below which optimum health may be jeopardized? Does the dietary fat requirement change throughout the life cycle? What type of diet results when fat calories are reduced? These questions are discussed in Chapter 23.

How do people reduce fat in their diets in real life when they are told about the major sources of dietary fat but are not given any rigid diet plans? This was the question addressed by the Women's Health Trial. Each person worked out her own diet plan. Overall, there was dramatic success in reducing fat intake. The purpose of Chapter 24 is to share some insights learned from the behavior of women in that study about techniques that help to lower dietary fat intake.

E. Reflections

Lowered prevalence of obesity is the bottom line of any discussion of the health consequence of low-calorie foods. Is it fair to ask whether commercial low-fat or artificially sweetened, low-calorie foods have, indeed, reduced the prevalence of obesity? This and the question of what it takes to change food preferences are the subject of this section.

Changes in dietary fat and sugar content and their consequences for public health are presented in Chapter 25. A key question is whether the availability of low-calorie foods "automatically" results in a change in the average diet or whether this additional variety of food choices is an adjunct to a comprehensive weight-reduction regimen. Another key question is whether the benefit from low-calorie foods has been stratified according to income.

If low-calorie foods are considered useful for improving health, then the problem is how to increase their acceptance and intake. This issue is addressed from a psychological perspective in Chapter 26.

The final chapter, Chapter 27, is an attempt to tie the chapters of this multiauthor volume together, at least to provide an approach to understanding the low-calorie foods and related phenomena. The enigma of the coexistence of low-calorie foods and extensive obesity is discussed, and comments are offered on what the individual and society can do to take better advantage of the proliferation of such foods.

REFERENCE

1. A. M. Altschul et al. Low-calorie foods. A scientific status summary by the Institute of Food Technologists' Expert Panel on Food Safety and Nutrition, *Food Technol., 42*(4): 113 (1989).

2
Adult Obesity

Aaron M. Altschul *Georgetown University School of Medicine, Washington, D.C.*

I. INTRODUCTION

Obesity in the United States is a major public health problem. Treatment of obesity or its prevention have had only limited success [1]. Approximately one-fifth of adult Americans—34 million people—were overweight in the period 1976–80; of this group 12.4 million were severely overweight [2].

The purpose of this chapter is to describe this problem and provide a perspective from which to view the possible public health influence of low-calorie foods.

II. PREVALENCE

A. Definition of Obesity

Obesity is a condition of higher than normal body fat content. An acceptable fat content is 15% for the reference man weighing 72 kg and 28% for the reference woman weighing 58 kg [3]. Body fat content can be estimated in many ways that include densitometry, measuring total body water, measuring bioelectrical impedance, and measuring skinfold thickness at one or several locations [4]. Another anthropometric measurement is body mass index (BMI).

Body mass index $\{(BMI) = \text{weight (kg)}/[\text{height (m)}]^2\}$ is the most likely measurement, since this is common to most surveys of large population numbers [5]. It has a relatively high correlation with the amount of body fat. Despite shortcomings [6], it is the best available measure and is used universally.

Overweight is defined in NHANES II (the American national survey taken in 1976–80) as the 85th percentile or more of the distribution of BMI for men and women ages 20–29; severely overweight as the 95th percentile and over of the same reference population [7]. The mean (50th percentile) BMI in that population for males was 24.3 and for females, 23.1; for overweight (85th percentile): males, 27.8; females, 27.3; for severe overweight (95th percentile): males, 31.1; females, 32.3 [7]. Must et al. provided reference data based on values derived from NHANES I (April 1971–June 1974); these are similar to those shown above [8].

The term *obese*, when used in a quantitative sense, is synonymous with or closely overlaps the term severe overweight. Morbid obesity is defined as excess weight per height of 100 lb or 100% or more above life insurance standards based on longevity [9]. The term *desirable weight* is used by Metropolitan Life to indicate weight associated with the lowest mortality. An index, the Metropolitan Relative Weight, is computed by forming the ratio of a person's body weight to the reference desirable weight for that height. Most adult American men have a Metropolitan Relative Weight above 120% [5].

B. Distribution In Population

1. By Sex

Slightly more women than men are overweight in the United States. About 14.5 million men (22.8%) and 18.1 million women (25.8%) were overweight when the NHANES II (1976–80) survey of persons aged 20–74 years was taken. Of these, about 8.4% men or 5.3 million and 8.8% women or 6.2 million were severely overweight [10].

2. By Age

The NHANES I study showed that weight of women increases with age; for men it increases to middle age and then levels off [8].

3. By Race and Ethnic Origin

Many minority populations in the United States have higher prevalences of overweight and obesity [11]. The prevalence of overweight among black women is 41.8%, much higher than of white women (24%). The prevalence of severe weight among black women is more than double that of white American women [10].

When Americans of different ethnic and racial groups were compared for age-adjusted overweight, no serious difference was found in the prevalence of overweight among the males. Prevalence of overweight was higher among females—the highest being among Mexican American, Puerto Rican, and non-Hispanic black, and the lowest among non-Hispanic white [12].

4. By Income and Education

The economic status of men does not affect their weight pattern, but overweight is markedly increased among poor women compared with those above the poverty level. Severe overweight follows pretty much the same pattern [12]. In girls older than 15 years and in adult women, fatness is *inversely* related to income [13].

5. In Other Countries

Obesity is a concomitant of industrial society. Hence, prevalence is high in Europe as well as in the United States. In Austria, for example, the prevalence of obesity increases with age to a maximum of about 19% at age 55 years for men and about 34% at 60 years for women [14]. An earlier seven-country study found that 13% of males aged 40–59 in northern Europe were above a BMI of 27; for southern Europe, the figure was 23%. The corresponding figure for Americans was 29.5% [15].

Compared to Canadian and British men, American men are more likely to be overweight, especially at the younger age levels. The United States has the highest proportion of excessively heavy women at all ages except 20–24 years [16].

But obesity is not confined solely to industrialized countries. High levels of obesity were noted among middle-aged women in Costa Rica, Nicaragua, and Trinidad [17].

6. Comment

Particularly for women, especially for black women, age, poverty, and low educational level increase the risk of being obese. But the place where you live also matters; anyone living in the United States runs a high risk of becoming obese.

C. Secular Trends

1. General Observations

When the entire population of the United States was considered, no consistent secular trend emerged for obesity [18,19]. But Bray [20] stated that in the decade 1975–85, both men and women of the same height became 2–8 lb heavier. Simopoulos [21] also found that both men and women were taller and heavier in 1971–74 and 1976–80 than in 1960–62.

2. Observations on Subgroups

When subgroups based on age, sex, body mass index, race, ethnic origin, income, and education were compared, secular trends emerged from the three national surveys covering the period 1960–80. The age-adjusted proportion of men and women severely overweight (BMI > 32) in 1976–80 significantly exceeded that in 1960–62 [22]. While mean value increased only modestly, the proportion of women classified as overweight or obese increased from one survey to the next [21,23,24]. The most striking secular trends were shown by adult females aged 25–34 years; mean BMI increased in each succeeding survey. The secular increase in mean BMI was greater at the lowest educational levels [25]. A greater proportion of black than white adult females were above the 85th percentile in the 1961 survey; this black-and-white difference increased in the later surveys [23].

3. Comment

Obesity increased in the United States between 1960 and 1980, particularly among women. Those already obese and at low educational and income levels were more likely to be effected. The more significant trends were not changes in the means or medians, which increased only modestly, but in the groups classified as overweight or obese. This means that individuals originally near the mean were moving into the higher weight categories, namely, the heaviest in any category were moving into the next.

III. HEALTH RISKS OF OVERWEIGHT AND OBESITY

A. Based on Total Body Fat

1. Risks to Disease

Obese individuals are at greater risk from surgery and anesthesia. They are at greater risk of having diabetes mellitus, hypertension, glucose intolerance, higher serum lipid values, and gallbladder disease, and suffer more from diseases of weight-bearing joints. They are in greater danger of sudden death; obesity and overweight are major causes of excess morbidity and mortality from coronary heart disease [115].

Overweight men show higher rates of prostatic and colorectal cancer; overweight women show higher rates of cancer of the gallbladder and biliary passages, breast, cervix, endometrium, uterus, and ovary [27,28].

Obesity is a predictor of cardiovascular disease independent of other risk factors [29]. Even mild to moderate overweight increases coronary risk in middle-aged women. Although a major portion of the excess coronary risk is attributable to the effect of adiposity on risk factors, a moderate residual effect remains that may be attributed to other mechanisms [30].

2. Mortality

It is not surprising that mortality data reflect this greater susceptibility to disease. Overweight persons, particularly those overweight at younger ages, tend to die sooner than average-weight persons [5].

The relationship between BMI and mortality takes the form of a "J" or "U" curve: the lowest mortality was at the desirable BMI, increased sharply as BMI increases, and increased as well at below-normal weights [31]. There was no evidence that weight gains during middle age increased longevity or that desirable weights increased with age [32].

B. Based on Regional Body Fat Distribution

1. The Concept

Much as body fat content and body mass index (a surrogate for body fat content) relate to risk of obesity, these indices are less sensitive indicators of risk than fat distribution. Central (or abdominal or truncal) body fat is more active metabolically than peripheral fat and is more related to mortality and morbidity of obesity. The relative proportions of abdominal fat to femoral-gluteal (thigh-hip) fat, measured as the ratio of waist-to-hip circumference (WHR), is a better predictor of risk in many instances [33].

Hence, one classification of obesity consists of two types: (1) android, or apple-shaped, characterized by a high WHR found mostly in men and in some women, and (2) gynoid, or pear-shaped, with a low WHR found in most women [34]. Vague (34) proposed that women with a more masculine distribution of body fat were at higher risk for diabetes, heart disease, and gout. Björklund et al. defined adiposity for women as having a BMI $\geq$ 30 or a WHR $\geq$ 0.82 or both [35].

2. Examples

A high WHR was associated with high rates of non–insulin-dependent diabetes mellitus, low HDL cholesterol values, and high triglyceride levels [36]; with an increased risk of coronary heart disease in middle-aged men [37]; with the end points of myocardial infarction, angina pectoris, stroke, and death in women [38]; and with the risk of coronary artery disease in older women [39]. Measures of total obesity had no or little predictive power in these cases.

WHR was the most powerful predictor of HDL_2 values in a population of healthy older individuals. BMI, total percentage of body fat, maximum oxygen uptake, and sex were not significant predictors when added to this model [40].

Women with increased central adiposity (as measured by the sum of the chest, abdomen, and subscapular skinfolds divided by the sum of triceps and thigh skinfolds) showed an elevated risk of breast cancer over a subsequent 28-year interval. This method of measuring central adiposity has characteristics similar to the waist-to-hip ratio [41].

3. Role of Genetics and Weight Fluctuation

Some elements of fat distribution are inherited [42]. Twenty-five percent of the extremity-to-trunk skinfold ratio is genetically transmitted [43].

Of particular interest is the suggestion that a history of repeated cycles of weight gain and loss may be associated with a more abdominally distributed fat. Repeated pregnancies (another instance of weight cycling) relate positively to WHR [44]. Hence, cycling not only makes weight reduction more difficult but increases the risk of disease as well.

4. Is There an Optimum Central Fat Content?

Although the plot of total mortality versus BMI is "U" shaped, no such shape exists for the relation of iliac-to-thigh circumference and mortality: the smaller the deposition of abdominal fat, the better seems the outlook for survival [45].

5. Comment

Fat distribution is now an important parameter for describing obesity. Epidemiologists must be concerned with both fat content and distribution as they seek associations between mortality and morbidity and body fat. Males at the same degree of overweight may be at more risk from the problems caused by obesity than females because male obesity favors a higher WHR.

IV. THE NATURE OF THE DISEASE

Greco-Roman physicians considered obesity as a disease requiring treatment, an idea that disappeared with the decline of antique medicine. Only in the second half of the nineteenth century was obesity rediscovered as a disease of nutritional imbalance, of an excess of energy intake over output [46].

Obesity is a heterogeneous disorder. A given body fat content can have various phenotypic characteristics. Body fat distribution, cited above, is one example. Another is the way in which fat is deposited under conditions of positive energy balance. As more fat is deposited, the adipocytes or fat cells enlarge (hypertrophy) up to a point. Continued positive energy balance causes cell numbers to rise (hyperplasia). This can go on as long as positive energy balance persists. The hypertropic/hyperplastic relationship is another phenotypic characteristic of body fat content. Various phenotypic characteristics can have different clinical consequences [47].

A. Controls for Normal Weight

Most adult humans are within the normal weight range. This is surely true when the amount of available food just balances the requirements. Even where there is more than enough to eat, it is also true. Consider the substantial number of people in the United States and other industrial societies who are at normal weight. The controls behind this weight homeostasis have intrigued scientists from the beginnings of modern biology.

1. What Is Regulated

The quantity and many aspects of the quality of food eaten are regulated [48]. Even though the food we eat varies considerably in protein content and in proportion of carbohydrate and fat, humans, given an adequate food supply, will eat 14–16% of dietary calories as protein. Rats regulate protein and carbohydrate intake under widely varying conditions of dietary choices. Fat intake is not as well regulated.

a. Hunger and Satiety [49–51]. Anyone seeking explanations for the regulation of hunger and satiety enters a maze of complexities. Part of the problem of unraveling the controls is their abundance and redundancy. Control of food intake involves both the brain and mechanisms originating in the peripheral organs such as the stomach, gut, liver, and adipose tissue. The hypothalamus is probably the brain region most involved in regulation of both quantity and quality of food intake. The hormones insulin and cholecystokinin have an important role but are not the only ones involved [52].

The regulatory event is recognition of the shift in the nature of the metabolic fuels. During the absorptive phase, after a meal, metabolic fuels are supplied by the recently consumed food; in the postabsorptive state metabolic fuels are supplied from stores of fat, carbohydrate, and protein accumulated on previous eating occasions. The shift from satiety to hunger occurs when the animal recognizes that the postabsorptive state has begun [52].

Onset of hunger could be explained as the time when the inhibitory signals generated by the previous meal have dissipated. Then the presence of palatable food could trigger a new eating episode [52]. Multiple metabolic signals such as a temporary fall in blood glucose level or decreased oxidation of fatty acids in the liver may also be involved [52]. Endogenous and exogenous opiate peptides stimulate eating. Hence, it may be that specific signals are required to initiate eating besides absence of inhibitor signals [48].

The digestion products of food can provide signals to the brain even before absorption of nutrients has begun by signaling the release of gastrointestinal hormones, which inhibit feeding. It may be that the caloric content of the food is monitored in the stomach to provide inhibitory signals. And chemoreceptors can detect utilization of metabolic fuels to provide additional inhibitory signals [52]. The net result is a feeling of satiety. There is no single metabolic signal for satiety [53].

Added to the complexity and redundancy of the metabolic controls over eating behavior is the influence of the specific food and the context in which it is presented. Culture influences eating habits. These general cultural effects are modified by each individual according to distinctive patterns established by past experience of sensory, social, and physiological correlates of eating [54]. Satiety is specific to the food that has been eaten [54,55].

Herman and Polivy [56] presented a boundary model that combines physiological and appetitive controls. Eating, according to this model, normally occurs to maintain the individual within boundaries corresponding to hunger and satiety, both subject to physiological controls. In between these boundaries is a region of biological indifference subject to appetitive control: social, cognitive, and other psychological controls. People will differ in the width of the zone of biological indifference, i.e., in the range between onset of physiological controls for hunger and satiety. This concept is somewhat satisfying because it makes sense of efforts to intervene by improving cognitive restraint.

b. Energy Balance. Energy is stored (weight is gained) when the energy intake exceeds energy output—the food energy lost in the urine and stool plus the heat production. Both thin and obese individuals fed excess food for a prolonged period will gain weight, but there is considerable variation between individuals in the amount of gain [57]. Some are more efficient in using excess energy intake to accumulate new tissue (fat and protein) than others. part of this variability is due to genetic differences, as will be discussed later.

Defective thermogenesis is often given as the reason for differences in ability to manage excesses of energy intake. Diet-induced thermogenesis arises from the energy costs of ingestion and digestion of food, increased activity of the food-processing tissues—the gut wall and the liver—and the cost of synthesis or turnover of body tissue. This can be measured as an increase in resting metabolic rate after a meal and is approximately 10% of the ingested calories. About one-third of obese women are said to have a defective therm-ogenic response [58], which could amount to a deficit in energy output of 130 kcal/day [59].

2. Cognitive Restraint

Some normal-weight individuals may have faulty controls over energy intake or energy output and yet manage to achieve energy balance. They do so by adding cognitive restraint to the somatic controls; they create artificial sig-nals—weight on the scale, size of dress, tightness of belt—and respond by deliberate restriction of food intake and/or increased physical activity [60–62]. Restrained eaters consumed less energy, took fewer meals, and preferred low-calorie foods compared to otherwise similar unrestrained eaters [63]. They were regulating their weight below the level that would have been reached without dietary restrictions [64].

3. Comment

Most people in the United States are at normal weight. They are so naturally, or they impose cognitive controls in addition to their residual natural con-trols over both energy intake and output. A very small number of restrained eaters lose control and engage in pathological behavior: they either become bulimic (binge and purge) or starve themselves voluntarily (anorexia nervosa). These are serious, and sometimes fatal, excesses of restraint; such individuals need professional psychological and psychiatric treatment.

B. When Controls Are Inadequate

Energy balance must be precise. An excess energy intake over output of 5% in a person who has an energy output of 2000 kcal/day results in a weight gain of 6–7 kg/yr (13.2–15.4 lb) [65].

Obesity can be found among both restrained or unrestrained eaters. Un-restrained obese persons allow their body weight to adjust to a level in equil-ibrium with their metabolic controls and their environment (food supply and opportunities for physical activity) without trying to intervene. Restrained eaters who are nevertheless obese have tried to intervene cognitively without success. It could be that their ability for restraint was limited or that what-ever capacity they had for restraint could not overcome the burden induced by their metabolic defects and the environment. Metabolic defects could have been genetically determined or may have been acquired as the result of the obese state itself, as will be discussed later; such acquired defects are dif-ficult to reverse [66].

But all agree that obesity is not an indication of indolence, gluttony, stupidity, or sloth. There are such individuals among the obese, but no more than in the general population. Obesity is truly a disease; its victims require a sympathetic hearing, the best possible treatment available, and a public health approach that makes it easier to maintain energy balance [67].

V. HEREDITY, INDUCED METABOLIC DEFECTS, AND ENVIRONMENT

This section deals with some factors, personal or environmental, that influence control of energy balance. It is not possible to predict the outcome of energy balance of a certain level of cognitive restraint. A person may be able to control energy balance through cognitive restraint in one environment but not in another. The same ability for cognitive restraint may succeed in preserving energy balance for one person and fail for another who has to overcome metabolic defects of genetic origin.

A. Heredity

Obesity runs along family lines [13]. The influence of genotype, apart from any common family environment, can be estimated by studying genetically unrelated individuals living in a single community, twins living apart, or twins subjected to a stress of overeating or overexercising.

1. Variability of Phenotype

Resting metabolic rate, which accounts for 60–70% of energy expenditure, is an individual characteristic independent of body size, age, and sex. In a community of Pima Indians it correlated with fat-free body mass; but even when adjusted for fat-free mass, age, and sex, there was considerable individual variation. Furthermore, the resting metabolic rate was aggregated in families, suggesting the presence of a genetic effect. This relates to obesity since a low resting metabolic rate was associated with a significantly increased risk for weight gain of 10 kg or more [68].

2. Genetic Component of Variability

Habitual physical activity, energy cost of submaximal exercise, resting metabolic rate, and thermic effect of a meal are influenced significantly by genetic characteristics, the heritability coefficient reaching, respectively, 25–30, 40, 40, and 40% of the variance [47]. Transmission from one generation to the next of body mass index and skinfold thicknesses is primarily cultural—customs and preferences about diet, social environment, or other activities [69]. The genetic component of the transmission is from 5% for body mass index to 30% for fat-free mass. These conclusions are at variance with those of Stunkard et al. [70], who stated that 70% of the variation in BMI was due to genetic influences.

There is no evidence of a significant genetic effect on energy intake per unit of body weight [47].

3. Interaction Between Genotypes and Chronic Overfeeding

Of more practical importance is the interaction between genotypes and the environment as measured by overfeeding. Individuals deliberately overfed in a controlled environment will *all* gain weight. But, as stated earlier, there is a fair amount of individual variability [57]. A combined environment and genetic effect of close to 90% for body fat content was derived from a study of twins who were overfed 1000 kcal/day. This is much higher than the genetic effect itself, which is about 30% [43,47,71].

Hence, a relatively small effect by itself becomes overwhelming when the environment is manipulated to cause overfeeding. The environment in Western society can be described as promoting overfeeding. Hence, we might expect that a genetic defect in energy expenditure could have major consequences for obesity in modern Western society.

B. Induced Metabolic Defects

The obese state itself may induce metabolic abnormalities. This can happen after obesity has persisted for long periods or could be the result of repeated cycles of weight loss and regain. Thus, reversibility of obesity in rats fed high-fat diets depends on the duration of the obese condition [72]. Human dieters find it more difficult to lose weight the second time after one cycle of weight loss [73]. Among the subjects participating in the Framingham Heart Study, those with highly variable body weights had higher total mortality and higher morbidity and mortality from coronary heart disease. These negative health consequences were independent for obesity and trend over time in body weight [74].

Explanations for the observations remain scarce. Following weight cycling, it is likely that the body composition after weight regain will not be the same as before dieting: more fat and less lean tissue would result, which would lead to a lower basal metabolic rate. Moreover, a formerly obese person may have a greater capacity for fat storage.

Prolonged obesity and weight cycling create more difficulties for the person who wants to maintain a more normal weight. Treatment of the problem at the very onset of obesity is more likely to succeed.

C. Environment

Earlier we stated that obesity is more prevalent in some countries than others. This points to something in the environment—the kinds of food available and eaten, the need and opportunities for physical activity—that overrides individual differences. The following section provides examples of how the environment could affect eating behavior.

1. Dietary Obesity in Animals

Laboratory rats raised ad libitum on nutritionally adequate chow (2–6% fat) under sedentary conditions will attain 10–20% body fat. But these rats can be converted into obese rats. When dietary fat is increased to 30–60%, the animals gain more weight and deposit more body fat than the normally fed animals. The most effective way to induce dietary obesity in otherwise normal-weight laboratory rats is to offer them a variety of high-fat, palatable foods. One "supermarket" or "cafeteria" diet provided chocolate chip cookies, salami, cheese, banana, marshmallows, milk chocolate, and peanut butter, in addition to regular chow. In every case when offered a choice, rats reject chow diets in favor of the more palatable high-fat and high-sugar diets and become obese [75,76].

2. Effect of Wartime Food Rationing

Food rationing during wartime, designed to provide equitable distribution of scarce food resources, limited intake of fat and sugar. The consequences for chronic diseases, particularly diabetes, were dramatic. Both diabetic mortality and fat intake decreased sharply in England and Wales in the periods of food rationing during World Wars I and II. In the interim period between the wars, mortality rose steadily to a slightly higher level than pre–World War I, only to drop sharply again within a year after beginning of World War II [77]. The death rate from arteriosclerosis (including diseases of the coronary arteries) during the years of World War II in Sweden and Finland declined sharply, to rise again after the war. Cases of diabetes treated in 22 medical clinics in Sweden dropped abruptly during the war years and returned to a higher level after the war [78]. Similar patterns for mortality from circulatory diseases were found in Norway [79] and for fat consumption and pulmonary embolism in Germany [80].

The caloric intake was such that a general lowering of weight would have been expected, but little information on this score is available. Grosse-Brockhoff (see Ref. 14) reported that the prevalence of obesity in patients of the Medical University Hospital, Bonn, reflected the reduction in available food energy during the years 1941–47.

3. Westernization and Chronic Disease

Migration from primitive, or at least greatly different, societies to Western-style cultures (e.g., Yemenite Jews who migrated to Israel [81] or Japanese living in Hiroshima and Nagasaki, Hawaii, and San Francisco, reviewed by Curb and Marcus [82]) offer an opportunity to relate changes in food availability to dietary and disease patterns. The Yemenite Jews acquired a diabetic disease pattern typical of the indigenous European-born Israeli population. Japanese living in Japan and Hawaii were followed for 25 years in a study begun in 1965. Those living in Japan had a lower BMI, one-third as much obesity, ate about 170 fewer kcal/day, and ate a diet containing 16% of the calories as fat compared with 33% fat calories in the diets of those of the same age (55 years) living in Hawaii.

Another approach is to study what happens following a cultural transition within a society. Diabetes is rare among Melanesians, and also among Polynesians and Micronesians who retain their traditional lifestyle; prevalence rates of adult-onset diabetes are high in those who have adopted a Western lifestyle. The traditional island diet of fresh fish, meat, and local fruits and vegetables has been replaced by a diet of imported goods such as rice, sugar, flour, canned meats, canned fruits and vegetables, soft drinks, and beer. Physical activity has declined. The prevalence of obesity is high [83].

Invariability when there is an increase in availability of foods rich in fat and sugar, whether by migration or by social change, this is accompanied by a dietary change that reflects their increased attractiveness.

4. Physical Activity

Resting metabolic rate accounts for 60–75% of an individual's 24-hour energy expenditure (ca. 1500 kcal/day in an individual expending 2500 kcal/day), the thermic effect of feeding provides another 10%, and physical activity, 15–30% [84]. The latter is the most variable component; it accounts for the large differences in energy expenditure when comparing various occupations and is the one over which the individual has the greatest control.

An analysis of activity in the United Kingdom found that coal miners, farmers, and forestry workers expended more than 3500 kcal/day; building workers and steel workers more than 3000 kcal/day; but for male office workers, 24-hour energy expenditure was about 2500 kcal/day. Middle-aged housewives used up 2000 kcal/day compared with female factory workers, who consumed 2300 kcal/day (85). The U.S. National Research Council calculated estimated daily energy allowances for 23-year-old adults [86]. On a very sedentary day, a male (70 kg) would require 2406 kcal compared with 3938 kcal for a very active day; a female (58 kg) would require 1856 kcal on a sedentary day and 3038 kcal when very active.

Consider the activities subsumed in the various categories of activity level [86]:

Very light: seated and standing activities, painting trades, driving, laboratory work, typing, sewing, ironing, cooking, playing cards, or playing a musical instrument.

Light: walking on a level surface at 2.5–3 mph, garage work, electrical trades, carpentry, restaurant trades, housecleaning, child care, golf, sailing, or table tennis.

Moderate: walking to 3.4–4 mph, weeding and hoeing, carrying a load, cycling, skiing, tennis, or dancing.

Most Americans are considered to be in the "light" or "moderate" category; many are in the "very light" category.

Hence, as the amount of physical labor associated with everyday living has declined, the energy requirements have declined as well. Instead of the physical activity of work, it now is necessary to engage purposely in athletic activity that will raise the level of daily energy expenditure. Otherwise there must be compensation by reduction in energy intake.

5. Discussion

It makes sense that the place where one lives determines in part the obesity pattern. Where the food supply is low and variety is limited, chronically or during a critical period, the chances for becoming obese are less. The reverse is true when food is abundant and variety is great. And this is even more true where human energy requirements are spared by mechanical devices.

VI. TREATMENT

A. Weight-Loss Strategies

A person intending to lose weight will undertake to reduce caloric intake and increase physical activity. The success of this endeavor will depend on how well and for how long the individuals are able to adjust their behavior to achieve and sustain this undertaking.

1. Behavioral Strategies

The cornerstone of any strategy to lose weight is to change behavior as it relates to eating and exercise [87]. This requires self-monitoring to identify settings in which eating occurs, particularly problem times. Once antecedents to problem eating are identified, techniques must be developed to break the chain between the stimulus to eating and eating itself. While there are general techniques for so doing, individuals must find or be helped to find the most suitable personal techniques and then learn to reward themselves for achieving appropriate behavior. Moreover, food is both a stressor and a stress reliever. Hence an important aspect of behavioral strategies is to learn how to deal with stress [90].

2. Diet

It is difficult to expect that exercise alone can cause weight loss unless one engages in hard physical labor or vigorous competitive sports. Hence, a weight-loss strategy must include serious reduction in caloric intake.

a. Dieting Strategies. The objective is to reduce energy intake to 800–1200 kcal/day to satisfy the first objective of losing weight, and then settle on a caloric intake just enough to support energy balance in order to maintain the new, lower weight. The types of foods eaten and the way they are eaten are the essence of most food strategies. Efforts to reduce portion size alone are not generally successful; more successful are changes in the types of food eaten—away from calorie-dense, fatty foods, towards more fruits and vegetables, towards a vegetarian diet. The following are some examples of techniques adopted by dieters [88,91,92].

The Main Meals. Limit amount of food taken at meals; choose foods and drinks low in calories; eat the same number of calories/day; eat meals at the same time each day; be strict about eating style—small mouthfuls, eat slowly; don't eat when doing something else; do not continue discussions at the table before the food is removed; substitute formulated meals for one or more of the regular meals.

The Snacks. Eat few nuts or high-fat snacks; avoid pastries as dessert or as snacks; avoid calories in drinks between meals.

Type of Foods. Drink little or no alcohol; add no salt to cooking; eat low-fat dairy foods; avoid unnecessary fat at meals (e.g., avoid fatty and red meats, avoid skin from poultry, avoid frying, remove fat before serving); eat foods high in fiber; use low-fat spreads instead of butter and margarine; avoid sugary foods; use low-calorie sweeteners in coffee or tea; wherever possible use foods labeled low-calorie or reduced calorie; eat more fresh fruits and vegetables and salads.

Food-Related Behaviors. Keep an eating diary; examine patterns in your eating; control cues that set off overeating; follow an eating schedule; do not clean your plate; serve and eat one portion at a time; learn what emotions or states set off overeating.

One can reduce caloric intake to 800–1200 kcal/day by selecting from among common foods. The availability of low-calorie analogs of common foods can help to achieve this goal.

b. Very Low-Calorie Diets. These provide 400–500 kcal/day in the form of formula diets designed to provide all essential nutrients daily. When properly supervised they are safe, but these programs can be abused and are reserved for the obese or severely overweight [93–96].

c. Bizarre Diets. Diet schemes, some clearly ridiculous, appear in books, magazines, and newspapers, new ones almost daily. They promise without reserve that they indeed are the cure for obesity. They highly restrict the number of allowable foods. Some restrict all fat; some all dairy products; some all carbohydrates. Sometimes the restrictions make no sense. Often the outcome is nutrient imbalance [97].

d. Comment. Weight can be lost, initially, provided that the individual is not ambivalent about the need to lose weight and persists in the effort. Brownell and Jeffery [98] observed that initial weight loss as reported in the literature has increased in the period 1974–1986, from 8.5 to 22 lb per attempt. Their explanation is that the later programs are better and last longer—lasting 16.7 weeks compared with 8.4 weeks for the earlier programs. Wing believes that the programs have also become more intensive [99].

3. Pharmacological Approaches

When drug treatment is combined with diet, weight loss is improved, but long-term maintenance of weight-loss is unchanged [89,100,101]. Fenfluramine is the drug most widely used in combined treatment studies. Rodin et al. [102] combined behavior treatment with administration of diethylpropion hydrochloride (Tenuate). The combined treatment showed a somewhat greater weight loss during the treatment period (20 weeks). But this weight differential disappeared 6 months after termination of treatment.

Over-the-counter and some prescription drugs are available to support weight loss. They are often abused, leading to serious side effects [103]. When several anorectic drugs were compared for abuse potential, amphetamine and diethylpropion had the greatest potential for abuse, fenfluramine and phenylpropanolamine the least [101]. But the use of appetite-suppressant medication is contraindicated unless one is prepared to continue the medication indefinitely [104].

4. Surgery

Another treatment that ensures rapid weight loss and carries over into the longer term is surgical treatment [105]. This procedure is reserved for the morbidly obese defined as having excess weight per height of 100 lb or more above life insurance standards based on longevity [9,105]. Despite numerous shortcomings and limitations, surgical methods are the only viable alternative for achieving and maintaining substantial weight loss in dangerously obese patients [104–106].

B. Evaluation of Treatment

Most of the information on effectiveness of treatment comes from analysis of organized programs. When participants who had lost weight in weight-loss programs were contacted after a year, it was found that they had gradually regained all or part of what they had lost. In one study, weight losses reported for sequential years of follow-up were 79, 69, 49, 33, and 47% of the original weight [98]. Jeffery [107] concluded that recidivism approximating 75–100% regain of initial weight losses is common among reports of follow-up beyond one year. As a rule, the more careful the methodology, the worse the results.

Of participants in a 15-week behaviorally oriented program, which included diet and exercise instruction, behavioral skills training, cognitive behavior modification, and relapse prevention training, only 0.9% of the men and 5.3% of the women maintained their initial weight loss during the 4-year follow-up period [108]. Some of them—3.5% of men and 10% women—showed significant recovery from relapse. Approximately 70% of the men showed a pattern of monotonic weight regain, while 15% interrupted the weight regain with a single weight loss; the comparable figures for women were 36.8 and 41.3%. Nearly 40% of the subjects gained weight up to the original values or above during the 4-year period. But 18.5% maintained at least one-half of their losses during follow up and 34% kept off at least one-quarter.

Volkmar et al. [109] reported that 50% of members in a commercial weight-loss program dropped out in 6 weeks and 70% in 12 weeks. Self-control is apparently difficult to master even when practiced under supervision over long periods of time. Then there is the failure of outreach. The number of individuals who are obese is much larger than the clinical resources currently available, and the cost of providing treatments in the current packages is excessive. It could be that the record is better than it seems to be. A similar control group (no intervention) might have gained additional weight during the same period [98,108].

Failure is not the universal outcome. Schacter [110] reported on the pattern of success of nonselected, nonclinical populations in dealing with smoking and obesity. He found that a considerably larger proportion of the general population may have given up smoking for long periods than may have been suspected from estimates based on therapeutic success. Of those with a history of obesity who had actively attempted to lose weight, 62.5% succeeded. Schacter concluded that the generally accepted professional and public impression that nicotine addiction, heroin addiction, and obesity are almost hopelessly difficult conditions to correct is wrong. He suggested that the analysis of therapeutic attempts is based on the results of a single attempt; the results in the general population represent a lifetime of effort. These multiple efforts are more likely to succeed than any single therapeutic attempt.

The main conclusion is that obesity is a chronic disease much like hypertension, diabetes, and cardiovascular disease. Instead, it has typically been treated as an acute illness.

C. Long-Term Management Strategies

If obesity is to be treated as a chronic disease, then the treatment strategies must be designed for a lifetime. The implications of quick and easy weight loss made by some commercial weight-loss organizations, by articles in magazines, and by some books are a disservice to the public. By keeping alive the hope of "magic bullets," quick and easy fixes, they distract the obese person from facing reality.

Obvious as it now seems, the recognition that obesity is a chronic condition requiring lifetime attention is a major step forward. No longer is the ability to achieve rapid initial weight loss of great significance. The objective now is to achieve and maintain a desirable weight over a lifetime. The initial weight loss is but the first step and can be rendered meaningless by weight regain because the conditions favoring weight loss were so artificial that they could not be sustained.

Hence, all current responsible strategies for dealing with obesity concentrate on long-term management. There is no perfect way that serves equally well for everyone. Obesity is a heterogeneous disease. Remedies must be tailored to the individual. We will review some factors that impact long-term maintenance and comment on the potential role of the food system.

1. Metabolic Disability

Those who seek therapeutic help—who have not been willing to undertake self-help or have failed in such attempts—are more likely to have a metabolic disability that requires a high degree of cognitive restraint to overcome. They may have a genetically reduced rate of metabolism or increased appetite, or both. Or they may have acquired such abnormalities in the obese state itself [73]. As a consequence, much of the effort of counselors must be to help the obese person exercise cognitive controls over powerful biological systems. It is like learning to live in a hungry state [104].

As was stated earlier, we are not dealing here with big numbers. An excess of 5% energy intake over output each day for a year is enough to induce a weight gain of about 6 kg (13.2 lb) [58]. This amounts to an error in energy balance of 75–100 kcal/day. A difference in resting metabolic rate of 70 kcal/day was sufficient to distinguish between gainers (gained more than 10 kg (22 lb) in 21 months) and nongainers [68].

That we are not dealing with big numbers is in itself worthy of comment. It illustrates how exquisitely well-tuned the energy balance system is in normal-weight individuals. It shows that an error of only 100 kcal/day is sufficient to create an obesity problem. But it also shows that those who can exercise cognitive restraint to reduce daily intake by 100 kcal/day will overcome most metabolic disabilities. This is not an impossible goal. Restrained eaters reported that they ate 410 kcal/day less than unrestrained eaters of same weight [64].

Some people have higher metabolic deficits. Bogardus et al. [68] reported a difference in resting metabolic rate of 500 kcal/day between the Pima Indian family that had the lowest value (ca. 1625 kcal/day) and the one with the highest (ca. 2115 kcal/day). For those with very low resting metabolic rates, cognitive restraint alone will probably not suffice. For some, surgery may be the only viable alternative.

2. Treatment

Any plan for improved long-term management must be built upon the best available combination of diet, exercise, and psychological counseling. Suggestions to improve long-term success include better screening, longer periods for initial weight loss, particular attention to snacks, and ongoing intervention following the initial weight loss [98,99,107,108].

Better screening would allow the counselor to tailor the program to suit individual needs. Screening for cognitive restraint and for resting metabolic rate would be helpful. Leon and Rosenthal (111) suggest that special efforts be made to identify individuals who are chronic dieters and who are engaging in food intake in response to emotional arousal.

Ideas for screening can come from comparison of successful maintainers to relapsers. Kayman et al. [112] found that correlates of successful maintenance of weight loss include exercise, positive self-statements related to weight-reduction efforts, and self-regulatory activities such as appropriate goal setting, self-monitoring of eating or weight, and early recognition of weight regain. Their own study found that maintainers exercised regularly, whereas most relapsers did not. Weight regain was frequently attributed to negative emotional states and unexpected or unpredictable stressful life events, but the maintainers believed themselves capable of handling their problems and used problem-solving skills to cope with their difficulties. Social or family support seemed significantly greater for maintainers.

The first result of a longer initial process of weight loss with adequate behavior counseling and therapy (as necessary) would be a greater initial weight loss. This in itself would lengthen the time required for weight regain. The longer initial process would also provide better training for the period ahead.

An idea of how programs can be improved is suggested by the finding that, in addition to program duration, weight loss is positively associated with the experience of the therapist and hours of therapist contact, a rigorous diet, practicing exercise, and involvement of the patient's family [113].

Booth [114] emphasized the difficulty likely to be created by energy taken in or with drinks between meals or by high-energy items taken towards the end of or after meals. Inappropriate snacks were, in his opinion, a major cause of excessive energy intake.

Finally, the strategy should include plans for ongoing intervention that could include formal and informal support groups, specific training in relapse and in stress management, refresher groups, hotlines, and provision for return to the original program when serious individual problems that threaten weight control develop [107].

The problem with all these ideas is the additional, overwhelming, cost of treatment that they impose. The benefits of improved treatment become even more skewed in favor of the affluent and against the poor, who suffer more from the problem of obesity and are in greater need of treatment. Therefore, more attention must be given to public health measures that might prevent or delay onset of obesity. Such measures as would promote more physical activity and reduce the amount of fat eaten could surely help a large part of the public at risk. But that may require a change in the physical and cultural environment [107].

3. The Food System

Earlier, we showed how the food supply could alter drastically the course of diseases related to obesity and overconsumption. Curtail it by rationing: people eat less total food energy, fat, and sugar; diseases related to overeating are reduced. Increase it by changing the social condition or by migration: people eat more, more fat, sugar, and fat; diseases of affluent malnutrition increase.

Now we face another phenomenon: low-fat and low-calorie choices added to a cornucopia of foods that contains anything a person may want to eat, from high- to low-calorie, from high- to low-fat, sweet or savory. Previous experience with rationing or with change to more affluence cannot predict what might happen in this new circumstance. Will this change make it easier to practice cognitive restraint or have no effect? Or, worse yet, will the presentation of more choice, albeit low-calorie or low-fat, require more cognitive restraint for energy balance?

Whether or not we can predict from previous experience, we can be sure that the nature of the food supply in some way must influence long-term management of energy balance. What we don't know is how the new situation, which includes low- and high-fat and low- and high-calorie choices, will play out. The mere fact of their existence may not be enough. Some type of education may be required to teach the public how to use them properly. The question then becomes: what other cultural changes are needed to convert the availability of new food choices into a positive public health benefit?

VII. STATUS AND PROSPECTS

Obesity is a chronic disease. Treatment is expensive and must take place regularly or episodically over a lifetime. Obesity is more frequent among the poor and less educated. Despite the recognition of the role of heredity, improvements in treatment modalities, the development of pharmacological aids to treatment, and of surgical procedures for the severely obese, opportunities for treatment are less available to the poor, who need it most and can least afford it. There has been no apparent decrease in the number of obese in the last several decades. Rather, obesity is increasing among children and adults.

Prevention is a socially more attractive option than is treatment. It is easier to deal with normal-weight individuals before they start to gain weight than with obese who seek to lose weight. Obese individuals may have acquired patterns of behavior and irreversible metabolic impairments that make it more difficult to maintain normal weight even if initial weight loss can be achieved.

But prevention means that we recognize that the prevailing cultural patterns as they impact on energy balance do not promote our best interests. The prevailing cultural patterns constitute a pressure for positive energy balance that strains the capacity of individual somatic and cognitive controls. Every day is a new day to wrestle again with the same environmental pressure to gain weight and to challenge once again the individual systems favoring energy balance. Then a stressful event comes along and resistance to the pressure to gain weight that worked yesterday fails today. Imagine, instead, living in a culture that does not promote weight gain or promotes it less. Failure to maintain energy balance would be less likely and recovery from an episodic weight gain would be much easier.

The cultural changes leading toward reduced pressure to overeat are no different than those now accepted by individuals undertaking to lose weight. The only difference is that now a person who seeks to lose weight must go against the grain of the prevailing social norms, whereas in a society with a more favorable cultural pattern, a person seeking to maintain energy balance would be going with the grain. Nor are they unlike the changes in lifestyle being promoted to reduce the risk of cardiovascular disease. The idea that the prevailing fat intake is too high and should be lowered to 30% of the calories or less is common to programs intended to reduce the incidence of obesity, cardiovascular disease, and cancer.

No one undertakes to change a basic cultural pattern lightly, nor is it easy to do, and only at great expense. Yet it is being attempted for cardiovascular disease [115]. Community programs to change lifestyle and eating patterns to reduce risk of cardiovascular disease were tested and evaluated [see Refs. 116,117]. It is too soon to project outcomes and costs. A change in social norms such as is advocated is never easy to achieve, especially since it goes against heavily ingrained hedonic desires. But it is an ongoing activity, one to be taken seriously by those interested in the public health problem that obesity presents. The alternative is longer and costlier treatments.

REFERENCES

1. T. B. VanItallie, The perils of obesity in middle-aged women, *N. Engl. J. Med.*, *322*: 929 (1990).
2. T. B. VanItallie, Health implications of overweight and obesity in the United States, *Ann. Intern. Med.*, *103*: 983 (1985).
3. G. B. Forbes, Body composition: Influence of nutrition, disease, growth, and aging, *Modern Nutrition in Health and Disease* (M. E. Shills and V. R. Young, eds.), Lea and Fabiger, Philadelphia, p. 546 (1988).
4. H. C. Lukaski, Methods for the assessment of human body composition: traditional and new, *Am. J. Clin. Nutr.*, *46*: 537 (1987).
5. A. P. Simopoulos and T. B. VanItallie, Body weight, health, and longevity, *Ann. Intern. Med.*, *100*: 285 (1984).
6. K. J. Smalley, A. N. Knerr, Z. V. Kendrick, J. A. Colliver, and O. E. Owen, Reassessment of body mass indices, *Am. J. Clin. Nutr.*, *52*: 405 (1990).
7. *The Surgeon General's Report on Nutrition and Health*, USDHHS, Public Health Service, DHHS(PHS) Publication No. 88–50210, Washington, D.C., 1988.
8. A. Must, G. A. Dallal, and W. H. Dietz, Reference data for obesity: 85th and 95th percentiles of body mass index (wt/ht²) and triceps skinfold thickness, *Am. J. Clin. Nutr.*, *53*: 839 (1991).
9. T. B. VanItallie, G. A. Bray, W. E. Connor, W. W. Faloon, J. G. Kral, E. E. Mason, and A. J. Stunkard, Guidelines for surgery for morbid obesity, *Am. J. Clin. Nutr.*, *42*: 904 (1985).

10. S. Abraham, M. D. Carroll, M. F. Najjar, and F. Robinson, *Obese and Overweight Adults in the United States*, Vital and Health Statistics, Publ. No. (PHS) 83–1680, PHS NCHS SERIES 11, No. 230, Hyattsville, MD: National Center for Health Statistics (1983).

11. N. D. Ernst and W. R. Harlan, guest editors, Obesity and cardiovascular disease in minority populations, *Am. J. Clin. Nutr.*, *53* (Suppl.): 1507S (1991).

12. Life Sciences Research Office. *Nutrition Monitoring in the United States: An Update Report on Nutrition Monitoring.* Prepared for the U.S. Department of Agriculture and the U.S. Department of Health and Human Services. DHHS Publication No. (PHS) 89–1225. Public Health Service, Washington, D.C., September 1989.

13. S. M. Garn, Family line and socioeconomic factors in fatness and obesity. *Nutr. Rev.*, *44*: 381 (1986).

14. R. Kluthe and A. Schubert, Obesity in Europe, *Ann. Intern. Med.*, *103*: 1037 (1985).

15. A. Keys, C. Aravanis, H. Blackburn, F. S. P. Van Buchem, R. Buzina, B. S. Djordjevic, F. Fidanza, M. J. Karvonen, A. Menotti, V. Puddu, and H. J. Taylor, Coronary heart disease: Overweight and obesity as risk factors, *Ann. Intern. Med.*, *77*: 15 (1972).

16. W. J. Millar and T. Stephens, The prevalence of overweight and obesity in Britain, Canada, and the United States, *Am. J. Public Health*, *77*: 38 (1987).

17. M. Gurney and J. Gorstein, The global prevalence of obesity—an initial overview of available data, *Wld. Hlth. Statist. Quart.*, *41*: 251 (1988).

18. T. B. VanItallie and S. Abraham, Some hazards of obesity and its treatment, *Recent Advances in Obesity Research IV* (J. Hirsch and T. B. VanItallie, eds.), John Libbey, London, p. 1 (1985).

19. U.S. Department of Health and Human Services and the U.S. Department of Agriculture, *Nutrition Monitoring in the United States.* Publication No. (PHS) 86–1255. Public Health Service, Washington, D.C. July 1986.

20. G. A. Bray, Obesity: Definition, diagnosis, and disadvantages, *Med. J. Australia*, *142* (Suppl.): 52 (1985).

21. A. P. Simopoulos, Characteristics of obesity: An overview, *Ann. N.Y. Acad. Sci.*, *499*: 4 (1987).

22. S. Abraham, M. D. Carroll, and M. F. Najjar, *Trends in Obesity and Overweight Among Adults Ages 20–74 years: United States 1960–1962, 1971–74, 1976–80*, Vital and Health Statistics, PHS NCHS SERIES 11, Hyattsville, MD: National Center for Health Statistics (1984).

23. W. R. Harlan, J. R. Landis, K. M. Flegal, C. S. Davis, and M. E. Miller, Trends in body mass in the United States, 1960–1980, *Am. J. Epidemiol.*, *128*: 1065 (1988).

24. K. M. Flegal, W. R. Harlan, and J. R. Landis, Trends in body mass index and skinfold thickness with socioeconomic factors in young adult men, *Am. J. Clin. Nutr.*, *48*: 544 (1988).

25. K. M. Flegal, W. R. Harlan, and J. R. Landis, Trends in body mass index and skinfold thickness with socioeconomic factors in young adult women, *Am. J. Clin. Nutr.*, *48*: 535 (1988).

26. F. X. Pi-Sunyer, Health implications of obesity, *Am. J. Clin. Nutr.*, *53*: 1595S (1991).
27. E. A. Lew and L. Garfinkel, Variations in mortality by weight among 750,000 men and women, *J. Chron. Dis.*, *32*: 563 (1979).
28. L. Garfinkel, Overweight and cancer, *Ann. Intern. Med.*, *103*: 1034 (1985).
29. H. B. Hubert, M. Feinleib, P. M. McNamara, and W. P. Castelli, Obesity as an independent risk factor for cardiovascular disease: A 26-year followup of participants in the Framingham Heart Study, *Circulation*, *67*: 968 (1983).
30. J. E. Manson, G. A. Colditz, M. J. Stampfer, W. C. Willett, B. Rosner, R. R. Monson, F. E. Speizer, and C. H. Hennekens, A prospective study of obesity and risk of coronary heart disease in women. *N. Engl. J. Med.*, *322*: 882 (1990).
31. G. A. Bray, *The Obese Patient*, Saunders, Philadelphia, p. 219 (1976).
32. R. J. Garrison and W. P. Castelli, Weight and thirty-year mortality of men in the Framingham study, *Ann. Intern. Med.*, *103*: 1006 (1985).
33. P. Bjorntorp, Regional patterns of fat distribution, *Ann. Intern. Med.*, *103*: 994 (1985).
34. J. Vague, The degree of masculine differentiation of obesities: A factor determining predisposition to diabetes, atherosclerosis, gout, and uric calculous disease, *Am. J. Clin. Nutr.*, *4*: 20 (1956).
35. C. V. Björkelund, C. B. Bengtsson, B. Carazo, L. Palm, G. Tarschus, and A. Wassen, Effects of a community risk factor reducing programme on weight, body fat distribution, and lipids in obese women, *Int. J. Obesity*, *15*: 251 (1991).
36. S. M. Haffner, M. P. Stern, H. P. Hazuda, J. Pugh, and J. K. Patterson, Do upper body and centralized adiposity measure different aspects of regional body-fat distribution? Relationship to non-insulin-dependent diabetes mellitus, lipids, and lipoproteins, *Diabetes*, *36*: 43 (1987).
37. B. Larsson, K. Svardsudd, L. Welin, L. Wilhelmsen, P. Bjorntorp, and G. Tibblin, Abdominal adipose tissue distribution, obesity, and risk of cardiovascular disease and death: A 13 year follow up of participants in the study of men born in 1913, *Br. Med. J.*, *288*: 1401 (1984).
38. L. Lapidus, C. Bengtsson, B. Larsson, K. Pennert, E. Rybo, and L. Sjostrom, Distribution of adipose tissue and risk of cardiovascular disease and death; a 12 year follow up of participants in the population study of women in Gothenburg, Sweden, *Br. Med. J.*, *289*: 1261 (1984).
39. A. Hartz, B. Grubb, R. Wild, J. J. Van Nort, E. Kuhn, D. Freedman, and A. Rimm. The association of waist hip ratio and angiographically determined coronary artery disease, *Int. J. Obesity*, *14*: 657 (1990).
40. R. E. Ostlund, Jr., M. Staten, W. M. Kohrt, J. Schultz, and M. Malley. The ratio of waist-to-hip circumference, plasma insulin level, and glucose intolerance as independent predictors of HDL$_2$ cholesterol level in older adults, *N. Engl. J. Med.*, *322*: 229 (1990).
41. R. Ballard-Barbash, A. Schatzkin, C. L. Carter, W. B. Kannel, B. E. Kreger, R. B. D'Agostino, G. L. Splansky, K. M. Anderson, and W. E. Helsel, Body fat distribution and breast cancer in the Framingham study, *J. Natl. Cancer Inst.*, *82*: 286 (1990).

42. J. V. Selby, B. Newman, C. P. Quesenberry Jr., R. R. Fabsitz, D. Carmelli, F. J. Meaney, and C. Slemenda, Genetic and behavioral influences in body fat distribution, *Int. J. Obesity*, *14*: 593 (1990).

43. C. Bouchard, Genetics of body fat, energy expenditure and adipose tissue metabolism, *Recent Advances in Obesity Research V*, (E. M. Berry, S. H. Blondheim, H. E. Eliahou, and E. Shafrir, eds.), John Libbey, London, p. 16 (1987).

44. J. Rodin, N. Radke-Sharpe, M. Rebuffe-Scrive, and M. R. C. Greenwood, Weight cycling and fat distribution, *Int. J. Obesity*, *14*: 303 (1990).

45. L. Cloarec-Blanchard, B. Darne, and P. Ducimetiere, Is there an ideal distribution of adipose tissue? *Lancet ii*, *336*: 1080 (Oct. 1970).

46. K. Y. Guggenheim, *Basic Issues in the History of Nutrition*, Akademia University Press, Jerusalem, p. 33 (1990).

47. C. Bouchard, Genetic factors in human obesity, *Med. Clin. North Am.*, *73*: 67 (1989).

48. G. H. Anderson, Metabolic regulation of food intake, *Modern Nutrition in Health and Disease* (M. E. Shills and V. R. Young, eds.), Lea and Febiger, Philadelphia, p. 561 (1988).

49. Thirteenth Marabou Symposium, Factors influencing food intake in man, *Nutr. Rev.*, *48*: 33 (1990).

50. M. Dallman, Neural and endocrine regulation of ingestive behavior, *Fed. Proc.*, *45*: 1383 (1986).

51. H. S. Koopmans and D. C. W. Lau (eds.), "The Joule, the Adipocyte, and Obesity," Symposia held at the 5th Annual NASSO Conference (Banff, 1988), *Int. J. Obesity*, *14* (Suppl. 3): (1990).

52. E. M. Stricker and J. G. Verbalis, Control of appetite and satiety: Insights from biologic and behavioral studies, *Nutr. Rev.*, *48*: 49 (1990).

53. D. A. York, Metabolic regulation of food intake, *Nutr. Rev.*, *48*: 64 (1990).

54. D. A. Booth, Sensory influences on food intake, *Nutr. Rev.*, *48*: 71 (1990).

55. B. J. Rolls, Sensory specific satiety, *Nutr. Rev.*, *44*: 93 (1986).

56. C. P. Herman and J. Polivy, A boundary model for the regulation of eating, *Eating and Its Disorders* (A. J. Stunkard and E. Steller, eds.) Raven Press, New York, p. 141 (1984).

57. G. B. Forbes, M. R. Brown, S. L. Welle, and B. A. Lipinski, Deliberate overfeeding in men and women: energy cost and composition of the weight gain, *Br. J. Nutr.*, *56*: 1 (1986).

58. E. Jequier and Y. Schutz, Does a defect in energy metabolism contribute to human obesity? *Recent Advances in Obesity Research*: *IV*, (J. Hirsch and T. B. VanItallie, eds.), Libbey, London, p. 76 (1985).

59. Y. Schutz, T. Bessard, and E. Jequier, Diet-induced thermogenesis measured over a whole day in obese and nonobese women, *Am. J. Clin. Nutr.*, *40*: 542 (1984).

60. J. Polivy and C. P. Herman, Diagnosis and treatment of normal eating, *J. Consult. Clin. Psychol.*, *55*: 635 (1987).

61. A. J. Stunkard and T. A. Wadden, Restrained eating and human obesity, *Nutr. Rev.*, *48*: 78 (1990).

62. A. J. Stunkard and S. Messick, A three-factor eating questionnaire to measure dietary restraint, disinhibition and hunger, *J. Psychosom. Res.*, *29*: 71 (1985).

63. R. G. Laessle, R. J. Tuschl, B. C. Kotthaus, and K-M. Pirke, Behavioral and biological correlates of dietary restraint in normal life, *Appetite, 12*: 83 (1989).

64. R. J. Tuschl, P. Platte, R. G. Laessle, W. Stichler, and K-M. Pirke, Energy expenditure and everyday eating behavior in healthy young women, *Am. J. Clin. Nutr.*, *52*: 81 (1990).

65. E. Jequier, Energy metabolism in obese patients before and after weight loss, and in patients who have relapsed, *Int. J. Obesity, 14* (Suppl. 1): 59 (1990).

66. C. Bogardus, Commentary on: 'Body weight regulation in obese and obese-reduced rats', *Int. J. Obesity, 14* (Suppl. 1): 46 (1990).

67. A. M. Altschul, Energy balance, *Weight Control: A Guide for Counselors and Therapists* (A. M. Altschul, ed.), Praeger, New York, p. 48 (1987).

68. C. Bogardus, S. Lillioja, and E. Ravussin, The pathogenesis of obesity in man: Results of studies on Pima Indians, *Int. J. Obesity, 14* (Suppl. 1): 59 (1990).

69. C. Bouchard, L. Perusse, C. Leblanc, A. Tremblay, and G. Theriault, Inheritance of the amount and distribution of human body fat, *Int. J. Obesity, 12*: 205 (1988).

70. A. J. Stunkard, J. R. Harris, N. L. Pedersen, and G. E. McClearn, The body-mass index of twins who have been reared apart, *N. Engl. J. Med., 322*: 1483 (1990).

71. C. Bouchard, A. Trembley, J-P. Depres, A. Nadeau, P. J. Lupien, G. Theriault, S. Moorjani, S. Pinault, G. Fournier, The response to long-term overfeeding in identical twins, *N. Engl. J. Med., 322*: 1477 (1990).

72. J. O. Hill, Body weight regulation in obese and obese-reduced rats, *Int. J. Obesity, 14* (Suppl. 1): 31 (1990).

73. G. L. Blackburn, G. T. Wilson, B. S. Kanders, L. J. Stein, P. T. Lavin, J. Adler, and K. T. Brownell, Weight cycling: The experience of human dieters, *Am. J. Clin. Nutr., 49*: 1105 (1989).

74. L. Lissner, P. M. Odell, R. B. D'Agostino, J. Stokes III, B. E. Kreger, A. L. Belanger, and K. D. Brownell, Variability of body weight and health outcomes in the Framingham population, *N. Engl. J. Med., 324*: 1839 (1991).

75. M. J. Stock and N. J. Rothwell, Criteria and experimental evidence for Luxuskonsumption, *Recent Advances in Obesity Research: IV* (E. M. Berry, S. H. Blondheim, H. E. Eliahou, and E. Shafrir, eds.), Libbey, London, p. 124 (1987).

76. A. Sclafani, Dietary obesity, *Obesity* (A. J. Stunkard, ed.). Saunders, Philadelphia, p. 166. (1980); Animal models of obesity: classification and characterization, *Int. J. Obesity, 8*: 491 (1984).

77. H. P. Himsworth, Diet in the aetiology of human diabetes. *Proc. Roy. Soc. Med., 42*: 323 (1949).

78. H. Malmros, The relation of nutrition to health: A statistical study of the effect of war-time on arteriosclerosis, cardiosclerosis, tuberculosis, and diabetes, *Acta Med. Scand. Suppl., 246*: 137 (1950).

79. A. Strom and R. A. Jensen, Mortality from circulatory diseases in Norway 1940-1945, *Lancet, i*: 126 (1951).

80. C. Schettler, Cardiovascular diseases during and after World War II: A comparison of the Federal Republic of Germany and other European countries, *Prev. Med., 8*: 581 (1979).
81. A. M. Cohen, S. Bavly, and R. Poznanski, Change of diet in relation to diabetes and ischemic heart disease, *Lancet, ii*: 1399 (1961).
82. J. D. Curb and E. B. Marcus, Body fat and obesity in Japanese Americans, *Am. J. Clin. Nutr., 53*: 1552S (1991).
83. P. Zimmet, Epidemiology of diabetes and its macrovascular manifestations in Pacific populations: The medical effects of social progress, *Diabetes Care, 2*: 144 (1979).
84. E. T. Poehlman and E. S. Horton, Regulation of energy expenditure in aging humans, *Annu. Rev. Nutr., 10*: 255 (1990).
85. F. I. Katch and W. D. McArdle, *Nutrition, Weight Control, and Exercise, 2nd ed.,* Lea and Febiger, Philadelphia, p. 97 (1983).
86. National Research Council (U.S.), *Recommended Dietary Allowances—10th rev. ed.,* Food and Nutrition Board, National Research Council, Washington, D.C. (1989).
87. G. T. Wilson, Behavior modification and the treatment of obesity, *Obesity* (A. J. Stunkard, ed.), Saunders, Philadelphia, p. 325 (1980).
88. K. D. Brownell, *The Learn Program for Weight Control*, University of Pennsylvania, Philadelphia, p. 157 (1988).
89. G. A. Bray and D. S. Gray, Treatment of obesity: An overview, *Diabetes/Metabolism Rev., 4*: 653 (1988).
90. S. A. Ramsey, Food as a stressor and as a stress reliever: Effectively managing stress, *Weight Control: A Guide for Counselors and Therapists* (A. M. Altschul, ed.), Praeger, New York, p. 181 (1987).
91. A. J. Blair, D. A. Booth, V. J. Lewis, and C. J. Wainwright, The relative success of official and informal weight reduction techniques: Retrospective correlational evidence, *Psychol. Health, 3*: 195 (1989).
92. R. B. Stuart and B. Davis, *Slim Chance in a Fat World: Behavior Control of Obesity*, Research, Champaign, IL (1972).
93. T. A. Wadden, T. B. VanItallie, and G. L. Blackburn, Responsible and irresponsible use of very-low-calorie diets in the treatment of obesity, *JAMA, 263*: 83 (1990).
94. D. L. Elliot, L. Goldberg, K. S. Kuehl, and W. M. Bennet, Sustained depression of the resting metabolic rate after massive weight loss, *Am. J. Clin. Nutr., 49*: 93 (1989).
95. G. D. Foster, T. A. Wadden, I. D. Feurer, A. J. Jennings, A. B. Stunkard, L. O. Crosby, J. Ship, and J. L. Mullen, Controlled trial of the metabolic effects of a very-low-calorie diet: Short- and long-term effects, *Am J. Clin. Nutr., 51*: 167 (1990).
96. J. U. Doherty, T. A. Wadden, L. Zuk, K. A. Letizia, G. D. Foster, and S. C. Day, Long-term evaluation of cardiac function in obese patients treated with a very-low-calorie diet: A controlled clinical study of patients without underlying cardiac disease, *Am J. Clin. Nutr., 53*: 854 (1991).

97. J. Dwyer, Sixteen popular diets: brief nutritional analyses, *Obesity* (A. J. Stunkard, ed.), Saunders, Philadelphia, p. 276 (1980).

98. K. D. Brownell and R. W. Jeffery, Improving long-term weight loss: Pushing the limits of treatment, *Behav. Ther., 18*: 353 (1987).

99. R. R. Wing, Behavior treatment of severe obesity, Gastrointestinal Surgery for Severe Obesity, Program and Abstracts, NIH Consensus Development Conference, Bethesda, MD, p. 49 (1991).

100. A. C. Sullivan and J. Triscari, Pharmacologic approaches to the regulation of metabolism and obesity, *Recent Advances in Obesity Research IV* (J. Hirsch and T. B. VanItallie, eds.), Libbey, London, p. 196 (1985).

101. M. Weintraub and G. A. Bray, Drug treatment of obesity, *Med. Clin. N. America, 73*: 237 (1989).

102. J. Rodin, M. Elias, L. R. Silberstein, and A. Wagner, Combined behavioral and pharmacologic treatment for obesity: Predictors of successful weight maintenance. *J. Consult. Clin. Psychol., 56*: 399 (1988).

103. J. M. Earll, Medical assessment of the patient with difficulty in weight management, *Weight Control: A Guide for Counselors and Therapists* (A. M. Altschul, ed.), Praeger, New York, p. 81 (1987).

104. Stunkard, A. J. The current status of treatment of obesity in adults, *Eating and Its Disorders* (A. J. Stunkard and E. Steller, eds.), Raven, New York, p. 157 (1984).

105. J. G. Kral, Surgical treatment of obesity, *Med. Clin. N. America, 73*: 251 (1989).

106. Gastrointestinal Surgery for Severe Obesity, Program and Abstracts, NIH Consensus Development Conference, Bethesda, MD, p. 49 (1991).

107. R. W. Jeffery, Behavioral treatment of obesity, *Ann. Behavioral Med, 9*: 20 (1987).

108. F. M. Kramer, R. W. Jeffery, J. L. Forster, and M. K. Snell, Long term follow-up of behavioral treatment for obesity: Patterns of weight regain among men and women, *Int. J. Obes. 13*: 123 (1989).

109. F. J. Volkmar, A. J. Stunkard, J. Woolston, and R. A. Bailey, High attrition rates in commercial weight reduction programs, *Arch. Intern. Med. 141*: 426 (1981).

110. S. Schacter, Recidivism and self-cure of smoking and obesity, *Am. Psychol., 37*: 436 (1982).

111. G. L. Leon and B. S. Rosenthal, Prognostic indicators of success or relapse in weight reduction, *Int. J. Eating Disorders, 3*: 15 (1984).

112. S. Kayman, W. Bruvold, and J. S. Stern, Maintenance and relapse after weight loss in women: Behavioral aspects, *Am. J. Clin. Nutr., 52*: 800 (1990).

113. G. A. Bennett, Behavior therapy for obesity: A quantitative review of the effects of selected treatment characteristics on outcome, *Behav. Ther., 17*: 554 (1986).

114. Booth, D. A. The zero-calorie drink break option. *Appetite, 11* (Suppl.): 94 (1988).

115. NCEP, Report of the National Cholesterol Education Program Expert Panel on Detection, Evaluation, and Treatment of High Blood Cholesterol in Adults. *Arch. Intern. Med., 148*: 36 (1988).

116. S. A. Norman, R. Greenberg, K. Marconi, W. Novelli, M. Felix, C. Schecter, P. D. Stolley, and A. J. Stunkard, A process evaluation of a two-year community cardiovascular risk reduction program: What was done and who knew about it, *Health Educ. Res., 5*: 87 (1990).
117. J. W. Farquhar, S. P. Fortmann, J. A. Flora, C. B. Taylor, W. L. Haskell, P. T. Williams, N. Maccoby, and P. D. Wood, Effects of communitywide education on cardiovascular disease risk factors. The Stanford Five-City Project. *JAMA, 264*: 359 (1990).

3
Childhood Obesity

Ramin Alemzadeh   *The University of Tennessee Medical Center at Knoxville, Knoxville, Tennessee*

Marie Fasano Ruggles   *North Shore University Hospital, Cornell University Medical College, Manhasset, New York*

Fima Lifshitz   *Maimonidies Medical Center, Brooklyn, New York*

I. INTRODUCTION

Obesity is a common disorder among children and adolescents in the United States, with an estimated prevalence of 25% as compared to 30% in adults. The prevalence of obesity appears to have risen by almost 50% among children and adolescents in the past two decades [1]. Obesity in childhood is not only accompanied by a greater risk for adult obesity, but also increasing risk for the development of hypertension [2], respiratory diseases [3], diabetes, many orthopedic conditions [4], and psychosocial disorders [5].

While obesity is a well-recognized medical entity, it remains a unique problem in that clinicians have difficulty determining who and how it should be treated. Moreover, it is still unclear to what extent the origin of obesity is linked to genetic, congenital, nutritional, metabolic, or behavioral factors. However, it is known that almost 10–20% of overweight infants will remain obese as children [6]. It has also been observed that 40% of obese children will continue to be overweight during adolescence. This risk increases to 70%

for an overweight adolescent continuing to be overweight as an adult. Also, the longer a child remains overweight, the chance of achieving normal weight later in life decreases. It has been observed that more than a third of overweight children will become obese adults [7].

This chapter reviews the potential risk factors for development of adipose tissue and the pathogenesis of obesity, evaluation and diagnostic criteria for obesity in children, causes of obesity, treatment and goals, and, finally, the role of preventive measures in the management of a child at risk.

II. GROWTH AND DEVELOPMENT OF ADIPOSE TISSUE

A. Cellular and Metabolic Events

The studies of cellular and metabolic processes during embryonic and fetal life unraveled the role of many factors involved in adipogenesis, which is accomplished by the transfer of maternal fatty acids in early gestation [8]. This is gradually followed by an increasing ability of the fetus to synthesize these fatty acids. There appear to be no gender differences in the rate of fat accumulation during the prenatal life. The rate of fetal fat deposition may be determined as a result of the balance that exists between adipogenesis and lipolysis. These processes are known to be modulated by sympathetic nervous system and hormonal influences. Indeed, catecholamines are known to be the most important acute stimulators of lipolysis [9]. Hormones like glucagon, adrenocorticotropic hormone (ACTH), and growth hormone (GH) have a lipolytic effect, wheras insulin appears to play a significant role in lipogenesis [10]. However, little is known about the role of these substances in prenatal growth of fat tissue. The study of large- and small-for-gestational-age infants suggests that the tissues may not be responsive to insulin until the early part of the third trimester [11], despite the presence of circulating insulin as early as 10–12 weeks gestation [11]. While the presence of some enzymes such as lipoprotein lipase (LPL) [12] and hormone-sensitive lipase [13], which are known to exist in the adipose tissue of children and adults, provided significant insights into their potential role in the pathogenesis of obesity [14–16], little is known about their role in fat metabolism during prenatal life.

Following birth, there is a significant increase in body fat content during the first 6 months of life, after which the rate of increase tapers off until the end of the first year [17]. However, the fat cell size increases rapidly and reaches the adolescent size within the first year of life. While the fat cell size remains relatively stable during childhood, it seems that from the first year to the onset of adolescence, the fat cell number increases steadily. However, between 2 and 6–8 years of life, the fat content decreases. This is followed by a characteristic substantial increase in adipocyte size and total number at puberty [18] and is accompanied by significant sex differences in the distribution, percentage, and duration of the growth of adipose tissue. For example, subcutaneous fat is predominantly distributed in the lower part of the body in females, whereas upper body subcutaneous fat deposits are seen in males. This difference seems to be related to the differences in their hormonal milieu. While girls show a steady increase in body fat content throughout puberty, boys tend to show a decrease in body fat content after their initial peak during early adolescence. Nevertheless, there is strong evidence that the growth of fat tissue is variable and differs from one fat deposit to another and between genders [17,19]. It is also believed that genetic and hormonal influences may play an important role in the growth of adipose tissue [20]. In addition, the pattern of feeding and overall feeding behavior is an important contributory factor in the development of adiposity. In fact, it has been shown that a very vigorous feeding pattern, as a genetically endowed behavior, may lead to an increase in adiposity, especially after 6 months of life [21]. However, further studies are indicated to better clarify the role of endocrine and metabolic processes and feeding behaviors in the postnatal adipogenesis.

B. Pathophysiology

The development of adiposity is a result of an energy imbalance over an extended length of time in which energy intake exceeds expenditure. However, calorie intakes have been reported to be comparable among obese and nonobese adults [22,23], therefore suggesting that overweight individuals have decreased energy expenditure. Indeed, evidence of an increase in metabolic "efficiency" and reduced caloric expenditure has been demonstrated in a genetic model of obesity, the Ob/Ob mouse [24].

The basal metabolic rate (BMR) is affected by fat-free mass (FFM), fat mass, age, stage of sexual development, and familial features. Nevertheless, the main determinant of BMR is FFM. It is believed that decreased obligatory energy expenditure, as reflected by the resting metabolic rate, could be the result of an incresed metabolic efficiency in obese individuals. However, Felig et al. demonstrated that BMR was, in fact, higher in the obese individual as compared to the nonobese subjects in fasting state as well as following a mixed meal [25]. They observed no defect in the thermogenic response in the postprandial state in the obese subjects. Also, in a more recent study among obese adolescents, BMR values corrected for FFM were relatively increased as compared to nonobese adolescents [26]. These observations, therefore, suggest that attainment of energy balance or weight maintenance in obese individuals requires a greater energy intake than in nonobese individuals.

The resting energy expenditure as corrected for FFM is believed to be genetically determined. Indeed, a study in Pima Indians showed decreased variability in BMR values among families as compared to the variance among the group studied [27]. This may suggest a genetic predisposition to enhanced metabolic efficiency of energy consumption in the resting state aggregated among some families. In fact, Ravussin et al. have shown that low BMR preceded significant weight gain [28]. However, this was followed by the elevation of metabolic rates, suggesting that weight gain may be a compensatory mechanism to normalize the BMR and raise energy expenditure. Heriditary decreases in the thermic effect of food over a protracted period of time could result in energy imbalance and an increase in body fat stores.

Decreased levels of physical energy expenditure have been observed in obese girls as compared to nonobese ones [29]. Similar findings have been observed in infants with excess weight gain who had decreased level of physical activity [30].

III. EVALUATION AND DIAGNOSTIC CRITERIA

A variety of measurements have been used to determine obesity and its severity. Definitions of excessive adiposity in children may be cosmetic, anthropometric, biochemical, and/or statistical. Obesity is usually considered to be an increase in body weight above some arbitrary standard usually defined in relation to height. Relative weight above 120% is a commonly used criterion of obesity in children. This is about the 95th percentile on the current weight-for-height charts [31]. Along with weight and height, body mass index, caliper skinfolds, and percent body fat have also been used as measures. Each method has its unique limitations as an index of childhood obesity. Weight and height charts can provide a ballpark range for normal weights but fail to take frame size and body composition into account. Similarly, body mass index (BMI, or weight-height^2 ratio) does not account for variations in musculature and could result in the classification of normal children as overweight.

The correlation of multiple skinfold measurements with total body adiposity is in the range of 0.7–0.8. However, obtaining accurate and reproducible caliper skinfold determinations in obese children can be a difficult task, especially when the skinfold exceeds 30 mm. Moreover, triceps skinfold, which is typically the site of measurement, is often difficult to grasp, and measurement reliability can be poor.

The determination of body adiposity can be accomplished by the measurement of body density derived from its specific gravity, that is, the weight of the body in and out of the water. This allows one to divide the body into fat and lean masses according their different densities. However, this tool requires appropriate facilities, therefore it remains a research method [32].

The use of isotopic and chemical dilution for measuring body compartments is another approach for determining body composition. Cyclopropane and krypton are two fat-soluble substances for measuring body fat content. Also, the determination of body fat from the measurement of body water can be estimated using tritiated deuterated water, or $H_2^{18}O$ or antipyrine, which equilibrate with body water [33].

Other techniques such as the use of ultrasound, electromagnetic conductivity, computerized tomography, and magnetic resonance imaging can provide information about the fat depth, quantity of fat versus lean tissues, as well as pictorial assessment of fat thickness, respectively.

Growth charts are the most useful tools for accurate individualized assessment of overweight children. By utilizing the growth chart, it is possible to locate a child's usual channel of growth. By 2–4 years of age most children's weight and height will consistently progress along one channel (i.e., 10th percentile for age, etc.). It is not uncommon for child's weight to be on a different percentile channel than his or her height. However, deviations from one's usual pattern represent a cause for concern.

In the following example, a growth chart is used to illustrate the pattern of true obesity in a 9-year-old girl (Lucy). The review of her growth chart (Fig. 1) revealed that her weight had been following the 50th percentile until age 4 years. She subsequently advanced to the 75th percentile within one year. In the following years, she continued to gain at an excessive rate, bringing her weight to above the 95th percentile. The final point on Lucy's chart (weight: 50 kg, height: 146 cm) represents 150% of her ideal body weight.

It is, however, important to differentiate true obesity from constitutional overweight. The latter is illustrated by the growth history in a 9-year-old girl (Terri) (Fig. 2). The review of her records reveal that Terri's weight has been above the 95th percentile since 2 years of age, indicating that this is her usual channel for weight advancement. The final point on Terri's growth chart (weight: 44.5 kg; height: 140 cm) represents 133% of her ideal body weight. However, the differences in weight progression between the two patients shown are more important than the degree of excess body weight for height and denote two distinct types of obesities.

Using the BMI classification system, the above two patients do not fall into separate categories of obesity (Table 1). For instance, Lucy, representing true obesity, has a BMI (23.4) above the 97th percentile for age. Similarly, Terri, classified as constitutionally overweight, has a very similar BMI (22.7) to the one obtained in Lucy, demonstrating that weight progression over time is a more valid clinical clue to detect the patient at risk for severe obesity

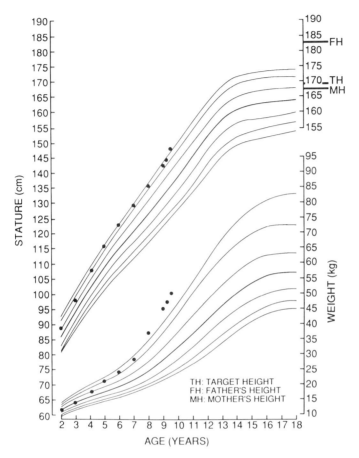

Figure 1 Growth chart illustrating pattern of true obesity in a 9-year-old girl. Notice the disproportionate amount of weight gained over time. Height progression also increased, with crossing of percentiles, but to a lesser degree than weight gain.

and for treatment. However, the BMI tables can be useful tools in those who are in their late adolescence and have almost completed their linear growth.

IV. CLASSIFICATION

Obesity in childhood can be of multiple etiologies and pathophysiological processes leading to excess accumulation of fat tissue. Obesity may be classified by etiology. The causes of obesity may be divided into nonorganic (genetic and environmental) and organic (endocrine and metabolic) categories.

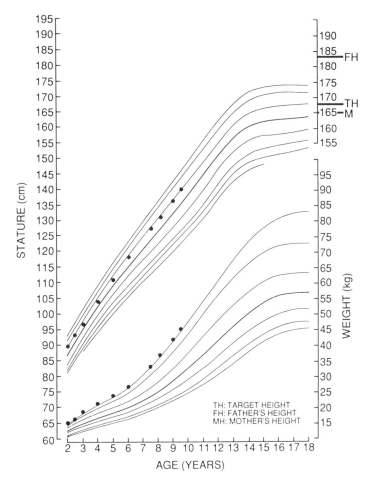

Figure 2 Growth chart illustrating pattern of constitutional overweight in a 9-year-old girl. Notice the constant body weight progression on the 95th percentile throughout the life of the child. The height progressed on the 75th percentile at a constant rate.

A. Nonorganic Causes

1. Genetic

To date no specific genetic defect responsible for disturbed energy balance and obesity has been identified. However, there are generally two groups of entities that lead to obesity. The first group is comprised of dysmorphic forms of obesity with possible underlying chromosomal defects, and the second

Table 1 Body Mass Index (BMI) Standards for Boys and Girls

Age (yr)	W/H² in percentile ranges[a]						
	3	10	25	50	75	90	97
Boys							
4–5	13.9	14.2	14.7	15.3	16.7	17	18
5–7	13.7	14.3	15	15.2	16.8	17	17.9
7–9	13.5	14	14.7	15	16.5	17.3	17.2
9–11	13.9	14.5	14.8	16	17	18.3	19.7
11–12	14.1	14.7	15	16.8	17.7	19.9	21
12–13	14.5	15	15.5	16.8	18.4	20.5	21.8
13–14	14.8	15	15.8	17	19	21	22
14–15	15.5	16	17	18.8	20.2	22	23
15–16	15.2	16.9	18	19	21	23	25
Girls							
4–5	13.3	14	14.8	15.9	16.3	17	18
5–7	13.5	14	14.8	15.2	16.2	17	18
7–9	14	14.2	15	15.5	16.5	17	18.5
9–11	14	14.9	15	16	17.5	19	20
11–12	14.9	15	16	17	18.8	20	21.5
12–13	14.4	15	16.4	16.8	19	20.8	22
13–14	14.6	15.5	16.8	18.7	19.1	21	22
14–15	14.5	16.5	17.2	19	20.6	22	25
15–16	15	17	18.2	19.2	20.5	22.5	25

[a]Weight in kilograms; height in meters.
Source: Ref. 78.

group is comprised of obesity that results from the interaction of environmental and familial genetic factors.

The dysmorphic forms of obesity are transmitted both by recessive and by dominant modes of inheritance. Prader-Willi syndrome is a genetic syndrome characterized by hyperphagia, hypotonia, developmental delay, hypogonadism, and short stature [34]. About half of these patients are said to have a translocation or deletion of chromosome 15. Obesity may start in infancy and becomes prominent in infancy, which in the presence of hyperphagia can lead to morbid obesity. The Lawrence-Moon-Biedl syndrome is another early-onset obesity, which is associated with retinitis pigmentosa, hypogonadism, mental retardation, and polydactyly [35]. It is transmitted by an autosomal recessive gene. It is believed that the obesity in these children is caused by a disturbance of appetite regulatory mechanism(s).

While monogenetic models of obesity have been described in both animals (i.e., fatty Zucker rats) and humans (i.e., Prader-Willi syndrome), most cases of obesity are generally believed to be the result of polygenic factors. Human twin studies, in fact, have provided strong evidence for genetic influences in obesity. This was initially demonstrated by Newman et al. [36], who examined the body weight of twins. There was a greater concordance of body fatness and weight for height among monzygotic twins with presumably identical genetic material as compared to dizygotic twins with genetic diversity [36]. Garn et al. studied the role of parental fatness in childhood fatness [37]. They demonstrated that children of two lean parents have about 14% likelihood of becoming obese. The offspring of a lean parent and an obese parent has a 40% risk of becoming obese, and the children of two overweight parents have up to an 80% likelihood of obesity. However, the latter study does not separate the genetic and environmental factors in a critical way. In a more distinctive approach, Stunkard et al. studied the role of genetic factors among adopted children [38]. They demonstrated that there was no relationship between indices of body fatness of the adoptive parents and their children, whereas body mass index of biological parents increased as the weight status of their children did. Additionally, the tendency for decreased rate of energy expenditure as a cause of excessive weight gain in obese patients has been found to aggregate in obese families [27,39], therefore reemphasizing the importance of genetic predisposition in the development of obesity.

2. Environmental

The impact of many environmental factors on the rate of weight gain with or without a genetic predisposition to obesity has been studied by some clinicians [37]. The environment interacts with genetic susceptibility to obesity.

The degree of body fatness of newborns has been directly related to maternal weight and weight gain during pregnancy [40], therefore providing evidence that newborn's fatness and growth was significantly influenced by intrauterine environment.

The determinants of weight gain and adiposity can vary from infancy to early childhood [41,42]. While birth weight, duration of breast feeding, sex (male), and age at the introduction of solid foods seems to significantly influence rate of weight gain during the first year of life, maternal relative weight also becomes a significant determinant for adiposity during the second year of life. The latter probably suggests that maternal environmental influences may play a significant role in the development of obesity as it determines the child's caloric intake and expenditure. In contrast, age at the introduction of solid foods does not seem to influence weight gain at 2 years. Also, male sex tends to retain its positive relationship with weight gain, but becomes negatively correlated with adiposity. Therefore, at 2 years boys are heavier, but girls are more obese. This relationship between sex and adiposity at 2 years may reflect the estrogenic or hormonal influences on body composition as early as 2 years of age.

Feeding behavior has been observed to influence the development of obesity in infants and children [21,43]. For example, significant differences in sucking frequency and formula consumption (if sweetened) has been observed among heavier infants as compared to ligher ones [44,45]. Similarly, obese children have been noted to eat more rapidly and chew their food less than those with normal weight [43]. These studies provide further evidence that vigorous eating behavior during infancy and childhood may set the ground for the development of adiposity.

Social behavior can also influence pattern of eating, which may be seen in situations where food may be used to reward behavior or to satisfy non-nutritional needs. Also, a familial pattern of overeating and decreasing level of physical activity may set the ground for the development of obesity in children.

It has been seen that socioeconomic status plays an important role in the development of obesity. Excess body weight is generally more common in lower-class females and upper-class males [46]. On the other hand, severe obesity does not appear to be related to socioeconomic status, which suggests that other factors such as genetic predisposition may play a role in its development.

The type and the amount of energy expenditures may also be different among obese individuals. Obese children and adults have often been characterized as slow or lazy individuals. Objective studies carried out in the past showed that obese children are less active [47,48]. Ravussin et al. measured differences of up to 500 kcal per day in energy expended as a result of spontaneous physical activity (i.e., fidgeting) [49].

Sedentary lifestyle also increases the risk for obesity. Children spend an average of 25 hours per week watching television; studies with adolescents have found that with each hour spent viewing television, the prevalence of obesity increases by 2% [50]. After following children through the 1970 and 1975 HANES surveys, child-obesity experts determined that "next to prior obesity, television viewing is the strongest predictor of subsequent obesity." They also agree that there exists a dose effect and that there is a very logical explanation for this correlation. Children tend to consume food in conjunction with the sedentary activity of television viewing. Their choices tend to reflect foods advertised in commercials—not the typical calorie-wise selections for the most part. Moreover, nearly everyone on television is thin; characters on prime-time television eat an average of eight times per hour. The messages that chidlren receive while viewing television are clearly inconsistent with reality.

B. Organic Causes

1. Metabolic and Endocrine

The occurrence of obesity in patients with hyperinsulinism, caused by islet-cell tumor or overinsulinization in an insulin-dependent diabetic patient with resultant increased food intake and fat storage, is well recognized. However, it is usually of small magnitude. Infants with hyperinsulinism due to islet-cell tumor or hyperplasia (nesidioblastosis) typically present with fasting hypoglycemia, not obesity. Hyperinsulinism may also be produced in response to excessive food intake in patients with exogenous obesity. This is usually associated with varying degrees of insulin resistance in some patients with obesity and non-insulin-dependent diabetes mellitus [51].

Hypercorticolism, secondary to pituitary overstimulation, adrenal adenoma, or exogenous steroid source, can result in a hyperinsulinemic state and excessive body fat accumulation with consequent altered body composition. The characteristic findings in a patient with Cushing's disease, secondary to glucocorticoid excess, are centripetal obesity, violaceous striae, glucose intolerance, and poor growth.

The presence of a hyperandrogenic state in a pubertal girl may be associated with excessive weight gain, signs of hirsutism or virilism, and irregularities of menstrual periods [52]. This may also be accompanied by hyperinsulinism and insulin resistance with or without glucose intolerance. Some patients may present with polycystic ovaries with abnormally elevated serum luteinizing hormone (LH), low follicle-stimulating hormone (FSH), and elevated free testosterone level.

Obesity is a well-recognized feature of primary hypogonadism. It is believed that hypogonadism results in excessive deposition of fat due to the deficiency of anabolic hormones, which are responsible for the growth of muscle. This effect is enhanced by the unopposed influence of estrogen leading to further fat accumulation in the hips and buttocks to produce the eunuchoid appearance.

Growth hormone (GH) deficiency is reported to result in a mild degree of obesity as compared to other causes of weight gain. It is believed that weight gain in a growth-deficient child is caused by diminished energy expenditure. Indeed, it has been observed that GH stimulates the growth of muscle tissue and breakdown of fat tissue, therefore affecting body composition [53]. Growth hormone levels are low in obese subjects, both in the fasted state and following stimulation [54,55].

Excessive weight gain secondary to an underactive thyroid gland is due to a combination of decreased metabolic rate and enhanced fluid retention [56]. However, it is not a common cause of obesity. Moreover, hypothyroidism in children is associated with sluggish linear growth. Therefore, a normally growing but overweight child is not likely to be hypothyroid.

2. Hypothalamic Obesity

This is a rare syndrome in humans (Fröhlich's syndrome) but can be produced in animals by injury to the ventromedial area of the hypothalamus. It was first described in a child with a pituitary tumor who was obese, hyperphagic, and sexually immature. Some believe that the hypothalamic injury leads to alterations in the appetite control center, which can result in hyperphagia and obesity. However, there is increasing evidence that the insulin hypersecretion seen in this syndrome may play a part in the development of obesity in this entity. Hypothalamic obesity has been reported under a variety of conditions [57] such as trauma, malignancy, and inflammatory disease.

TREATMENT

Prior to institution of any form of therapy, a comprehensive medical evaluation is indicated. This includes information on the rate of growth, developmental milestones, and family history. The latter is helpful to identify those with parental obesity, hypertension, diabetes mellitus, hyperlipidemia, and thyroid dysfunction. Furthermore, the evaluation should include nutritional, psychological, and physical fitness assessments.

The physical examination should consist of measuring blood pressure, looking for signs of insulin resistance (acanthosis nigricans), hypothyroidism, and/or Cushing's syndrome.

A. Goals of Therapy

In general, any therapeutic modality for childhood obesity is designed to induce decreased energy intake, while preserving normal growth at the same time. Intervention to induce weight loss must take into account all of the factors known to cause obesity and the forms of therapy that have been effective. Our present experience in the treatment of childhood obesity has identified environmental and behavioral factors as primary areas of intervention. Since genetic factors are known to influence the development of childhood obesity, early intervention in a child predisposed to obesity is indicated before it reaches extreme proportions. Moreover, any form of treatment for obesity should take into consideration potential underlying medical conditions (i.e., hypotonia) that may frustrate or render it ineffective. Therefore, the therapeutic plan should be individualized to reach its desired goal.

Both eating and exercise behavior are influenced by a number of physiological, psychological, social, and cultural factors. Therefore, in order to sufficiently achieve the desired therapeutic effect, a multifaceted approach is needed. Half-hearted attempts to treat obesity lead to failure and frustration and can set the stage for a lifelong struggle with obesity and weight cycling.

Long-term use of medications to suppress the appetite or other pills are not indicated in the treatment of pediatric obesity. The effectiveness of appetite-suppressant drugs appears to decrease with time, and there may be more side effects. Although these drugs are by no means the solution to weight loss, they may help people in the beginning of weight-loss programs by suppressing appetite, but these must be used with caution and for a very limited time [58].

Bulking agents and nonprescription diet aids, such as methylcellulose and other noncaloric bulk materials, have also been used in experimental and clinical attempts to inhibit food intake. The rationale for the use of such agents is that they swell in the stomach and supposedly give a feeling of satiety. However, the use of such agents as appetite suppressants works on a principle that has not proved to be effective in reducing feelings of hunger in patients on weight-loss programs. The use of pectin has been shown to reduce gastric emptying and increase satiety, but no long-term trial for obesity treatment has been carried out [59].

B. Dietary Management

Many special diets and dietary regimens have been used in the management of obesity. However, the best approach is appropriate reduction of energy intake combined with physical exercise. A well-balanced, normal diet that provides all the necessary nutrients is the most effective and safest treatment for obesity. The modification of caloric intake should be based upon the weight history of the child in conjunction with the usual caloric intake. Rate of growth, degree of adiposity, desired weight, and estimated exercise in a day should also be taken into consideration.

In general, moderately obese children should be placed on an energy-intake and exercise level that will slow weight gain or induce a slight weight loss. In order to accomplish this goal, it can be assumed that for every pound of weight loss 3500 kcal need to be used up. This is demonstrated in the following example.

In the case of Lucy (see Fig. 1), who was 50 kg (110 lb), weight loss was considered an important goal of treatment. Her caloric intake was reported to be 3400 kcal per day. An appropriate goal for Lucy would be to lose 2–5 kg (5–11 pounds) and then to maintain her weight until her height caught up to normalize the height-to-weight ratio. Once the initial weight loss was accomplished, Lucy would be at 130–140% of her ideal body weight. Although this still represents a weight excess, it is a safe goal at this time since additional weight loss may affect linear growth.

Applying the above guidelines, for Lucy to lose 1% of her body weight per week she would have to restrict her intake by enough calories to lose 0.5 kg/week (1.1 lb/week). She would attain this weight loss if she consumes 550 kcal/day less than her usual intake (3500 kcal/per pound of weight loss). Furthermore, if she would enhance her energy expenditures with exercise by 100–200 kcal/day she would only need to reduce her caloric intake by 300–400 kcal/day. In fact, this would allow her to eat a substantial amount during the day (2850 kcal/day) and still lose weight.

Overweight children often desire immediate rewards. Severe dietary restriction may lead to loss of lean body mass [60] and many other unphysiological changes [58] as well as to nutritional deficiencies. This can also lead to noncompliance and frustration with repeated attempts. Sufficient counseling and reassurance will set the goals straight between therapist, patient, and parent for long-lasting results and avoidance of failure and frustration.

It is important to realize that weight loss may not occur every week. As weight changes are monitored, the caloric value of the diet and the exercise level can be further modified accordingly. Obese children, especially those who have gone through dieting in the past, may have adjusted to a lower level of dietary consumption while maintaining weight. If there is no weight loss for 3 weeks, with no obvious noncompliance factor, then a reduction in the energy intake or an increase in physical activity level may be necessary.

The diet should be modified according to appropriate nutritional guidelines. This should include the reduction of fat to about one-third of the calories while increasing complex carbohydrates. The patient, Lucy, was managed by increasing vegetables in the diet and eating other low-calorie snacks, which subsitiuted for the high-fat foods. She was given three meals and two snacks instead of her one larger meal (supper). It is well recognized that frequent meals are more effective for weight control than one large meal [61, 62].

Daily variations in caloric intake are characteristic of normal eating patterns and should be allowed as long as they are within an acceptable range. For instance, it would be appropriate for Lucy, on a 2850 kcal food plan, to have a range of intakes from approximately 2500 to 3200 kcal. While the assessment of the rate of weight loss and growth is important, periodic evaluation of nutrient composition of the diet is essential. This is particularly important for such micronutrients like calcium, iron, magnesium, copper, zinc, folacin, and vitamin B_6, since these nutrients are very likely to be deficient on a restricted intake [63].

1. Low-Calorie Diets

Many types of low-calorie diet programs have become popular in attempts to speed up the process of weight loss. They include total fasting, very low-calorie diets, low-carbohydrate diets, protein-sparing diets, and high-protein diets. None of these are recommended for children as a routine treatment for obesity.

These aggressive weight-loss regimens are not appropriate for obese children since they may cause negative nitrogen balance, altered body composition, and eventually retard proper growth and development. A summary of many of these diets that are currently in use, with the associated nutrient deficiencies and possible side effects, is presented in Table 2.

Low-carbohydrate diets are usually high in protein and fat. They encourage consumption of large quantities of meat and restrict carbohydrate-containing foods such as fruits, vegetables, and grain products. The high intake of fat in such diets can increase the risk of coronary heart disease and other problems like gallstones and high cholesterol. The body relies heavily on its fat stores for energy while on a low-carbohydrate diet. This can lead to *ketosis* (the breakdown of fats for energy). The rapid weight loss on these diets is composed of 60–70% water, and the dieters often regain weight rapidly once normal eating is resumed.

Severe calorie restriction using protein-sparing, modified fast (PSMF) diets (400–700 kcal/day) can generate a rapid weight loss, up to 5 pounds (2.3 kg) per week. The protein is supplied either as food such as lean meat or fish, or in a milk- or egg-based liquid formula. This is associated with increased risk of medical complications. It has long been suggested that these diets spare body protein by decreasing insulin levels and enhancing fat breakdown [64], while inhibiting the release of amino acids from muscle [65]. However, several deaths have been associated with the use of these formulas [66], and there is little evidence that it produces a safer and more effective weight loss than a mixed diet. Moreover, these quick-fix weight-loss schemes are inappropriate for use in children and do not promote healthy eating behaviors for life-long weight control.

2. Weight Cycling

Recently, research has shed light onto the question of what happens when a person's weight continuously goes up and down. Weight cycling has a profound effect on body composition and its metabolic efficiency. Weight loss followed by weight gain results in negative consequences:

Weight loss from muscle
Regained weight as fat

Table 2 Nutrient Deficiencies and Side Effects Associated with Nutritionally Inadequate Diets

Diet	Examples	Potential nutrient deficiencies	Possible side effects

Low-carbohydrate diet	Air Force Diet
	Banting Diet
	Boston Police Diet
	Brand Name Carbohydrate Diet
	Calories Don't Count Diet
	Cormillot Thin Forever Diet
	Dr. Atkins Diet Revolution
	Dr. Cooper's Fabulous 14-Day
	  Fructose Diet
	Dr. Stillman's Quick Weight Loss Diet
	Dr. Yudkin's Lose Weight Feel Great Diet
	Drinking Man's Diet
	DuPont Diet
	Fat-Destroyer Foods Diet
	Paul Michael Weight Loss Plan
	Pennington Diet
	Scarsdale Diet
	Ski Team Diet
	Woman Doctor's Diet for Women
		Calcium
		Fiber
		Folic acid
		Magnesium
		Niacin
		Pantothenic acid
		Potassium
		Riboflavin
		Thiamin
		Vitamins
			Fatigue
			Apathy
			Dizziness
			Nervousness
			Ketosis
			Postural hypotension (fall in
			  blood pressure when standing
			  or getting up)
			Elevated blood lipid
			  (cholesterol and
			  triglycerides) levels
			Accelerated atherosclerosis
			Kidney problems
			Dehydration
			Damage to vision
			Scurvy
			Calcium depletion

High-carbohydrate diet	Best Chance Diet Beverly Hills Diet Beverly Hills Medical Diet Carbohydrate Cravers Diet Diet of a Desperate Housewife Dr. Stillman's Quick Inches Off Diet Hollywood Emergency Diet Kempner Rice Diet Macrobiotic Rice Diet	Calcium Copper Fatty acids Iron Potassium Protein Sodium Vitamin A Vitamin B_{12}	Weakness Dizziness Bloating Diarrhea Abnormally high and low swings in blood sugar levels Drop in blood pressure Fever Hair loss

Diet	Nutrient deficiencies	Effects
Pritikin Diet		
Quick Weight Loss Program	Vitamin D	Gout
200 Calorie Solution	Vitamin E	Kidney stones
	Zinc	Abnormal heart rhythms
Fasting	Calcium	Weakness
	Magnesium	Dizziness
	Nitrogen	Bad breath
	Phosphorus	Dry mouth
	Potassium	Irritability
	Sodium	Nausea
	Multiple vitamin deficiencies	Vomiting
		Diarrhea
		Fainting
		Ketosis
		Postural hypotension
		Sleeplessness
		Muscle cramps
		Dry skin
		Anemia
		Intolerance to cold
		Lowered blood pressure and heart rate
		Metabolic rate drops
		Apathy
		Depression
		Decreased sex drive
		Severe headaches
		Nervous tremors
		Hallucinations
		Amenorrhea
		Decreased muscle strength
		Speech impairment
		Loss of hearing

Table 2 (*Continued*)

Diet	Examples	Potential nutrient deficiencies	Possible side effects
Fasting (continued)			Blurred vision
			Hair loss
			Ulcerated mouth
			Retarded growth in children
			Erosion of bone mineral
			Unconsciousness
			Abnormal heart rhythms
			Coma
			Death
Protein-sparing modified fast	Cambridge Diet	Calcium	Fatigue
	Last Chance Diet	Copper	Irritability
	Oxford Diet	Electrolytes	Weakness
	University Diet	Magnesium	Fainting
	Optifast	Phosphorus	Nausea
		Potassium	Constipation
		Protein	Diarrhea
		Selenium	Vomiting
		Sodium	Muscle cramps
			Dry skin
			Cold intolerance
			Hair loss
			Amino acid imbalance
			Kidney damage
			Abnormal heart rhythms
			Dehydration
			Death

Source: Modified from *Weight Management: A Summary of Current Theory and Practice*, National Dairy Council, Copyright © 1985 National Dairy Council.

Body learns to cope with dieting
Increased risk of heart disease
Increased frustration

In essence, repeat dieters learn to cope with dieting. They develop a very efficient metabolism and maintain their weight with fewer and fewer calories with each diet cycle. This leads to the loss of muscle mass, which is replaced by fat. Similarly, repeated cycles of food restriction and overeating resulting in weight loss and regain in rats are associated with changes in levels of lipoprotein lipase, increased basal insulin, and selective deposition of fat in the intraabdominal region [67]. Along with changes in the body composition, the patient becomes psychologically frustrated as he or she fails to achieve the desired weight loss. The outcome is a patient who ingests very few calories and yet remains obese.

Appropriate strategies to avoid weight cycling should be considered at the beginning of a child's weight-reduction program. When a child is ready to undertake a weight-reduction program, it should represent a serious commitment of the child and his or her family to produce a successful outcome.

3. Growth Failure

In planning the dietary management of an obese child, growth should also be considered. A child who loses weight is in a negative energy balance and, therefore, may not grow in height [68]. This is observed in obese children who are very "motivated" and rapidly lose weight. If the weight loss continues for a long time, growth retardation due to dieting may become a potential problem. Dieting during periods of rapid growth like infancy or adolescence results in a higher risk of interfering with height advancement than when dieting occurs during periods of slow growth.

In the management of childhood obesity, an appropriate balance should exist between the needs of a patient to lose weight and the nutritional requirements for linear growth. However, since this balance can be difficult to achieve, the goals for weight loss should be conservative in order to preserve normal growth. Occasionally, it may be adequate if a child just ceases to gain weight and allows the height to catch up with his or her present weight. Since most obese children are above average for height for their age and demonstrate rapid growth rate and earlier sexual maturity than normal-weight children, some clinicians may not be concerned with slowing down the growth velocity during management of obesity. However, if a child's height velocity slows too drastically, the individual should be reassessed, including an evaluation of daily energy intake. A new dietary regimen should be considered to allow for growth to take place. Therefore, accurate assessment of linear growth is essential in the dietary management of childhood obesity.

Dietary restriction and weight reduction can only be considered successful if there is a normal growth in height proceeding simultaneously with weight loss.

C. Exercise

Dietary and behavioral treatments of obesity are based on the assumption that the energy intake of obese children exceeds their needs. However, it is clear that interventions using diet alone have left a trail of failure. To achieve desired weight loss can be extremely difficult and even more difficult to maintain over a long period of time. Furthermore, the composition of weight loss on low-calorie regimens (without exercise) comprises a relatively larger loss of lean body mass [69].

Physical activity has a significant influence on energy expenditure, and the energy cost for most activities is generally greater for heavier people. Regular aerobic exercise combined with energy restriction will result in greater reductions in body weight than dieting alone [70].

Dietary management of childhood obesity treatment should always be combined with exercise. An exercise program based upon the initial fitness level with a slow progression of the intensity, frequency, and duration is required to achieve the goal of weight control.

D. Psychological/Psychiatric Factors

Evaluation and management of psychological, social, and cultural factors that influence eating behavior is an essential aspect of the treatment of childhood obesity. It is believed that this aspect of treatment should be based on the assumption that overweight people eat in response to emotional states such as depression. In contrast, behavioral approaches focus primarily on how food cues in the environment stimulate overeating. The expertise of a social worker, psychologist, or psychiatrist, preferably with a special interest in obesity, should be utilized to address pertinent issues in this area of treatment. Topics frequently focused on with obese children include techniques such as relaxation for coping with emotions, obtaining social support, and self-control.

Dietary management and physical exercise are essential components for the development of effective treatments, and the area of greatest concern for psychologists is how to get children to alter food intake and activity behaviors. Because the primary focus is on changing the chlid's behavior, parenting skills represent an integral component of the intervention. Family support has been shown to influence the degree of immediate and continued weight loss in children, with parental participation repeatedly showing a positive impact.

E. Behavior Modification

Stimulus-control procedures in the behavioral control of overeating have led to the development of several behavioral techniques for the treatment of obesity, which include (1) self-monitoring of body weight and/or food intake, (2) goal setting, (3) reward and punishment, (4) aversion therapy, (5) social reinforcement, and (6) stimulus control. Several of these modifications have been found to be effective with children [71–73].

These interventions are based on the assumptions that the obese child is an overeater who is hypersensitive to food stimuli and can be trained to behave like a nonobese person and subsequently lose weight. Moreover, parental involvement and positive reinforcement by family and friends have been found to have a positive outcome on weight loss.

VI. THE PREVENTION OF OBESITY

The increasing problem of overweight constitutes a major public health problem in the United States. Very few studies have been conducted on the effectiveness of preventive measures, especially in regard to the effect of infant feeding practices on weight patterns throughout life. However, there is some evidence that feeding practices play an important role in infant weight gain and obesity. In fact, a study by Pisacano et al. revealed that less than 3.0% of 3-month-old infants who were maintained on a lowered-fat and lowered-total calorie diet (skim milk and solids) became overweight by 3 years of age [74]. This is a pertinent fact to be considered in the prevention of obesity in a high-risk group of children.

Early intervention in the management of obesity is critical from a treatment standpoint. Initial calorie excess results in enlarged fat cells. Once the fat cells have reached their capacity for size, the actual number of fat cells will begin to increase to provide for excess energy (triglyceride) stores. As an individual moves into this second stage, called "hyperplastic obesity," the condition becomes more refractory to treatment [75].

The diet from which children make choices has been called a "cafeteria" or "supermarket" diet. With relatively free access to highly palatable choices, the chances for overeating are increased. In fact, obesity occurred among rats given a "cafeteria" diet rather than their usual feed [76]. Thus, free access to highly palatable, nutritionally weak foods may encourage the development of obesity in susceptible individuals.

The availability of a variety of nutritious foods will set the ground for the development of healthy eating practices in children and adolescents. These foods should include an assortment of fresh or frozen vegetables and legumes; dairy products (low-fat for at-risk children above age 2); fresh fruits;

breads (preferably whole grain); and pastas, rice, cereals, and other grain products. Children should not be coaxed to eat everything on their plates and should not be expected to like all foods introduced to them. Deciding how *much* food to consume should be the perogative of the child. Sweets and other nutrient-poor foods should be allowed in limited amounts that will not interfere with the child's consumption of basic foods. Overzealous attempts to avoid "junk food" and/or to prevent obesity should be discouraged, as they may lead to other problems and even failure to thrive [77].

On a larger scale, the schools, the government, and the food industry should support measures that can improve the food habits and exercise patterns of children and adults. The government and local authorities should play a more active role in promoting physical activity through the provision of more community facilities for exercise affordable to all residents. The government should also regulate commercial slimming organizations and provide standards of treatment to reduce deception and fradulent practices to which obese persons so frequently fall victim. The media should assume a responsible position in regard to idealized concepts of beauty by appropriate programming and feeding messages passed through to children and to society at large. Finally, health insurance companies should assume responsibility in paying for obesity treatment before it leads to more costly long-term complications.

REFERENCES

1. S. L. Gortmaker, W. H. Dietz, A. M. Sobol, and C. A. Wehler, Increasing pediatric obesity in the United States, *Am. J. Dis. Child., 141*: 535 (1987).
2. L. K. Rames, W. R. Clarke, W. E. Connor, M. A. Reiter, and R. M. Laurer, Normal blood pressure and the evaluation of sustained blood pressure elevation in childhood: The Muscatine Study, *Pediatrics, 61*: 245 (1978).
3. V. V. Tracey, N. C. De, and J. R. Harper, Obesity and respiratory infection in infants and young children, *Br. Med. J., 1*: 16 (1971).
4. J. L. Kelsey, R. M. Acheson, and K. J. Keggi, The body build of patients with slipped capital femoral epiphysis. *Am. J. Dis. Child., 124*: 276 (1972).
5. L. F. Monello and J. Mayer, Obese adolescent girls: An interdisciplinary study of adolescent obesity, *J. Pediatr., 13*: 35 (1972).
6. J. Merritt and S. Russel, Obesity, *Curr. Probl. Pediatr., 12*: 1 (1982).
7. D. Stark, E. Alkins, D. H. Wolff, and J. W. B. Douglas, Longitudinal study of obesity in the National Survey of Health and Development, *Br. Med. J., 282*: 12 (1981).
8. J. F. Roux and T. Yoshioka, Lipid metabolism in the fetus during development, *Clin. Obstet. Gynecol., 13*: 595 (1970).
9. U. Smith and L. Sjostrom, Adipose tissue development and metabolism, *Int. J. Obesity, 5*: 545,720 (1981).

10. M. A. Sperling, Insulin and glucagon, *Perinatal Physiology*, 2nd ed. (U. Stave, ed.), Plenum Medical Book Co., New York and London, p. 813 (1978).
11. D. E. Hill, Fetal effects of insulin, *Obstet. Gynecol. Annu.*, *11*: 133 (1982).
12. A. Cryer, Tissue lipoprotein lipase activity and its action in lipoprotein metabolism, *Int. J. Biochem.*, *13*: 525 (1981).
13. F. O. Adebonojo, P. M. Coates, and J. A. Cortner, Hormone-sensitive lipase in human adipose tissue, isolated adipocyte, and cultured adipocytes. *Pediatr. Res.*, *16*: 982 (1982).
14. P. A. Kern, S. Marshall, and R. H. Eckel, Regulation of LPL in primary cultures of isolated human adipocytes, *J. Clin. Invest.*, *75*: 199 (1985).
15. L. Jonasson, G. K. Hansson, G. Bondjers, G. Bergtsson, and T. Olivecrona, Immunohistochemical localization of lipoprotein lipase in human adipose tissue, *Atherosclerosis*, *51*: 313 (1984).
16. P. Bjorntorp, M. Karlsson, P. Patterson, and G. Sypniewska, Differentiation and function of rat adipocyte precursor cells in primary culture, *J. Lipid. Res.*, *21*: 714 (1980).
17. D. C. Sinclair, Human growth after birth, *Human Growth After Birth,* 3rd ed. (D. C. Sinclair, ed.), Oxford University Press, New York, p. 48 (1978).
18. F. P. Bonnet, D. Rocour-Brumioul, and A. Heuskin, Regional variations of adipose cell size and local cellularity in human subcutaneous fat during normal growth, *Acta. Paediatr. Belg.*, *32*: 17 (1979).
19. C. G. D. Brook, Composition of human adipose tissue from deep and subcutaneous sites, *Br. J. Nutr.*, *25*: 377. (1971).
20. F. Ginsberg-Fellner, Growth of adipose tissue in infants, children and adolescents: Variations in growth disorders, *Int. J. Obesity*, *6*: 605 (1981).
21. W. S. Agras, H. C. Kraemer, R. I. Berkowitz, A. F. Korner, and L. D. Hammer, Does a vigorous feeding style influence early development of adiposity? *J. Pediatr.*, *110*: 799 (1987).
22. R. Beardin and R. J. Mayer, Food intakes of obese and non-obese women, *J. Am. Diet. Assoc.*, *29*: 29 (1953).
23. E. Maxfield and F. Konishi, Patterns of food intake and physical activity in obesity, *J. Am. Diet. Assoc.*, *49*: 406 (1966).
24. P. Trayhur, P. L. Thurlby, and W. P. T. James, Thermogenic defect in pre-obese Ob/Ob mice, *Nature*, *266*: 60 (1977).
25. P. Felig, J. Cunningham, M. Levitt, R. Hendler, and E. Nadel, Energy expenditure in obesity in fasting and postprandial state. *Am. J. Physiol.*, *244* (1): E45 (1983).
26. L. G. Bandini, D. A. Schoeller, and W. H. Dietz, Energy expenditure in obese and non-obese adolescents, *Pediatr. Res.*, *27*: 198 (1990).
27. C. Bogardus, S. Lillioja, E. Ravussin, W. Abbott, K. Zawadzki, A. Young, W. C. Knowles, R. Jacobowitz, and P. P. Moll, Familial dependency of resting metabolic rate, *N. Engl. J. Med.*, *315*: 96 (1986).
28. E. Ravussin, S. Lillioja, W. C. Knowles, L. Christin, D. Freymond, W. G. H. Abbot, V. Boyce, B. V. Howard, and C. Bogardus, Reduced rate of energy expenditure as a risk factor for body-weight gain, *N. Engl. J. Med.*, *318*: 467 (1988).

29. E. Ravussin, B. Burnand, Y. Schutz, and E. Jequier, Twenty-four hour energy expenditure and resting metabolic rate in obese, moderately obese, and control subjects, *Am. J. Clin. Nutr., 35*: 566 (1982).
30. S. B. Roberts, J. Savage, W. A. Coward, B. Chew and A. Lucas, Energy expenditure and intake in infants born to lean and overweight mothers, *N. Engl. J. Med., 318*: 461 (1988).
31. P. V. Hamill, T. A. Drizd, C. L. Johnson, R. B. Reed, A. F. Roche, and W. M. Moore, Physical growth: National Center for Health Statistics percentiles, *Am. J. Clin. Nutr., 32*: 607 (1979).
32. J. L. Leonard, C. S. Leach, and P. C. Rambaut, Quantitation of tissue loss during prolonged space flight, *Am. J. Clin. Nutr., 38*: 667 (1983).
33. G. A. Bray, *The Obese Patient, Major Problems in Internal Medicine*, Vol. 9, W. B. Saunders Company, Philadelphia, p. 18 (1976).
34. G. A. Bray, The Prader-Willi Syndrome. A study of 40 patients and a review of the literature, *Medicine, 62*: 59 (1983).
35. M. L. Bauman and G. R. Hogan, Laurence-Moon-Biedel Syndrome, *Am. J. Dis. Child., 126*: 119 (1973).
36. H. H. Newman, F. N. Freeman, and K. H. Holzinger, *Twins: A Study of Heredity and Environment*, University of Chicago Press, Chicago (1937).
37. S. M. Garn, T. V. Sullivan, and V. M. Hawthorne, Fatness and obesity of the parents of obese individuals, *Am. J. Clin. Nutr., 50*: 1380 (1989).
38. A. J. Stunkard, T. I. A. Sorensen, C. Hanis, T. W. Teasdale, R. Chakraborty, W. J. Scholl, and F. Schulsinger, Adoption study of human obesity, *N. Engl. J. Med., 314*: 193 (1986).
39. C. Bogardus, S. Lillioja, E. Ravussin, W. C. Abbott, J. K. Zawadzki, A. Young, W. C. Knowler, R. Jacobwitz, P. P. Moll, Familial dependence of the resting metabolic rate, *N. Engl. J. Med., 315*: 96 (1986).
40. J. N. Udall, G. G. Harrison, Y. Vaucher, D. D. Walson, and G. Morrow, 3rd., Interaction of maternal and neonatal obesity, *Pediatrics, 62*: 17 (1978).
41. M. S. Kramer, R. G. Barr, D. G. Leduc, C. Boisjoly and I. B. Pless, Determinants of weight and adiposity in the first year of life, *J. Pediatr., 106*: 10 (1985).
42. M. S. Kramer, R. G. Barr, D. G. Leduce, C. Boisjoly, and I. B. Pless, Infant determinants of childhood weight and adiposity, *J. Pediatr., 107*: 104 (1985).
43. R. S. Drabman, G. Cordua, D. Hammer, G. J. Jarvie, and W. Horton, Developmental trends in eating rates of normal and overweight preschool children, *Child. Dev., 50*: 211 (1979).
44. T. Engen, L. P. Lipsitt, and D. O. Robinson, The human newborn's sucking behavior for sweet fluids as a function of birth weight and maternal weight, *Infant Behav. Dev., 1*: 118 (1968).
45. R. M. Milstein, Responsiveness in newborn infants of overweight and normal weight parents, *Appetite, 1*: 65 (1980).
46. P. B. Goldblatt, M. E. Moore, and A. J. Stunkard. Social factors in obesity, *JAMA, 192*: 1039 (1965).
47. B. A. Bullen, R. B. Reed, and J. Mayer, Physical activity of obese and non-obese girls appraised by motion picture sampling, *J. Clin. Nutr., 14*: 211 (1964).

48. H. E. Rose and J. Mayer, Activity, calorie intake, fat storage, and the energy balance of infants, *Pediatrics, 41*: 18 (1968).
49. E. Ravussin, S. Lillioja, T. E. Anderson, and L. Christin, Determinants of 24 hour energy expenditure in man: Methods and results using a respiratory chamber, *J. Clin. Invest., 78*: 1568 (1986).
50. W. H. Dietz and S. L. Gortmaker, Do we fatten our children at the TV set. Television viewing and obesity in children and adolescents, *Pediatrics, 75*: 807 (1985).
51. J. M. Olefsky, O. G. Kolterman, and J. A. Scarlett, Insulin action and resistance in obesity and non-insulin-dependent type II diabetes mellitus, *Am. J. Physiol., 243*: E15 (1982).
52. H. J. Hartz, P. N. Barboriak, A. Wong, K. P. Katayama, and A. A. Rimm, The association of obesity with infertility and related menstrual abnormalities in women. *Int. J. Obesity, 3*: 57 (1979).
53. L. P. Novak, A. B. Hayles, and M. D. Cloutier, Effect of HGH on body composition of hypopituitary dwarfs, *Mayo Clin. Proc., 47*: 241 (1972).
54. M. T Meistas, G. V. Foster, S. Margoles, and A. A. Kowarski, Integrated concentration of growth hormone, insulin, C-peptide and prolactin in human obesity, *Metabolism, 31*: 1224 (1982).
55. E. A. H. Sims, E. Danforth Jr., E. S. Horton, G. Bray, J. Glennon, and L. Salans, Endocrine and metabolic effects of experimental obesity in man, *Recent Prog. Horm. Res., 29*: 457 (1973).
56. J. H. Kyle, M. F. Ball, and P. D. Dolan, Effect of thyroid hormone on body composition in myxedema and obesity, *N. Engl. J. Med., 275*: 12 (1965).
57. G. A. Bray, Syndromes of hypothalamic obesity in man, *Pediatr. Ann., 13*: 525 (1984).
58. G. A. Bray and D. S. Gray, Treatment of obesity: An overview. *Diabetes/Metabolism Rev., 4*: 655 (1988).
59. C. DiLorenzo, C. M. Williams, F. Hajnal, and J. Valenzuela. Pectin delays gastric emptying and increases satiety in obese subjects, *Gastroenterology, 95*: 1211 (1988).
60. J. O. Hill, P. B. Sparling, T. W. Shields, and P. Heller, Effects of exercise and food restriction on body composition and metabolic rate in obese women, *Am. J. Clin. Nutr., 46*: 622 (1987).
61. G. A. Bray, Lipogenesis in human adipose tissue: Some effects of nibbling and gorging, *J. Clin. Invest., 51*: 537 (1972).
62. H. L. Metzner, The relationship between frequency of eating and adiposity in adult men and women in the Tecumseh Community Health Study, *Am. J. Clin. Nutr., 30*: 712 (1989).
63. Nationwide Food Consumption Survey of Food Intakes by Individuals, Women 19–50 years and their children 1–5 years, 1 day, *NCFS, CSFII Report No. 85-1*, U.S. Department of Agriculture, Human Nutrition Service, Nutrition Monitoring Division, Washington, D. C. (1985).
64. J. P. Flatt and G. L. Blackburn, The metabolic fuel regulatory system: Implications for protein-sparing therapies during caloric deprivation and disease, *Am. J. Clin. Nutr., 27*: 175 (1974).

65. R. S. Sherwin, R. G. Hendler, and P. Felig, Effect of ketone infusions on amino acid and nitrogen metabolism in man, *J. Clin. Invest.*, *55*(6): 1382 (1975).
66. H. E. Sours, V. P. Frattali, C. D. Brand, R. A. Feldman, A. L. Forbes, R. C. Swanson, and A. L. Paris. Sudden death associated with very-low-calorie weight reduction regimens, *Am. J. Clin. Nutr.*, *34*: 453 (1981).
67. K. Brownell, M. R. C. Greenwood, E. Stellar, and E. Shrager, The effects of repeated cycles of weight loss and regain in rats, *Physiol. Behav.*, *38*: 459 (1987).
68. W. H. Dietz and R. Hartung, Changes in height velocity of obese preadolescents during weight reduction, *Am. J. Dis. Child.*, *139*: 704 (1985).
69. S. R. Newmark and B. Williamson, Survey of very-low-calorie weight reduction diets. II. Total fasting, protein-sparing modified fasts, chemically defined diets, *Arch. Intern. Med.*, *143*: 1423 (1983).
70. R. D. Hagars, S. J. Upton, L. Wong, and J. Whittam, The effects of aerobic conditioning and/or caloric restriction in overweight men and women, *Med. Sci. Sports Exerc.*, *18*: 87 (1986).
71. L. D. Brownell and A. J. Stunkard. Behavioral treatment of obesity in children, *Am. J. Dis. Child.*, *132*: 403 (1978).
72. L. H. Epstein, Review of behavioral treatments for childhood obesity, *Eating Disorders* (K. D. Brownell, J. P. Foreyt, eds.), Basic Books, Inc., New York, pp. 159–179 (1986).
73. L. H. Epstein, R. W. Rena, R. Koeske, and A. Valoski, Long-term effects of family-based treatment of childhood obesity, *J. Consul. Clin. Psy.*, *55*: 91 (1987).
74. J. C. Pisacano, H. Lichter, J. Ritter, and A. P. Siegal, An attempt at prevention of obesity in infancy, *Pediatrics*, *61*: 360. (1978).
75. L. Buckmanster and K. Brownell, Behavior modification: the state of the art, *Obesity and Weight Control* (R. Frankle and M. Yang, eds.), Aspen Publishers, Inc., Rockville, Maryland (1988).
76. A. Sclafani, Dietary obesity, *Obesity* (A. J. Stunkard, ed.), W. B. Saunders Co., Philadelphia pp. 166–181 (1980).
77. M. Pugliese, M. Weyman-Daum, N. Moses, and F. Lifshitz, Parental health beliefs as a cause of non-organic failure to thrive, *Pediatrics*, *80*: 175 (1987).
78. M. F. Roland-Cachera, M. Sempe, M. Guilloud-Bataille, E. Patois, F. Pequig-not-Guggenbuhl, and V. Fautrad, Adiposity indices in children, *Am. J. Clin. Nutr.*, *36*: 178 (1982).

4

Trends in Eating Patterns
in the United States

D. Elizabeth Randall and Susan McCann   *State University of New York at Buffalo, Buffalo, New York*

I. INTRODUCTION

To understand the changes that have occurred in the diets of Americans in this century is to understand what has happened to American society itself. Since the federal government began tracking the food supply in 1909 to the present time, we have experienced several wars and a major economic depression, a shift from an agriculture-dominated to an industrially based economy driven by technological innovation, and a migration within the population to urban and metropolitan communities and away from rural areas. A sophisticated system of highways has been built intentionally to support a national distribution of commercial goods, including foods. The United States has become trading partners with many foreign nations, who are adding to our food supply, which is now more plentiful and less affected by seasonal variability.

Personal disposable income has increased dramatically, as has the proportion of the population graduating from high school and, more recently, from college [1]. Household structure has changed away from the extended and towards the nuclear family in response to the mobility of the population. Increasing numbers of women, traditionally responsible for food decision-making, work outside the home and spend fewer hours in meal preparation. They make important economic contributions to households that frequently translate into acquisition of services, including the purchase of prepared and other convenience foods.

The population is currently in the process of growing older. Fewer children die in the first years of life, the development of antibiotics has decreased the number of persons dying of infectious diseases dramatically, and as a result chronic diseases have replaced them as the major causes of death [2,3]. Further advances in medical technology have extended the duration of life for persons developing these chronic diseases.

Diets result from the complexity of behaviors whereby foods are combined into meals in patterns directed not only by physiological need and cultural heritage, but also by such additional parameters as availability, cost, taste, age, preferences of other household members, demands of daily activities, and values placed on health and social status [4]. Given the plethora of changes in factors known to shape food behaviors, it is not surprising that diets in the United States have undergone major adjustments concurrent to the social changes witnessed in the twentieth century.

II. MEASURING DIETS

We in the United States are fortunate in having a wealth of data available for tracking these changes in our diets over time. Since 1909 the U.S. Department of Agriculture (USDA) has collected information on foods acquired by the population for consumption, referred to as food disappearance data [5,6]. Quantities of food disappearing from commercial sources are adjusted to account for losses in storage and preparation prior to consumption and divided by the population size to generate estimates of per capita availability of foods as well as energy and macronutrients supplied by these foods [7].

The USDA enhanced these data beginning approximately 65 years ago when it began surveying food use within households in this country. Over the last 25 years it has expanded the surveys to support the study of regional and seasonal differences in consumption, as well as assessments of dietary intakes of individual household members [5,6]. Until recently, these USDA surveys of households and individuals were conducted approximately every 10 years; since 1985 the surveys have been designed to be continuously in the field. These USDA surveys of food use within households provide the strongest base for examining impacts of socioeconomic forces and the effects of governmental policies on food consumption in this country over the past 25 years.

Since the 1970s, the U.S. Department of Health and Human Services (DHHS) has had responsibility for the National Health and Nutrition Examination Surveys (NHANES). Dietary data are collected from representative individuals in the U.S. population, along with other parameters that support examinations of diet and health relationships [6,8,9], in contrast to the economic analyses supported by USDA surveys. NHANES data support nutrition status assessments for major subgroups in the population, defined by such demographic variables as ethnicity, age, gender, and income.

Because of history of concern for food consumption in this country, we have data available to use for assessing current diets, as well as the capability for tracking changes over time and for predicting future trends [3]. Unfortunately, the various surveys provide data differing in level of measurement, regional and seasonal specificity, and relevant time periods [6,10,11]. Per capita food disappearance data have been collected annually since 1909. These data are applicable to the entire population, but they cannot support studies of food distribution within finer divisions of the population. Data for household food use began in approximately 1935, but the samples were not regionally or seasonally representative of all households, and data adequate for assessing intakes of individual household members were not obtained until the 1977–78 survey. In the USDA household surveys, diets of individuals are measured with a 24-hour recall method supplemented with multiple days of diet records. Since they began in 1971, the NHANES surveys rely on the 24-hour recall for dietary assessments. Although such differences in dietary methodology do not prevent comparisons, they do restrict linkages between the surveys and demand care in any interpretation of changes in diet over time, if more than one of these data sources is used.

III. CHARACTERIZING THE AMERICAN DIET

The food industry provides consumers in this country with literally thousands of options from which to select the relatively few foods that will be combined to create the diets of individual Americans. The majority of Americans have access to an ample diet, and many suffer from the problems of a surfeit of food [12,13].

Food disappearance data for 1985 indicate that (1) fats and oil, (2) grain products, (3) meat, fish and poultry, and (4) sweeteners, in that order, are the top-ranked *food types* in terms of their contributions of energy in the American diet [6]. Block et al. [14] identified actual *foods* that make the greatest contributions to the intakes of specific nutrients in the United States using the 24-hour recall data collected in the NHANES II (1976–80). Nutrient intakes of the total survey sample were calculated and individual foods reported as being consumed by subjects were rank-ordered according to their percent contributions to the intakes of nutrients for the entire sample. Fifty foods accounted for 88.5% of the energy intake; Table 1 lists those foods, ranked by their contributions to energy within important groups of foods.

According to these NHANES data, the groups making the greatest contributions of energy are animal proteins, legumes, and nuts; grains; dairy products; and other beverages (excluding milk and soft drinks and juices).

Table 1   Major Food Sources of Energy in the Diets of Americans, NHANES II, 1976–80

Food group	Food item	Percent energy contributed
Meat and alternates	Ground beef (including meatloaf and hamburgers)	4.39
	Beef (steaks, roasts)	4.14
	Hot dogs, luncheon meats, ham	3.19
	Eggs	2.53
	Pork (chops, roasts)	2.28
	Dried beans	1.17
	Poultry (excluding fried)	1.12
	Fried fish	0.91
	Peanuts and peanut butter	0.89
	Fried chicken	0.84
	Bacon	0.64
	Sausage	0.57
	Tuna (including salad, casserole)	0.51
	Total	23.18
Breads and cereals	White bread, rolls and crackers	9.59
	Donuts, cakes, cookies	5.70
	Whole grain breads	1.70
	Salty snacks	1.41
	Pies (excluding pumpkin)	1.31
	Cornbread, grits, tortillas	0.99
	Cold cereals (excluding bran and super-fortified cereals)	0.86
	Rice	0.64
	Bran and granola cereals	0.59
	Total	22.79

Table 1 (Continued)

Food group	Food item	Percent energy contributed
Dairy products	Whole milk and beverages made with whole milk	4.72
	Cheeses (excluding cottage cheese)	2.45
	Ice cream and frozen desserts	1.71
	2% milk	1.67
	Skim milk and buttermilk	0.78
	Total	11.33
Beverages (excluding milk, soft drinks, and juices)	Alcoholic beverages	5.70
	Coffee, tea	1.31
	Hi-C and fortified fruit drinks	0.52
	Total	7.53
Fruits and vegetables	French fries and fried potatoes	2.53
	Other potatoes	1.47
	Orange juice	1.38
	Other fruit juices	0.73
	Apples and applesauce	0.57
	Total	6.68
Sweeteners	Soft drinks	3.63
	Sugar	1.48
	Candy, chocolate	0.85
	Jellies, jams, honey	0.48
	Total	6.44
Fats and oils	Mayonnaise and salad dressings	1.67
	Margarine	1.64
	Salad and cooking oils	0.94
	Butter	0.87
	Gravy and other meat sauces	0.53
	Total	5.65
Mixed dishes	Spaghetti and tomato sauce	1.61
	Pizza	0.87
	Chili	0.77
	Soups (excluding vegetables and tomato)	0.60
	Mixed dishes with cheese	0.54
	Beef stew, pot pie	0.53
	Total	4.95
Total		88.55

Source: Ref. 14.

White bread, rolls, and crackers, specifically, supply the greatest amount of food energy in this country; they provide almost 10% of the calories consumed. Beef in its various forms is also a dominant source of food energy, accounting for another approximately 10% of food energy. Additional sources of energy, in descending order of their contributions to intakes, are baked goods, alcoholic beverages, whole milk, soft drinks, processed meats, eggs, fried potatoes, cheese, and pork.

Using such an approach to identifying major food sources of energy permits two factors in food use to be expressed: the percentage of the population consuming a given food and the relative contribution of energy made by a serving of the food. Most of the foods listed as important sources of energy are calorically dense items. Others such as juices, white bread, and lowfat milks are not, but are consumed by a sufficiently large number of people that they make important contributions to the aggregate intake of food energy in the population. As a consequence of this phenomenon, fruits and vegetables that tend not to be calorically dense but that are consumed by a large proportion of the population are important sources of energy in this country. This finding reinforces the concept that an individual food does not have to contain a large number of calories in order to be a major source of energy if it is eaten often or in large amounts.

National cross-sectional surveys provide a snapshot of the diets of individuals at a single point in time. But diets are dynamic, constantly responding to such forces as economic and political pressures, changing social values, and technological advances in food product development. The food disappearance data available for the United States since 1909 can provide a longitudinal perspective but can provide data on only per capita consumption. They cannot address changes in the diets of individuals or of segments of the population.

Based on food disappearance data, the percent contribution of foods in the animal protein group (meat, poultry, fish, and eggs) to energy availability declined between 1909 and 1939, then increased between 1947 and 1969 before experiencing slight decreases in recent decades [6,10,11]. This food group is dominated by red meats, whose individual consumption patterns mirror the trends apparent for the food group as a whole. The contribution of eggs to energy intake also displays similar trends, although their contributions to energy peaked earlier, in 1959 rather than 1969. Fish and shellfish consumption has increased in importance gradually over the century, until experiencing its current rise in popularity, resulting in a 41% increase in per capita use between 1966 and 1987 [15]. Poultry, on the other hand, has displayed steadily increasing popularity since 1947.

Dairy products display trends that are highly similar to these animal protein foods [6,10] in that their contributions to energy availability peaked in mid-century [1947–1959] and have declined subsequently. Their decline can be linked to the reduced significance of whole milk to energy consumption, a decrease not compensated for fully by increased contributions from low-fat milks that are less calorically dense. The steady increase in the contributions of cheeses is noteworthy in contrast to the trends to lower reliance on high-fat animal products as food sources of energy in the latter half of this century; its use has been linked to its complementary function with wine, which has experienced significantly increased use over this time period and to a surge in popularity of Italian cuisine, especially pizza [15,16].

Grains have consistently decreased in importance as a source of energy; the rate of this decrease has slowed in recent decades. Sweeteners, on the other hand, have increased dramatically in their importance as energy sources [6,10,17,18].

The role of food technology in changing the fat composition of the food supply up to this point may be no more evident than for such fats as butter, margarine, shortening, lard, beef tallow, and edible oils used in cooking or as additions to foods. There has been an overall increase in the contribution of such fats to energy intake in this century, but the development of the ability to extract oils from vegetable sources in the post–World War II era has dramatically changed the relative importance of saturated and unsaturated fatty acids in the diets of Americans [6,10,18,19]. The total contribution of spreads (butter and margarine) to energy consumption has been stable until recently, when it declined slightly, despite the fact that margarine has interchanged with butter as the dominant spread in current use [6,7,10,18]. Both shortening and edible oils currently contribute a greater proportion of energy than they did prior to World War II. We now are on the brink of another technological revolution in dietary fat composition as food manufacturers prepare to introduce fat substitutes to the food supply [19,20].

Given these trends in food sources of energy as well as in increases in overall availability of energy [6], nutrient composition of diets would be expected to exhibit changes between early and late phases of the twentieth century. Protein consistently has contributed 11–12% of calories in the U.S. diet. The contribution of fat to caloric intake has increased from 33 to 43% and that of carbohydrate has decreased from 58 to 46% [10]. Not only have carbohydrates decreased as sources of energy, but such decreases are attributable predominantly to complex carbohydrates, since the contributions of sweeteners, being simple carbohydrates, have actually increased over this time period [6,17].

Based on data from national surveys, it can be stated that, despite the consumption of foods with lower fat densities in recent decades, Americans are consuming a higher proportion of their calories from fat than they did early in this century [10]. Since 1977 the general population has gained greater awareness of the importance of fat intake to health [21]. Within the population, a greater proportion of college graduates became aware of the relationship than did less well-educated persons. Such awareness has tranlated only modestly into more prudent fat intakes, which have dropped from approximately 41% of calories to 37% in 1986. However, the diets of college graduates were no less fat dense than those of persons with less education [21]. It has been suggested that individual Americans are making changes towards less saturated fats without decreasing intakes of total fat to the extent advocated by the various dietary guidelines [12].

Epidemiological studies focused on selected populations demonstrated variability in fat intake expressed as a percentage of caloric intake. Persons whose diets are most compliant with recommended dietary guidelines have fat intakes approaching 30% of calories; less prudent eating styles obtain approximately 40% of calories from fat [22].

Block et al. [23] compared intakes of macronutrients based on gender, age, income, and ethnic differences. Those patterns apparent for energy were observed for fat and saturated fat intakes as well. Consistently, men exhibit higher intakes than do women; whites have higher intakes than do blacks; and older persons (55–74 years) consume less than younger adults (19–34 years). The effects of income were less consistent except in the oldest age group, in which case there were linear, positive associations between income and intakes of each of energy, total fat, and saturated fatty acids. For other age groups, the relationships with income were inconsistent, several of them appearing to be bimodal with highest intakes expressed by moderate income individuals.

IV. RECENT CHANGES IN THE AMERICAN DIET

A. General Observations

To this point the emphasis has been placed on trends in food use over this century. By focusing on the last quarter century, specifically, a clearer picture can be drawn of contemporary trends in dietary practices as well as more accurate projections for the future. When the focus of attention is on the diets of Americans in the time period since 1965, relevant data sources include not only food disappearance data, but also data for individuals included in the household food consumption surveys (USDA) since 1965 and from the NHANES surveys [6,19].

The population has developed preferences for foods that are fresh, low in fat, or sweet [15,18,24,25]. For example, there have been large increases in the consumption of soft drinks, specifically, as well as for an array of sweeteners and sweetened foods [17,20]. Per capita consumption and mean portion sizes for red meats have declined, while intakes of poultry and fish have increased, as have the intakes of mixed dishes in which these animal proteins predominate [6,26]. The implication is that we are substituting leaner sources of protein for the more traditional red meats, which, when they are consumed, are done so in reduced portion sizes. These reductions are being achieved, in part, by combining foods to create mixed dishes of lower overall fat content. Low-fat dairy products have much greater popularity with an ongoing interchange of low-fat milks for whole milk and a burgeoning in the availability of fat-modified cheeses, sour cream, yogurt, and frozen dairy desserts. Consumption of fresh and frozen vegetables has increased, as has that of fresh fruit, especially noncitrus fruits [25,26]. The use of some grain products is increasing, especially pasta and rice [26].

These trends to continued reliance on fats composed of more unsaturated fatty acids [10,18] lend credence to the belief that Americans are placing greater value on health [21]. Hard cheeses with their high saturated fatty acid content continue to increase in popularity; this trend appears to be dominated by greater consumption of Italian cheeses [18]. The apparent paradox can be explained if it is recognized that health is only one of several values shaping food choices. Allocation of the resources of money and time also shape choices.

In the past quarter century these latter values appear to be expressed in increased use of convenience foods and a greater proportion of the diet supplied by foods consumed away from home. Disposable personal incomes have increased over the interval, while the food expenditures expressed as a percentage of this figure have decreased [1,26]. Subdividing food expenditures into those made for foods consumed at home and away from home indicate that a greater proportion of income is being spent on the latter. In 1959 only 26 cents of every food dollar was spent on foods consumed away from home; in 1969, this figure reached 34 cents, and by 1989, 44 cents of each food dollar were so allocated [1]. In 1958, 5% of dollars spent on foods consumed away from home were spent on fast foods.

There are also trends in the type of fast foods being consumed [1,26]. The number of fast food establishments specializing in the sale of beef, hamburgers specifically, and chicken have increased; but the rate of increase is greater for those serving chicken. And this rate is surpassed by pizza franchises, which actually quadrupled in number between 1973 and 1985, perhaps explaining why cheese, especially Italian cheeses, have demonstrated increased contributions of calories to the American diet during that time period.

These data are valuable, not only for their economic significance, but for their nutritional implications as well. Foods consumed away from home tend to be higher in energy, fat, saturated fat, and sodium; they also tend to be lower in dietary fiber and several of the micronutrients [27,28]. Dietary trends apparently motivated by concerns for health are presented here deliberately juxtaposed with those shaped by economics to emphasize two trends coexisting in society that appear to lack consistency. Food service industries, food technologists, and marketers, as well as consumers appear to be trying to resolve this conflict.

B. Eating Away from Home

Data concerning the extent of use of foods acquired and eaten away from home and their contributions to energy intakes are presented in Table 2 for various subgroups within the population. USDA's Continuing Survey of Food Intake by Individuals (CFSII) for 1986, which emphasized the intakes of women 19–50 years of age and their children who were 5 years old or younger, provides relevant information [26].

Eating away from home has become a part of the American way of life; 81% of the children and 90% of the women surveyed in 1986 acquired and consumed food away from home on at least one of the 4 days on which diet records were kept. These data imply that such behavior is almost universal in the population. Only 11% of children expressed this behavior on all 4 days, whereas almost one-quarter of the women did so; 19% of the food energy consumed by children and 30% of that of women was contributed by foods eaten away from home. A slightly larger percentage of fat intake and lower proportions of protein and carbohydrate were obtained from foods from these sources.

The practice of consuming foods from sources other than household supplies is expressed differently within various segments of the population. It is less common among the younger children (1–3 years) than among the older ones (4–5 years) in terms of both the proportion of children expressing the behavior and also in the contribution made to nutrient intakes. Such foods made greater contribution to the diets of black children than to those of whites, despite similarity in the number of children consuming foods away from home. These statistics may reflect ethnic differences in arrangements for child care. Although eating foods away from home is more prevalent among children in households with higher incomes, differences in the contributions made to nutrient intake are small. Consuming food away from home relates to the type of community in which the child lives. The practice is most prevalent in suburban households and is expressed as a greater proportion of children eating foods outside the home at any time in the 4 days of record-keeping, in the proportion of children eating such foods daily, as well as in the contributions these foods make to nutrient intakes.

Table 2 Mean Percent of Energy, Carbohydrate, Fat, and Protein per Individual Provided by Foods Obtained and Eaten Away from Home, Among Children and Women in the CSFII, 1986

	Persons eating out at least once in four days (%)	Percent of daily intake as:			
		Food energy	Total fat	Carbo-hydrate	Protein
Children					
All children	81.1	19.1	20.3	18.6	18.4
Age					
1–3 yr	77.2	16.9	17.9	16.6	15.9
4–5 yr	85.9	22.0	23.3	21.2	21.6
Income[a]					
Low	75.3	19.2	19.4	19.5	18.2
Middle	78.8	18.6	19.9	18.0	17.9
High	91.9	20.8	22.6	19.7	20.0
Race					
White	82.8	19.1	20.3	18.6	18.3
Black	83.1	25.4	26.1	25.2	24.9
Urbanization					
Central City	75.1	17.4	18.5	17.1	16.8
Suburban	84.6	20.5	21.8	19.9	19.5
Non-Metro	78.8	17.8	18.7	17.3	17.5
Women					
All women	90.1	29.6	30.9	28.4	27.9
Age					
19–34 yr	90.8	31.9	32.9	30.6	29.9
35–50 yr	89.4	27.1	28.7	26.0	25.8
Income					
Low	78.2	23.0	23.1	23.1	22.2
Middle	89.4	27.4	28.5	26.8	25.3
High	96.0	33.7	36.0	31.6	32.1
Race					
White	92.0	30.9	32.4	29.5	29.4
Black	81.1	23.5	22.8	23.7	19.8
Urbanization					
Central City	85.0	29.2	30.1	28.2	27.8
Suburban	92.9	31.1	32.8	29.7	29.1
Non-Metro	89.4	26.2	27.2	25.2	25.0

[a]Household income: low < 131%; high > 300% of poverty level as defined by USDA.
Source: Ref. 27.

These trends in children are not consistent with the data for the adult sample. Eating food acquired away from home is similar among younger (18–34 years) and older (35–50 years) women, although younger women obtain more of their nutrients from these foods. The effect of income on this practice is more linear. Women in highest income households consume more foods away from home, express this behavior on a daily basis more commonly, and obtain more of their nutrients from such foods. As with children, subjects living in suburban households are most reliant on foods from sources outside the home.

Based on data collected in the 1981 National Restaurant Association survey, men eat out even more frequently than do women [28]. Younger persons are more likely to eat out at fast food establishments, whereas young adults (23–34 years) are more likely to acquire foods from sources in the workplace, and older adults are more heavily reliant on restaurants.

C. Changes in Food Use

Data on the use of specific foods currently undergoing change in society [27] are presented in Tables 3 through 7 for children and women included in the CFSII in 1986 broken down by age group and income level. With the exceptions of milk and fruit that predominate in the diets of very young children, older children have larger intakes of most foods, presumably because of their larger capacity and need for food. Differences in portion sizes among the women would be more reflective of preferences.

Adoption of new foods could be expressed, first, among more affluent persons because of lower opportunity costs in adopting change [29]; income can be expected to be higher among middle-aged persons, who are closer to the ages of peak earning potential, than among younger adults. On the other hand, change may occur faster among younger adults since they have less firmly developed traditions and have lives that are undergoing other changes that could impact on food choices, such as beginning independent living, marriage, childbirth, and job changes during career development.

1. Meat, Poultry, and Fish

The trends observed in the U.S. population towards the substitution of leaner foods for red meat, and towards a greater reliance on food mixtures containing animal protein are not observed consistently among children. Although children from higher-income households ate smaller amounts of beef and greater amounts of fish and seafood than did other children, the consumption of mixtures appears to be universal among children. The consumption trends for poultry may be bimodal, with children in both lowest and

Table 3 Differences in Mean Daily Intakes of Meat, Poultry, and Fish Among Children (1–5 years) and Women (19–50 years) by Age and Income[a] in the CFSII, 1986

	Mean intake in grams (% using in 4-day period)			
	Beef	Poultry	Fish and shellfish	Mixtures[b]
Children				
All Children	14 (60)	15 (61)	5 (22)	40 (75)
Age				
1–3 yr	11 (55)	13 (59)	5 (22)	35 (71)
4–5 yr	17 (68)	17 (64)	5 (22)	47 (81)
Income				
Low	15 (63)	18 (69)	4 (23)	39 (79)
Middle	16 (65)	13 (54)	5 (21)	41 (73)
High	11 (55)	15 (66)	6 (25)	39 (75)
Women				
All Women	27 (63)	21 (57)	12 (30)	64 (73)
Age				
19–34 yr	25 (60)	21 (56)	11 (30)	68 (73)
35–50 yr	29 (67)	21 (58)	12 (31)	60 (73)
Income				
Low	28 (64)	22 (54)	8 (22)	53 (64)
Middle	28 (67)	22 (59)	12 (31)	64 (73)
High	24 (60)	20 (57)	12 (34)	69 (78)

[a]Household income: low < 131%, high > 300% of poverty level as defined by USDA.
[b]In which meat, fish, or poultry predominate.
Source: Ref. 27.

highest income households having the greatest intakes. Poultry could be an inexpensive choice for children in less affluent households as well as a low-fat alternative to red meat. The percentage of children reporting the consumption of beef is lower in higher-income homes as is the average daily intake of beef. The intakes of poultry and fish are greater in higher-income homes than observed among children from households with moderate incomes. These observations provide some support for the hypothesis that change will occur earlier among affluent persons.

Both older and younger women consume comparable amounts of poultry and fish. Older women, however, consume more beef and less mixtures composed of these items. Women in higher income households consume less beef and more fish and protein mixtures. The implication, here, is that the

Table 4   Differences in Mean Daily Intakes of Dairy Products Among Children (1–5 years) and Women (19–50 years) by Age and Income[a] in the CFSII, 1986

| | Mean intake in grams (% using in 4-day period) | | | |
| | Milk | | | |
	Whole	Lowfat	Cheese	Yogurt
Children				
All children	176 (68)	173 (62)	13 (77)	7 (13)
Age				
1–3 yr	187 (64)	176 (64)	14 (78)	6 (14)
4–5 yr	162 (74)	170 (60)	13 (75)	7 (11)
Income				
Low	229 (86)	105 (43)	11 (74)	1 (4)
Middle	142 (64)	200 (66)	14 (76)	4 (9)
High	186 (62)	177 (72)	14 (80)	15 (26)
Women				
All women	57 (44)	91 (49)	17 (71)	8 (12)
Age				
19–34 yr	70 (46)	100 (51)	18 (73)	8 (13)
35–50 yr	45 (42)	81 (47)	17 (69)	8 (11)
Income				
Low	76 (59)	53 (33)	13 (57)	4 (6)
Middle	60 (46)	105 (49)	18 (72)	7 (12)
High	49 (37)	102 (56)	19 (78)	11 (16)

[a]Household income: Low < 131%, high > 300% of poverty level as defined by USDA.
Source: Ref. 27.

trend towards leaner animal proteins is occurring in women and is being expressed among younger and higher-income persons.

2. Dairy Products

Milk and cheese are popular items in the diets of children. Whole milk is consumed less extensively by children in moderate- and high-income households than in low-income homes, while the use of low-fat milk is more common among them (Table 4). These observations are suggestive of the trend towards lower fat dairy products being expressed within this young age group; the data indicate a substantially greater use of yogurt among children from the most affluent homes, supporting the belief that affluence facilitates the adoption of change [29]. Cheese seems to be universally popular among children.

Table 5 Differences in Mean Daily Intakes of Juices, Soft Drinks, and Other Beverages Among Children (1–5 years) and Women (19–50 years) by Age and Income[a] in the CFSII, 1986

	Mean intake in grams (% using in 4-day period)					
	Fruit drinks, ades		Juices		Soft drinks	
	Reg.	Low-cal	Citrus	Other	Reg.	Low-cal
Children						
All children	60 (52)	13 (13)	59 (64)	69 (48)	67 (58)	14 (17)
Age						
1–3 yr	60 (51)	15 (14)	54 (60)	83 (54)	53 (52)	11 (15)
4–5 yr	60 (54)	11 (12)	65 (68)	51 (40)	85 (65)	17 (20)
Income						
Low	64 (54)	8 (9)	49 (59)	32 (33)	76 (60)	4 (11)
Middle	58 (53)	15 (16)	58 (65)	78 (49)	79 (60)	9 (13)
High	58 (51)	16 (15)	72 (67)	94 (61)	45 (51)	30 (30)
Women						
All women	29 (24)	9 (7)	48 (48)	14 (15)	153 (61)	28 (44)
Age						
19–34 yr	34 (27)	13 (9)	52 (48)	16 (16)	181 (66)	127 (45)
35–50 yr	25 (21)	5 (5)	45 (48)	11 (13)	124 (55)	128 (44)
Income						
Low	36 (31)	6 (6)	49 (38)	11 (12)	189 (67)	68 (24)
Middle	36 (26)	12 (7)	50 (48)	11 (14)	166 (64)	106 (42)
High	22 (19)	9 (8)	53 (54)	16 (16)	129 (55)	172 (57)

[a]Household income: low < 131%, high > 300% of poverty level defined by USDA.
Source: Ref. 27.

Older women consume less milk, regardless of its fat content, than do younger women; the use of low-fat milk is greater than whole milk in both age groups. Income is associated negatively with the use of whole milk and positively with that of low-fat milks. There are no differences in the use of yogurt and cheese in the two age groups, but the intakes of both these foods are higher among women of greater affluence.

3. Juices, Soft Drinks, and Other Beverages

Beverages represent a major source of sweeteners, both caloric and noncaloric, in the diets of Americans. Children from higher-income households are more likely to consume juices and less likely to consume their alternatives, namely fruit drinks and carbonated beverages (Table 5). Although sugared beverages predominate over those containing artificial sweeteners in the diets

Table 6 Differences in Mean Daily Intakes of Fruits and Vegetables Among Children (1–5 years) and Women (19–50 years) by Age and Income[a] in the CFSII, 1986

| | Mean intake in grams (% using in 4-day period) | | | |
| | | Vegetables | | |
	Fruits	Dark green	Deep yellow	Salad dressings
Children				
All children	208 (94)	7 (26)	5 (29)	2 (51)
Age				
1–3 yr	219 (94)	6 (27)	6 (30)	2 (46)
4–5 yr	195 (95)	8 (24)	4 (27)	2 (56)
Income				
Low	131 (89)	9 (34)	3 (20)	2 (44)
Middle	228 (97)	5 (20)	7 (33)	2 (56)
High	262 (98)	6 (27)	4 (30)	2 (49)
Women				
All women	127 (81)	12 (32)	6 (31)	9 (74)
Age				
19–34 yr	123 (79)	12 (31)	6 (28)	9 (71)
35–50 yr	131 (83)	12 (34)	7 (34)	9 (76)
Income				
Low	89 (67)	9 (26)	3 (23)	6 (61)
Middle	128 (81)	10 (26)	6 (27)	9 (72)
High	147 (87)	15 (38)	8 (38)	11 (80)

[a]Household income: low < 131%, high > 300% of poverty level as defined by USDA.
Source: Ref. 27.

of children, the use of artificially sweetened drinks is more common among children of more affluent households than among those from households with lower incomes.

Income also appears to be an important factor in the selection of beverages by adults. Consumption of juices is more extensive among women with higher incomes; the use of fruit drinks as well as soft drinks is less extensive. Age does not appear to be a determinant of the use of artificial sweeteners in these products. On the other hand, women from higher-income households are much more likely to consume artificially sweetened soft drinks than are women with lower incomes.

Table 7 Differences in Mean Daily Intakes of Grain Products Among Children (1–5 years) and Women (19–50 years) by Age and Income[a] in the CFSII, 1986

	Mean intake in grams (% using in 4-day period)	
	Cereals and pasta	Baked goods
Children		
All children	57 (96)	42 (96)
Age		
1–3 yr	56 (97)	40 (96)
4–5 yr	58 (94)	45 (96)
Income		
Low	82 (97)	38 (92)
Middle	50 (96)	44 (98)
High	45 (94)	42 (98)
Women		
All women	40 (66)	44 (89)
Age		
19–34 yr	41 (68)	41 (89)
35–50 yr	40 (63)	48 (89)
Income		
Low	51 (66)	43 (84)
Middle	39 (62)	43 (90)
High	36 (69)	48 (91)

[a]Household income: low < 131%, high > 300% of poverty level as defined by USDA.
Source: Ref. 27.

4. Fruits and Vegetables

Use of dark green and deep yellow vegetables is examined in Table 6 as a means of investigating current trends towards consumption of fresh fruits and vegetables as constituents of a healthful, contemporary eating style. Other categories of vegetables included in the CFSII are suggestive of more traditional eating styles incorporating the less nutrient-dense starchy vegetables [30]. The use of salad dressing implies a consumption of salads.

Children from low-income households were more likely to eat dark green vegetables, and less likely to consume deep yellow ones; this finding may reflect the use of greens in ethnic eating styles. But there is little evidence that the trend to fresh produce is being expressed in children. Fruit, on the other hand, is more likely to be consumed, and consumed in larger portions, by children from more affluent households. This observation is reinforced by their greater intakes of fruit juices as well (Table 5).

Women's use of dark green and deep yellow vegetables and fruits appears to be influenced only weakly by age; older women may be more likely to consume fruit. Income is strongly related both to portion size and to the proportion of women consuming these fruits and vegetables. These data suggest the likelihood of a continuation of this trend to increased use of fresh fruits and vegetables.

5. Grain Products

Cereals and pasta are more popular among lower-income children and less so among their moderate- and high-income counterparts (Table 7). Baked goods show the reverse pattern. Data published by USDA does not separate the use of pasta and cereals, both of which are consumed commonly by children. Perhaps, as a result of the aggregation of the two food types, a trend towards greater use of pasta, specifically, is obscured. Neither can such a trend be seen among women. Their use of baked goods is suggestive of a positive association with income and age.

V. DISCUSSION

After almost a century of commitment to maintaining sound information about food consumption in this country, we have extensive data on the foods eaten by Americans and the nutrients derived from those foods. What we are not yet able to do is to identify patterns, or eating styles, existing in the population. In other words, we do not understand how, or why, foods are combined in predictable ways shaped by underlying values. The ability to do so would provide a better understanding of dietary *structures* that direct food choices and support investigations of the role of the *mixed* diet, with its composite of risk-elevating and protective factors, in the etiologies of major diseases.

Currently such diseases are the leading causes of death in the population. Obesity, cardiovascular disease, cancer, and hypertension develop over an extended period of time and exhibit multiple risk factors. Diet as it is linked to lifestyles that in turn emanate from underlying values is being studied in efforts to lower mortality statistics and extend the length of independent life.

Measures of patterns in food use approach diet multidimensionally; they incorporate nutrient intakes as well as underlying behaviors, both dietary and nondietary. Various investigators have established associations between diet and changes in cardiovascular disease risks [11–13]. More recently we have been attempting to lower cancer risks with nutrition interventions. Using data collected in a case-control study of diet and cancer, we in Buffalo have used factor analysis to identify various eating styles among the normal, healthy free-living control subjects in a case-control study of cancer at various sites, and then link them to other health-related behaviors [30]. Both prudent and imprudent eating styles emerged in terms of intakes of energy, as well as total and saturated fat [30,31]. These patterns displayed distinctive gender differences. More than one eating style is associated with high fat intake, and these patterns were further distinguishable by intakes of other nutrients, namely energy, dietary fiber, sodium, and vitamins A and C. The patterns were found to be associated also with such health-related behaviors as trimming fat from meat, choice of fat used in cooking or as additions to foods, ingestion of salt-cured and smoked foods, alcohol consumption, and both current and past smoking [31].

Risk factors clearly coalesce within eating styles, with persons relying on lean foods being more prudent in other health behaviors as well. These results are preliminary because of the developmental nature of the multidimensional measures of diet employed. However, they do provide insights for disease risks incorporated into mixed diets and highlight the potential for understanding how dietary choices are made, how they ultimately impact on health status, and how nutrition interventions can be designed for maximum effect. The current distinctive changes in the nation's food supply and in consumer concern for health need such a multidimensional approach if they are to capitalize on understanding of diet as it influences health. The ultimate goal is to enter the twenty-first century with good health status throughout the population, having profited from our long-term investment in dietary study.

REFERENCES

1. J. J. Putnam, *Food Consumption, Prices, and Expenditures*, 1967–88, Statistical Bulletin No. 804, Commodity Economics Division, Economic Research Service, U.S. Department of Agriculture, Washington, D.C. (1990).
2. U.S. Department of Health and Human Services, *Healthy People. National Health Promotion and Disease Prevention Objectives.* (PHS)91-50212, Public Health Service Washington, D.C. (1991).
3. E. Sills-Levy, U.S. trends leading to the year 2000, *Food Technol.*, (*Apr*): 128 (1989).
4. D. Sanjur, *Social and Cultural Perspectives in Nutrition,* Prentice-Hall, Englewood Cliffs, NJ (1982).
5. E. M. Pao, K. E. Sykes, and Y. S. Cypel, *USDA Methodological Research for Large-Scale Dietary Intake Surveys, 1976–88.* Home Economics Research Report 49, U.S. Department of Agriculture, Human Nutrition Information Service, Washington, D.C. (1989).

6. Life Sciences Research Office, Federation of American Societies for Experimental Biology, *Nutrition Monitoring in the United States—An Update Report on Nutrition Monotoring*, Prepared for the U.S. Department of Agriculture and the U.S. Department of Health and Human Services, DHHS Publication No. (PHS)89-1255, Public Health Service, U.S. Government Printing Office, Washington, D.C. (1969).

7. R. M. Marston and N. R. Raper, Counting America's food. Nutrient content of the U.S. food supply, *National Food Review 29* (*winter*): 5 (1986).

8. U.S. Department of Health and Human Services, *Plan and Operation of the Second National Health and Nutrition Examination Survey. 1976*–1980, DHHS Publication No. (PHS)81-1317, Washington, D.C. (1981).

9. M. D. Carroll, S. Abraham, and C. M. Dresser, *Dietary Intake Source Data: United States. 1976*–80. DHHS Publication No. (PHS)83-1681, U.S. Department of Health and Human Services, National Center for Health Statistics, Vital and Health Statistics, Series 11-No. 231, Public Health Service, Washington, D.C. (1983).

10. N. R. Raper and R. M. Marston, Levels and Sources of fat in the U.S. food supply, *Dietary Fat and Cancer* (C. Ip, ed.), Alan R. Liss, Inc., New York (1986).

11. M. L. Slattery and D. E. Randall, Trends in coronary heart disease mortality and food consumption in the United States between 1909 and 1980, *Am. J. Clin. Nutr., 47*: 1060 (1988).

12. U.S. Department of Health and Human Services, *The Surgeon General's Report on Nutrition and Health,* DHHS (PHS) Publication No. 88-50210, Public Health Service, Washington, D.C. (1988).

13. Committee on Diet and Health, National Research Council, *Diet and Health, Implications for Reducing Calorie Disease Risk,* Food and Nutrition Board, Commission on Life Sciences, National Academy Press, Washington, D.C. (1989).

14. G. Block, C. M. Dresser, A. M. Hartman, and M. D. Carroll, Nutrient sources in the American diet: Quantitative data from the NHANESII survey, *Am. J. Epidemiol. 22*: 27 (1985).

15. J. Putnam, Food Consumption, *Natl. Food Rev., 12* (2): 1 (1989).

16. R. Haidacher and J. Blaylock, Why has dairy product consumption increased? *Natl. Food Rev., 11* (4): 28 (1988).

17. Institute of Food Technologies, Sweeteners. Consumption trends, *Food Technol., 40* (1): 112 (1986).

18. L. Bailey, L. Duewer, F. Gray, R. Hoskin, J. Putnam, and S. Short, Food consumption, *Natl. Food Rev., 11* (2): 1 (1988).

19. R. M. Morrison, Food policy and research. The market for fat substitutes, *Natl. Food Rev., 13* (2): 24 (1990).

20. A. M. Altschul, Low-calorie foods, *Food Technol.* (*April*): 113 (1989).

21. D. Putler and E. Frazao, Linking agriculture to the economy. Diet/health concerns about fat intake, *Natl. Food Rev., 14* (1): 16 (1991).

22. E. Randall, J. R. Marshall, J. Brasure, and S. Graham, Patterns in food use and their compliance with NCI dietary guidelines, *Nutr. and Cancer 15*: 141 (1991).

23. G. Block, W. F. Rosenberger, and B. H. Patterson, Calories, fat and cholesterol: Intake patterns in the U.S. population by race, sex and age, *Am. J. Pub. Health, 78*: 1150 (1988).
24. K. Bunch, Counting America's: Consumption trends favor fresh, lowfat, and sweet, *Natl. Food Rev., 29* (winter): 1 (1986).
25. C. Greene, The food industry heading into 1990. A new look for supermarket produce sections, *Natl. Food Rev., 11* (4): 1 (1988).
26. J. Blaylock and H. Elizak, A review of the decade. Food expenditures, *Natl. Food Rev., 13* (3): 17 (1990).
27. U.S. Department of Agriculture, *Nationwide Food Consumption Survey, Continuing Survey of Food Intakes by Individuals. Women 19-50 Years and their Children 1-5 Years.* 4 Days, NCFCS CSFII Report No. 86-3, Human Nutrition Information Service (1988).
28. C. P. Ries, K. Kline, and S. O. Weaver, Impact of commercial eating on nutrient adequacy, *J. Am. Dietet. Assoc., 87*: 463 (1987).
29. E. M. Rogers, *Diffusion of Innovation*, 3rd ed., Free Press, New York (1983).
30. E. Randall, J. R. Marshall, S. Graham, and J. Brasure, Patterns in food use and their associations with nutrient intakes, *Am. J. Clin. Nutr., 52*: 739 (1990).
31. E. Randall, J. R. Marshall, S. Graham, and S. Brasure, High risk health behaviors associated with various dietary patterns, *Nutr. and Cancer, 16*: 135 (1991).

5
Fat in Foods

Aaron M. Altschul   *Georgetown University School of Medicine, Washington, D.C.*

I. INTRODUCTION

Much will be said throughout this volume about fat in foods. High-fat foods have high caloric density; low-fat foods have low caloric density. Weight control is not the only issue. Advice on how to lower serum cholesterol values includes the recommendation to eat less fat: total fat less than 30% of calories; saturated fatty acids less than 10% of calories; cholesterol less than 300 mg/day [1,2].

The purpose of this chapter is to present a panorama of fat in foods, from the highest to the lowest. Examples will be chosen to illustrate the range; more details will be found in the ensuing chapters.

II. PERCENTAGE OF CALORIES FROM FAT

The percentage of calories furnished by fat is a convenient way to describe the fat content of a diet. Thus a 2000 kcalorie diet containing 100 g of fat provides 45% of the calories as fat:

$$100 \times 9 = 900 \text{ kcalories}$$

$$\frac{900}{2000} \times 100 = 45\%$$

Americans eat a diet that provides about 37% of the calories as fat [3] (see also Chapter 4). If an individual now eating an average diet wishes to reduce fat intake to less than 30% of the calories as fat, it becomes necessary to shift from foods with a higher percentage of calories as fat to those with a lower percentage. An essential part of reading and understanding a label, then, is to be able to translate the figures into percentage of calories as fat. The calculation is simple:

$$\frac{\text{Grams fat per serving}}{\text{kcalories per serving}} \times 900 = \text{percentage of calories as fat}$$

A nomogram for the same purpose is given in Figure 1.

III. CATEGORIES OF FOODS BASED ON FAT CONTENT

Our food supply might be segregated on the basis of fat content into three arbitrary categories: (1) those that provide more than 40% of the calories as fat; (2) those providing 25–40% of fat calories; and (3) those containing less than 25% of the calories as fat. Anyone wishing to reduce fat intake to less than 30% of the calories as fat will eat less of foods in group (1) and more of foods in group (3). Tables 1–3 give examples of foods in each of the categories.

Margarine and mayonnaise were not included in Table 1 because they are a special case. Practically 100% of their energy content is from fat. Even when they are modified to have less than normal fat, the percentage of fat calories remains the same because all that was done was to dilute the fat with water and/or air. For example:

Regular margarine: 101 calories/tbsp, 100% fat calories
Light margarine, imitation: 50 calories/tbsp, 100% fat calories
Regular mayonnaise: 98 calories/tbsp, 100% fat calories
Light mayonnaise: 50 calories/tbsp, 90% fat calories

Yet there is much to be gained toward reducing fat intake by choosing the lower-fat product. Potato salad made with light mayonnaise contained 54% calories from fat compared with 71% in a potato salad made with regular mayonnaise (M. A. Bieber, private communication). A slice of toast and regular margarine (1 tsp) provides 42% calories as fat; toast with diet margarine-like spread provides 29% of calories as fat (M.A. Bieber, private communication). One can spread the margarine more thickly or more thinly; the differential remains.

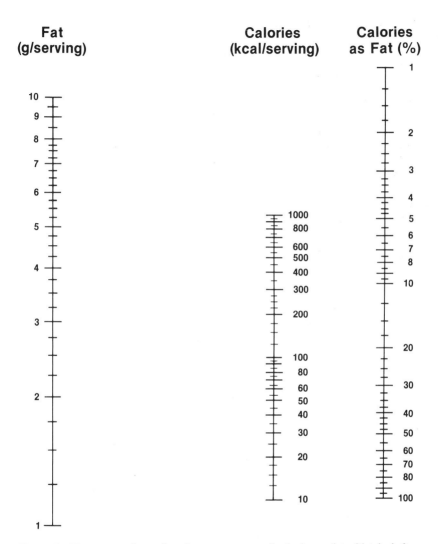

Figure 1 Nomogram for estimating percentage of calories as fat. Obtain information on grams of fat and calories per serving of a particular food or recipe from the label, recipe, or table of composition. Put a dot for grams of fat/serving at the appropriate location on the left-hand scale; put a dot for kcalories per serving at the appropriate location on the middle scale. Connect the two dots and read the approximate percentage of calories as fat on the right-hand scale. If the amount of fat per serving is greater than 10, divide the serving by 2 or 3 to reach a range between 1 and 10 grams of fat. Example: Baked cheese ravioli, a frozen entree, contains 310 kcal/serving and 12 g fat/serving. Divide by 2 to yield a serving size that contains 155 kcal and 6 g fat. The line connecting 6 g fat and 155 kcal crosses the right-hand scale at approximately 35% of calories as fat.

Table 1 Foods with More than 40% Fat Calories (High-Fat)

Food item	Percent calories as fat	Ref.
Nuts, mixed	85	4
Sausage, pork, cooked	84	4
Bacon, fried	77	5
Duck, roasted, meat with skin	76	8
American cheese, pasteurized	75	6
Mozzarella cheese	69	6
Eggs, chicken, whole, poached	64	6
Potato chips	62	4
Ice cream, 16% fat	61	6
Mozzarella cheese, part skim	56	6
Chocolate bar	56	4
Soup, canned, cream of celery	56	4
Ground beef, broiled, extra lean	54	7
Yeast-leavened donuts	54–64	See ch. 13
Duck, roasted, meat only	50	8
Milk, whole, 3.3% fat	49	6
Ice cream, regular, 10% fat	48	6
Yogurt, plain, whole milk	48	6
French fries	47	4
Ham, cured, roasted, 11% fat	46	5
Fried chicken, with skin	46	8
Haddock, breaded, fried	46	9
Apple pie	43	4

Table 2 Foods with 25–40% Fat Calories (Medium-Fat)

Food item	Percent calories as fat	Ref.
Cheese, creamed, cottage	39	6
Beef, eye of round, prime, broiled	37	7
Tuna, canned, light, oil pack	37	9
Chicken, with skin, breast, roasted	36	8
Milk, 2% fat	34	6
Ham, extra lean (5% fat), roasted	34	5
Soup, canned, beef noodle	34	4
Dinner, frozen, chicken cacciatore	28	9
Ice milk, 4% fat	28	6
Dinner, frozen, Oriental beef with vegetables and rice	27	9
Pork, tenderloin, roasted	26	5

Table 3   Foods with Less than 25% of Calories as Fat (Low-Fat)

Food item	Percent calories as fat	Ref.
Chicken, without skin, light meat, roasted	23	8
Milk, 1% fat	23	6
Halibut, broiled	19	9
Cheese, cottage, 2% fat	19	6
Turkey, without skin, light meat, roasted	18	8
Cocoa mix, hot, sugar free	18	[a]
Tuna, canned, water-packed	17	9
Dinner, frozen, shrimp primavera with fettucine	14	10
Cheese, cottage, 1% fat	13	6
Soup, canned, bean, black	12	4
Yogurt, low-fat, fruit flavored	12	6
Bread, wheat etc.	11	6
Shrimp, steamed	9	9
Cereal, All-Bran	8	4
Soup, canned, chicken gumbo	5	4
Yogurt, light, artificially sweetened	4	[a]
Milk, skim	5	6
Yogurt, plain, from skim milk	3	6
Spaghetti, cooked	3	4
Beans, lima, frozen, cooked, drained solids	2	4
Rice, cooked	1	4
Potato, baked with skin	1	4
Egg Beaters	0	[a]
Gelatin dessert	0	4
All fruits and most vegetables	0	4

[a]Manufacturer's nutrition label

Another example is cream cheese:

Regular: 99 calories/oz, 90% fat calories
Light Philadelphia: 60 calories/oz, 75% fat calories

Both are high-fat foods, but there is an advantage to using the "light" version as a spread.

"Processed" foods are found in all three tables; so are "natural" foods. Any strategy to reduce fat intake likely involves changes in consumption of both "processed" and "natural" foods, shifting to lower-fat versions. The choice of how to shift, of what high-fat foods to discourage, and what low-fat foods to encourage is complicated. It depends on tastes to be missed or enjoyed, on cost, on availability, and on each individual's diet philosophy: to shift to more low-fat "natural" foods or to be willing freely to interchange "natural" and "processed" foods as a way of lowering fat intake.

REFERENCES

1. NCEP, Report of the National Cholesterol Education Program Expert Panel on Detection, Evaluation, and Treatment of High Blood Cholesterol in Adults, *Arch. Intern. Med., 148*: 36 (1988).
2. Food and Nutrition Board. *Recommended Dietary Allowances*, 10th rev. ed. National Research Council, Washington, D.C., p. 49 (1989).
3. A. M. Stephen and N. J. Wald, Trends in individual consumption of dietary fat in the United States, 1920–1984, *Am. J. Clin. Nutr., 52*: 457 (1990).
4. G. A. Leveille, M. E. Zabik, and K. J. Morgan, *Nutrients in Foods*, The Nutrition Guild, Cambridge, MA (1983).
5. Composition of Foods: Pork Products, *Agriculture Handbook No. 8-10*, U.S. Department of Agriculture, Washington, D.C. (1983).
6. Composition of Foods: Dairy and Egg Products, *Agriculture Handbook No. 8-1*, U.S. Department of Agriculture, Washington, D.C. (1976).
7. Composition of Foods: Beef Products, *Agriculture Handbook No. 8-13*, U.S. Department of Agriculture, Washington, D.C. (1986).
8. Compositon of Foods: Poultry Products, *Agriculture Handbook No. 8-5*, U.S. Department of Agriculture, Washington, D.C. (1979).
9. *Designing Foods*: *Animal Product Options in the Marketplace*, Committee on Technological Options to Improve the Nutritional Attributes of Animal Products, Board on Agriculture, National Research Council, National Academy Press, Washington, D.C. (1988).
10. A. M. Altschul, Low-calorie foods: A scientific status summary by the Institute of Food Technologists' Expert Panel on Food Safety and Nutrition, *Food Technol., 43*: 113 (1989).

6

History of the Commercial Development of Low-Calorie Foods

Lyn O'Brien Nabors and Russell Lemieux   *Calorie Control Council, Atlanta, Georgia*

I. INTRODUCTION

What we now refer to as low-calorie, low-fat, and, often, light foods and beverages were originally known as dietetic or "diet" foods. These products were developed for diabetics or others with specific medical conditions, including obesity. They were found in health food stores or on obscure shelves in the special dietetic section of the grocery. They were not known for their variety or taste but for their high prices. Today, these products are found in virtually every department of the supermarket, are greatly improved in taste, and are priced competitively with comparable full-calorie products.

What has been the role of low-calorie ingredients in the tremendous growth of the low-calorie food and beverage category? How has the number of individual product categories expanded? What can be expected in the future? This chapter is designed to answer these questions.

II. CONSUMPTION OF LOW-CALORIE FOODS AND BEVERAGES IN THE UNITED STATES

In 1991, 141 million adult Americans (three out of four) consumed low-calorie and/or low-fat foods and beverages. These light-product consumers include 81% of adult women and 71% of men. No single age category, including 18-to-24-year-olds and even those over 60, has an incidence rate of product use below 71%. Also, more than 100 million people consume sugar-free, low-calorie products. Over half (52%) consume these low-calorie products daily [1] (Fig. 1).

   These data are from the latest of five national surveys the Calorie Control Council conducted to gauge consumer attitudes and behavior in the marketplace over the past 12 years. The survey completed in January 1991 examined trends in dieting and the use of low-calorie, sugar-free products and low-fat products.

   Qualified respondents in the survey were males and females age 18 or older. A total of 1511 telephone interviews were completed for the 1991 survey utilizing a national random probability sample. These data were then weighted by sex and region to produce a sample that would be projectable to the entire U.S. population. The study was carefully designed to ensure valid comparisons and trend analyses with past Council surveys.

   The most dominant segment of the light consumer market today is the consumer of reduced-fat foods and beverages. Two-thirds of the adult pop-

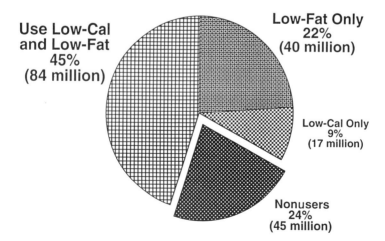

Figure 1   Proportion of adult users and nonusers of low-calorie foods in the United States. (From Ref. 1.)

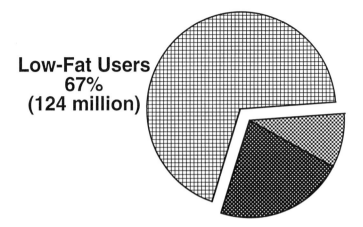

Low-Fat Users
67%
(124 million)

Figure 2 Proportion of adult users and nonusers of low-fat foods in the United States. The identification of the segments is the same as in Figure 1: 17 million (9%) low-cal only and 45 million (24%) nonusers. (From Ref. 1.)

ulation, 124 million Americans, are using products low or reduced in fat (Fig. 2, Table 1). The most popular low-fat products are low-fat dairy products, including cheese, yogurt, and sour cream. Nearly half (49%) of the adult population consume these products, followed by low-fat beverages at 43%, low-fat ice cream and frozen desserts at 34%, and low-fat chips and snack food at 31%.

Eighty-two percent of low-fat product consumers say that they use these products for better overall health, 80% to reduce cholesterol, 73% to reduce fat, and 64% to reduce calories. Weight maintenace was mentioned by 61%, maintaining an attractive appearance by 59%, and losing weight by 43%. Note, however, that only 38% said they are consuming low-fat products because they taste good (Table 2).

Table 1 The Most Popular Reduced-Fat Products

	% Total population	% Low-fat consumers
Cheese/dairy products	49	74
Beverages	43	64
Ice cream/frozen desserts	34	51
Chips/snack foods	31	46
Cakes/baked goods	25	37
Dinner entrees	23	34

Source: Ref. 1.

Table 2 Reasons for Using Reduced-Fat Products

	% Low-fat consumers
Stay in better overall health	82
Reduce cholesterol	80
Reduce fat	73
Reduce calories	64
Maintain weight	61
Maintain attractive appearance	59
Lose weight	43

Source: Ref. 1.

The 1991 study found that 101 million adult Americans, age 18 and over (60 million women and 41 million men), regularly consume low-calorie, sugar-free foods and beverages (i.e., products containing a low-calorie sweetener) [1]. Over the past 5 years, incidence of use of these products increased from 45% of the adult population to 54%. In projectable terms, that is an increase of 23 million people, from 78 to 101 million adult Americans [2]. This is more than half the adult population and 2.4 times the 42 million consumers using sugar-free products in 1978 [3] (Figure 3).

Women are more likely to consume low-calorie, sugar-free products than men. In fact, of the increase of 8 million consumers since 1989, 7 million were women [4]. These findings conflict with trends identified between

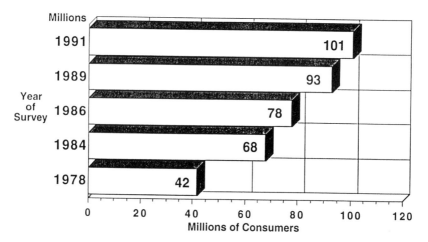

Figure 3 Number of Americans who consume low-calorie foods and beverages—1978–1991. (From Refs. 1, 2, 4.)

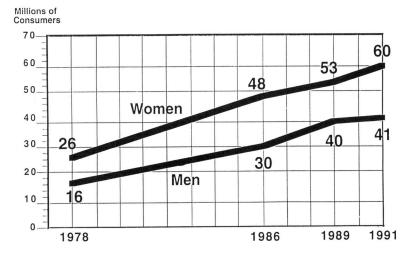

Figure 4 Trend by sex in consumption of low-calorie foods and beverages—1978–1991. (From Refs. 1, 2, 4.)

1986 and 1989. In 1986, the incidence of low-calorie, sugar-free product usage among women was 53%, and 36% among men. From 1986 to 1989, however, only a modest increase was found among women (to 57% incidence), while a very significant 25% increase was found among men, to 45% incidence (Fig. 4).

During the past 5 years, low-calorie, sugar-free product usage has increased most dramatically among older respondents, in particular those age 60 and over. As shown in Table 3, in 1986, this age category was clearly the least penetrated by low-calorie foods and beverages. Since then, the incidence of use among these consumers has increased 62%, bringing it in line with the incidence rates for the rest of the adult population.

Table 3 Users of Low-Calorie Products Arranged According to Age, 1986–1991

| Year | % use at age: | | | | |
	18–24	25–34	35–49	50–59	60+
1991	49	52	56	56	54
1989	45	53	51	57	47
1986	53	47	48	46	33

Source: Refs. 1, 2, 4.

Sugar-free soft drinks continue to be the most popular low-calorie food and beverage—consumed by nearly half of the population, including 78% of low-calorie consumers. Other product categories in order of their popularity are sugar substitutes, sugar-free gums and candies, "other," sugar-free puddings and gelatins, frozen desserts, yogurt, and powdered drink mixes. The category of "other low-calorie foods and beverages" scored an impressive 45% incidence, making it the fourth most mentioned low-calorie product category. This is likely due to popular "light" entrees and dairy products (Table 4).

The 1991 survey found, as have previous studies, that the number one reason for using low-calorie or light foods and beverages is to stay in better overall health—not weight control. In fact, more than two-thirds of the low-calorie consumers are *not* on a diet. Maintaining current weight was the second most mentioned reason for using low-calorie, sugar-free products, followed by maintaining an attractive physical appearance (an especially popular reason among women). Rounding out the top five reasons for using low-calorie products are reducing weight and refreshment or taste. Weight maintenance and weight reduction are also of particular importance to women [1] (Table 5).

The 962 calorie-reduced foods introduced in 1989 were more than double the number introduced in 1988. Introduction of new products claiming reduced fat content increased 127% to 626. Overall, products claiming reduced fat and/or calories accounted for 10% of the new products introduced in 1989 [5]. A $3 billion dollar business in 1976, Americans spent more than $22 billion by 1990 on reduced-calorie and reduced-fat products [6]. These figures are a further indication of the tremendous continuing growth of the low-calorie, low-fat, light foods and beverages market.

Table 4 The Most Popular Low-Calorie Products

	% Total population	% Low-cal consumers
Sugar-free carbonated soft drinks	42	78
Sugar substitutes	31	57
Sugar-free gum, candy	28	51
Sugar-free pudding, gelatin	18	34
Sugar-free frozen desserts	15	27
Sugar-free yogurt	12	22
Sugar-free powdered drink mixes	12	21
Sugar-free cakes, cookies	9	17
Other low-calorie or "light" foods/beverages	24	45

Source: Ref. 1.

Table 5 Reasons for Using Low-Calorie Products

	% Low-calorie consumers
Stay in better overall health	67
Maintain current weight	60
Maintain attractive physical appearance	53
Reduce weight	48
Refreshment or taste	43
Prevent/Control dental cavities	38
Help with a medical condition	33

III. THE IMPACT OF LOW-CALORIE INGREDIENTS

The development and approval of a variety of low-calorie sweeteners, fat replacers, and other low-calorie ingredients play a critical role in the availability and success of low-calorie foods and beverages. Having a variety of low-calorie foods and beverages. Saccharin was discovered in 1878 and ingredient, or combination of ingredients, best suited for a given product—"the multiple ingredient approach" to calorie control. A more detailed treatment of these ingredients is found in Chapters 8–11.

A. Intense Sweeteners

Historically, intense sweeteners have been the basis for the development of low-calorie foods and beverages. Saccharin was discovered in 1878 and introduced to the U.S. food supply around the turn of the century. With the availability of saccharin, consumers could continue to consume sweet products while reducing their calories from sugar. It was initially used in canned corn, peas, and tomatoes, and to sweeten sarsaparilla, cream soda, and other summer "soft" beverages that had a tendency to ferment with sugar [7].

The benefit of saccharin in place of sugar for diabetics and the obese was recognized before 1910. Although saccharin use increased during World Wars I and II, as did the number of products in which it was incorporated, saccharin use remained limited in the general population for several decades [8].

The development of cyclamates during the 1950s accelerated the growth of the diet industry and provided the first application of the multiple ingredient approach for low-calorie foods and beverages. The use of cyclamate and saccharin in combination had both taste and cost advantages. When used together the two sweeteners act synergistically, thereby providing increased sweetening power and masking any off-taste that might be apparent if the sweeteners were used alone.

Cyclamate use in foods and beverages increased from 0.5 million pounds in 1958 to 16 million pounds in 1968. Saccharin use was approximately 3 million pounds in 1968 [9]. Saccharin is 300 times sweeter than sugar and cyclamate 30 times sweeter. The mixture most commonly used contained 10 parts cyclamate to one part saccharin.

By the time cyclamate was banned, the diet market had become a significant one. A number of brands were well established and, consequently, the diet food industry suffered losses of over $150 million when the cyclamate ban became effective in 1970. During the 4-week period after the announcement of the ban of cyclamate, total diet food sales were down more than 50% over the preceding year. Sales for all types of diet foods declined [10].

Throughout the 1970s, saccharin again was the only intense sweetener available and was used in a number of products. The growth of the diet foods and beverages industry during this period, however, was limited. However, the remarkable success of cyclamate/saccharin-sweetened products fostered the development of new sweeteners, which would ignite a market explosion in the next decade.

Aspartame was introduced into the U.S. food supply in 1981 and became available for use in soft drinks in 1983. It became the driving force behind the booming popularity of low-calorie products. Aspartame was responsible for more new products in the 1980s than any other new ingredient [11]. By 1989, more than 500 new products containing aspartame had been developed in the United States alone, with a 70% success rate [12]. It is currently available in over 5000 brand products worldwide with reported sales in 1990 of more than $970 million in the United States alone [13].

Acesulfame-K received approval by the Food and Drug Administration (FDA) for a number of dry uses in 1988. Petitions are pending for its use in carbonated soft drinks, as well as confections and baked goods—categories for which it is especially well suited. Currently, petitions also are pending for three additional low-calorie sweeteners—alitame, cyclamate, and sucralose.

During the 1980s, U.S. per capita consumption of intense sweeteners almost tripled to an all time high of 22 pounds of sugar equivalent (by actual weight, approximately 1.5 ounces per person). The market for low-calorie sweeteners has increased from 5% of total sweeteners in 1983 to 12–14% in 1990. Low-calorie sweetener sales are projected to be $1.3 billion by 1993 [14].

B. Fat Replacers

Fats are a tremendous source of hidden calories with more than twice the number of calories as carbohydrates (9 vs. 4 calories per gram). With the

Surgeon General, National Institutes of Health, the American Heart Association, and others all recommending reducing fat intake, fat replacers have received significant public interest in the last few years. Current technology could *theoretically* reduce fat content and calories in daily diets by almost 100 and 50%, respectively [15].

The ideal fat replacer would duplicate all the attributes of fat while also significantly reducing both the fat and calorie content. Unfortunately, the "ideal" fat replacer (like the "ideal" sweetener) does not exist. Therefore, the type of fat replacer(s) used in a given product depends on which of the diverse properties of fat are required.

Although Simplesse and Olestra are the two fat replacers that have generated the most public attention, a number of additional ingredients are currently being used to replace fat in the American food supply. Most of the low-fat products introduced in recent years contain carbohydrate-based fat replacers such as cellulose, maltodextrins, gums, modified starch, and polydextrose.

Today's fat replacer market is reported to be worth about $40 million and growing at an annual rate of 15–20% percent [16]. In the United States, 0.5% of new food and beverage products were low or no fat in 1986, compared to 1.6% in 1987, 6.5% in 1988, 9.4% in 1989, and 11.0% in 1990 [17]. Retail sales of reduced-fat/reduced-calorie food products in the United States reached about $6 billion in 1989. Projections indicate that some food categories, such as reduced-fat margarines and salad and cooking oils, could generate ingredient markets exceeding $500 million per year in the United States alone by the year 2000 [15].

IV. DEVELOPMENT OF LOW-CALORIE FOODS BY CATEGORY

A. Soft Drinks

Diet soft drinks were introduced in the late 1950s. With the explosive growth of cyclamate/saccharin-sweetened products between 1962 and 1965, the soft drink industry was transformed. Diet Rite Cola, the first diet soft drink, captured 50% of the diet cola market. Tab was introduced in May 1963. Diet soft drink sales doubled in three consecutive years—1962, 3%; 1963, 7.5%; and 1964, 14.6% [18].

When cyclamate was taken off the market, diet soft drink sales declined somewhat. By 1977, they accounted for 12% of total soft drink sales. With the approval of aspartame for use in soft drinks in 1983, diet soft drink sales increased tremendously. By 1989, they had captured 26.6% of the market [19]. Diet Coke recorded $1 billion in sales its first year [12]. By 1990, four of the top 10 brands of soft drinks fell into the diet category [20].

B. Baked Products

"Low-calorie" bread has been around for years. The calories were reduced in many of these products by simply slicing the bread thinner than the comparable full-calorie product, and more recently by the addition of fiber. Significant changes, however, were seen in low-calorie baked goods in the late 1980s. By 1990, 279 (or 48.4% of the new bakery products introduced) were positioned as "healthy." Of these, 62 were low-calorie/low-fat and nine were no-fat products [21].

In October 1989, Entenmann's, a division of Kraft General Foods, introduced a line of fat-free products. In the first year, Entenmann's light line sales reached more than $200 million and was named new product of the year by *Adweek* magazine [22].

Sara Lee's Free & Light line of no- or low-fat baked products was unveiled in October 1990. Ten years earlier, Sara Lee introduced "light" products, which the company reportedly withdrew from the market because they were not well received by consumers [23]. Sara Lee has also recently introduced Sara Lee Lights, a line of low-calorie, single-serving desserts.

The latest low-calorie introductions in the baked goods category are low-calorie, low-fat cake and brownie mixes and frostings. Duncan Hines, Betty Crocker, and Pillsbury all have products in this category [24]. Approval of pending low-calorie sweetener petitions coupled with the use of bulking agents and fat replacers will make baked goods an area of significant growth in the future.

C. Dairy Products

The dairy category is responsible for as many new reduced-fat products as any single category. Retail sales of fat-reduced dairy products and frozen desserts in 1990 totaled about $19.4 million [16]. Skim milk is both an end product and an ingredient as many reduced fat foods are made by replacing whole milk with skim milk.

Per capita sales of whole milk declined from 191 pounds in 1972 to 92 pounds in 1989. Low-fat and skim milk rose from approximately 42 to 116 pounds. Low-fat cottage cheese sales increased from 60 million pounds in 1970 to 300 million pounds in 1989, while creamed cottage cheese sales declined from 984 to 570 million pounds [25]. Purchases of low-fat/low-calorie cheeses increased 22% in volume between 1986–87 and the previous year [26]. Reduced-fat sour cream was first introduced in 1988 and reduced-fat yogurt soon afterward.

Numerous low-fat dairy desserts have been introduced over the past 5 years. For example, during a 15-month period of 1989–90, 56 different ice cream lines or extensions, over 260 flavors, were introduced. More than one-third of these were marketed as low-fat ice milks and frozen desserts [27]. In mid-1991 the first sugar-free, low-fat frozen dessert, Simple Pleasures Light, was introduced. In addition, low-calorie frozen novelty sales increased 52% between 1988 and 1989.

Essentially all yogurt companies introduced nonfat yogurts between 1986 and 1989. Approximately 11% of all yogurt sold in 1989 was nonfat. With the approval of aspartame for yogurt in 1988, the nonfat category has experienced even greater expansion [28]. In 1991, the packaged yogurt market in the United States was roughly 40% low-fat or light; for the overall U.S. market, including frozen yogurts, the percentage was 80% [29].

D. Entrees

Low-calorie, high-quality frozen entree/dinners are extremely popular with consumers. Although available for a couple of decades, this category experienced massive growth in 1981 with the introduction of Stouffer's Lean Cuisine. Sales were reported to be $120 million during the first year. Weight Watcher's quickly reformulated its 13-year-old frozen entree line and doubled its sales in 1981.

By 1987, the low-calorie frozen entree and dinner market was estimated at $1.5 billion with Lean Cuisine and Weight Watchers controlling 70% of that market [30]. More than a third of U.S. households purchased low-calorie frozen entrees in 1988, up from 25% of households in 1986. In 1988, low-calorie frozen entrees/dinners were among the fastest-growing frozen food segments, with sales growth averaging 24% per year over the previous 5 years [31].

Portion control was initially responsible for the caloric reduction in most low-calorie entrees/dinners. The introduction and success of ConAgra's Healthy Choice frozen entrees and dinners in 1989 changed that. Healthy Choice products claiming reduced cholesterol, fat, and sodium reportedly became a $150 million product in its first year and now produces more than $200 million in annual sales. Other companies moved quickly to compete with Healthy Choice. Stouffer's completely reformulated its Lean Cuisine and Heinz its Weight Watchers dinners/entrees. For example, the 1991 reformulated Weight Watchers entrees contained 20% less sodium, 19% less cholesterol, and 14% less fat than in 1990 [32–34].

The newest players in this market are the Ultra Slim-Fast entrees. These entrees are being billed as "the first weight control meal that combines nutritious, satisfying 12 oz. portions, calorie control, low fat, low cholesterol in great tasting, popular varieties" [32].

E. Meat Products

Recent research shows that today's beef is 27% leaner than the U.S. Department of Agriculture (USDA) handbook values of the mid-1980s, and pork is 43% leaner at retail compared to the early 1980s. Fat is now routinely trimmed from meat by many retailers, and in some cases meat is even being grown leaner [35].

In March 1988, USDA issued a new regulation allowing meat processors to produce reduced-fat sausages using higher levels of added water. For example, under earlier cooked sausage regulations the fat content of frankfurters was 29–30% with 9–10% added water. Today, frankfurters are being formulated with about 18–22% fat and 16–19% added water. New technologies have been developed to bind the water in these products to replace flavor lost with fat reduction [36].

More than 3 billion pounds of ground beef products are consumed in the United States each year. This is 44% of the total fresh beef cuts available for consumption. Lean ground beef products have been developed recently to meet the demands of diet-conscious consumers. Consumer-acceptable products with 20% fat content (a 40% reduction) are now available [37]. McDonald's McLean Deluxe hamburger, for example, contains less than half the fat of regular hamburger. Water and carrageenan, as a product stabilizer, are added to defatted lean cuts of beef [33].

F. Confections

"Sugarless" confections made their debut in the U.S. market in the late 1950s and early 1960s. Since that time the two key product lines have been chewing gum and pressed tablets [38].

The "sugarless" or "sugar-free" descriptors are not, however, synonymous with low- or reduced-calorie. Most sugarless confections are marketed as not promoting tooth decay and/or useful for diabetics and contain polyols rather than sugar. Gums and breath mints are, however, now available with the low-calorie sweeteners aspartame, saccharin, or acesulfame-K.

Few low-calorie confections are available in the United States at this time. Polydextrose, a low-calorie bulking agent, is used for caloric reduction in some products.

The development and marketing of low-calorie candies in the United States has been severely hampered by the regulatory situation, which prevents the use of nonnutritive sweeteners in confectionery. (Aspartame, which is considered a nutritive sweetener, is not yet approved for hard or soft candies.) Under section 402(d)(3) of the Federal Food, Drug and Cosmetic Act, confectionery is adulterated if it contains any nonnutritive substance, unless the nonnutritive substance has some practical functional purpose in manufacturing, packaging, or storage of the product, and the use of the substance does not otherwise deceive the consumer. The same section also authorizes the FDA to promulgate regulations interpreting this subsection of the Act to avoid or resolve uncertainty as to its application.

On October 1, 1980, FDA issued a Compliance Policy Guide, which specifically stated that "the use of nonnutritive artificial sweeteners in confectionery for the purpose of caloric reduction is not considered to be a practical functional purpose." In response to numerous requests, the FDA is expected to amend or revoke Compliance Policy Guide No. 7105.01 and permit the use of nonnutritive sweeteners in confection [39]. Petitions for the use of acesulfame-K and aspartame in confections are pending before FDA.

G. Canned Fruit

Canned fruit was a major category for cyclamate use during the 1960s and was one of the few categories in which cyclamate was used as the sole sweetener. California Canners & Growers, considered in the 1960s the largest grower-owned cooperative of its type in the world, controlled 65% of the diet fruit market. When the FDA banned cyclamate, California Canners had 7 million cases of its "Diet Delight" products on store shelves and in warehouses. "Diet Delight" immediately became unsellable, leading to the demise of California Canners [40].

Since cyclamate's removal from the market, saccharin has been used to sweeten some special dietetic canned fruits, but most "light" canned fruit today consists of products packed in their own juice. Sales of light fruit accounted for 24% percent of total canned fruit sales in 1986 and continues to be a significant subsegment [41].

H. Salad Dressings

By the end of the 1970s, the technology was available for producing low-calorie salad dressings. A gum system for producing no-oil salad dressings and a stabilizer system for no-oil pourable dressings had both been reported [42]. By 1981 low-calorie salad dressings were well established as a major subcategory. Supermarket sales for dietetic and low-calorie sauces and dressings reportedly were $53 million in 1980 and $63.6 in 1982. Although the sauces and dressings category experienced a 20% increase overall, sales of dressings rose by as much as 30–40%. Part of this growth was due to a shift in marketing emphasis from consumers with special medical needs to diet-conscious consumers [43].

By 1986, significant sales increases were still occurring in the low-calorie dressing category, while sales of higher-calorie dressings were falling. Low-calorie dressing sales were $146 million in 1986, $170 million in 1987, $204 million in 1988, and $252 million in 1989 [44–46]. By 1990, light salad dressings accounted for almost one-third of the market [47].

Low-fat, no-cholesterol dressings hit the shelves in 1990 with the introduction of a number of fat-free products as well. Kraft Free ranch salad dressing (0 grams of fat, 16 calories per tablespoon) became the nation's most popular dressing only 5 months after its introduction [33].

Gums continue to be used to thicken many of these products. Most contain caloric sweeteners, with the reduction in fat content being responsible for the significant reduction in calories.

I. Snack Products

So-called healthy snacks (e.g., oat bran added, no cholesterol, etc.) have been around for some time, but only recently have salty snack foods become available in low-calorie or "lite" versions. In 1989, light products accounted for 2.4% of all potato chip and 3.1% of microwave popcorn sales [48]. Interestingly, in making popcorn microwavable, manufacturers substantially increased the caloric content of the popcorn. In 1989 microwave popcorn accounted for 80% of popcorn sales and light popcorn was the hottest subsegment of the hottest snack segment.

In early 1990, Frito-Lay Inc., the world's largest manufacturer and marketer of salty snack foods, introduced nationwide its Light line of low-oil snacks (one-third less oil). The line is reportedly doing very well and is expected to be Frito-Lay's most successful product introduction in recent years [49].

V. RESTAURANTS

A major trend in restaurants during the past several years has been the incorporation of healthy, light items on menus. Responsible for this trend are the increased popularity of grilled rather than fried foods, the proliferation of salads, pastas, fish, and chicken, and the availability of nutritional and caloric information for menu items.

Wendy's led fast-food restaurants with the introduction of its salad bar in 1979 [50]. The emphasis on salads in other restaurants came soon after. Also trimming the fat and calories from its menu, McDonald's recently replaced shredded cheese on salads with grated carrots [51].

In a 1991 Food Marketing Industry Speaks survey, over 60% of retailer respondents said their menu planning had been influenced by consumers' nutrition concerns and awareness. In addition to adding poultry and switching to vegetable oils used in frying, products with lower salt, cholesterol, and calorie counts topped retailers' lists of new menu items [52].

VI. CONCLUSION

The H.J. Heinz Company purchased Weight Watchers and its related companies in 1978 for $100 million. In 1989 the brand's operating income to Heinz exceeded the purchase price [53]. In 1989, over 600 new reduced-fat foods were introduced in the United States and more than 10% of all new products had reduced-fat and/or reduced-calorie claims [54].

According to a 1990 Gallup Survey, 74% of consumers say they are reducing their fat intake, and a 1990 Harris Poll found that 48% of consumers had purchased a reduced-fat product within the last 30 days. These are but a few indicators of the growth and potential growth for low-calorie products [55].

Although a 1991 survey conducted for the Calorie Control Council found that 101 million Americans consume low-calorie, sugar-free products, and 124 million use products low or reduced in fat, only 42.6 and 38%, respectively, say they use these products because they taste good [1]. A market for new and improved products really exists.

Low-calorie products have become part of the American diet. Once known strictly as dietetic products, and then diet products, today they are perceived as mainstream products that can help people live more healthfully. As the food and beverage industry moves closer to meeting consumer expectations, low-calorie product sales will continue to increase.

REFERENCES

1. Dieting and Low-Calorie/Reduced-Calorie Products Survey, Booth Research Services, Inc., Atlanta, GA (1991) (unpublished).
2. Dieting and Low-Calorie Products Survey, Booth Research Services, Inc., Atlanta, GA (1989) (unpublished).
3. An Assessment of the Benefits of Saccharin to the American Population, Market Facts, Inc., Chicago, IL (1978) (unpublished).
4. Dieting and Low-Calorie Products Survey, Booth Research Services, Inc., Atlanta, GA (1986) (unpublished).
5. D. Best, Health perceptions preoccupy product developers, *Prep. Foods New Prod. Annu.*, *159*(8): 47 (1990).

6. M. A. Kantor, Light dairy products: The need and the consequences, *Food Technol.*, *44*(10): 81 (1990).

7. T. Smith, *Saccharin*, American Council on Science & Health, New York, pp. 11-13 (1979).

8. G. J. Walter and M. L. Mitchell, Saccharin, *Alternative Sweeteners* (L. O'Brien Nabors and R. C. Gelardi, eds.), Marcel Dekker, Inc., New York, pp. 15-41 (1986).

9. Sweeteners: Capacity, troubles, competition all growing, *Oil, Paint, Drug, Rep.* (Feb. 22, 1965).

10. *SAMI Report*, The Cyclamate Ban: Its Effect Upon Sales of Diet Foods, Selling Areas-Marketing, Inc. (April 1970).

11. M. Friedman, Twenty-five years and 98,900 new products later . . . , *Prep. Foods New Prod. Annu.*, *159*(8): 23 (1990).

12. B. Gorman, New products: What's your next move?, *Prep. Foods New Prod. Annu.*, *158*(8): 20 (1989).

13. A. Ghazaii, Sweetening the pot, *Food Additives '91—A CMR Special Report*, p. SR18 (June 3, 1991).

14. A. Ghazaii, Sweeteners gain from calorie cuts, *Food Additives '90—A CMR Special Report*, p. SR33 (June 18, 1990).

15. M. J. Rudolph, C. G. Greenwald, and R. P. Flesch, Fat replacers: U.S. markets and technologies, *Spectrum*, Decision Resources, Inc., Burlington, MA (Feb. 12, 1991).

16. A. Naude, Getting out the fat, *Food Additives '91—A CMR Special Report*, p. SR13 (June 3, 1991).

17. R. Lawrence, Marketing intelligence, *Food Bus.*, *3*(19): 40 (1990).

18. W. T. Miller, The legacy of cyclamate, Symposium presented by the IFT Toxicology and Safety Evaluation Division at the 46th Annual Meeting of the Institute of Food Technologists, Dallas, TX (1986).

19. *Jesse Meyer's Beverage Digest*, *18*(3) (1991).

20. *Jesse Meyer's Beverage Digest*, *18*(2) (1991).

21. C. E. Morris, P. M. Dillon, and L. Moore, Light bakery, *Food Eng.*, *63*(3): 77 (1991).

22. J. Neff, Sara Lee shakes high-fat image, *Food Bus.*, *3*(21): 14 (1990).

23. K. Springen, J. Schwartz, and A. Miller, How low can they go?, *Newsweek*, pp. 66-67 (August 20, 1990).

24. Fat falls from bake mixes, *Food Bus.*, *4*(6): 37 (1990).

25. *Milk Facts*, Milk Industry Foundation, Washington, D.C., pp. 11-20 (1990).

26. State of the food industry, dairy products, *Food Eng.*, *60*(6): 80 (1988).

27. J. Umhoeffer, A. trimming tradition, *Prep. Foods New Prod. Annu.*, *158* (8): 87 (1989).

28. *The Food Industry Newsletter 18(7)*, Newsletters, Inc., Fairfax, VA, pp. 1-2 (1989).

29. Personal Communication from Sandy Wood of the National Dairy Council, (October, 1990).

30. M. Magiera and J. L. Erickson, All American set to serve low-cal line, *Ad Age*, pp. 3, 47 (July 1988).

31. State of the food industry, frozen foods, *Food Eng.*, *61*(6): 98 (1989).

32. M. Friedman, New products round-up, *Prep. Foods*, *160*(5): 60 (1991).
33. J. Mullich, Healthy foods shaping up profits, *Food Bus.*, *3*(20): 30 (1990).
34. State of the food industry, frozen foods, *Food Eng.*, *62*(6): 78 (1990).
35. L. C. Gilbert and S. M. Starr, Red meat trims the fat, *Food Bus.*, *4*(6): 39 (1991).
36. D. G. Murray, Formulating lower-fat and lower-salt . . . . processed meats, *Food Eng.*, *61*(9): 46 (1989).
37. D. L. Huffman and W. R. Egbert, *Advances in Lean Ground Beef Production, Bulletin 606*, Alabama Agricultural Experiment Station, Auburn University, AL (1990).
38. W. Vink, Applications in confectionery: Tableted confections, *Manuf. Confect.*, *70*(11): 77 (1990).
39. L. O'Brien Nabors, Intense sweeteners: Acesulfame K, alitame, aspartame, saccharin, sucralose, *Manuf. Confect.*, *70*(11): 65 (1990).
40. *Picks and Packs*, University of California Cooperative Extension, Berkeley, CA (October, November, December 1986).
41. E. Sullivan, Canning a bad image, *Prog. Grocer*, *66*(7): 95 (1987).
42. D. D. Duxbury, Specialty/Functional ingredients, *Food Process.*, *5*(11): 102 (1990).
43. Half of America pounds away, *Chain Store Age/Supermarkets*, pp. 105–106 (July 1982).
44. State of the food industry, dressings and sauces, *Food Eng.*, *60*(6): 92 (1988).
45. State of the food industry, dressings and sauces, *Food Eng.*, *61*(6): 96 (1989).
46. State of the food industry, confections, *Food Eng.*, *62*(6): 88 (1990).
47. L. Therrien, Kraft is looking for fat growth from fat-free foods, *Business Week*, pp. 100–101 (March 26, 1990).
48. News in a Minute, *The Food Institute Report, 22*: 6 (June 1990).
49. B. Salvage, Lighten up, say snack food manufacturers, *Food Bus.*, *4*(2): 32 (1991).
50. D. Long, Food trends: menus for the '80's, *Restaurant Bus.*, *85*: 165 (November 1, 1986)
51. B. M. Dawson and B. Lorenzini, On the light side, *Restaurants & Institutions, 101*(13): 133 (1991).
52. M. Williams, Food service must address nutrition, *Supermarket News, 41*(20): 57 (1991).
53. Marketplace, Weight Watcher line expands 20% in sales, *Food Eng., 61*(6): 32 (1989).
54. S. M. Starr and L. M. Gilbert, Lighter, healthier foods: Coming soon to a supermarket near you, *Food and Nutr.*, pp. 10–11 (January 1991).
55. R. J. Bannar, Free food: Fat-free, that is, *Dairy & Frozen Foods*, *2*(1): 43 (1991).

7
Regulation of Low-Calorie Foods

John E. Vanderveen *Food and Drug Administration, Washington, D.C.*

I. BACKGROUND

The Federal Food, Drug and Cosmetic (FD&C) Act, which provided authority to regulate claims on food labels, was signed into law on June 30, 1938. It replaced the Pure Food and Drug Act of June 30, 1906, which focused mainly on the safety of food and drug products. Before the passage of the FD&C Act, the provision of the law that restricted claims on food labels was limited; therefore, many claims were unsubstantiated. This lack of restraint on the part of some manufacturers contributed to the enactment of the legislation [1].

In 1940 the Food and Drug Administration (FDA) held hearings on foods for special dietary use. There was considerable participation by industry and members of the academic community. Although the official record of the meeting that contains the original presentations is no longer available, it is clear from the findings of fact published by the agency in 1941 that the issue of foods for weight control was an important part of the record. The relevant findings of fact associated with the calorie content of foods are found in Appendix A.

The conclusions relative to calorie intake from the 1940 hearings were that (1) the sources and the amounts of calories consumed are important to controlling body weight, (2) the value of a food for special dietary use may depend on the regulation of intake of protein, fat, carbohydrates, or calories, (3) the calories in some carbohydrates are not available to humans, (4) the use of such carbohydrates and other nonnutritive ingredients such as mineral oil and saccharin can reduce calorie intake, and (5) label information is necessary for the purchaser to evaluate a food for use in the control of body weight.

The 1941 regulations, established in response to the 1940 hearing, included labeling requirements for foods purported to be or represented for use as a means of controlling body weight [2]. These regulations, shown in Appendix B [2], required that the percent of protein, fat, and carbohydrates, and the number of available calories supplied by a specified quantity of a food be given on the product label. The regulation also required that nondigestible carbohydrates from plant origin be labeled as crude fiber and that other nondigestible substances such as nonnutritive sweeteners be listed on the label. These requirements were to remain in effect for more than 37 years.

II. CURRENT REGULATIONS

On June 20, 1962, the FDA published a notice of proposed rulemaking for foods for special dietary use that included revision of requirements for the labeling of foods purporting to be for, or represented for, controlling body weight [3]. Final regulations were published on June 18, 1966, with an effective date of December 15, 1966 [4]. A number of objections and requests for a public hearing was filed during the 30-day period provided by the order. The Commissioner stayed the regulation pending a hearing. A hearing was convened on May 21, 1968, and continued for 2 years, closing on May 14, 1970. This hearing made history by being the longest administrative hearing ever held and resulted in many hundreds of thousands of pages of evidence. On July 19, 1977, the agency published a document in the *Federal Register* that included proposed findings of fact, proposed conclusions, and a tentative order on the labeling of foods for special dietary use because of their usefulness in reducing or maintaining calorie intake or body weight [5]. A final order was published on September 22, 1978, with an effective date of July 1, 1979 [6].

This regulation required that any food that purports to be or is represented for special dietary use because of its usefulness in maintaining or reducing calorie intake or body weight, including, but not limited to, any food that bears representations that it is low or reduced in calories, shall (1) bear nutrition labeling, (2) contain a statement that explains the basis on which the food claims special dietary usefulness or identifies the food as a low- or a reduced-calorie food, and (3) bear a label statement that the food contains a nonnutritive ingredient to achieve its effect or the presence of a nonnutritive sweetener. The regulation defined low calorie as a food containing fewer than 40 calories per serving and less than 0.4 calorie per gram or a sugar substitute. A reduced-calorie food was defined as a substitute food having one-third fewer calories per specified serving than the food that it replaces; the substitute food may not be nutritionally inferior under the regulations defining substitute foods [7]. The regulations also required that foods not meeting the definitions for low calorie or reduced calorie could not use such terms as "sugar-free," "sugarless," or "no sugar" unless such terms were accompanied by the statement "Not a reduced-calorie food," "Not a low-calorie food," "Not for weight control," "Useful only in not promoting tooth decay," or any other term indicating that the sole special usefulness of the food is for a specified purpose other than weight control.

Foods that are naturally low in calories without having any fabrication or alteration may be labeled as low-calorie foods, but the term low calorie may not precede the name of the food because such terminology would imply that the food had been altered to lower its calories.

There was strong opposition from the baking industry and others because such products as bread made with added fiber were thought to be unable to achieve the necessary one-third reduction in calories required for labeling as a reduced-calorie product. Because a meaningful reduction in calories for a high-volume food such as bread would have a major public health significance, the agency decided to have a petition process that would permit decisions on a case-by-case basis [5].

The agency published a proposed rule [8] that would have provided an exception for bread in the same issue of the *Federal Register* that contained the final regulation on label statements relating to usefulness in reducing or maintaining calorie intake or body weight. This proposal was later withdrawn when it became evident that a satisfactory product could be made that achieved a one-third reduction in calories [9]. Part of the success in reaching this conclusion was due to the fact that the agency allowed the use of dietary fiber methods in place of the crude fiber analysis previously used [10,11].

One other footnote is worthy of comment. Early in the 1980s, a manufacturer of a cooking spray became aware that the term low calorie could no longer be used because such products contain more than 0.4 calorie per gram. The firm undertook extensive research to demonstrate that the use of cooking sprays in place of traditional frying fats would reduce the calories of fried foods by one-third. Although a substantial reduction in calories was achieved for the use of cooking sprays in frying vegetables, the use of such sprays resulted in no reduction of calories for frying meats and other food when compared with foods fried with traditional fats and oils.

III. FUTURE REGULATIONS FOR CALORIE CONTENT CLAIMS

The Nutrition Labeling and Education Act (NLEA) of 1990 [12] requires that total calories and calories from fat be included as part of mandatory nutrition labeling and a review be made of all regulations that control nutrient content claims such as low calorie and reduced calorie. NLEA permits only content claims defined by regulation to be used on the food label. The new law also requires that any content claim be accompanied by the statement "See _____ for nutrition information" in which the blank shall identify the panel on which the information described in the claim may be found. The absence of a nutrient in a food can be claimed only if the nutrient is usually present in the food, unless the Secretary by regulation permits the claim on the basis of a finding that such a statement would assist consumers in maintaining a healthy diet, and the claim discloses that the nutrient is not usually present in the food. Finally, the new law requires that if a food bearing a nutrient content claim contains another nutrient at a level that will increase the risk of a disease, then the amount of that nutrient must be disclosed in the immediate proximity to such a claim and with appropriate prominence (in type not less than one-half the size of that used in the claim). For example, if a food having a low-calorie claim also contains a level of fat that increases the risk of a disease, then the level of fat would have to be disclosed next to the claim.

The agency proposed regulations to implement the provisions of NLEA on November 27, 1991 [13]. The proposed regulations included mandatory nutrition labeling for most packaged foods, defined terms for nutrient content claims, and listed rules for implementing the use of disease-related claims on food labels. The proposed regulation on mandatory nutrition labeling included the revision of U.S. Recommended Daily Allowances (U.S. RDAs) for vitamins and essential mineral elements, and proposed the creation of Daily Reference Values (DRVs) for major components of foods, including total fat, saturated fat, cholesterol, total carbohydrates, dietary fiber, sodium, and potassium, and the establishment of reference amounts customarily consumed per eating occasion, which are to be used by manufacturers to establish serving sizes for their products as described below.

It was difficult for the agency to establish the levels of nutrients in a single food that increased the risk of a disease. After much deliberation, the agency proposed that 11.5 grams of fat, 4 grams of saturated fat, 45 mg of cholesterol, or 360 mg of sodium per serving or per 100 grams were the levels at which there was an increased risk of disease. When these levels are used in conjunction with the nutrient content claims assessed for a food, they are called disclosure levels.

The NLEA required that certain terms used in conjunction with nutrient content claims on foods be defined. These include "free," "low," "light," "lite," "reduced," "less," and "high." All of these terms, with the exception of "less" and "high," have been used by manufacturers to describe the calorie content of foods. The agency has proposed definitions for "reduced" "fewer" in a proposed rule published in the *Federal Register* on November 27, 1991. All of these definitions are included in Appendix C [13]. The comment period for this proposed rule extended to February 25, 1992. NLEA requires that unless the agency publishes a final rule by November 8, 1992, the proposed rule will become the final rule.

The proposed rule does not change the basic definitions for low calorie and reduced calorie that were established in 1978. A low-calorie food is defined as a food having a level of fewer than 40 calories per serving and less than 0.4 calorie per gram. A reduced-calorie product is defined as a food having at least one-third fewer calories than the same food without the fabrication or alteration to reduce the calorie level. A reduced-calorie food must also be accompanied by a comparative statement and be nutritionally equivalent to the original food to which it is being compared. There is a new requirement, however, that the calorie reduction must be at least 40 calories per serving.

The proposed rule also contains definitions not previously used for "free," "fewer," and "light or lite." A calorie-free food is defined as having fewer than 5 calories per serving. The term "fewer" can be used as a comparative claim if the reduction in calories is at least 25% and more than 40 calories per serving. A food described as having "fewer" calories must also be nutritionally equivalent and have a comparative statement describing the reduction relative to the food that it resembles and for which it substitutes. The term "light or lite" is defined as containing one-third fewer calories with a minimum reduction of 40 calories per serving. In the case where the original food contains more than 50% of the calories derived from fat, the proposed rule would require a fat reduction of 50% with a minimum reduction of more than 3 grams per serving.

It should be noted that in all these definitions the claim is based on serving size. Traditionally the serving size of a food was established by the manufacturer. The NLEA now requires that standards be established to define serving sizes in common household units based on amounts commonly consumed. The agency has proposed values, by categories of foods, for reference amounts customarily consumed. The manufacturers must use these values in establishing serving sizes for nutrition labeling. These reference amounts are based in part on data obtained from the 1978–1979 Nation-wide Food Consumption Survey, which was conducted by the United States Department of Agriculture. Adjustments in these reference amounts will be made from time to time because the amounts commonly consumed of some food items are likely to change. There will probably be a continued concern that serving sizes will not be perfect for all foods. However, the proposed regulations are expected to help consumers make more meaningful compar-isons between similar foods and create an equitable environment for manu-facturers.

Not all government agencies responsible for coordinating with FDA on the proposed regulations concurred with the requirements for nutrient con-tent descriptors prepared by FDA. However, there was insufficient time to consider alternatives and meet the statutory deadline imposed by NLEA. Therefore, it was announced in the November 27, 1991, proposal [13] that a proposal for an alternative approach on the nutrient content claims would be published at a later date.

IV. NUTRIENT-DISEASE CLAIMS

The NLEA authorizes FDA to approve nutrient-disease claims on food la-beling provided certain criteria are met. These criteria include that (1) the claim is based on the totality of publicly available scientific evidence, (2) there is significant scientific agreement among experts qualified by scienti-fic training and experience to evaluate the claim, (3) the claim is supported by the evidence, and (4) the food does not contain a level of any nutrient in an amount that increases the risk to persons in the general population of a disease or health-related condition that is diet related. The agency has pro-posed general principles for implementing these criteria [13] (see Appendix D). The agency has proposed to define the levels at which nutrients increase the risk of a diet-related disease or condition to be the same as those proposed as disclosure levels for nutrient content claims. Although the relationship between calorie intake and obesity is well known, as is the relationship be-tween obesity and the prevalence of several disease conditions, the NLEA did not require the FDA to determine the appropriateness of a calorie-dis-ease claim, and this was not accomplished. However, the NLEA requires that a petition process by established for manufacturers to petition the agency to permit nutrient-disease claims.

V. SUMMARY

Since 1938, the Federal Food, Drug, and Cosmetic Act has required that information on labels of food be truthful and not misleading. For more than 50 years, FDA has required that foods claiming to be useful in controlling body weight be labeled to indicate the composition of carbohydrate, fat, and protein. In addition, the label had to indicate the percentages of nondigestible substances present. Since 1978, the content claims of "low calorie" and "reduced calorie" have been defined by regulation. The Nutrition Labeling and Education Act of 1990 has imposed new restrictions on the use of nutrient content claims. These restrictions require FDA to repropose all nutrient content claims. Proposed regulations published in response to the NLEA provide definitions for "calorie free," "low calorie," "reduced calorie," and "fewer calories." Two alternatives were proposed for comparative claims such as "reduced calories" and "fewer calories." The use of calorie content claims requires that additional information accompany the claim when the levels of fat, saturated fat, cholesterol, and sodium in the product exceed levels determined to increase the risk of disease. The NLEA permits FDA to authorize the use of claims for nutrient and disease relationships provided that such claims meet specific requirements concerning the existence of scientific data and substantial agreement among knowledgeable scientists that the claims are appropriate. However, no calorie-disease claims have been proposed.

APPENDIX A.   REQUIREMENTS FOR CALORIE-INTAKE STATEMENTS, 1941

The regulations published by FDA in 1941 in conjunction with the findings of fact included requirements relating to label statements for foods used in control of body weight and to label statements regarding nonnutritive constituents used in foods for the purpose of lowering calories. Statements relating to calorie intake included:

87. The value of a food for special dietary use may depend on its suitability for use in the control of body weight through regulating the intake of protein, fat, carbohydrates, or calories.
88. The quantity and relative proportions of protein, fat, and carbohydrates, and the number of calories consumed are important factors in the regulation of body weight.
89. The value of a food for special dietary use may depend on its suitability for use in dietary management with respect to disease through

regulating the intake of protein, fat, carbohydrates, or calories: such management is an important factor in the treatment of many diseases.

90. Some carbohydrate substances are not digested or assimilated by the human organism and supply no food energy. Only the carbohydrates which may be digested and assimilated are available to the metabolic processes of the organism.

91. Carbohydrates which are non-available to the metabolic processes have a theoretical calorie value but supply no calories to the human organism.

92. Information necessary for the purchaser to evaluate a food for use in the control of body weight, or in dietary management with respect to disease, includes a statement on the label of the percent by weight of protein, fat, and available carbohydrates in such food and a statement on the label of the number of available calories supplied by a specified quantity of the food.

93. The value of a food for special dietary use may depend on the presence therein of a constituent which is not utilized in normal metabolism and which consequently has no nutritive value.

94. Its use may be for the reduction of caloric intake as in the case of mineral oil; for the promotion of laxation, as in the case of fibrous plant matter; or for the satisfaction of taste desires without increasing food value, as in the case of saccharin.

95. Information necessary to inform the purchaser of the value of a food for special dietary use by reason of its content of such a constituent includes a statement of the percent by weight of the constituent in the food, preceded or followed by the word "nonnutritive", except as hereinafter noted in Finding 98 with respect to saccharin.

96. If such constituent is fibrous plant matter it is commonly determined as and expressed as crude fiber.

97. Saccharin, alone or in combination in a saccharin salt, is a nonnutritive, synthetic sweetening substance sometimes used to satisfy the psychological desire for sweets in the diets of persons who must restrict their intake of carbohydrates. It has no other use as a food and is not utilized in normal metabolism.

98. Information necessary to inform the purchaser of the value of a food for special dietary use by reason of its saccharin content is a statement that it contains a specified percent by weight of saccharin, a nonnutritive, artificial sweetener which should be used only by persons who must restrict their intake of ordinary sweets.

APPENDIX B.   FDA REGULATIONS
ESTABLISHED IN 1941

Section 125.06. Label statements relating to certain food used in control of body weight or in dietary management with respect to disease. If a food purports to be or is represented for special dietary use by man by reason of its use as a means of regulating the intake of protein, fat, carbohydrate, or calories, for the purpose of controlling body weight, or for the purpose of dietary management with respect to disease, the label shall bear a statement of—

(a)   the percent by weight of protein, fat, and available carbohydrates in such food; and

(b)   the number of available calories supplied by a specified quantity of food.

Section 125.07. Label statements relating to nonnutritive constituents. If a food purports to be or is represented for special dietary use by man by reason of the presence of any constituent which is not utilized in normal metabolism, the label shall bear a statement of the percent by weight of such constituent, and in juxtaposition with the name of such constituent, the word "nonnutritive." If such constituent is fibrous plant matter, it shall be considered to be crude fiber and its percent expressed as such. But if such constituent is saccharin or a saccharin salt, the label shall bear, in lieu of such statement and word, the statement "Contains—saccharin (or saccharin salt, as the case may be), a nonnutritive, artificial sweetener which should be used only by persons who must restrict their intake of ordinary sweets," the blank to be filled in with the percent by weight of saccharin or saccharin salt in such food. The provisions of this section shall not be construed as authorizing the use of saccharin or its salts in any food other than one for use by persons who must restrict their intake of carbohydrates, or as relieving any food from compliance with any requirement of sections 402 (b) or (d), 403 (g), or other provisions of the Act.

APPENDIX C.   PROPOSED RULE FOR NUTRIENT CONTENT
CLAIMS, NOV. 27, 1991

§ 101.13 *Nutrient content claims—general principles.*

(a)   This section and the regulations in Subpart D of this part apply to foods that are intended for human consumption and that are offered for sale.

(b)   A claim that expressly or implicitly characterizes the level of a nutrient (nutrient content claim) of the type required in nutrition labeling under

§ 101.9 may not be made on the label or in labeling of foods unless the claim is made in accordance with this regulation and with the applicable regulations in Subpart D of this part.

(1) An expressed nutrient content claim is any direct statement about the level (or range) of a nutrient in the food, e.g., "low sodium."

(2) An implied nutrient content claim is any claim that describes the food or an ingredient therein in such a manner that leads a consumer to assume that a nutrient is absent or present in a certain amount (e.g., "high in oat bran") or that the food because of its nutrient content may be useful in achieving a total diet that conforms to current dietary recommendations (e.g., healthy").

(3) No nutrient content claims may be made on food intended specifically for use by infants and toddlers less than 2 years of age.

(c) Information that is required or permitted by § 101.9 to be declared in nutrition labeling, and that appears as part of the nutrition label, is not a nutrient content claim and is not subject to the requirements of this section. If such information is declared elsewhere on the label or in labeling, it is a nutrient content claim and is subject to the requirements for nutrient content claims.

(d) A "substitute" food is one that may be used interchangeably with another food that it resembles, i.e., that it is organoleptically, physically, and functionally (including shelf life) similar to, and that it is not nutritionally inferior to; unless it is labeled as an "imitation."

(1) If there is a difference in performance characteristics, the food may still be considered a substitute if the label includes a disclaimer adjacent to the most prominent claim as defined in paragraph (j) (2) (ii) of this section, informing the consumer of such difference (e.g., not for use in cooking).

(2) This disclaimer must be in easily legible print or type and in a size no less than one-half the size of the type of the descriptive term but in no case less than one-sixteenth of an inch in height.

(e) (1) Because the use of a "free" or "low" claim before the name of a food implies that the food has been altered compared to other foods of the same type to lower the amount of the nutrient in the food, only foods that have been specially processed, altered, formulated, or reformulated so as to remove the nutrient from the food may bear such a claim (e.g., low sodium potato chips).

(2) Any claim for the absence of a nutrient in a food, or that a food is low in a nutrient, when the food has not been specially processed, altered, formulated, or reformulated to qualify for that claim, shall indicate that the food inherently, meets the criteria and shall clearly refer to all foods of that type and not merely to the particular brand to which the labeling attaches (e.g., "corn oil, a sodium free food").

(f)   A nutrient content claim shall be in type size and style no larger than that of the statement of identity.

(g)   The label or labeling of a food for which a nutrient content claim is made shall contain prominently and in immediate proximity to such claim the following referral statement: "See _____ for nutrition information" with the blank filled in with the identity of the panel on which nutrition labeling is located.

(1)   The referral statement "See [appropriate panel] for nutrition information" shall be in easily legible boldface print or type, in distinct contrast to other printed or graphic matter, that is no less than one-half the size of the type of the nutrient content claim but in no case less than one-sixteenth of an inch in height.

(2)   The referral statement shall be immediately adjacent to the nutrient content claim and may have no intervening materal other than, if applicable, other information in the statement of identity or any other information that is required to be presented with the claim under this section (see, e.g., paragraph (j)(2) of this section or under a regulation in Subpart D of this part (see, e.g., §§ 101.54 and 101.62)). If the nutrient content claim appears on more than one panel of the label, the referral statement shall be adjacent to the claim on each panel except for the panel that bears the nutrition information.

(3)   If a single panel of a food label or labeling contains multiple nutrient content claims or a single claim repeated several times, a single referral statement may be made. The statement shall be adjacent to the claim that is printed in the largest type on that panel.

(h)   In place of the referral statement described in paragraph (g) of this section, if a food contains more than 11.5 grams (g) of fat, 4.0 g of saturated fat, 45 milligrams (mg) of cholesterol, or 360 mg of sodium per reference amount customarily consumed, per labeled serving size, or per 100 grams, then that food must disclose, as part of the referral statement, that the nutrient exceeding the specified level is present in the food as follows: "See [appropriate panel] for information about [nutrient requiring disclosure] and other nutrients," e.g., "See side panel for information about fats and other nutrients."

(i)   Except as provided in paragraph (o) (3) of this section, the label or labeling of a product may contain a statement about the amount or percentage of a nutrient that implies that the food is high or low in that nutrient only if the food actually meets the definition for either "high" or "low" as defined for the nutrient that the label addresses. Such a claim might be "contains 100 mg of sodium per serving."

(j)   Products may bear a statement that compares the level of a nutrient in the product with the level of a nutrient in a reference food. These statements shall be known as "relative claims" and include "reduced," "light" and comparative claims.

(1)   To bear a relative claim about the level of a nutrient, the amount of that nutrient in the food must be compared as specified below to a reference food. Such foods are:

(i)   For all relative claims, an industry wide norm, i.e., a composite value weighted according to a national market share on a unit or tonnage basis of all the foods of the same type as the food for which the claim is made;

(ii)   For reduced and comparative claims only, a manufacturer's regular product that has been offered for sale to the public on a regular basis for a substantial period of time in the same geographic area by the same business entity or by one entitled to use its trade name; or

(iii)   For comparative claims only, a food or class of food whose composition is reported in a current valid data base such as U.S. Department of Agriculture's Handbook 8, *Composition of Foods, Raw, Processed, Prepared*.

(2)   For foods bearing relative claims:

(i)   The label or labeling must bear, immediately adjacent to the claim that is in the most prominent location on the labeling or labeling and in type no less than one-half the size of the type of the claim but no less than one-sixteenth of an inch, the following accompanying information:

(A)   The identity of the reference food;

(B)   The percentage (or fraction) of the amount of the nutrient in the reference food by which the nutrient has been modified, (e.g., "50% less fat," "1/3 fewer calories"); and

(C)   Clear and concise quantitative information comparing the amount of the subject nutrient in the product per labeled serving with that of the reference food.

(ii)   The determination of which use of the claim is in the most prominent location on the label or labeling will be made based on the following factors, considered in order:

(A)   A claim on the principal display panel adjacent to the statement of identity;

(B)   A claim elsewhere on the principal display panel;

(C)   A claim on the information panel; or

(D)   A claim elsewhere on the label or labeling.

(iii)   Relative claims for decreased levels of nutrients may be made on the label or in labeling of a food only if the nutrient content for that nutrient differs from that of the reference food by more than the amount specified in the definition of "low" for that nutrient.

(k) The term "modified" may be used in the statement of identity of a food that bears a comparative claim that complies with the requirements of this part, followed immediately by the name of the nutrient whose content has been altered (e.g., "Modified fat cheesecake"). This statement of identity must be immediately followed by the comparative statement such as "Contains 35% less fat than _____" and all other information required in paragraph (j)(2) of this section for comparative claims.

(1) For purposes of making a claim, a "meal-type product" shall be defined as a food that:

(1) Makes a significant contribution to the diet by:

(i) Providing at least 200 calories per serving (container); or

(ii) Weighing at least 6 ounces per serving (container); and

(2) Contains ingredients from 2 or more of the following 4 food groups:

(i) Bread, cereal, rice and pasta group;

(ii) Fruits and vegetables group;

(iii) Milk, yogurt, and cheese group;

(iv) Meat, poultry, fish, dry beans, eggs, and nuts group; and

(3) Is represented as, or is in a form commonly understood to be, a breakfast, lunch, dinner, meal, main dish, entree, or pizza. Such representations may be made either by statements, photographs, or vignettes.

(m) Nutrition labeling shall be provided for any food for which a nutrient content claim is made in accordance with §§ 101.9 and 101.36.

(n) Compliance with requirements for nutrient content claims in this section and in regulations in Subpart D of this part, will be determined using analytical methodology prescribed for determining compliance with nutrition labeling in § 101.9 of this chapter.

(o) The following exemptions apply:

(1) Nutrient content claims that have not been defined by regulation and that appear as part of a brand name that was in use prior to October 25, 1989, may continue to be used as part of that brand name, provided they are not false or misleading under section 403(a) of the Federal Food, Drug, and Cosmetic Act (the act).

(2) A soft drink that used the term "diet" as part of its brand name before October 25, 1989, and whose use of that term was in compliance with § 105.66 of this chapter as that regulation appeared in the Code of Federal Regulations on that date, may continue to use that term as part of its brand name, provided that its use of the term is not false or misleading under section 403(a) of the act.

(3) A statement that describes the percentage of a vitamin or mineral in the food in relation to a reference daily intake (RDI) as defined in § 101.9 may be made on the label or in labeling of a food without a regulation auth-

orizing such a claim for a specific vitamin or mineral unless such claim is expressly prohibited by regulation under 403(r)(2)(A)(vi) of the act.

(4)   The requirements of this section do not apply to:

(i)   Infant formulas subject to section 412(h) of the act; and

(ii)   Medical foods defined by section 5(b) of the Orphan Drug Act.

(5)   A nutrient content claim used on food that is served in restaurants or other establishments in which food is served for immediate human consumption or which is sold for sale or use in such establishments shall comply with the requirements of this section and the appropriate definition in Subpart D of this part, except that such claim is exempt from the requirements for disclosure statements in paragraphs (g) and (h) of this section and §§ 101.54(d), 101.62(c), (d)(1)(ii)(C), (d)(2)(ii)(C), (d)(3), (d)(4)(ii)(C), and (d)(5)(ii)(C).

(6)   Nutrient content claims that were part of the common or usual names of foods that were subject to a standard of identity on November 8, 1990, are not subject to the requirements of paragraphs (b), (g), and (h) of this section or to definitions in Subpart D of this part.

(7)   Implied nutrient content claims may be used as part of a brand name, provided that the use of the claim has been authorized by the Food and Drug Administration. Petitions requesting approval of such a claim may be submitted under § 101.50(h).

(8)   The terms "sugar free," "sugarless," and "no sugar" may be used on the label and in labeling of chewing gums containing no sucrose provided that when the product is not "low calorie" or "reduced calorie" under § 101.60(b), the label also bear immediately adjacent to the claim each time it is used, the statement "Not a reduced-calorie food," "Not a low-calorie food," "Not for weight control," or "Useful Only in Not Promoting Tooth Decay."

5.   Subpart D is added to read as follows:

Subpart D—Specific Requirements for Nutrient Content Claims Sec.

101.54   Nutrient content claims for "source," "high," and "more."

101.56   Nutrient content claims for "light" or "lite."

101.60   Nutrient content claims for the calorie content of foods.

101.61   Nutrient content claims for the sodium content of foods.

101.62   Nutrient content claims for the fat, fatty acids, and cholesterol content of foods.

101.69   Petitions for nutrient content claims.

Subpart D—Specific Requirements for Nutrient Content Claims

§ 101.54   *Nutrient content claims for "source," "high," and more."*

(a) *General requirements.* Except as provided in paragraph (e) of this section, a claim about the level of a nutrient in a food in relation to the Reference Daily Intake (RDI) established for that nutrient in § 101.9(c)(11)(iv) or Daily Reference Value (DRV) established for that nutrient in § 101.9(c)(12)(i), (excluding total carbohydrates and unsaturated fatty acids) may only be made on the label and in labeling of the food if:

(1) The claim uses one of the terms defined in this section in accordance with the definition for that term;

(2) The claim is made in accordance with the general requirements for nutrient content claims in § 101.13; and

(3) The food for which the claim is made is labeled in accordance with § 101.9 or, where applicable, § 101.36.

(b) *"High" claims.*

(1) The terms "high," "rich in," or "major source of" may be used on the label and in the labeling of a food except meal-type products as defined in § 101.13(1), provided that the food contains 20 percent or more of the RDI or the DRV per reference amount customarily consumed and per labeled serving size.

(2) These terms may be used on the label and in the labeling of a meal-type product as defined in § 101.13(1), provided that it contains per 100 grams (g) of product, an amount of the nutrient that is equal to 20 percent or more of the RDI or DRV.

(c) *"Source" claims.*

(1) The terms "source," "good source of," or "important source of" may be used on the label or in the labeling of a food when the food except meal-type products as described in § 101.13(1) contains 10 to 19 percent of the (RDI) or the (DRV) per reference amount customarily consumed and per labeled serving size.

(2) These terms may be used on the label and in the labeling of a meal-type product as defined in § 101.13(1), provided that it contains per 100 g of product, an amount of the nutrient that is equal to 10 to 19 percent of the RDI or DRV.

(d) *"Fiber" claim.* If a nutrient content claim is made with respect to the level of dietary fiber, that is, that the product is high in fiber, a source of fiber, or that the food contains "more" fiber, and the food is not low in total fat as defined in § 101.62(b)(2), then the label shall disclose the level of total fat per labeled serving. The disclosure shall appear in immediate proximity to such claim and precede the referral statement required in § 101.13(g) (e.g., "Contains [*X amount*] of total fat per serving. See [*appropriate panel*] for nutrition information.")

(e)(1) *"More."* A comparative claim using the term "more" may be used on the label and in the labeling to describe the level of protein, vitamins, minerals, dietary fiber, or potassium in a food, including meal-type products as defined in § 101.13(1), provided that:

(i) The food contains at least 10 percent more of the RDI for protein, vitamins, or minerals or of the DRV for dietary fiber or potassium (expressed as a percent of the Daily Value) than the reference food that it resembles and for which it substitutes as specified in § 101.13(j)(1)(i), (j)(1)(ii), and (j)(1)(iii);

(ii) Where the claim is based on a nutrient that has been added to the food, that fortification is in accordance with the policy on fortification of foods in § 104.20 of this chapter; and

(iii) As required in § 101.13(j)(2) for relative claims, the identity of the reference food; the percentage (or fraction) that the nutrient was increased relative to the RDI or DRV; and quantitative information comparing the level of the nutrient in the product per labeled serving size, with that of the reference food that it replaces are declared in immediate proximity to the most prominent such claim (e.g., "Contains 10% more of the daily value for fiber than white bread. Fiber content of white bread is 1 g per serving; (this product) 3.5 g per serving.")

(2) A comparative claim using the term "more" may be used to describe the level of complex carbohydrates in a food, including meal-type products as defined in § 101.13(1), provided that the food contains at least 4 percent more of the DRV for carbohydrates than the reference food, and the difference between the two foods is only complex carbohydrates as defined in § 101.9(c)(6)(i). The identity of the reference food and quantitative information comparing the level of complex carbohydrates with that of the reference food that it replaces shall be declared in immediate proximity to the most prominent such claim.

(3) A comparative claim using the term "more" may be used to describe the level of unsaturated fat in a food including meal-type products as defined in § 101.13(1) provided that the food contains at least 4 percent more of the DRV for unsaturated fat than the reference food, the level of total fat is not increased, and the level of *trans* fatty acids does not exceed 1 percent of the total fat. The identity of the reference food and quantitative information comparing the level of unsaturated fat with that of the reference food that it replaces shall be declared in immediate proximity to the most prominent such claim.

§ 101.56 *Nutrient content claims for "light" or "lite."*

(a) *General requirements.* A claim using the term "light" or "lite" to describe a food may only be made on the label and in labeling of the food if:

(1)   The claim uses one of the terms defined in this section in accordance with the definition for that term;

(2)   The claim is made in accordance with the general requirements for nutrient content claims in § 101.13; and

(3)   The food is labeled in accordance with § 101.9 or, where applicable, § 101.36.

(b)   The terms "light" or "lite" may be used on the label and in the labeling without further qualification to describe a food, except meal-type products as defined in § 101.13(1). provided that:

(1)   The food has at least a 1/3 (33 1/3 percent) reduction in the number of calories compared to a reference food as specified in § 101.13(j)(1)(i) with a minimum reduction of more than 40 calories per reference amount customarily consumed and per labeled serving size;

(2)   If the food derives 50 percent or more of its calories from fat, its fat content is reduced by 50 percent or more compared to the reference food that it resembles or for which it substitutes as specified in § 101.13(j)(1)(i) with a minimum reduction of more than 3 grams (g) per reference amount customarily consumed and per labeled serving size; and

(3)   As required in § 101.13(j)(2) for relative claims, the identity of the reference food; the percent (or fraction) that the calories, and, if appropriate, the fat, were reduced; and quantitative information comparing the level of calories and, if appropriate, fat content, in the product per labeled serving size, with that of the reference food that it replaces are declared in immediate proximity to the most prominent such claim (e.g., "1/3 fewer calories and 50% less fat than our regular cheese cake: lite cheese cake—200 calories, 4 grams fat; regular cheese cake—300 calories, 8 grams fat per serving").

(c)   A product, other than a salt substitute, that is low, reduced or otherwise altered in sodium content cannot use the term "light" solely because of this alteration but rather shall use, as appropriate, the term "reduced sodium" or "low sodium."

(d)   The term "light" or "lite" may be used to describe a salt substitute if the sodium content of the product has been reduced by at least 50 percent compared to ordinary table salt.

(e)   The term "light" or "lite" may not be used to refer to a food that is not reduced in calories by 1/3 and, if applicable, in fat by 50 percent, unless:

(1)   It describes some physical or organoleptic attribute of the food such as texture or color and the qualifying information (e.g., "light in color" or "light in texture") so stated clearly conveys the nature of the product; and

(2)   The qualifying information is in the same type size, style, color, and prominence as the word "light" and in immediate proximity thereto.

(f)   If a manufacturer can demonstrate that the word "light" has been associated, through common use, with a particular food (e.g., light brown sugar, light corn syrup, or light molasses) to the point where it has become part of the statement of identity, such use of the term "light" shall not be considered a nutrient content claim subject to the requirements in this part.

§ 101.60 *Nutrient content claims for the calorie content of foods.*

(a) *General requirements.* A claim about the calorie content of a food may only be made on the label and in the labeling of the food if:

(1) The claim uses one of the terms defined in this section in accordance with the definition for that term;

(2) The claim is made in accordance with the general requirements for nutrient content claims in § 101.13; and

(3) The food for which the claim is made is labeled in accordance with § 101.9 or, where applicable, § 101.36.

(b) *"Calorie content claims."*

(1) The terms "calorie free," "free of calories," "no calories," "zero calories," "trivial source of calories," "negligible source of calories," or "dietarily insignificant source of calories" may be used on the label and in the labeling of a food provided that:

(i) The food contains less than 5 calories per reference amount customarily consumed and per labeled serving size; and

(ii) As required in § 101.13(e)(2), if the food meets this condition without the benefit of special processing, alteration, formulation, or reformulation to lower the caloric content, it is labeled to disclose that calories are not usually present in the food (e.g., "soda water, a calorie free food").

(2) The terms "low calorie," "few calories," "contains a small amount of calories," "low source of calories," or "low in calories" may be used on the label and in labeling of foods except meal-type products as defined in § 101.13(1) provided that:

(i) The food does not provide more than 40 calories per reference amount customarily consumed, per labeled serving size, and, except for sugar substitute, per 100 grams (g); and

(ii) If a food meets these conditions without the benefit of special processing, alteration, formulation or reformulation to vary the caloric content, it is labeled to clearly refer to all foods of its type and not merely to the particular brand to which the label attaches (e.g., "celery, a low calorie food").

(3) The terms listed in paragraph (b)(2) of this section may be used on the label or in labeling of meal-type products as defined in § 101.13(1) provided that:

(i) The product contains 105 calories or less per 100 g; and

(ii)   If the product meets this condition without the benefit of special processing, alteration, formulation, or reformulation to lower the calorie content, it is labeled to clearly refer to all foods of its type and not merely to the particular brand to which it attaches.

(4)   The terms "reduced calorie," "reduced in calories" or "calorie reduced" may be used to describe a food, except meal-type products as defined in § 101.13(1), provided that:

(i)   The food has been specifically processed, altered, formulated, or reformulated, to reduce its caloric content by 33 1/3 percent or more with a minimum reduction of more than 40 calories per reference amount customarily consumed and per labeled serving size from the reference food that it resembles and for which it substitutes as defined in § 101.13(j)(1)(i) and (j)(1)(ii); and

(ii)   As required in § 101.13(j)(2) for relative claims, the identity of the reference food, the percent (or fraction) that the calories have been reduced, and quantitative information comparing the level of the nutrient in the product per labeled serving size with that of the reference food that it replaces are declared in immediate proximity to the most prominent such claim (e.g., Reduced calorie cupcakes "33 1/3% fewer calories than regular cupcakes. Calorie content has been reduced from 150 to 100 calories per serving").

(5)   A comparative claim using the term "fewer" may be used on the label or in labeling of a food, including meal type products as defined in § 101.13(1), provided that:

(i)   The food contains at least 25 percent fewer calories, with a minimum reduction of more than 40 calories per reference amount customarily consumed and per labeled serving size, then the reference food that it resembles and for which it substitutes as defined in § 101.13(j)(1)(i), (j)(1)(ii), and (j)(1)(iii); and

(ii)   As required in § 101.13(j)(2) for relative claims, the identity of the reference food, the percent (or fraction) that the calories have been reduced, and quantitative information comparing the level of the calories in the product per labeled serving size with that of the reference food that it replaces are declared in immediate proximity to the most prominent such claim (e.g., "This cheese cake contains 25 percent fewer calories than our regular cheese cake. Calorie content has been lowered from 200 to 150 calories per serving").

(c)   *Sugars content claims.*

(1)   *Use of terms such as "sugars free," "no sugars," or "zero sugars."* Consumers may reasonably be expected to regard terms that represent that the food contains no sugars or sweeteners e.g., "sugar free," or "no sugars," as indicating that a product which is low in calories or significantly reduced in calories. Consequently, except as provided in paragraph (c)(2) of this section, a food may not be labeled with such terms unless:

(i)   The food contains less than 0.5 g of sugars, as defined in § 101.9(c)(6)(ii)(A), per reference amount customarily consumed and per labeled serving size;

(ii)   The food contains no added ingredients that are sugars; and

(iii)(A)   It is labeled "low calorie" or "reduced calorie" or bears a comparative claim of special dietary usefulness labeled in compliance with paragraphs (b)(2), (b)(3), or (b)(4) of this section; or

(B)   Such term is immediately accompanied, each time it is used, by either the statement "not a reduced calorie food," "not a low calorie food," or "not for weight control."

(2)   The terms "no added sugars," "without added sugars," or "no sugars added" may be used only if:

(i)   No amount of sugars as defined in § 101.9(c)(6)(ii)(A) is added during processing or packaging;

(ii)   The product does not contain ingredients containing added sugars such as jam, jelly, and concentrated fruit juice;

(iii)   The sugars content has not been increased above the amount naturally present in the ingredients by some means such as the use of enzymes;

(iv)   The food that it resembles and for which it substitutes normally contains added sugars; and

(v)   The product bears a statement indicating that the food is not low calorie or calorie reduced (unless the food meets the requirements for a low or reduced calorie food) and directing consumers' attention to the nutrition panel for further information on sugars and calorie content.

(3)   Paragraph (c)(1) of this section shall not apply to a factual statement that a food is unsweetened or contains no added sweeteners in the case of a food that contains apparent substantial inherent sugar content, e.g., juices.

(4)   A comparative claim using the term "less" may be used on the label or in labeling of a food, including meal type products as defined in § 101.13(1), provided that:

(i)   The food contains at least 25 percent less sugars per reference amount customarily consumed and per labeled serving size than the reference food that it resembles and for which it substitutes as defined in § 101.13(j)(1)(i), (j)(1)(ii), and (j)(1)(iii); and

(ii)   As required in § 101.13(j)(2) for relative claims, the identity of the reference food, the percent (or fraction) that the sugars have been reduced, and quantitative information comparing the level of the sugars in the product per labeled serving size with that of the reference food that it replaces are declared in immediate proximity to the most prominent such claim (e.g., "These corn flakes contain 25 percent less sugars than our sugar coated corn flakes. Sugars content has been lowered from 8 g to 6 g per serving").

APPENDIX D.   PROPOSED GENERAL PRINCIPLES TO IMPLEMENT CRITERIA FOR LABELING HEALTH CLAIMS, NOV. 27, 1991

§ 101.14   *Health claims: general requirements.*

(a)   *Definitions.* For purposes of this section, the following definitions apply:

(1)   "Health claim" means any claim made on the label or in labeling of a food, including a dietary supplement, that expressly or by implication, including "third party" endorsements, written statements (e.g., a brand name including a term such as "heart"), symbols (e.g., a heart symbol), or vignettes, that characterizes the relationship of any substance to a disease or health-related condition. Implied health claims include only those statements, symbols, vignettes, or other forms of communication that a manufacturer intends, or would be likely to be understood, to assert or direct beneficial relationship between the presence or level of any substance in the food and a health or disease-related condition.

(2)   "Substance" means a component of a conventional food or of a dietary supplement of vitamins, minerals, herbs, or other nutritional substances.

(3)   "Nutritive value" means a value in sustaining human existence by such processes as promoting growth, replacing loss of essential nutrients, or providing energy.

(4)   "Dietary supplement" means a food, other than a conventional food, that supplies a component with nutritive value to supplement the diet by increasing the total dietary intake of that substance. A dietary supplement includes a food for special dietary use within the meaning of § 101.9 (a)(2) that is in conventional food form.

(5)   "Disqualifying nutrient levels" means the levels of total fat, saturated fat, cholesterol, or sodium in a food above which the food will be disqualified from making a health claim. These levels are 11.5 grams (g) of fat, 4.0 g of saturated fat, 45 milligrams (mg) of cholesterol, or 360 mg of sodium, per reference amount commonly consumed, per label serving size, and per 100 g. Any one of the levels, on a per reference amount commonly consumed, a per label serving size, or a per 100 g basis, will disqualify a food from making a health claim.

(b)   For a substance to be eligible for a health claim:

(1)   The substance must be associated with a disease or health-related condition for which the general U.S. population, or an identified U.S. population subgroup (e.g., the elderly) is at risk, or, alternatively, the petition submitted by the proponent of the claim otherwise explains the prevalence

of the disease or health-related condition in the U.S. population and the relevance of the claim in the context of the total daily diet and satisfies the other requirements of this section.

(2) If the substance is to be consumed as a component of a conventional food at decreased dietary levels, the substance must be a nutrient listed in 21 U.S.C. 343(q)(1)(C) or (D), or one that FDA has required to be included in the label or labeling under 21 U.S.C. 343(q)(2)(A); and

(3) If the substance is to be consumed at other than decreased dietary levels:

(i) The substance must be consumed as a component of a conventional food or of a dietary supplement and contribute taste, aroma, or nutritive value, or any other technical effect listed in § 170.3(o) to the food and must retain that attribute when consumed at levels that are necessary to justify a claim; and

(ii) The substance must be a food ingredient or a component of a food ingredient whose use at the levels necessary to justify a claim has been demonstrated by the proponent of the claim, to FDA's satisfaction, to be safe and lawful under the applicable food safety provisions of the act.

(c) *Validity requirements.* FDA will promulgate regulations authorizing a health claim only when it determines, based on the totality of publicly available scientific evidence (including evidence from well-designed studies conducted in a manner which is consistent with generally recognized scientific procedures and principles), that there is significant scientific agreement, among experts qualified by scientific training and experience to evaluate such claims, that the claim is supported by such evidence.

(1) It must be supported by the totality of publicly available scientific evidence (including evidence from well-designed studies conducted in a manner which is consistent with generally recognized scientific procedures and principles); and

(2) There must be significant scientific agreement among experts qualified by scientific training and experience to evaluate such claims that this support exists.

(d) *General health claim labeling requirements.* (1) When FDA determines that a health claim meets the validity requirements of paragraph (c) of this section, FDA will propose a regulation in Subpart E of this part to authorize the use of that claim. If the claim pertains to a substance not provided for in §§ 101.9 or 101.36, FDA will propose amending these regulations to include declaration of the substance.

(2) When a regulation has been established in Subpart E of this part providing for a health claim, firms may make claims based on the regulation in Subpart E of this part, provided that:

(i)   All label or labeling statements about the substance-disease relationship that is the subject of the claim are based on, and consistent with, the conclusions set forth in the summary of scientific information and model health claims provided in regulations in Subpart E of this part;

(ii)   The claim is limited to describing the value that ingestion (or reduced ingestion) of the substance, as part of a total dietary pattern, may have on a particular disease or health-related condition;

(iii)   The claim is complete, truthful, and not misleading. Where factors other than dietary intake of the substance affect the health benefit, such factors may be required to be addressed in the claim by a specific regulation in Subpart E of this part;

(iv)   All information required to be included in the claim appears in one place, in the same type size, without other intervening material: Except that the label may bear the statement "See _____ for information about the relationship between _____ and _____," with the blanks filled in with references to the location of the labeling containing the health claim, the name of the substance, and the disease or health-related condition (e.g., "See attached pamphlet for information about calcium and osteoporosis"), with the entire claim appearing on the other labeling;

(v)   The claim enables the public to comprehend the information provided and to understand the relative significance of such information in the context of a total daily diet; and

(vi)   If the claim is about the effects of consuming the substance at decreased dietary levels, the level of the substance in the food is sufficiently low to justify the claim. To meet this requirement, if a definition for use of the term "low" has been established for that substance under this part, the substance must be present at a level that meets the requirements for use of that term, unless a specific alternative level has been established for the substance in Subpart E of this part. If no definition for "low" has been established, the level of the substance must meet the level established in the regulation authorizing the claim; or

(vii)   If the claim is about the effects of consuming the substance at other than decreased dietary levels, the level of the substance in the food is sufficiently high and in an appropriate form to justify the claim. To meet this requirement, if a definition for use of the term "high" for that substance has been established under this part, the substance must be present at a level that meets the requirements for use of that term, unless a specific alternative level has been established for the substance in Subpart E of this part. If no definition for "high" has been established, the level of the substance must meet the level established in the regulation authorizing the claim.

(3)   Nutrition labeling shall be provided in the label or labeling of any food for which a health claim is made in accordance with §§ 101.9 and 101.36.

(e) *Prohibited health claims.* No expressed or implied health claim may be made on the label or in labeling for a food unless:

(1)   The claim is specifically provided for in Subpart E of this part; and

(2)   The claim conforms to all general provisions of this section as well as to all specific provisions in the appropriate section of Subpart E of this part;

(3)   None of the disqualifying levels identified in paragraph (a)(5) of this section is exceeded in the food, unless specific alternative levels have been established for the substance in Subpart E of this part; or unless FDA has permitted a claim despite the fact that a disqualifying level of a nutrient is present in the food based on a finding that such a claim will assist consumers in maintaining healthy dietary practices, and, in accordance with the regulation in Subpart E that makes such a finding, the label bears a referral statement that complies with § 101.13(h) highlighting the nutrient that exceeds the disqualifying level;

(4)   No substance, other than one for which a "disqualifying nutrient level" is established, is present at an inappropriate level as determined in specific provisions of Subpart E of this part; and

(5)   The label does not represent or purport that the food is for infants and toddlers less than 2 years of age.

(f)   The requirements of this section do not apply to:

(1)   Infant formulas subject to section 412(h) of the Federal Food, Drug, and Cosmetic Act, and

(2)   Medical foods defined by section 5(b) of the Orphan Drug Act.

(g)   *Applicability.* The requirements of this section apply to foods intended for human consumption that are offered for sale.

(6)   Subpart E consisting of § 101.70 is added to read as follows:

Subpart E—Specific Requirements for Health Claims

§ 101.70   *Petitions for health claims.*

(a)   Any interested person may petition the Food and Drug Administration (FDA) to issue a regulation regarding a health claim. The petition shall be submitted in quadruplicate. If any part of the material submitted is in a foreign language, it shall be accompanied by an accurate and complete English translation. The petition shall state the petitioner's post office address to which any correspondence required by section 403 of the Federal Food, Drug, and Cosmetic Act may be sent.

(b)   Pertinent information may be incorporated in, and will be considered as part of, a petition on the basis of specific reference to such information submitted to and retained in the files of FDA. Any reference to published information shall be accompanied by reprints, or easily readable copies of such information.

(c) If nonclinical laboratory studies are included in a petition, the petition shall include, with respect to each nonclinical study contained in the petition, either a statement that the study has been conducted in compliance with the good laboratory practice regulations as set forth in Part 58 of this chapter, or, if any such study was not conducted in compliance with such regulations, a brief statement of the reason for the noncompliance.

(d) If clinical or other human investigations are included in a petition, the petition shall include a statement that they were either conducted in compliance with the requirements for institutional review set forth in Part 56 of this chapter, or were not subject to such requirements in accordance with § 56.104 or § 56.105, and a statement that they were conducted in compliance with the requirements for informed consent set forth in Part 50 of this chapter.

(e) All data and information in a health claim petition are available for public disclosure after the notice of filing of petition is issued to the petitioner, except that clinical investigation reports, adverse reaction reports, product experience reports, consumer complaints, and other similar data and information shall only be available after deletion of:

(1) Names and any information that would identify the person using the product.

(2) Names and any information that would identify any third party involved with the report, such as a physician or hospital or other institution.

(f) Petitions for a health claim shall include the following data and be submitted in the following form:

(Date)
Name of petitioner_____
Post office address_____
Subject of the petition_____
Food and Drug Administration, Regulatory Affairs Staff (HFF-204), Office of Nutrition and Food Sciences, 200 C St. SW., Washington, DC 20204,

The undersigned, _____ submits this petition pursuant to section 403(r) (4) or 403(r)(5)(D) of the Federal Food, Drug and Cosmetic Act with respect to (statement of the substance and its health claim).

Attached hereto, in quadruplicate, and constituting a part of this petition, are the following:

A. Model health claim. One or more model health claims that represent label statements that may be used on a food label or in labeling for a food to characterize the relationship between the substance in a food to a disease or health-related condition that is justified by the summary of scientific data provided in section C of the petition. The model health claim shall include:

1. A brief capsulized statement of the relevant conclusions of the summary, and

2. A statement of how this substance helps the consumer to attain a total dietary pattern or goal associated with the health benefit that is provided.

B. Preliminary requirements. A complete explanation of how the substance conforms to the requirements of § 101.14(b). For petitions where the subject substance is a food ingredient or a component of a food ingredient, the petitioner should compile a comprehensive list of the specific ingredients that will be added to the food to supply the substance in the food bearing the health claims. For each such ingredient listed, the petitioner should state how the ingredient complies with the requirements of § 101.14(b)(3)(ii), e.g., that its use is GRAS, listed as a food additive, or authorized by a prior sanction issued by the agency, and what the basis is for the GRAS claim, the food additive status, or prior sanctioned status.

C. Summary of scientific data. The summary of scientific data provides the basis upon which authorizing a health claim can be justified as providing the health benefit. The summary must establish that, based on the totality of publicly available scientific evidence (including evidence from well designed studies conducted in a manner which is consistent with generally recognized scientific procedures and principles), there is significant scientific agreement among experts qualified by scientific training and experience to evaluate such claims, that the claim is supported by such evidence.

The summary shall state what public health benefit will derive from use of the claim as proposed. If the claim is intended for a specific group within the population, the summary shall specifically address nutritional needs of such group and shall include scientific data showing how the claim is likely to assist in meeting such needs.

The summary shall concentrate on the findings of appropriate review articles, National Institutes of Health consensus development conferences, and other appropriate resource materials. Issues addressed in the summary shall include answers to such questions as:

1. Is there an optimum level of the particular substance to be consumed beyond which no benefit would be expected?

2. Is there any level at which an adverse effect from the substance or from foods containing the substance occurs for any segment of the population?

3. Are there certain populations that must receive special consideration?

4. What other nutritional or health factors (both positive and negative) are important to consider when consuming the substance?

In addition, the summary of scientific data shall include a detailed analysis of the potential effect of the use of the proposed claim on food consumption, specifically any change due to significant alterations in eating habits and corresponding changes in nutrient intake resulting from such changes in food consumption. The latter item shall specifically address the effect on the intake of nutrients that have beneficial and negative consequences in the total diet.

If the claim is intended for a significant subpopulation within the general U.S. population, the analysis shall specifically address the dietary practices of such group, and shall include data sufficient to demonstrate that the dietary analysis is representative of such group (e.g., adolescents or the elderly).

If appropriate, the petition shall explain the prevalence of the disease or health-related condition in the U.S. population and the relevance of the claim in the context of the total daily diet.

Also, the summary shall demonstrate that the substance that is the subject of the proposed claim conforms to the definition of the term "substance" in paragraph (a)(2) of § 101.14.

D.   Analytical data that show the amount of the substance that is present in representative foods that would be candidates to bear the claim should be obtained from representative samples using methods from the Association of Official Analytical Chemists (AOAC), where available. If no AOAC method is available, the petitioner shall submit the assay method used and data establishing the validity of the method for assaying the substance in food. The validation data should include a statistical analysis of the analytical and product variability.

E.   The petition shall include the following attachments:

1.   Copies of any computer literature searches done by the petitioner (e.g., Medline).

2.   Copies of articles cited in the literature searches and other information as follows:

a.   All information relied upon for the support of the health claim, including copies of publications or other information cited in review articles and used to perform meta-analyses.

b.   All information concerning adverse consequences to any segment of the population (e.g., sensitivity to the substance).

c.   All information pertaining to the U.S. population.

F.   The petitioner is required to submit either a claim for categorical exclusion under § 25.24 of this chapter or an environmental assessment under § 25.31 of this chapter.

> Yours very truly,
> Petitioner _____
> By_____
>   (Indicate authority)

(g)   The data specified under the several lettered headings should be submitted on separate pages or sets of pages, suitably identified. If such data have already been submitted with an earlier application from the petitioner or any other final petition, the present petition may incorporate it by specific reference to the earlier petition.

(h)   The petition shall include a statement signed by the person responsible for the petition that, to the best of his/her knowledge, it is a representative and balanced submission that includes unfavorable information as well as favorable information, known to him/her to be pertinent to the evaluation of the proposed health claim.

(i)   The petition shall be signed by the petitioner or by his/her attorney or agent, or (if a corporation) by an authorized official.

(j)   *Agency action on the petition.* (1) Within 15 days of receipt of the petition, the petitioner will be notified by letter of the date on which the petition was received. Such notice will inform the petitioner that the petition is undergoing agency review and that the petitioner will subsequently be notified of the agency's decision to file for comprehensive review or deny the petition.

(2)   Within 100 days of the date of receipt of the petition, FDA will notify the petitioner by letter than the petition has either been filed for comprehensive review or denied. The agency will deny a petition without reviewing the information contained in C. *Summary of Scientific Data* if the information in B. *Preliminary Requirements* is inadequate in explaining how the substance conforms to the requirements of § 101.14(b). If the petition is denied, the notification will state the reasons therefor, including justification of the rejection of any report from an authoritative scientific body of the U.S. Government. If filed, the date of the notification letter becomes the date of filing for the purposes of this regulation. A petition that has been denied will not be made available to the public. A filed petition will be available to the public to the extent provided under paragraph (e) of this section.

(3)   Within 90 days of the date of filing, FDA will by letter of notification to the petitioner:

(i)   Deny the petition, or

(ii)   Inform the petitioner that a proposed regulation to provide for the requested use of the health claim will be published in the FEDERAL REGISTER. If the petition is denied, the notification will state the reasons therefore, including justification for the rejection of any report from an authoritative scientific body of the U.S. Government. FDA will publish the proposal to amend the regulations to provide for the requested use of the health claim in the FEDERAL REGISTER within 90 days of the date of filing. The proposal will also announce the availability of the petition for public review.

REFERENCES

1. *A Legislative History of the Food, Drug, and Cosmetic Act and Its Amendments*, Vol 6, U.S. Department of Health, Education, and Welfare, Public Health Service, Food and Drug Administration, Rockville, MD, p. 339 (1979).
2. Label statements concerning dietary properties of foods purporting to be or represented for special dietary uses, *Fed. Reg., 6*: 5921 (1941).
3. Dietary foods, *Fed. Reg., 27*: 5815 (1962).
4. Foods for special dietary uses, *Fed. Reg., 31*: 8521 (June 15, 1966).
5. Proposed statement of reasons, proposed findings of fact, proposed conclusions, and tentative order, *Fed. Reg., 42*: 37166 (1977).
6. Foods for special dietary use, *Fed. Reg., 43*: 43248 (1978).
7. Identity labeling of food in packaged form, *Fed. Reg., 42*: 14308 (1977).
8. Special dietary foods label statements, misleading statements: Reduced calorie labeling for bread, *Fed. Reg., 43*: 43261 (1978).
9. Special dietary foods label statements; withdrawal of proposed statement on reduced calorie labeling of bread, *Fed. Reg., 45*: 41652 (1980).
10. Food labeling; nutrition labeling of food: Calorie content, *Fed. Reg., 49*: 32216 (1984).
11. Nutrition labeling of food: Caloric content; correction, *Fed. Reg., 49*: 36405 (1984).
12. Nutrition Labeling and Education Act of 1990, Public Law 101-535, *21 U.S. Code 301* (1990).
13. Food labeling; general provisions; nutrition labeling; nutrient content claims; health claims; ingredient labeling; state and local requirements, and exemptions; proposed rules, *Fed. Reg., 56*: 60366 (1991).

8
Sugar Substitutes

Rosetta Newsome *Institute of Food Technologists, Chicago, Illinois*

I. INTRODUCTION

Sugar substitutes are important components of low-calorie foods. Studies with adults, as well as infants, have demonstrated that a preference for sweetness in foods is "an unlearned preference present from birth" [1]. Consumers select low-calorie foods sweetened with sugar substitutes for a variety of reasons, primarily to decrease or control calorie intake and thus body weight and to aid control of certain health/medical conditions such as diabetes and hypoglycemia. An added benefit of some sugar substitutes available in low-calorie foods is their noncariogenicity or cariostatic properties.

Sugar substitutes may be either caloric or noncaloric, depending on their metabolism in the body. High-intensity nutritive or caloric sugar substitutes do not contribute significant calories to the products they sweeten because very small quantities of the substances are required to impart sweetness. For example, aspartame provides the same number of calories as sucrose gram for gram, but because it is approximately 200 times sweeter than sucrose it may be used in very small quantities, thereby contributing negligible calories to the products it sweetens. The relative sweetness of sugar substitutes currently available or under development or regulatory review within the United States is listed in Table 1. Sweetness is a subjective measurement that is dependent on several factors, including the concentration of the sweetener, temperature, pH, type of medium used, and sensitivity of the taster [2]. Evaluation of sweetness is made on a weight basis and compared to sucrose, the usual standard [2].

The bulk of high-intensity sweetener use is concentrated in Western Europe, North America, and Japan, where there is a high level of diet consciousness and where uses go beyond use in soft drinks to use in "light foods"—one of the fastest growing segments of many food industries [3]. Of 10,301 new products introduced in 1990, 1165 were reduced-calorie, low-calorie, or "lite" products, a 21% increase compared to 1989 [4,5].

Global consumption of high-intensity sweeteners by region is shown in Table 2. In some developing countries the presence of caloric sweeteners such

Table 1 Sweetness Intensity of Sugar Substitutes

Substitute	Sweetness[a]
Currently available in the United States	
Acesulfame-K	200
Aspartame	180–220
Saccharin	300–500
Mannitol	0.5
Sorbitol	0.54–0.7
Xylitol	1
Crystalline fructose	1.2–1.8
Glycyrrhizin[b]	50–100
Thaumatin[b]	2,000–3,000
Under development or regulatory review in the United States	
Alitame	2,900
Cyclamate	30
Hydrogenated starch hydrolysates	0.7–0.9
Isomalt	0.45–0.65
Lactitol	0.4
L-sugars	<1
Maltitol	0.85–0.95
Sucralose	600

[a]The sweetness value indicated is an approximation relative to an approximate sweetness index for sucrose of 1.
[b]Approved for use in the U.S. as a flavorant and outside the U.S. as a sweetener.

Table 2 Global Consumption of High-Intensity Sweeteners, by Region[a]

Region	Year			
	1975	1980	1985	1988
Americas	1.65	2.3	3	3.8
Asia	1.5	1.9	2.5	2.75
Europe	0.75	0.9	1.11	1.2
Africa and Oceania	0.03	0.09	0.08	0.1

[a]Million tons/sugar sweetness equivalent.
Source: Ref. 6.

as sugar or starch in soft drinks is seen by health authorities as an important energy source [6]. Nevertheless, there are large segments of the populations of many developing countries where diet consciousness and health concerns make the attractiveness of diet products containing low-calorie sweeteners potentially lucrative markets [6].

Overall caloric sweetener consumption has risen in the United States (reaching nearly 135 lb per capita in 1990, up from 124 lb in 1980 and 130 lb in 1985), and low-calorie sweetener consumption has risen in a fashion complementary to that of caloric sweeteners [7]. However, it appears that high-intensity sweeteners are growing faster than the other two segments of the U.S. sweetener market—sugar and corn sweeteners [3].

The chemical properties/technical aspects, food product applications, and safety/regulatory aspects of sugar substitutes currently available or under development in the United States are reviewed in this chapter. Examples of beverages and foods that utilize sugar substitutes are given in Chapters 15 and 16.

II. SUGAR SUBSTITUTES CURRENTLY AVAILABLE IN THE UNITED STATES

A. Acesulfame-K

1. Chemical Properties and Technical Aspects

Discovered in 1967 by a scientist at Hoechst Celanese Corporation, Somerville, New Jersey, acesulfame-K is marketed under the brand names Sunette and Sweet One. A derivative of acetoacetic acid, it is the potassium salt of 6-methyl-1,2,3-oxathiazine-4(3H)-one-2,2-dioxide.

Acesulfame-K is approximately 200 times sweeter than a 3–4% solution of sucrose. The sweetness intensity of acesulfame-K is inversely related to its concentration [8]. The sweet taste of acesulfame-K is perceived quickly but often fades rapidly [9,10]. The sweetener does not exhibit an aftertaste except at elevated concentrations [11]. Acesulfame-K, which is freely soluble in water and is stable in aqueous solutions in the pH range of 3–7, does not decompose at temperatures and conditions normally encountered in food manufacture or in storage of the raw material, thus allowing its use in cooked, baked, and other heat-processed foods [12,13]. Acesulfame-K is synergistic with other sweeteners, and when used in combination with other sweeteners, it reduces the undesirable effects of other sweeteners and balances the overall sweetener profile [14].

Acesulfame-K is not metabolized and is thus noncaloric [10]. The majority of the sweetener is excreted by the kidneys with no tissue accumulation [15]. In metabolism studies, no indication of the formation of metabolites was found in the excreta of rats, dogs, pigs, and humans [8].

2. Applications

Mixtures of acesulfame-K with sugar alcohols, in particular, have a full and well-balanced sweetness particularly suitable for products, such as sugarless confectionery, that require a bulking agent [9]. Acesulfame-K was approved in the United States in July 1988 for use in table-top sweetener formulations, gums, and dry bases for imitation dairy products, gelatins, and beverages [16]. Petitions for expanded use in the United States (in hard and soft candies, baked goods, baking mixes, and soft drinks, including nonalcoholic beverages and beverage bases, yogurt and yogurt-type products, frozen and refrigerated desserts, and syrups and toppings) are pending. Several other food applications of acesulfame-K, such as pickles, marinated fish, and delicatessen products, exist in other countries that have approved the sweetener [12].

3. Safety and Regulatory Aspects

The U.S. Food and Drug Administration allocated an Acceptable Daily Intake (ADI) of 15 mg/kg body weight [16]. ADI has been defined as "an estimate of the amount of the food additive, expressed on a body weight basis that can be ingested daily over a lifetime without appreciable health risk" [17]. Several other countries approved the use of acesulfame-K. Petitions for approval are pending in Canada and the European Community [3].

The sweetener has been subjected to extensive research, including pharmacological, mutagenicity, reproductive, and acute, subchronic, and chronic toxicity studies, many of which involved human subjects. Reviews of these studies are available [8,9]. Except for cecal enlargement observed in rats fed 3% or more of the diet, which was attributed to the presence of the osmotically active potassium salt [8], no untoward effects were observed.

In 1982, the Food Additives and Contaminants Committee in Great Britain accepted acesulfame-K for use in food [18]. The Joint Expert Committee on Food Additives of the World Health Organization (WHO) and the Food and Agriculture Organization (FAO) of the United Nations concluded in 1983 that acesulfame-K does not exhibit mutagenic, carcinogenic, or toxicological effects and set an ADI of 0-9 mg/kg body weight [19]. Evaluation of additional data made available since 1983 resulted in a revision of the ADI to 0-15 mg/kg [20]. The committee also reviewed extensive toxicological studies on the breakdown products, acetoacetamide and acetoacetamide-N-sulfonic acid, and concluded that these compounds have a low toxicity and are not mutagenic [20]. The Scientific Committee for Foods of the EC accepted acesulfame K for use in foods and beverages and allocated an ADI of 0-9 mg/kg, on the basis of lack of dose-related increases in specific tumors and treatment-related pathological changes of significance [21].

B. Aspartame

1. Chemical Properties and Technical Aspects

Aspartame is a dipeptide consisting of aspartic acid and phenylalanine (N-L-α-aspartyl-L-phenylalanine-1-methyl ester). It is commonly known in the United States by the trade name NutraSweet™ (The NutraSweet Co., Mount Prospect, IL). Because aspartame contains phenylalanine, which must be controlled in the diets of individuals with the rare disease phenylketonuria (PKU), products that contain aspartame must be labeled: "Phenylketonurics: contains phenylalanine."

Aspartame was discovered in 1965 by a scientist at G.D. Searle and Co. (Skokie, IL). It is a nutritive sweetener 180-220 times sweeter than sucrose and metabolized similarly to peptides. Because aspartame is a high-intensity sweetener, permitting use of very small amounts to sweeten foods, it does not provide significant calories to the products it sweetens.

Aspartame is slightly soluble in water (dependent upon temperature and pH) and is susceptible to hydrolysis to aspartylphenylalanine and methanol and cyclization to diketopiperazine (DKP) under certain conditions of moisture, extreme temperature, and pH [22], resulting in loss of sweetness, but without development of off-flavors [23]. Aspartame can withstand high-temperature, short-time or ultra-high-temperature processing with minimal degradation, but the nonprotected form currently available is susceptible to temperatures encountered in baking [22]. Aspartame's susceptibility to degradation at elevated temperatures is greater at neutral pH than at acidic pH. A newly developed heat-protected version is encapsulated with a special polymer coating to protect it—in a time/temperature release manner—against moisture exposure during heat treatment [24]. Approval by FDA will allow use of aspartame in areas such as baked goods, baking mixes, and possibly fried products and certain confections once thought not to be feasible [22].

Aspartame has a taste similar to sugar, without a bitter aftertaste [25–29]. In addition to its intense sweetness, aspartame also has a flavor-enhancing property for certain food and beverage flavors, particularly acid fruit flavors [22].

2. Applications

Aspartame is currently approved for use as a free-flowing sugar substitute or in tablet form for table-top use. Food applications include carbonated beverages, powdered soft drinks and beverages, ready-to-eat cereal, dry-mix gelatins, puddings, and fillings, refrigerated gelatins, fruit spreads, refrigerated or frozen fruit/juice drinks, wine coolers, aseptic juice/fruit drinks, frozen or refrigerated fruit toppings, and refrigerated, frozen, and fermented dairy products [22]. Other applications recently approved include malt beverages of less than 7% ethanol by volume and containing fruit juice, hot and instant breakfast cereals, and refrigerated ready-to-serve gelatins, puddings and fillings [126]. Petitions for use in hard candy, confections and soft candy, baked goods and baking mixes, and nonrefrigerated and noncarbonated beverages are pending.

3. Safety and Regulatory Aspects

Aspartame has been approved for use in more than 80 countries, including the United States, and is available in more than 1700 products worldwide [6]. Before its approval in the United States, extensive metabolic, pharmacological, toxicological, and clinical studies were done in animals and in normal humans as well as certain subpopulations such as heterozygous phenylketonurics, diabetics, obese individuals, and lactating females [30]. Since aspartame's approval, research has continued; consumption data are monitored and evaluation of anecdotal reports is conducted. Detailed reviews of the safety issues and research conducted on aspartame, its constituents, and its metabolites—methanol and diketopiperazine—are available [22,31–33].

Aspartame has been reviewed and approved for use by the Joint Expert Committee on Food Additives of the FAO/WHO and the Scientific Committee for Foods of the European Community (EC) [31].

Aspartame is metabolized in the gastrointestinal tract to aspartic acid, phenylalanine, and methanol. Studies indicate that the sweetener does not exert pharmacological effects at doses substantially above those possible for human consumption [22,31]. Infants as young as one year of age and children metabolize aspartame at rates similar to those of adults [32]. Acute, chronic, and developmental toxicological studies indicate that the sweetener is safe for use by PKU heterozygotes and pregnant females [31]. Giving its approval in 1981, the FDA Commissioner announced, after evaluating all of the relevant data regarding aspartame, that the sweetener is safe for the general population, including pregnant women and children [30]. FDA established an ADI of 50 mg/kg body weight—a sweetness equivalent of approximately 600 g (1.3 lb) of sucrose consumed daily by a 60-kg person [34].

Concern has been expressed by some individuals that because of the substantial number and variety of aspartame-containing products available, individuals—particularly children, because of their lower body weights— might consume quantities of the sweetener above the ADI. When aspartame was approved, FDA noted that if the sweetener replaced all the sucrose in our diets, consumption would be approximately 8.3 mg/kg/day [30]. Aspartame has remained considerably below 10 mg/kg at the 90th percentile of consumption in adults and children [31]. Upon evaluation of the adverse reactions reported as part of the postmarketing surveillance process, the Centers for Disease Control (CDC) and the FDA reported that there were no symptoms that were clearly related to aspartame consumption that would suggest a public health hazard [35-37].

C. Saccharin

1. Chemical Properties and Technical Aspects

The name for this sugar substitute is derived from *saccharum*, Latin for sugar [2]. Discovered by chemists in 1879, saccharin is a cyclized derivative of *ortho*-sulfamoylbenzoic acid. It is only slightly soluble in water, is 300-500 times as sweet as sucrose, and is stable under many conditions encountered in food preparation (up to 125 °C, pH 3.3-8.0) [38]. Saccharin is commercially available in three forms: as the sodium salt (the most commonly used form), as the calcium salt, and in the acid form [39]. In aqueous solutions, saccharin has a slighly bitter aftertaste, detectable by about 25% of the population [40].

Saccharin is not metabolized. It is excreted unchanged, predominantly in the urine [41], and thus does not provide any calories to the products it sweetens.

2. Applications

Saccharin is used in table-top sweeteners in tablet, powder, and liquid form and is used in soft drinks, fruit juice drinks, other beverages and beverage bases or mixes, processed fruits, chewing gum, confections, gelatin desserts, juices, jams, toppings, sauces, and dressings [39]. Prior to the U.S. ban of cyclamate in 1969, saccharin was used in combination with cyclamate. Now it is frequently used in combination with aspartame [13] in fountain beverage bases or mixes, where it provides thermal stability and enhances shelf life.

Saccharin works well in combination with other sweeteners and is synergistic with many of them [42]. The continued use of saccharin is due at least in part to its longer shelf life, lower price, and greater thermal stability than aspartame [13]. At its current low cost (approximately $3.00/lb), saccharin is by far the least costly of the three high-intensity sweeteners [39]. About a penny's worth of saccharin has the sweetening power of 1 pound of sugar [3].

The sole U.S. producer of saccharin is PMC Specialties Group (Cincinnati, OH), which markets saccharin under the trade name Syncal™. This trade name, however, is not used at the retail level to the same extent as is NutraSweet [13].

3. Safety and Regulatory Aspects

Saccharin has been in use in the United States since the early 1900s and was originally classified in 1958 as Generally Recognized as Safe (GRAS). However, research conducted by the Canadian Health Protection Branch, FDA, and the Wisconsin Alumni Research Foundation showed evidence of bladder cancer in rats at levels of 5 and 7.5% of the diet [43–45]. Consequently, saccharin was removed from the GRAS list in 1972, and a ban was proposed in 1977 in the United States. Saccharin was also banned from general use in Canada in 1979. However, the U.S. Congress passed the Saccharin Study and Labeling Act in 1977, declaring a moratorium on the ban in the United States until further research on its safety was completed.

The act and its extensions require more toxicological research and a warning label on all saccharin-containing foods stating, "Use of this product may be hazardous to your health. This product contains saccharin which has been determined to cause cancer in laboratory animals." Saccharin's continued use in the United States is permitted under an interim food additive regulation (21 CFR 180.37) in special dietary foods.

Recent toxicological studies in animals indicate that saccharin indeed increases the incidence of bladder tumors, but only under certain specific conditions (i.e., when fed to male rats, from birth, at dietary concentrations, equal to or greater than 3%—levels that produce profound biochemical and physiological changes in the urinary and gastrointestinal tracts) [45]. The relevance to humans of this effect (a dose equivalent to a human intake of 450 liters of saccharin-sweetened beverage every day of life from birth) is questionable [45].

Unlike typical carcinogens, which interact with DNA, sodium saccharin is not genotoxic but leads to an increase in cell proliferation of the urothelium, the only target tissue, and it appears that the effect of saccharin is modified by the salt form in which it is administered [46]. Dose-response, tumor-promoting activity by sodium saccharin but not by acid saccharin and similar tumor-promoting activity by sodium chloride and sodium ascorbate were observed [47]. Furthermore, the bladder tumor–promoting activity of sodium saccharin was completely eliminated upon lowering the rats' elevated urinary pH by coadministration of a buffering agent [47]. The research suggests that the human bladder is more likely to be resistant to the effects of saccharin than the rat's and that if humans are susceptible at all, an extremely high threshold level is likely to exist [46].

Epidemiological studies (some of which were very large and which included expected heavy users of saccharin and expected neonatal exposure) have failed to show a definitive link between saccharin and bladder cancer (or any other cancers) in humans. The safe use of saccharin has been affirmed by the American Medical Association [48], the American Dietetic Association [49], and the American Diabetes Association [50], and its continued use has been approved by the Joint FAO/WHO Expert Committee on Food Additives [51] and the EC's Scientific Committee for Food [52].

D. Sugar Alcohols

The chemical properties and technical aspects such as production of the sugar alcohols—mannitol, sorbitol, and xylitol—are discussed in Chapter 11. The sucrose sweetness equivalence, dietary importance, safety, and regulatory aspects of these sweeteners are discussed here.

1. Mannitol

a. Dietary Importance. Mannitol is a naturally occurring sweetener in fruits and certain plants. It is half as sweet as sucrose. Mannitol is converted to fructose after absorption. It is not metabolized as well as sorbitol and provides only 2 kcal/g [53].

b. Safety and Regulatory Aspects. Approved for use in a number of other countries, mannitol has interim food additive status in the United States (21 CFR 180.25) [54] and may be used at levels not to exceed the following: pressed mints (98%), hard candies (5%), cough drops (5%), chewing gum (31%), soft candies (40%), confections and frostings (8%), nonstandardized jams and jellies (15%), and others (2.5%) [53]. Because mannitol has a laxative effect when large amounts are consumed, FDA requires that foods whose "reasonably foreseeable consumption" may result in a daily ingestion of 20 g of mannitol bear the label statement, "Excess consumption may have a laxative effect" (CFR 21.180. 25(e)). Because of this low laxative threshold, mannitol is less desirable in the diabetic diet than sorbitol [53].

2. Sorbitol

a. Dietary Importance. Sorbitol has been used as a sweetening agent in the diets of diabetics since the first report, in the late 1920s, that moderate amounts of sorbitol taken by normal or diabetic subjects caused only a slight rise in blood sugar concentration [53]. The polyalcohol, which occurs naturally in a variety of fruits, is absorbed slowly in the intestine, is converted in the liver to fructose, and is believed to be metabolized independently of insulin. For this reason, sorbitol is considered to be valuable in foods designed for consumption by diabetics and others requiring special diets. Sorbitol provides the same number of calories per gram as sucrose but is only 0.54–0.7 times as sweet. It is generally considered to be noncariogenic, but some evidence has been presented which indicates that the polyalcohol is not necessarily inert in caries formation [55].

b. Safety and Regulatory Aspects. Permitted for use in a number of countries, sorbitol is considered Generally Recognized as Safe (GRAS) in the United States [56] and may be used in foods at levels which do not exceed good manufacturing practices (GMPs). Current GMPs (21 CFR 184.1835) permit the use of sorbitol up to the following maximum levels: hard candy and cough drops (99%), chewing gum (75%), soft candy (98%), nonstandardized jams and jellies (30%), baked goods and baking mixes (30%), frozen dairy desserts and mixes (17%), and other foods (12%) [53].

Sorbitol has a laxative and diuretic effect when more than 25–80 g/day is consumed [57–59], although as little as 5 g may cause gastrointestinal distress [60]. This laxative effect may be particularly encountered among small children who swallow dietetic chewing gum [33]. FDA requires that food whose "reasonably foreseeable consumption" may result in a daily ingestion of 50 g of sorbitol bear the following label statement, "Excess consumption may have a laxative effect" (CFR 21.184.1835 (e)).

3. Xylitol

a. Dietary Importance. Xylitol, a naturally occurring sweetener in a variety of fruits and vegetables, has been used in foods since the 1960s [61]. It is metabolized either directly, mainly in the liver, or indirectly, via fermentation by intestinal bacteria independently of insulin [61,62]. The rise in blood glucose and the insulin response are lower after xylitol ingestion than after ingestion of sucrose or glucose [63–65]. Moreover, a limited number of short-term clinical trials in the dietary management of diabetes suggest that xylitol as a substitute for rapidly absorbed simple carbohydrate sweeteners may, in proper dosage, be of value in prevention of postprandial fluctuations of blood glucose levels [63].

Xylitol is as sweet as sucrose and may be used in comparable amounts in foods, thus providing sugar substitution with bulk. Although xylitol is fermentable by one type of bacteria comprising dental plaque [55], numerous studies indicate that it is not fermented by caries-causing bacteria [66–69] and is cariostatic [70–74]. Xylitol may be safely used in foods for special dietary uses, provided the amount used is not greater than that required to produce its intended effect (CFR 172.395).

b. Safety and Regulatory Aspects. In October 1971, FDA proposed to revoke xylitol's approval for use, but no further action has been taken. An ad hoc Expert Panel of the Federation of American Societies for Experimental Biology reviewed the experimental protocols and results of chronic and short-term feeding studies of xylitol (and other alcohols) in response to a series of questions posed by FDA on certain effects that were observed in the studies [75]. The effects in question were adrenal hyperplasia and pheochromocytoma lesions observed in rats fed sugar alcohols, urinary bladder hyperplasia in mice fed xylitol, and hepatic responses in dogs fed xylitol.

The Expert Panel concluded that the effects in question resulted from high dietary levels of the sugar alcohols in the studied species and strains, which, unlike humans, exhibit high spontaneous incidences of lesions (rats) and greater insulin secretory responses (dogs) [75]. Subsequent research has confirmed that the adverse effects questioned by FDA lack relevance to humans because of the species specificity of the underlying mechanisms [76, 77]. Results of studies of human tolerance to high oral doses of xylitol, with both healthy and diabetic subjects, show good tolerance to intakes up to 200 g/day [61]. The only side effect occasionally noted was transient laxation and gastrointestinal discomfort [78–80].

Xylitol is approved for use in foods in many countries [81]. The Joint FAO/WHO Expert Committee on Food Additives has allocated an ADI of "not specified" (the most favorable category possible) for xylitol [82]. The EC's Scientific Committee for Food also determined xylitol "acceptable" for dietary uses [81].

E. Other Sugar Substitutes

Other sweet substances described below include crystalline fructose, a sugar that, because it is sweeter than sucrose, can play a role in low-calorie foods, and glycyrrhizin and thaumatin, two high-intensity sweeteners used in the United States as flavorants and in countries outside the United States as sweeteners.

1. Crystalline Fructose

Although crystalline fructose is a sugar, its higher sweetening power and slower metabolism in the human body compared to other sugars enables it to play a role in low-calorie or dietetic foods and beverages. Crystalline fructose has been commercially available in the United States since 1975. It is produced from liquid dextrose by enzymatic isomerization. This sweetener is 1.2–1.8 times or up to 70% sweeter than sugar, depending on its anomeric state, temperature, pH, and solution concentration [83]. It provides 3.7 kcal/g, but because of its sweetness, it can be used at lower levels than other sugars. The sweetener is also hygroscopic and functions as a humectant, which is advantageous in moisture retention in products such as breads and cakes.

Crystalline fructose may be successfully applied in dietetic foods such as cake mixes, candies, and beverages, as well as in gelatins and puddings, gums, table-top sweeteners, frozen desserts, energy drinks, dietary meal replacers, powdered beverage bases, and chocolate and carob candies. It is synergistic with saccharin and aspartame and may provide additional specific advantages when used in conjunction with these sweeteners. A more detailed review of this sweetener is provided by Osberger [83].

2. Glycyrrhizin

Glycyrrhizin is a noncaloric extract of licorice root (*Glycyrrhiza*) that is 50–100 times sweeter than sucrose [84]. The compound has a slow onset of sweetness and, depending on the exact commerical form, may exhibit a prolonged licorice aftertaste. Ammoniated glycyrrhizin, a form that exhibits increased solubility and stability, is GRAS and approved in the United States for use as a flavor and flavor enhancer. It may be used in some confectionery products, baked goods, dairy products, soups, salad dressings, meats and meat seasonings, desserts, and beverages [84]. Glycyrrhizin is widely used in Japan as a sweetener in foods and beverages and as a flavorant in tobacco products and cosmetics [84].

3. Thaumatin

Thaumatin is a protein extract of the fruit of the West African plant *Thaumatococcus daniellii*. It is marketed under the trade name Talin™ by Tate and Lyle Specialty Products (Reading, England). The extract exhibits a sweetness level 2000–3000 times higher than that of sucrose but has a delayed sweetness development and a licorice aftertaste [85]. Thaumatin is approved for use in Japan, Australia, and the United Kingdom and is undergoing review in a number of other countries [85]. Thaumatin is considered GRAS in the United States and is approved for use as a flavor adjunct in chewing gum. Applications in other countries include beverages and desserts. Applications requiring a significant heat treatment at neutral pH, such as baked goods, are precluded because of its instability to heat above pH 6.0. [85]

III. SUGAR SUBSTITUTES UNDER DEVELOPMENT OR REGULATORY REVIEW IN THE UNITED STATES

A. Alitame

1. Chemical Properties and Technical Aspects

Developed by Pfizer, Inc. (Groton, CT), alitame is a dipeptide composed of L-aspartic acid, D-alanine, and the amide 2,2,4,4-tetra-methylthienanyl amine. Alitame is approximately 2900 times sweeter than sucrose at sweetness levels of 2–3% sucrose [86]. This high potency enables use at very low levels, probably in the 20–200 ppm range [13].

Alitame has a clean taste similar to that of sucrose, with no unpleasant bitter or metallic aftertaste. The sweetness of alitame develops rapidly in the mouth and lingers slightly, in a manner similar to that of aspartame [87]. Alitame is readily water soluble, stable in solution over a broad pH range, and heat stable. Alitame and structurally related peptide sweeteners have been patented [88].

The majority (77–96%) of alitame is metabolized to aspartic acid and a mixture of metabolites (alanine amide fragments, sulfoxide isomers, and sulfone). The aspartic acid then undergoes normal amino acid metabolism, resulting in a caloric contribution of 1.4 kcal/g; the metabolites are excreted in the urine; and the remainder of the alitame is excreted unchanged in the feces [87].

2. Applications

The sweetener's heat stability would permit its potential use in baked goods and baking mixes, hard and soft candies, and heat-pasteurized foods [87]. Pfizer petitioned FDA in 1986 for use of alitame in 16 categories of food [86,89]; baked goods and baking mixes (restricted to fruit; custard- and pudding-filled pies; cakes; cookies, and similar baked products); presweetened, ready-to-eat breakfast cereals; milk products (restricted to flavored milk- or dairy-based beverages and mixes for their preparation, yogurt, and dietetic milk products); frozen desserts and mixes; fruit and water ices and mixes; fruit drinks, ades, and mixes, including diluted juice beverages and concentrates (frozen and nonfrozen) for dilute juice beverages; confections and frostings; jams, jellies, preserves, sweet spreads; sweet sauces, toppings and mixes; gelatins, puddings, custards, fillings, and mixes; beverages, nonalcoholic beverage mixes; dairy product analogs (restricted to toppings and topping mixes); sugar substitutes; sweetened coffee and tea beverages, including mixes and concentrates; candy (including soft and hard candies and cough drops); and chewing gum [87].

Pfizer has also sought approval for use of alitame in the United Kingdom, the Netherlands, France, Switzerland, Sweden, Australia, and Canada. Approval has also been requested from the EC's Scientific Committee for Food and the Joint FAO/WHO Expert Committee on Food Additives.

3. Safety and Regulatory Aspects

A number of studies were conducted in animals and humans to establish alitame's safety prior to petition for approval. The research includes toxicology, teratology, reproductive, and oncogenicity studies in rats, mice, rabbits, dogs, and humans. The data indicate that the sweetener has an extremely low order of toxicity and a no-observed-effect level (NOEL) above 100 mg/kg; this is more than 300 times the estimated mean chronic human exposure (assuming that alitame serves as the only sweetener in all food categories) [87]. Moreover, no evidence of carcinogenicity, embryotoxicity, teratogenicity, genotoxicity, or negative effects on reproductive or physiological function were observed [87].

At levels above the NOEL, alitame resulted in a dose-related increase in liver weight. This was attributed to the induction of hepatic microsomal metabolizing enzymes—a common adaptive response of the liver to xenobiotics—and was not observed in the human studies at doses of 12 and 18 liters of alitame-sweetened beverage consumed per day by a 60-kg individual [88].

B. Cyclamate

1. Chemical Properties and Technical Aspects

Cyclamate was discovered in 1937 and was first marketed as a dietetic aid by Abbott Laboratories (Abbott Park, IL) in the early 1950s. Produced and marketed in three forms—cyclamic acid, calcium cyclamate, and sodium cyclamate—cyclamate is currently available in more than 50 countries [90].

Cyclamate is heat stable, exhibits good shelf life in solution, an ability to enhance some flavors, to mask the bitterness of saccharin, and to enhance the sweetness intensity of other sweeteners [90]. It is approximately 30 times sweeter than sucrose.

Cyclamate, which is not metabolized by the majority of consumers, is noncaloric. Only some individuals can metabolize cyclamate (60% of which is available for conversion) to cyclohexylamine, which is formed in the large intestine by gut microflora [91]. Approximately 89% of 363 individuals studied converted de minimis amounts (less than 1% of the ingested dose) of cyclamate, and the average conversion rate for all subjects was approximately 2.1% of the dose [92].

2. Applications

During the 1960s, cyclamate was widely used, primarily blended with saccharin, in beverages and other low-calorie foods and chewing gum. It was also extensively used as a table-top sweetener. Cyclamate is used in numerous food and beverage products and as a table-top sweetener in other countries [90].

3. Safety and Regulatory Aspects

Cyclamate was classified as GRAS until October 1969, when evidence from a rat study [93] of a cyclamate/saccharin mixture (2500 mg/kg/day throughout the lifetime) implicated an association with bladder tumors. However, both calcification and parasites were observed in the test animals, and six of the nine reported tumors occurred in rats with consecutive numbering, a highly improbable event, suggesting that the tumors were caused by something other than the treatment [91]. FDA then removed cyclamate from the GRAS list for foods, beverages, and pharmaceuticals [94]. In Canada, its use was restricted to table-top sweeteners, but it was approved again in 1978 for use in pharmaceuticals [33].

FDA is currently considering a petition submitted in 1982 by the Calorie Control Council and Abbott Laboratories following availability of additional scientific evidence. The new petition noted, among other items, that new scientific evidence confirmed the safety of cyclamate and assisted in determining safe consumption levels, that the Joint FAO/WHO Expert Committee on Food Additives had consistently approved cyclamate, and that the sweetener was available in more than 40 countries [127].

FDA's Cancer Assessment Committee reviewed cyclamate and issued a report in 1984 concluding that the "collective weight of many experiments . . . indicates that cyclamate is not carcinogenic" [95]. In 1985, the National Academy of Sciences reported that "the totality of the evidence from studies in animals does not indicate that cyclamate or its major metabolite cyclohexylamine is carcinogenic by itself" [96]. The NAS report, however, suggested that cyclamate might be a promoter; FDA then contracted with the MITRE Corporation to study this possibility. In 1987, the corporation reported on its assessment of the relevance of direct bladder exposure studies to the estimation of human carcinogenic risk and concluded that cyclamate promotion studies are unsuitable for predicting human carcinogenic risk [97].

The short-term, acute, subchronic, and chronic studies of cyclamate and cyclohexylamine in animals and the extensive data on pharmacokinetics and metabolism in humans and animals, combined with epidemiological evidence, support the safety of cyclamate for human use [91].

C. Hydrogenated Starch Hydrolysates

1. Chemical Properties and Technical Aspects

Hydrogenated starch hydrolysates (HSHs), first developed by the Swedish company Lyckeby in the 1960s, are produced by enzymatic hydrolysis of starch, resulting in syrups of varying proportions of oligosaccharides [98]. In the United States, two types of HSHs are available [98]: Lycasin™, manufactured and marketed by Roquette Corp. (Gurnee, IL) and Hystar™, manufactured and marketed by Lonza Inc. (Fairlawn, NJ). Lycasin consists of 52% maltitol, 18% maltotriitol, 6% sorbitol, and other polyols. A number of Hystar HSHs are available. Composition of these HSHs includes 8–60% maltitol, 7–15% sorbitol, 10–12% maltotriitol, and 22–68% other polyols. HSHs exhibit 0.7–0.9 times the sweetness of sucrose [2].

HSHs are metabolized to glucose, maltitol, and sorbitol. The more recently developed and improved version of HSHs, Lycasin 80/55, is noncariogenic and "safe for teeth," although it is slightly fermentable [98–101]. The noncariogenicity of Hystar HSHs, however, has not been clearly established.

HSHs are not particularly suitable for the diabetic because they are metabolized to glucose and sorbitol [98], with proportionally more glucose released than sorbitol [102]. For the same reason, HSHs are considered to be caloric, contributing approximately 4 kcal/g [98].

Lycasin and Hystar both exhibit laxation, because of the presence of sorbitol. However, estimates of potential average daily consumption are far below the level expected to cause laxation [98]. The laxative effect of Hystar HSHs varies depending on the levels of sorbitol and hydrogenated oligosaccharides. An acceptable range of consumption for Hystar was determined to be 50–100 g/day [98].

2. Applications

HSHs can directly substitute for sugar and corn syrup in many applications such as caramels, gummy bears and nougats, taffy, chewing gum, hard-boiled candy, and pan-coated candy. They cannot be easily substituted for sugar in chocolates or pressed tablets where their water content would pose problems [98]. HSHs can also be used to partially replace sugar or corn syrup in baked goods [98]. In applications where sweetness profiles equal to that of sucrose are required, addition of high-intensity sweeteners is necessary [98].

3. Safety and Regulatory Aspects

A GRAS affirmation petition seeking approval for use of Lycasin in candies and confections was submitted by the Roquette Corp. and accepted for filing by FDA in 1983 [98]. A similar petition seeking approval for use of Hystar was submitted in 1985.

The GRAS affirmation petition for Lycasin indicated that none of the acute, subacute, chronic and subchronic, carcinogenic, mutagenic and teratogenic studies of HSH have shown any evidence of adverse effects [98].

The Joint FAO/WHO Expert Committee on Food Additives has assigned an ADI of "not specified" [103]. Lycasin is approved for use in 12 countries, including France, Japan, the United Kingdom, and the Netherlands. A petition for approval has been filed in three other countries as well as in the United States [98].

D. Isomalt

1. Chemical Properties and Technical Aspects

Isomalt, which consists of α-D-glycopyranosyl-1, 6-D-sorbitol, and α-D-glucopyranosyl-1, 1-D-mannitol, and 5% water, has 0.45–0.65% the sweetness of sucrose. The sweetness is similar to that of sucrose and is without any undesirable aftertaste. Isomalt is manufactured by the enzymatic transglucosidation of α-D-glucopyranosyl $(1\rightarrow2)$-D-fructofuranoside (sucrose, saccharose) into α-D-glucopyranosyl $(1\rightarrow6)$ fructose (isomaltulose, Palatinose® [104,105]. The sweetener is manufactured by Palatinit SuBungsmittel GmbH (Mannheim, Germany) and is sold under the tradename Palatinit™. Isomalt is synergistic with other sugar alcohols and intense sweeteners [104]. A sweetening power comparable to that of sucrose can be obtained with a mixture of 90% isomalt and 10% other sugar alcohols [104].

The $1\rightarrow6$ glycosidic bond is very stable under acidic or alkaline conditions and is resistant to enzymatic hydrolysis. As a result, isomalt does not readily provide a substrate for most bacteria and is thus noncariogenic [104]. Isomalt is only partially hydrolyzed [104] and absorbed in the small intestine [106]. A caloric value of 2 kcal/g has been adopted by various government agencies that regulate the caloric value of specific food substances in countries such as Switzerland, France, Austria, Luxembourg, and Australia [104]. Clinical trials indicate that the sweetener is easily tolerated by diabetics because its ingestion results in insignificant changes in serum glucose and insulin levels [106,107].

2. Applications

Isomalt can substitute for sucrose in many applications [106]. The sweetener is being used in Europe in a wide variety of confectionery products such as chocolates, caramels, hard candy, tablets, pan-coated products, and chewing gum [106]. Isomalt could also be successfully applied in baked goods; breakfast cereals; fillings, frostings, and icings; frozen dairy desserts; fruit and water ices; jams, jellies, and fruit; puddings and gelatin desserts; sauces; snack foods; spreads; and table-top sweeteners [104].

3. Safety and Regulatory Aspects

The Joint FAO/WHO Expert Committee on Food Additives has reviewed the available chronic and embryotoxicological studies and assigned an ADI of "not specified" [108]. Approval for use of isomalt has been obtained in most European countries and a number of countries in the Far East and Australia, and petitions for approval are pending in other countries in the Far East, New Zealand, and the United States. The GRAS affirmation petition in the United States was submitted in September 1986 and was accepted for filing in October 1990 [104].

E. Lactitol

1. Chemical Properties and Technical Aspects

Lactitol (4,0-(β-D-galactopyranosyl)-D-glucitol) is a bulk sweetener marketed under the trade name Lacty® by Purac, Inc., The Netherlands. A detailed review of lactitol is available [109]. It is produced by hydrogenation of lactose. In most applications, it has a sweetness level 0.4 times that of sucrose. It has a clean sweet taste without an undesirable aftertaste.

Lactitol exhibits sufficient solubility not to cause inconveniences during processing. The sweetener has a molecular weight almost identical to that of sucrose and therefore exhibits a similar water activity and freezing-point depression in ice cream. Because of the absence of a carbonyl group, lactitol is chemically more stable than lactose [109]. Its stability in the presence of alkali is much higher, and its stability in acid is similar to that of lactose [109]. Lactitol also exhibits excellent storage stability.

Lactitol is not metabolized as a carbohydrate because it is not hydrolyzed or absorbed in the intestine. However, it is fermented by bacteria in the intestine and converted into biomass, organic acids, carbon dioxide, and hydrogen, resulting in a caloric value of 2 kcal/g [109]. Because lactitol does not increase blood glucose or insulin levels, it is suitable for use by diabetics [109]. Lactitol is slowly converted to lactic acid by tooth plaque bacteria and thus does not cause dental caries [109].

2. Applications

Lactitol could play a role in any application in which carbohydrates are used. When used for its bulking properties, it may be substituted on an equal-weight basis; but when used for its sweetness only, substitution at a level of 2.5 times that of the replaced sweetener may be required [109]. Lactitol has applications in baked goods, chocolates, confectionery products (in combination with other sweeteners), ice cream, preserves, and chewing gum [109].

3. Safety and Regulatory Issues

Required studies for use as a food additive have been conducted; these include long-term feeding studies at high dietary levels for 2½ years in rats and 2 years in mice [109]. No deleterious effects at levels of up to 10% of the diet were observed. The Joint FAO/WHO Expert Committee on Food Additives approved lactitol in 1983 and set an ADI of "not specified" [110]. The EC's Scientific Committee on Food evaluated lactitol and concluded that it was a safe product [111]. The sweetener has been approved for use in a number of countries, including France, Japan, the Netherlands, and the United Kingdom. Approval is expected in Canada during 1991 and in all EC countries after 1992 [109]. Applications for approval are pending in many other countries, including the United States.

F. L-Sugars

1. Chemical Properties and Technical Aspects

L-sugars are left-handed sugars with "levo" configurations instead of their asymmetric "dextro" or right-handed counterparts (D-hexoses). Biospherics, Inc. (Beltsville, MD) has patented 10 L-sugars under the name of Lev-O-Cal™ for use in low-calorie foods, beverages, and drugs. Lev-O-Cal is produced by a variety of proprietary processes, which are the subject of a number of patent applications [112].

The L-sugars are identical in physical and chemical properties to their "dextro" counterparts. Unlike the high-intensity sugar substitutes currently available in the United States, L-sugars brown upon baking. Although the taste profiles of L-sugars are similar to those of D-hexoses, their sweetness intensity is somewhat less than that of sucrose. Depending on product sweetness requirements, L-sugars may be used either alone or in conjunction with intense sweeteners [112]. L-sugars provide the same bulk and crystallinity as their dextro counterparts. Because of their levo configuration, however, L-sugars are expected to be nonmetabolizable and thus noncaloric [112].

2. Applications

The initial target markets for Lev-O-Cal include confectionery products, baked goods, heat-processed foods, frozen desserts, ice cream, and gum [112].

3. Safety and Regulatory Aspects

The U.S. patent for Lev-O-Cal was issued in April 1981. Biospherics also filed similar patents in a number of other countries.

The toxicological testing required by FDA for approval of L-sugars is underway. Studies conducted to date indicate that the L-sugars tested do not exhibit toxicity or mutagenicity [112]. The findings of the human testing support the expected low-caloric dietary contribution but indicate that the sweeteners may be subject to acceptable daily intake limitations, as are the sugar alcohols [112]. Preliminary tests also indicate that the L-sugars are noncariogenic [112].

G. Maltitol

1. Chemical Properties and Technical Aspects

Maltitol ($\alpha(1 \rightarrow 4)$-glucosylsorbitol) is produced by the hydrogenation of maltose (manufactured by the enzymatic hydrolysis of corn starch) using a process developed by Hayashibara Biochemical Laboratories (Okayama, Japan). Maltitol, which has been in use in Japan since about 1964, may be produced in the form of a syrup containing more than 50% maltitol and low levels of sorbitol, maltotriitol, and other hydrogenated oligosaccharides, or in the form of a crystalline powder with up to 99% maltitol [98]. The crystalline form has a sweetness level 85–95% of that of sucrose and is sweeter than all other polyols except xylitol [98].

Crystalline maltitol and maltitol syrup are manufactured and marketed under the brand names Amalty and Mabit by Towa Chemical Industry, Co., Ltd., and affiliate of Mitsubishi (Tokyo, Japan) in the United States and several other countries including Japan; Malbit by ANIC and its subsidiary Melida, SpA (Milan, Italy); and Maltisorb Crystalline by Roquette Frères (Lestrem, France).

Maltitol is a bulk sweetener (in contrast to high-intensity sweeteners such as aspartame, saccharin, and acesulfame-K) which has a sweetness profile similar to that of sucrose and is noncariogenic [98,113]. The exact caloric value of maltitol is a matter of controversy [98]. Research has indicated that the intestinal microflora play a role in fermentation in the large intestine, and studies have suggested caloric values of 50–100% of that of other fully metabolized carbohydrates [98].

Maltitol is metabolized to glucose and sorbitol. Because hydrolysis of maltitol is slower than that of sucrose and because the sweetener does not appear to produce marked elevations in blood glucose levels, maltitol may have utility in diabetic diets [98]. As with other polyols, maltitol may produce a laxative effect if consumed in excessive quantities but the laxation effect is less than that exhibited by sorbitol [98]. FDA requires that foods that may result in a daily ingestion of 50 g of sorbitol be labeled with the statement, "Excess consumption may have a laxative effect" (21 CFR 184. 1835 (e)); thus, such a label for maltitol, which is metabolized into sorbitol, may be required in certain applications.

2. Applications

Applications of maltitol include confections such as chocolates, hard candy, pressed tablets, caramels, jellies and jams, gums, pastilles, table-top sweeteners (in combination with a high-intensity sweetener such as aspartame), cookies, cakes, and ice cream analogs [98].

3. Safety and Regulatory Aspects

Towa Chemical Industry filed a petition with FDA to reaffirm the GRAS status of maltitol in 1986. The petition seeks approval for use of maltitol as a nutritive sweetener and in a variety of other applications such as flavoring agent, formulation and processing aid, humectant, sequestrant, stabilizer and thickener, surface-finishing agent, and texturizer [98].

The petition indicates that none of the acute, subacute, chronic and subchronic, carcinogenic, mutagenic, and teratogenic studies of maltitol have shown any evidence of adverse effects [98]. The Joint FAO/WHO Expert Committee on Food Additives has set the ADI of maltitol at "not specified" [109]. The EC's Scientific Committee for Food reported in 1984 that maltitol is "acceptable" and that it deemed establishment of an ADI for this sweetener inappropriate [98]. Maltitol is approved for use in 11 countries, including France, Japan, and the United Kingdom [98].

H. Sucralose

1. Chemical Properties and Technical Aspects

Sucralose was developed in the 1970s by Tate and Lyle (London, England). The sweetener (1,6-dichloro-1,6-dideoxy-D-fructofuranosyl-4-chloro-4-deoxy-α-D-galactopyranoside) is made by a patented process involving the selective chlorination of sucrose, which results in intense sweetness and stability. The development of sucralose as well as its potential applications and research conducted during its development have been reviewed [114].

Sucralose is approximately 600 times sweeter than sucrose. It is heat stable and highly soluble in water; has a sweet taste and flavor profile similar to those of sucrose; and does not leave an unpleasant aftertaste [114, 115]. Sucralose is not metabolized and thus is noncaloric. Studies indicate that it is also noncariogenic [114].

2. Applications

The food additive petition for approval in the United States was filed with FDA in 1987 by McNeil Specialty Products Co. (New Brunswick, NJ, a subsidiary of Johnson & Johnson) under a licensing agreement with Tate and Lyle [116]. The petition requests approval for use in baked goods and baking mixes, beverages and beverage bases, chewing gum, coffee and tea, confections and frostings, dairy product analogs, fats and oils (salad dressings), frozen dairy desserts and mixes, fruits and water ices, gelatins and puddings, jams and jellies, milk products, processed fruits and fruit juices, sugar substitutes, sweet sauces, toppings, and syrups.

3. Safety Issues and Regulatory Aspects

One hundred studies were conducted to establish the safety of sucralose [114]. The sweetener was determined to be nontoxic following acute exposure in rodents at levels up to 16,000 mg/kg/day—equal to consumption of approximately 4000 carbonated soft drinks/day. In three lifetime animal studies with doses of up to 3% of the diet, sucralose showed no evidence of carcinogenicity. Further, it did not exhibit teratological or genetic toxicity or central nervous system effects. Human studies have also been conducted without any negative physiological, biochemical, hematological, or blood sugar effects [114].

Sucralose was approved in September 1991 in Canada where it will be marketed under the name "Splenda" by Tate and Lyle. It was approved for a number of applications, including use in table-top sweeteners. The Joint FAO/WHO Expert Committee on Food Additives reviewed sucralose, as well as 6-chlorfructose, one of its potential breakdown products dependent upon pH, temperature, and time, when exposed to acid hydrolysis and set an ADI of 15 mg/kg [20].

The sweetener is being reviewed by regulatory authorities in the United Kingdom, the EC, Denmark, and Australia as well as the United States.

I. Other Sugar Substitutes

A number of naturally occurring and synthetic sugar substitutes are available in countries outside the United States. These include the more common neohesperidin dihydrochalcone (II) and stevioside. A brief description of these sweeteners is provided. More detailed reviews may be found in Higgenbotham [85], Horowitz and Gentili [117], and Kinghorn and Soejarto [118].

1. Neohesperidin Dihydrochalcone (II)

This compound, a derivative of citrus flavones, is synthesized from naringin or extracted from citrus peel. The substance is approximately 1800 times sweeter than sucrose and has an estimated caloric value of no more than 2 kcal/g [117]. It is approved in a number of countries for use in chewing gum and some beverages.

2. Stevioside

Stevioside is a glycoside obtained from the leaves of the *Stevia rebaudiana* plant native to northeastern Paraguay. It is approximately 300 times sweeter than a 0.4% sucrose solution [118]. The extract is stable and provides a long-lasting taste; however, it exhibits some bitterness and aftertaste. Stevioside is used in Paraguay, Japan, South Korea, Brazil, and China. Applications include soft drinks, chewing gum, fish sauces, syrups, and table-top use [118].

IV. OUTLOOK

A number of sugar substitutes are currently available, or are under development or regulatory review, for the manufacture of low-calorie foods and beverages. A number of sweeteners are also available to consumers for sweetening foods and beverages at home.

Additional substances have been recently discovered or patented in the United States. These include D-tagatose (a low-calorie substance that provides bulk) [119], two heat-stable, amino acid–based substances [120], suosan-related substances up to 20,000 times sweeter than sucrose [121]; heat-stable "Sweetener 2000," which is 10,000 times sweeter than sugar [122]; and erythritol, a polyalcohol that provides only 0.3 kcal/g [123]. These recent developments and a few of the most noted characteristics of the sweeteners are listed in Table 3.

It is clear that the perfect sugar substitute does not yet exist. While each sweetener has certain advantages, each also has disadvantages—such as bitter aftertaste, instability during heating and/or storage, or lack of bulk—which are undesirable to the consumer or to food manufacturers.

Sugar substitutes are typically synergistic in combination, providing a similar sweetness level with less total sweetener. Combinations of sweeteners also exhibit improved taste profiles. Taste panels of table-top preparations conducted by ABIC International Consultants (Fairfield, NJ) have confirmed

Table 3 Potential Sugar Substitutes Recently Discovered or Patented

Substance	Source/Manufacture	Characteristics
D-tagatose	D-galactose, process patented by Biospherics, Inc., Beltsville, MD	Low-calorie, same bulk as sucrose
Amino acid–based	Dipeptide ester compounds patented by General Foods	Heat stable, 2000–5000 times sweeter than sucrose
"Sweetener 2000"	Developed by Nutra-Sweet from aryl ureas and trisubstituted guanidines, patented by researchers at Claude Bernard University, Lyon, France	Heat stable, 20,000 times sweeter than sucrose
Suosan-related	Derived from β-substituted β-amino acids, developed by NutraSweet	Up to 20,000 times sweeter than sucrose
Erythritol	Developed by Cerestar, United Kingdom, Belgium, enzymatic hydrolysis and yeast fermentation	Polyalcohol, no laxative effect, 0.3 kcal/g

Source: Refs. 120–124.

the superiority of combinations of aspartame with saccharin, cyclamate, and acesulfame-K over the individual sweeteners [124].

Combinations of sweeteners—a "multiple-sweeteners approach"—is beneficial in minimizing or overcoming the undesirable characteristics of individual sweeteners [2]. Having a variety of low-calorie sweeteners to choose from allows manufacturers to use the ingredient or combination of ingredients best suited for a given product [125].

Increased interaction is expected among the three major components of sweeteners available in the United States and throughout the world—sugar, high-fructose corn syrups and/or high-fructose starch syrups and high-intensity sweeteners—either as complementary sweeteners in different uses, as sugar substitutes, or perhaps as "blends" in the same product [6]. Consumer interest in sugar substitutes is also expected to increase as additional table-top sugar substitutes become available, thus allowing broader uses of them in the home and more choices among a greater variety of low-calorie products in the marketplace.

REFERENCES

1. J. A. Desor, O. Maller, and L. S. Greene, Preference for sweet in humans: Infants, children, and adults, *Taste and Development: The Genesis of Sweet Preference* (J. M. Weiffenbach, ed.), U.S. Department of Health, Education, and Welfare, Washington, D.C., p. 171 (1977).
2. L. O'Brien Nabors and R. C. Gelardi, eds., *Alternative Sweeteners*, 2nd ed., Marcel Dekker, Inc., New York, p. 1 (1991).
3. ERS, Sugar and Sweeteners, "Situation and Outlook Report," United States Department of Agriculture, Economic Research Service, Washington, D.C. (Dec., 1990).
4. B. Gorman, New products, new realities, *Prep. Foods, 160*(4): 14 (1991).
5. K. Hochberg, Health claims shift into high gear, *Prep. Foods, 160*(4): 47 (1991).
6. P. J. Buzzanell, World and U.S. outlook for sweeteners, Presented at the Annual Agricultural Outlook Conference, United States Department of Agriculture, Washington, D.C., Nov. 28 (1990).
7. R. D. Barry, The U.S. and world sugar markets in transition, Presented at the Fifth Annual Agribusiness Outlook Forum, New York, Jan. 23 (1991).
8. G.-W. von Rymon Lipinski and D. Mayer, Acesulfame-K, *Comment. Toxicol.* 3(4): 279 (1989).
9. G.-W. von Rymon Lipinski, Acesulfame-K, *Alternative Sweeteners* (L. O'Brien Nabors and R. C. Gelardi, eds.), 2nd ed., Marcel Dekker, Inc., New York, p. 11 (1991).
10. M. Volz, O. Christ, H. G. Eckert, J. Herok, H.-M. Kellner, and W. Rupp, Kinetics and biotransformation of acesulfame-K, *Acesulfame-K* (D. G. Mayer and F. N. Kemper, eds.), Marcel Dekker, Inc., New York, p. 7 (1991).
11. G.-W. von Rymon Lipinski, The new intense sweetener acesulfame K, *Food Chem., 16*: 259 (1985).
12. G.-W. von Rymon Lipinski, Properties and applications of acesulfame-K, *Acesulfame-K* (D. G. Mayer and F. N. Kemper, eds.), Marcel Dekker, Inc., New York, p. 209 (1991).
13. J. A. Stamp, Sorting out sweeteners, *Cereal Foods World, 35*(4): 395 (1990).
14. G.-W. Von Rymon Lipinski, Sensory properties of acesulfame-K, *Acesulfame-K* (D. G. Mayer and F. N. Kemper, eds.), Marcel Dekker, Inc., New York, p. 197 (1991).

15. A. G. Renwick, The fate of intense sweeteners in the body, *Food Chem., 16*: 281 (1985).

16. FDA, Food additives permitted for direct addition to food for human consumption; acesulfame potassium, *Fed. Reg., 53*(145): 28379 (1988).

17. WHO, Principles for the safety assessment of food additives and contaminants in food, *Environmental Health Criteria*, No. 80, World Health Organization, Geneva, p. 75 (1987).

18. Report on the Review of Sweeteners in Food, Food Additives and Contaminants Committee, Her Majesty's Stationery Office, London (1982).

19. WHO, "WHO Food Additives Series," No. 18, World Health Organization, Geneva, p. 12 (1983).

20. WHO, Evaluation of certain food additives and contaminants, "Report of the 37th meeting of the Joint FAO/WHO Expert Committee on Food Additives," World Health Organization, Geneva (1991).

21. EC, Sweeteners, "Report of the Scientific Committee for Food," Commission of the European Communities, No. 16, Luxembourg, p. 8 (1985).

22. B. E. Holmer, R. C. Deis, and W. H. Shazer, Aspartame, *Alternative Sweeteners* (L. O'Brien Nabors and R. C. Gelardi, eds.), 2nd ed., Marcel Dekker, Inc., New York, p. 39 (1991).

23. C. I. Beck, Application potential for aspartame in low calorie and dietetic foods. *Low Calorie and Special Dietary Foods* (B. K. Dwivedi, ed.), CRC Press, West Palm Beach, FL, p. 59 (1978).

24. D. Pszczola, Applications of aspartame in baking, *Food Technol., 42*(1): 56 (1988).

25. M. R. Cloninger and R. E. Baldwin, L-Aspartyl-L-phenylalanine methyl ester (aspartame) as a sweetener, *J. Food Sci., 39*: 347 (1974).

26. N. Larson-Powers and R. M. Pangborn, Paired comparisons and time-intensity measurements of the sensory properties of beverages and gelatins containing sucrose or synthetic sweeteners, *J. Food Sci., 43*: 41 (1978).

27. N. Larson-Powers and R. M. Pangborn, Descriptive analysis of the sensory properties of beverages and gelatins containing sucrose or synthetic sweeteners, *J. Food Sci., 43*: 47 (1978).

28. R. H. Mazur, J. M. Schlatter, and A. H. Goldkamp, Structure-taste relationships of some dipeptides, *J. Amer. Chem. Soc., 91*: 2684 (1969).

29. S. S. Schiffman, Comparison of taste properties of aspartame with other sweeteners, *Aspartame: Physiology and Biochemistry* (L. D. Stegink and L. J. Filer, Jr., eds.), Marcel Dekker, Inc., New York, p. 207 (1984).

30. FDA, Aspartame: Commissioner's final decision, *Fed. Reg., 46*: 38284 (1981).

31. H. H. Butchko, and F. N. Kotsonis, Aspartame: Review of recent research. *Comment. Toxicol., III*(4): 253 (1989).

32. L. D. Stegink and L. J. Filer (eds.), *Aspartame: Physiology and Biochemistry*, Marcel Dekker, Inc., New York (1984).

33. IFT, Sweeteners: Nutritive and non-nutritive, A Scientific Status Summary by the Institute of Food Technologists' Expert Panel on Food Safety and Nutrition, Chicago, IL, *Food Technol., 40*(8): 195 (1986).

34. FDA, Food additives permitted for direct addition to food for human consumption: Aspartame, *Fed. Reg. 49*: 6672 (1984).
35. M. K. Bradstock, J. S. Serdula, R. J. Marks, N. T. Barnard, P. L. Crane, P. L. Remington, and F. L. Trowbridge, Evaluation of reactions to food additives: The aspartame experience, *Am. J. Clin. Nutr., 43*: 464 (1986).
36. L. Tollefson, R. J. Barnard, and W. H. Glinsmann, *Dietary Phenylalanine and Brain Function* (R. J. Wurtman and E. Ritter-Walker, eds.), Birkhauser, Boston, p. 317 (1988).
37. L. Tollefson, Monitoring adverse reactions to food additives in the U.S. Food and Drug Administration, *Reg. Tox. Pharm., 8*: 438 (1988).
38. D. L. Arnold, D. Krewski, and I. C. Munro, Saccharin: A toxicological and historical perspective, *Toxicology, 27*: 179 (1983).
39. M. L. Mitchell and R. L. Pearson, Saccharin, *Alternative Sweeteners* (L. O'Brien Nabors and R. C. Gelardi, eds.), 2nd ed., Marcel Dekker, Inc., New York, p. 127 (1991).
40. F. J. Helgren, M. J. Lunch, and F. J. Kirchmeyer, A taste panel study of the saccharin off-taste. *J. Am. Pharm. Assoc.* (Sci. ed.), *44*: 353 (1955).
41. T. W. Sweatman and A. G. Renwick, The tissue distribution and pharmacokinetics of saccharin in the rat, *Toxicol. Appl. Pharmacol., 55*: 18 (1980).
42. A. Porter, Effectiveness of multiple sweeteners and other ingredients in food formulation. *Chem. Ind., 18*: 696 (1983).
43. J. M. Taylor, M. A. Weinberger, and L. Friedman, Chronic toxicity and carcinogenicity to the urinary bladder of sodium saccharin in the in utero-exposed rat, *Toxicol. Appl. Pharmacol., 54*: 57 (1980).
44. M. O. Tisdel, P. O. Nees, D. L. Harris, and P. H. Derse, Long-term feeding of saccharin in rats, *Symposium: Sweeteners* (G. E. Inglett, ed.), AVI Pub. Co., Westport, CT, p. 145 (1974).
45. A. G. Renwick, Saccharin: A toxicological evaluation. *Comment. Toxicol. III* (4): 289 (1989).
46. L. B. Ellwein and S. M. Cohen, The health risks of saccharin revisited, *Toxicology, 20*(5): 311 (1990).
47. S. M. Cohen, L. B. Ellwein, T. Okamura, T. Masui, S. L. Johansson, R. A. Smith, J. M. Wehner, M. Khachab, C. I. Chappel, G. P. Schoenig, J. L. Emerson, and E. M. Garland, Comparative bladder tumor promoting activity of sodium saccharin, sodium ascorbate, related acids and calcium salts in rats, *Cancer Res., 51*: 1766 (1991).
48. AMA, Saccharin, review of safety issues, Council on Scientific Affairs, American Medical Association. *J. Am. Med. Assoc., 254*: 2622 (1985).
49. ADA, Position of the American Dietetic Association: Appropriate use of nutritive and non-nutritive sweeteners, *J. Am. Diet. Assoc., 87*: 1689 (1987).
50. ADA, Use of noncaloric sweeteners, Council on nutrition sciences and metabolism, American Diabetes Association, *Diabetes Care, 10*: 526 (1987).
51. WHO, Evaluation of certain food additives and contaminants, 28th Report of the Joint Expert Committee on Food Additives, Food and Agriculture Organization/World Health Organization, Geneva (1984).

52. EEC, Sweeteners, Report of the Scientific Committee for Food, Commission of the European Economic Communities, (Dec. 1987).

53. B. K. Dwivedi, Polyalcohols: Sorbitol, mannitol, maltitol and hydrogenated starch hydrolysates, *Alternative Sweeteners* (L. O'Brien Nabors and R. C. Gelardi, eds.), Marcel Dekker, New York, p. 165 (1986).

54. FDA, Mannitol: removal from GRAS status and establishment of interim food additive regulation for direct human food use, *Fed. Reg. 39*: 34178 (1974).

55. I. H. C. Gallagher and E. I. F. Pearce, The fermentation of sucrose, sorbitol, and xylitol by *Propionibacterium avidum,* resulting in the formation of caries-like lesions in enamel, *New Zealand J. Dent., 79*: 357 (1983).

56. FDA, Sorbitol: affirmation of GRAS status as direct human food ingredient, *Fed. Reg., 39*: 3418C (1974).

57. F. W. Ellis and J. C. Krantz, Sugar alcohols XXIV. The metabolism of sorbitol in diabetes. *Ann. Int. Med., 18*: 792 (1943).

58. L. O'Brien and R. C. Gelardi, Alternative sweeteners, *Chemtech:* 274 (May 1981).

59. R. Peters and R. H. Loch, Laxative effects of sorbitol, *Brit. Med. J., 2*: 677 (1958).

60. J. S. Hyams, Sorbitol intolerance: An unappreciated cause of gastrointestinal complaints, *Gastroenterology, 84*(1): 30 (1983).

61. A. Bar, Xylitol, *Alternative Sweeteners* (L. O'Brien Nabors and R. C. Gelardi, eds.), 2nd ed., Marcel Dekker, Inc., New York, p. 349 (1991).

62. T. Pepper and P. M. Olinger, Xylitol in sugar-free confections, *Food Technol., 42*(10): 98 (1988).

63. FASEB, Dietary Sugars in Health and Disease. II. Xylitol. A report prepared for the Food and Drug Administration, Life Sciences Research Office, Federation of American Societies for Experimental Biology, Bethesda, MD (1978).

64. W. Hassinger, G. Sauer, U. Cordes, U. Kruse, J. Beyer, and K. H. Baessler, The effects of equal caloric amounts of xylitol, sucrose and starch on insulin requirements and blood glucose levels in insulin-dependent diabetics, *Diabetologia, 21*: 37 (1981).

65. J. S. Skyler and N. E. Miller, The use of sweeteners by diabetic patients, *Pract. Cardiol., 6*: 119 (1980).

66. W. Edgar and M. Dobbs, The effect of sweeteners on acid production in plaque, *Int. Dent. J., 35*: 18 (1985).

67. M. Hayes and K. Roberts, The breakdown of glucose, xylitol and other sugar alcohols by human dental plaque bacteria, *Arch. Oral. Biol., 23*: 445 (1978).

68. D. Platt and S. R. Werrin, Acid production from alditols by oral streptococci, *J. Dent. Res., 58*: 1733 (1979).

69. D. Kandelman and G. Gagnon, Clinical results after 12 months from a study of the incidence and progression of dental caries in relation to consumption of chewing gum containing xylitol in school preventive programs, *J. Dent. Res., 66*: 1407 (1987).

70. D. Kandelman, A. Bar, and A. Hefti, Collaborative WHO xylitol field study in French Polynesia, *Caries Res. 22*: (1988).

71. A. Scheinin, K. Makinen, and K. Ylitalo, Turku sugar studies V, Final report on the effect of sucrose, frustose and xylitol diets on the caries incidence in man, *Acta Odont. Scand., 33*(Suppl. 70): 67 (1975).

72. A. Scheinin, K. Makinen, and K. Ylitalo, Turku sugar studies. XVIII. Incidence of dental caries in relation to 1-year consumption of xylitol chewing gum, *Acta Odont. Scand., 33*(Suppl. 70): 307 (1975).

73. A. Scheinin, J. Banoczy, J. Szoke, I. Esztari, K. Pienihakkinen, U. J. Scheinen, J. Tiekso, P. Zimmerman, and E. Hada, Collaborative WHO xylitol field studies in Hungary. I. Three-year caries activity in institutional children, *Acta Odont. Scand., 43*: 327 (1985).

74. W. J. Loesche, The effect of sugar alcohols on plaque and saliva level of *Streptococcus mutans, Swed. Dent. J., 8*: 125 (1984).

75. FASEB, Health Aspects of Sugar Alcohols and Lactose. A report prepared for the Food and Drug Administration, Life Sciences Research Office, Federation of American Societies for Experimental Biology, Bethesda, MD, (1986).

76. A. Baer, Safety assessment of polyol sweeteners—some aspects of toxicology, *Food Chem., 16*: 231 (1985).

77. A. Baer, Sugars and adrenomedullary proliferative lesions: The effects of lactose and various polyalcohols, *J. Am. Coll. Toxicol., 7*: 71 (1988).

78. H. K. Akerblom, T. Koivukangas, R. Punka, and M. Mononen, The tolerance of increasing amounts of dietary xylitol in children, *Int. J. Vit. Nutr. Res., 22*(Suppl.): 53 (1981).

79. K. K. Maekinen, Biochemical principles of the use of xylitol in medicine and nutrition with special consideration of dental aspects, *Experientia. Suppl., 30*: 1 (1978).

80. WHO/FAO, Summary of toxicological data of certain food additives and contaminants, Twenty-second Report of the Joint FAO/WHO Expert Committee on Food Additives, Technical Report Series No. 631, World Health Organization, Geneva, p. 28 (1978).

81. A. Bar, Xylitol, *Alternative Sweeteners* (L. O'Brien Nabors and R. C. Gelardi, eds.), 2nd ed., Marcel Dekker, Inc., New York, p. 341 (1991).

82. WHO/FAO, Evaluation of certain food additives and contaminants, Twenty-seventh Report of the Joint FAO/WHO Expert Committee on Food Additives, WHO Technical Report Series No. 696, World Health Organization, Geneva, p. 23 (1983).

83. T. F. Osberger, Crystalline fructose, *Alternative Sweeteners* (L. O'Brien Nabors and R. C. Gelardi, eds.), 2nd ed., Marcel Dekker, Inc., New York, p. 219 (1991).

84. A. D. Kinghorn and C. M. Compadre, Less common high-potency sweeteners, *Alternative Sweeteners* (L. O'Brien Nabors and R. C. Gelardi, eds.), 2nd ed., Marcel Dekker, Inc., New York, p. 197 (1991).

85. J. D. Higgenbotham, Talin protein (thaumatin), *Alternative Sweeteners* (L. O'Brien Nabors and R. C. Gelardi, ed.), Marcel Dekker, New York, p. 103 (1986).

86. J. T. Liebrand, Alitame, Presented at the 23rd Annual Symposium of the Western New York Section of IFT and the Institute of Food Science, Cornell University, Ithaca, New York, Nov. 1988, Special Report Number 63 (1989).

87. M. E. Hendrick, Alitame, *Alternative Sweeteners* (L. O'Brien Nabors and R. C. Gelardi, eds.), 2nd ed., Marcel Dekker, Inc., New York, p. 29 (1991).

88. T. M. Brennan and M. E. Hendrick, Branched amides of L-aspartyl–D-amino acid dipeptides, U.S. Patent No. 4,411,925 (Oct. 25, 1983).

89. FDA, Food additives permitted for direct addition to food for human consumption; alitame, *Fed. Reg., 51*(188): 34503 (1986).

90. B. A. Bopp and P. Price, Cyclamate, Alternative Sweeteners (L. O'Brien Nabors and R. C. Gelardi, eds.), 2nd ed., Marcel Dekker, Inc., New York, p. 71 (1991).

91. L. O'Brien Nabors and W. T. Miller, Cyclamate—a toxicological review, *Comment. Toxicol., III*(4): 307 (1989).

92. CCC and Abbott Laboratories, Supplement to Food Additive Petition 2A 3672, June 4, Calorie Control Council, Atlanta, Georgia and Abbott Laboratories, Abbott Park, IL (1986).

93. B. L. Oser, S. Carson, G. E. Cox, E. E. Vogin, and S. S. Sternberg, Chronic toxicity study of cyclamate: Saccharin (10:1) in rats, *Toxicology, 4*: 315 (1975).

94. FDA, Cyclamic acid and its salts, *Fed. Reg., 34*: 17063, Oct. 21 (1969).

95. CAC, Scientific review of the long-term carcinogenic bioassays performed on the artificial sweetener, cyclamate, Cancer Assessment Committee, Center for Food Safety and Applied Nutrition, Food and Drug Administration, Washington, D.C. (1984).

96. NAS/NRC, Evaluation of cyclamate for carcinogenicity, Committee on the Evaluation of Cyclamate for Carcinogenicity, National Academy of Sciences/National Research Council, National Academy Press, Washington, D.C. (1985).

97. J. M. DeSesso, J. M. Kelley, and B. B. Fuller, MITRE Corporation report to U.S. Food and Drug Administration, FDA Contract No. 223-86-2104 (May 1987).

98. A. H. Moskowitz, Maltitol and hydrogenated starch hydrolysate, *Alternative Sweeteners* (L. O'Brien Nabors and R. C. Gelardi, eds.), 2nd ed., Marcel Dekker, Inc., New York, p. 259 (1991).

99. T. Imfeld and H. R. Muhlemann, Addendum to acid production from Swedish Lycasin® (candy quality) and French Lycasin® (80/55) in human dental plaques (G. Frostell and D. Birkhed), *Caries Res., 12*: 262 (1978).

100. G. Frostell and D. Birkhed, Acid production from Swedish Lycasin® (candy quality) and French Lycasin® (80/55) in human dental plaques, *Caries Res., 12*: 256 (1978).

101. T. H. Grenby, Dental effects of Lycasin® in the diet of laboratory rats, *Caries Res., 22*: 288 (1988).

102. S. C. Ziesenitz and G. Siebert, Polyols and other bulk sweeteners, *Developments in Sweeteners—3* (T. H. Grenby, ed.), Elsevier-Applied Science Publisher, London and New York, p. 109 (1987).

103. WHO, Toxicological evaluation of certain food additives and contaminants. Twenty-ninth report of the FAO/WHO Expert Committee on Food Additives and Contaminants, Cambridge University Press, Cambridge, United Kingdom, p. 179 (1987).

104. P. J. Strater and W. E. Irwin, Isomalt, *Alternative Sweeteners* (L. O'Brien Nabors and R. C. Gelardi, eds.), 2nd ed., Marcel Dekker, Inc., New York, p. 309 (1991).
105. W. E. Irwin and P. J. Strater, Isomaltulose, *Alternative Sweeteners* (L. O'Brien Nabors and R. C. Gelardi, eds.), Marcel Dekker, Inc., New York, p. 299 (1991).
106. W. E. Irwin, Isomalt-A sweet, reduced-calorie bulking agent, *Food Technol., 44*(6): 128 (1990).
107. D. Thiebaud, E. Jacot, H. Schmitz, M. Spengler, and J. P. Felber, Comparative study of Isomalt and sucrose by means of continuous indirect calorimetry, *Metabolism, 33*(9): 808 (1984).
108. WHO, Isomalt, Toxicological evaluation of certain food additives and contaminants, Joint FAO/WHO Expert Committee on Food Additives, WHO Food Additive Series, No. 20, Cambridge University Press, Cambridge, United Kingdom, p. 207 (1987).
109. J. A. Van Velthuijsen and I. H. Blankers, Lactitol: A new reduced calorie sweetener, *Alternative Sweeteners,* (L. O'Brien Nabors and R. C. Gelardi, eds.), 2nd ed., Marcel Dekker, Inc., New York, p. 283 (1991).
110. WHO, Toxicological evaluation of certain food additives and contaminants: Lactitol, Joint FAO/WHO Expert Committee on Food Additives, 27th report, WHO Food Additives Series, Geneva, p. 82 (1983).
111. EEC, Sweeteners, Report of the Scientific Committee for Food, Commission of the European Economic Communities, EC-Document III/1316/84/CS/EDUL/27 rev. (1984).
112. G. V. Levin and L. R. Zehner, L-Sugars: Lev-O-Cal™, *Alternative Sweeteners* (L. O'Brien Nabors and R. C. Gelardi, eds.), 2nd ed., Marcel Dekker, Inc., New York, p. 127 (1991).
113. J. Rundgren, T. Koulourides, and T. Encson, Contribution of maltitol and Lycasin to experimental enamel demineralization in the human mouth, *Caries Res., 14*: 67 (1980).
114. G. A. Miller, Sucralose, *Alternative Sweeteners* (L. O'Brien Nabors and R. C. Gelardi, eds.), 2nd ed., Marcel Dekker, Inc., New York, p. 173 (1991).
115. R. L. Barndt, Sucralose: A review of the features and benefits of this new high-potency sweetener, Presented at the 23rd Annual Symposium of the Western New York Section of IFT and the Institute of Food Science, Cornell University, Ithaca, New York, Nov. 1988, Special Report Number 63 (1989).
116. FDA, McNeil Specialty Products Co., Filing of food additive petition, *Fed. Reg., 52*(89): 17475 (1987).
117. R. M. Horowitz, and B. Gentili, Dihydrochalcone sweeteners from citrus flavanones, *Alternative Sweeteners* (L. O'Brien Nabors and R. C. Gelardi, eds.), 2nd ed., Marcel Dekker, Inc., New York, p. 97 (1991).
118. A. D. Kinghorn and D. D. Soejarto, Stevioside, *Alternative Sweeteners* (L. O'Brien Nabors and R. C. Gelardi, eds.), 2nd ed., Marcel Dekker, Inc., New York, p. 157 (1991).
119. Patent awarded for method of making sugar substitute, *Wall Street Journal* (April 9, 1991).

120. General Foods receives patent on two new sweeteners, *Prep. Foods, 157*(12): 27 (1988).
121. W. W. Orthy, Synthetic sweeteners developed by design, *Chem. Eng. News*, April 30, p. 8 (1990).
122. A. M. Freedman and R. Gibson, Monsanto touts new sugar substitutes as sweetest yet, *Wall Street Journal,* March 29 (1991).
123. L. Tuley, The sweet option, *Food Manuf., 66*(1): 16 (1991).
124. A. I. Bakal, Mixed sweetener functionality, *Alternative Sweeteners* (L. O'Brien Nabors and R. C. Gelardi, eds.), 2nd ed., Marcel Dekker, Inc., New York, p. 381 (1991).
125. G. Gelardi, Low calorie sweeteners outlook, Presented at the Sweeteners Session, U.S. Dept. of Agriculture Outlook Conference, Nov. 28, Washington, D.C. (1990).
126. FDA, Food additives permitted for direct addition to food for human consumption; aspartame, *Fed. Reg. 57*: 3701 (1992).
127. CCC and Abbott Laboratories, Food Additive Petition for Cyclamate, 2A3672, Sept. 22, Calorie Control Council, Atlanta, Georgia and Abbott Laboratories, Abbott Park, IL (1982).

9

Microparticulated Proteins as Fat Substitutes

Norman S. Singer and Robert H. Moser   *The NutraSweet Company, Mount Prospect, Illinois*

I. INTRODUCTION

The scientific evidence is compelling that a high-fat diet (at least in the United States) is a significant health risk. The average American consumes excessive dietary fat relative to dietary carbohydrate and protein. The direct relationship between a high-fat diet and coronary heart disease, obesity, and some forms of cancer is accepted by most health professionals [1].

Marketing surveys indicate that the average American consumer understands the message now communicated by many health-care organizations and desires a healthful, low-fat diet. But marketing data also show that most consumers are unwilling to sacrifice good taste for healthfulness [2–4]. The persistent perception is that a food that is "good for you" probably tastes bad [5]. Therefore, consumers are less willing to try alternative foods instead of their traditional favorites. Health-care professionals play a crucial role in educating people about the importance of a low-fat diet. They dispense information to promote health, to prevent disease, and to translate dietary recommendations into practice in the supermarket and the kitchen. The consumer, confused by conflicting messages in the media, frequently turns to his or her health-care provider for advice. Consumer consternation is understandably the result of the historical failure to express the fat content in foods in a comprehensive manner in addition to an array of frequently questionable health claims.

The food industry employs various methods to reduce the fat content of foods. Using leaner cuts of meats, adding fillers such as rice or soy protein, substituting milk for cream, etc., are common-sense ways to reduce fat through ingredient substitution and formulation. The majority of food manufacturers, however, use fat substitutes in addition to other methods. Fat substitutes are generally derived from carbohydrate, fat, or protein starting materials. The ingredients that are most commonly sold as fat substitutes are carbohydrates that have been used for many years as stabilizers and thickeners. Cellulose, gums, modified starches, polydextrose, and maltodextrins are well known and widely used. However, the effective replacement of fat requires more than such materials can deliver. A number of low- or no-calorie fat replacers derived from fats are under development but are not approved for use (see also Chapters 10 and 11).

Simplesse®, made by the NutraSweet Co., is a pioneering breakthrough in the search for a healthful fat substitute. It was the first fat substitute to be affirmed by the Food and Drug Administration (FDA) as GRAS (generally recognized as safe) [6]. It is an all-natural protein ingredient which is highly effective in replacing fat in many foods. This effectiveness is a consequence of the novel physical form in which the protein has been caused to gel. This gel is in the form of microparticles, about 0.001 mm in diameter. Each microparticle is made of many millions of intact protein molecules. The use of protein microparticles to replace fat is a new approach which makes it possible to retain traditional sensory quality while reducing the fat. The discovery, development, and application of microparticulated protein are described below.

II. MICROPARTICULATED PROTEIN AS A FAT SUBSTITUTE

Like many scientific breakthroughs, the discovery that protein can mimic certain properties of fat was the result of serendipity, keen observation, and extrapolation. While working on a project unrelated to fat substitution, it was discovered that a combination of cooking and blending could convert solutions of whey protein into a product that was found to have the sort of creaminess normally associated with high fat levels [7].

The necessary fatlike properties were obtained when pasteurization and homogenization were performed simultaneously instead of sequentially as is usually done during food processing. Under microscopic examination, an abundance of uniformly round particles was found. Essentially all were approximately 1 μm in diameter [8].

Protein microparticles occur naturally in foods such as milk, egg, grains, and legumes, but are not found in the necessary size, shape, or sufficient abundance to function as fat replacers [9]. Casein micelles, which occur in all dairy foods, are much smaller than 1 μm in diameter and are, therefore, too small to produce the required effect. By contrast, microparticles from vegetable proteins such as soy may be as large as 80 μm in diameter and are too large to function as fat substitutes.

The simple patented process called microparticulation is unique in that it produces a large quantity of protein microparticles that are uniformly the necessary size and shape [7]. Each protein particle consists of several million loosely packed protein molecules. The particles are so small that 50 billion would fit on a teaspoon [10]. A study of the structure and function of the protein microparticulates revealed that the size and shape of the particles were essential in providing fat-like mouthfeel.

Based on the above discoveries, microparticulated protein as a fat substitute was patented, developed, and commercialized internationally by its registered trademark Simplesse.

III. SIMPLESSE

Simplesse is the first fat substitute that replaces fat with protein. The protein can be derived, for example, from egg whites, skim milk, and/or whey protein. Protein particles prepared by microparticulation deliver the taste and texture of high-fat foods.

Rigorous scientific examination demonstrated that the highly nutritive quality of the egg white and dairy proteins is unchanged during Simplesse production. The protein particles were subjected to extensive analyses by independent research investigators in an evaluation more typical of the pharmaceutical industry than the food industry. The organization of protein molecules in the particles was examined by transmission electron microscopy. Gel electrophoresis, amino acid assays, protein efficiency ratios, and in vitro allergenicity tests confirmed that the amino acid sequence and three-dimensional structure of the proteins were unchanged by the microparticulation process [12–15]. The only difference was in the physical way in which the protein molecules aggregated.

In February 1990, following a thorough examination of all the data, the FDA affirmed Simplesse prepared from egg white and/or skim milk to be

GRAS for use in frozen desserts [6]. A second form of Simplesse prepared from whey protein concentrate was approved by FDA in August 1991 for use in a wide range of food applications.

Simplesse can, in fact, be made from a variety of proteins. Different products may require different source proteins. The desired taste and textural characteristics of the end product determine which form of Simplesse is used.

IV. SENSORY PROPERTIES AND USE OF SIMPLESSE

For many consumers, the sensory properties of Simplesse products are probably more important than the substitution of protein for fat. Fat performs many functions in food. Fat solubilizes flavor components that are essential for good taste. Because of complex chemical and physical factors, lowering the fat content of food while fulfilling consumer expectations for flavor is a challenge.

Fat also provides texture, primarily creaminess. Smoothness is an important component of creaminess. People sense smoothness by rubbing the food between the tongue and the palate or between the tongue and the back of the teeth. The round shape and uniform size of the Simplesse protein particles allows them to roll easily over one another [11]. The tongue does not perceive the particles individually but rather as a creamy fluid with the smoothness and richness typically associated with fat.

In the mouth, particles that are too large are sensed as powdery or gritty. Particles that are too small are often perceived as gelatinous, slippery, or sticky with "insubstantial" mouthfeel [11]. Most consumers who have experimented with a variety of other reduced-fat products have experienced both of the above extremes in sensory perception.

Simplesse particles have the correct size and shape to provide the necessary sensory attributes in replacing fat. Simplesse can be used in the formulation of a wide variety of cooked and baked foods including cheesecakes, cakes, pie crusts, pie fillings, puddings, soups, and sauces. Sour cream, yogurt, and a variety of cheese products will soon be available throughout the country. Mayonnaise, salad dressings, dips, and spreads prepared with Simplesse are available in grocery stores or are in development.

Simplesse products can also be used in traditional home food preparation. Pizza and lasagna, for example, can be prepared substituting Simplesse cheeses for the usual high-fat cheeses. Baked potatoes can be topped with sour cream or microwaveable cheese sauce, both made with Simplesse. Many other creative alternatives are obviously possible.

V. IMPLICATIONS FOR HEALTH AND NUTRITION

The National Institutes of Health estimate that 100,000 lives could be saved per year if dietary fat intake were reduced [16]. The dietary guidelines recommended by the National Heart, Lung, and Blood Institute, the U.S. Departments of Health and Human Services and Agriculture, the American Dietetic Association, and the American Heart Association all state that no more than 30% of total calories should come from fat [1,17-19]. Studies indicate, however, that the average proportion of calories derived from fat is 36% for American men and 37% for American women [20-23]. Because products made with Simplesse provide the same good taste of foods high in fat, their availability may help people reduce their dietary fat intake and, therefore, reduce their risk for medical conditions such as obesity, atherosclerosis, and some types of cancer.

Replacement of unwanted fat in the diet with protein is an excellent nutritional exchange. The digestive pathways for fats, carbohydrates, and proteins differ in both the products and energy derived. The "energy content" of foods is expressed in calories, which is really a measure of heat. For example, when fats are metabolized, the energy or heat derived from 1 gram of fat is approximately 9 calories. Proteins and carbohydrates are digested by different reactions and "contain" less energy. One gram of either protein or carbohydrate is approximately equivalent to 4 calories [24]. Hence, the exchange of protein or carbohydrate for fat is an excellent way to reduce both caloric intake and the percentage of calories derived from fat.

Simplesse provides an additional caloric advantage. The proteins that make up Simplesse are hydrated during the manufacturing process so that the final caloric value is actually only 1-2 calories per gram. Therefore, the use of Simplesse results in a significant reduction in fat and a 50-80% reduction in calories in many products (Figs. 1,2). In those products where Simplesse replaces animal fat, a significant reduction in saturated fat and cholesterol content is also achieved.

Theoretically, if Simplesse were used in all products for which it is applicable, it would replace approximately 19% of total dietary fat, about 21% of dietary saturated fat, and approximately 9% of dietary cholesterol [25]. This would produce a theoretical reduction in total calories (from fat) from 37% to 30%, the proportion recommended by many health authorities.

Furthermore, there is no reason for concern that the maximal use of Simplesse would unbalance the diet by providing excessive protein. Research indicates that projected daily consumption of all product categories made with Simplesse, even by heavy users (i.e., those in the 90th percentile of consumption), would add an amount of protein approximately equal to that

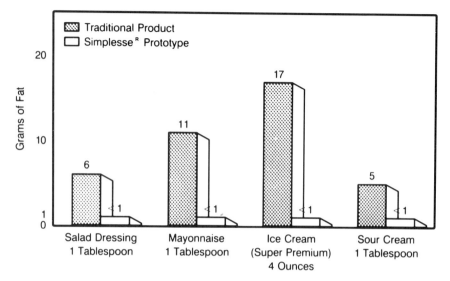

Figure 1   Role of Simplesse in fat reduction. (From Ref. 28 and Hazelton Laboratories.)

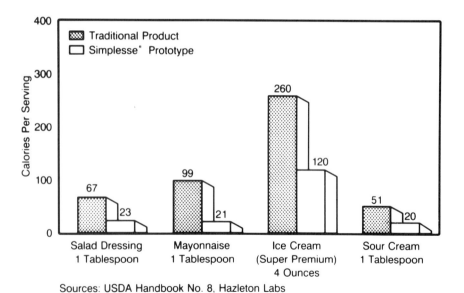

Figure 2   Role of Simplesse in calorie reduction. (From Ref. 28 and Hazelton Laboratories.)

present in 8 fluid ounces of milk [26]. Given normal daily fluctuations in dietary protein intake, this is an insignificant amount.

A comprehensive literature review of more than 5000 articles and a number of laboratory tests have identified no safety-related issues regarding the use of Simplese [6]. Evaluation of the protein quality of Simplesse has demonstrated that the microparticulation process does not alter the quality or nutritional value of the protein in the final product [8,13,15,27]. Microparticulation neither creates new proteins nor results in changes in protein structure or quality different from those that occur with conventional cooking [8,13,27].

When recommending Simplesse products as reduced-fat alternatives, health-care professionals should remember that people who are allergic to egg or milk proteins can be expected to be allergic to Simplesse made from those proteins. Studies of the antibody responses of patients allergic to cow's milk and/or egg proteins indicate that allergic individuals had no greater antibody response to proteins in the Simplesse samples than to the proteins from egg or cow's milk [14].

Experts recommend that to maintain good nutrition, people should focus on the total diet and eat a variety of foods. Simplesse cannot solve all of the problems with fat in the American diet. But by incorporating foods made with Simplesse as part of a well-balanced daily regime, individuals can reduce dietary fat intake without sacrificing taste and pleasure in a long-term strategy for successful dietary change.

VI. SUMMARY

Most health-care professionals believe that the high-fat American diet is a significant factor in the development of coronary heart disease, obesity, and some forms of cancer. While many consumers understand and agree with this message, they are unable to sustain long-term dietary changes. Exchanging high-fat food favorites for low-fat alternatives is frequently perceived as an unacceptable sacrifice in sensory enjoyment.

Most fat substitutes are made from carbohydrates. Only one available protein-based fat substitute has been approved by the FDA. Simplesse is an all natural fat substitute which replaces fat with nutritious protein from egg whites, skim milk, and/or whey. The microparticulated protein delivers the taste and texture of high-fat foods.

Foods made with Simplesse allow the consumer to lower dietary fat without sacrificing sensory quality. By incorporating Simplesse products into a balanced diet, consumers may be more successful in achieving dietary change without the feeling of sacrifice which appears to threaten the long-term success of dietary strategies.

REFERENCES

1. USDA, *Dietary Guidelines for Americans*, 3rd ed., U. S. Department of Health and Human Services, Washington, DC (1990).
2. A. Drewnowski. Dietary fats: Perceptions and preferences, *J. Am. Coll. Nutr.*, *9*: 431 (1990).
3. FDA, *Health and Diet Survey, 1988,* National Heart, Lung, and Blood Institute, Washington, DC (December 1988).
4. *Trends 1988: Consumer Attitudes and the Supermarket*, Food Marketing Institute, Washington, DC (1988).
5. F. Rose, If it feels good, it must be bad, *Fortune*, p. 91 (October 21, 1991).
6. Direct food substances affirmed as generally recognized as safe; microparticulated protein product, (CFR Part 184). *Fed. Reg., 55*: 6384 (February 23, 1990).
7. N. S. Singer, S. Yamamoto, and J. Latella, *Protein Product Base*, U. S. Patent 4,734,287 (March 29, 1988).
8. J. M. Dunn, N. Singer, and H. H. Chang, Electron microscopic characterization of microparticulared protein (Simplesse®). (Abstract). Presented at the Federation of American Societies for Experimental Biology (FASEB), New Orleans (March 1989).
9. M. Kalab, Microparticulate protein in foods. *J. Am. Coll. Nutr., 9*: 374 (1990).
10. N. S. Singer and J. M. Dunn, Protein microparticulation: The principle and the process, *J. Am. Coll. Nutr., 9*: 38 (1990).
11. G. V. Civille, The sensory properties of products made with microparticulated protein, *J. Am. Coll. Nutr., 9*: 427 (1990).
12. M. Kretchmer, Summary: Microparticulated protein. *J. Am. Coll. Nutr., 9*: 371 (1990).
13. R. Dudley, M. Dunn, J. Hjelle, F. Kotsoris, and B. Dickie, Microparticulation of protein in Simplesse® does not alter protein efficiency ratio. (Abstract). Presented at the Federation of American Societies for Experimental Biology (FASEB), New Orleans (March 1989).
14. H. A. Sampson and S. K. Cooke, Food allergy and the potential allergenicity-antigenicity of microparticulated egg and cow's milk proteins, *J. Am. Coll. Nutr., 9*: 410 (1990).
15. P. S. Tang, H. H. Chang, J. M. Dunn, and N. Singer, A gel electrophoretic study of microparticulated protein (Simplesse®), (Abstract). Presented at the Federation of American Societies for Experimental Biology (FASEB), New Orleans (March 1989).
16. The Expert Panel, Report of the National Cholesterol Education Program Expert Panel on detection, evaluation, and treatment of high blood cholesterol in adults, *Arch. Intern. Med., 148*: 36 (1988).
17. National Cholesterol Education Program, *Report of the Expert Panel on Population Strategies for Blood Cholesterol Reduction*, U.S. Department of Health and Human Services, Public Health Service, National Institutes of Health, National Heart, Lung, and Blood Institute, NIH Publication 90-3046, Bethesda, MD (November 1990).
18. Dietary guidelines for healthy American adults, A statement for physicians and health professionals by the Nutrition Committee, American Heart Association, *Circulation, 77*: 721A (1988).

19. ADA timely statement on Nutrition and Your Health: Dietary Guidelines for Americans, *ADA Rep., 90*: 1720 (1990).
20. Human Nutrition Information Service, *Nationwide food consumption survey: Continuing survey of food intakes by individuals. Women 19-50 and their children 1-5, 1 day,* U.S. Department of Agriculture, CSFII Report, No. 85-1, Hyattsville, MD (November 1985).
21. Human Nutrition Information Service *Nationwide food consumption survey: Continuing survey of food intakes by individuals. Men 19-50, 1 day,* U.S. Department of Agriculture, CSFII Report, No. 85-3, Hyattsville, MD (1985).
22. Human Nutrition Information Service, *Nationwide food consumption survey,* U.S. Department of Agriculture, CSFII Report, No. 85-4, Hyattsville, MD (1985).
23. Human Nutrition Information Service, *Nationwide food consumption survey,* U.S. Department of Agriculture, CSFII Report, No. 86-3, Hyattsville, MD (1986).
24. L. Stryer, Part III: Generation and Storage of Metabolic Energy, *Biochemistry,* 3rd ed., W. H. Freeman & Co., New York, pp. 313–544 (1988).
25. The NutraSweet Company, Deerfield, IL. Data on file, Calculated from NHANES II data.
26. Market Research Corporation of America (MRCA) Survey, Data on file, The NutraSweet Company, Deerfield, IL.
27. J. W. Erdman, The quality of microparticulated protein, *J. Am. Coll. Nutr., 9*: 398 (1990).
28. USDA, Composition of foods: Raw, processed, and prepared, *Agriculture Handbook No. 8*, U.S. Government Printing Office, Washington, DC (1963).

10
Fat Substitutes: Sucrose Polyesters and Other Synthetic Oils

Kathleen A. Harrigan and William M. Breene   *University of Minnesota, St. Paul, Minnesota*

I. INTRODUCTION

A. Overview

Other chapters described the importance of reducing the consumption of fat calories in the American diet from a current level of 37% to 30% of total calories. Dietary fat reduction can be achieved by consuming a balanced diet that limits the amount of fat calories ingested. However, most consumers are looking for convenient low-calorie alternatives that are tasty and healthy. The food industry has responded with a plethora of new food products and even some new foods, so let us begin with definitions for both.

Foods such as fruits, vegetables, and meats are naturally complete biological entities that are basically unadulterated except where some form of processing has been used to preserve them, in which case chemical and structural changes may occur (e.g., canned peaches, frozen broccoli). Fat in foods can be reduced by genetic manipulation, as in lean red meat and low-cholesterol poultry, or by limiting the introduction of fat during processing in the plant (lean ground beef, 1% milk) or in the home (broiled skinless chicken, unbuttered popcorn). Methods of reducing fat and cholesterol in meat and dairy foods were recently reported [1] and are reviewed in Chapters 12 and 17.

Food products, on the other hand, can be seen as mixtures of distinct chemical compounds (proteins, carbohydrates, lipids, water) blended and processed together to achieve a desired flavor, texture, and/or caloric profile. Look at almost any manufactured food product label and you will see a dizzying array of food constituents. Limiting the fat in food products can be accomplished by reducing the amount of fat used in the formulation and/ or by substituting a fatlike compound for the real thing. Both of these methods can reduce fat levels, but they create flavor, texture, and functionality problems that must be overcome. For example, reduced fat in cheese was initially accomplished by lowering the amount of fat and adding more water, a formulation unacceptable to most consumers because the product lacked richness. No matter how you rearrange it, water does not feel like fat, and low-calorie cheese will not be eaten if it doesn't taste right. However, the tongue can be fooled. If we are to reduce the amount and types of fat in our diet, we must know what functions lipids serve, how they interact with other food components, and how they can be replaced or substituted and still achieve a quality product.

Reduced-calorie formulations can be achieved by extending the properties of traditional ingredients such as air, oils, gums, starches, and proteins [2–4]. The types of fat replacers currently employed and researched can be classified into three groups: protein-based substitutes (e.g., Simplesse) (see Chapter 9), oil compounds, and carbohydrate-based substitutes (see Chapter 11). These categories can be confusing, because some synthetic oils have carbohydrate backbones and some carbohydrate-based substitutes are known as bulking agents. Ingredients in each of the three categories have been referred to as fat substitutes, fat replacers, fat analogs, and fat mimics, and the products they are added to range from fat-free to calorie-reduced types [5,6]. However, this nomenclature does not clearly distinguish between the types of fat substitutes, some of which have GRAS status (Simplesse®, Maltrin®, N-Oil®, Stellar), others of which are awaiting FDA spproval (olestra, Trailblazer). The rapid proliferation of fat-reduced food products has certainly given consumers healthier options, but it has also created confusion about labeling standards, concern about long-term fat-free eating patterns, and fear about synthetic ingredients completely replacing real food [7,8].

The fat substitutes discussed in this chapter will focus on the synthetic oil compounds and specifically on sucrose polyesters (SPEs). SPEs are nonabsorbable and, therefore, noncaloric polymers that can be used in all types of food products (frozen and heated) and thus constitute true fat replacement —functional fat without the calories. Although they are not considered a separate class of food compounds, final FDA approval of any synthetic oils (none of which have yet been approved) may warrant such a classification. Since most of the research on SPEs has focused on Procter & Gamble's product called olestra, much of the section on SPEs refers specifically to olestra, even though it was originally called sucrose octaester. There are other sucrose-based synthetic oils (e.g., Colestra™), but information on them is considered proprietary until FDA approves olestra.

B. Lipids and Fatty Acids

The terms "fats" and "oils" have been used interchangeably with "lipids" to describe that complex group of substances [9,10]. The term lipid refers to a naturally occurring heterogeneous class of compounds insoluble in water but soluble in hydrocarbon solvents. Included in this group are large high molecular weight alcohols, such as cholesterol and its esters, as well as phospholipids, steroids, and terpenes. Also included are dietary fats and oils, esters of glycerol, and carboxylic acids (acyl lipids) generally containing an even number of 4–20 carbon atoms in an unbranched chain. Carboxylic acids were first isolated from fats, which led to the use of the term fatty acid. Acids found in fats (solids) are mostly saturated (no double bonds), while those in oils (liquids) tend to be unsaturated with one or more double bonds.

The behavior of a lipid is determined by the chemistry and structure of its predominant fatty acids, specifically by chain length, degree of saturation, and polymorphic or crystalline form. The importance of the first two features will become apparent when fat substitution using synthetic oil is discussed. Chain length is characteristic of the fatty acid source. For example, short-chain acids predominate in the milk fats of ruminants and in coconut and palm kernel oils. A diverse mixture of long-chain acids occurs in fish oils, while monounsaturated acids are predominant in olive oil. These characteristics directly affect the melting properties of a lipid; unsaturated fatty acids impart melting points consistent with their degree of unsaturation because double bonds cause bends (*cis* conformation) in the fatty acid chains making association between the chains difficult, resulting in lower melting points. The double-bond carbons of unsaturated fatty acids can be hydrogenated (saturated with hydrogen atoms) to convert liquid oil into solid fat, as in the case of margarine, which may contain partially hydrogenated fats. Saturated fats are solid at room and body temperatures and have higher melting points because straight chains of fatty acids align themselves into crystalline structures. The beta-crystalline form has a high degree of order, which makes the crystals relatively large and thermally stable. With the introduction of double bonds, the melting point decreases.

Triglycerides—glycerol esters of fatty acids—account for 90% of the lipids in our diet, and they exist in naturally occurring fats and oils as mixtures of simple and mixed fatty acid residues. Simple triglycerides contain three identical fatty acids, whereas mixed triglycerides have more than one fatty acid species. Not only are the fatty acids mixed, they occur in relative proportions at positions 1, 2, and 3 on the triglyceride molecule, depending on the lipid. Lard has a definite tendency for unsaturated fatty acids to occupy the outer positions of the triglyceride, whereas the reverse is true for cocoa butter. The choices of fatty acid, chain length, and degree of saturation are important in most food formulations but especially in those requiring fat substitution in order to achieve a desirable pattern of physical properties.

C. Functionality

Aside from their essential nature in the diet, fats and oils are highly valued for two critical properties—satiety and flavor. Due to their high energy content, lipids produce a feeling of fullness because it takes more time to hydrolyze, emulsify, and transport them across intestinal membranes; by slowing down the emptying rate of the stomach, the early recurrence of hunger can be prevented [11]. Food products with fat replacement should provide the same level of satiety as full-fat systems.

Flavor is probably the most highly regarded quality of fat in the diet because lipids contribute to mouthfeel, aroma, and texture by providing creaminess, richness, aroma precursors, and flavor retention to food and food products. Fatty acids form volatile flavor compounds via beta oxidation, hydroxyacid cleavage, and oxidation by lipoxygenase enzymes. While the primary products of these pathways include aldehydes and ketones, various oxidations, reductions, and esterifications also yield substantial quantities of acids, alcohols, lactones, and esters [12]. Many of these flavor compounds are formed or released during fermentation by microbial action (e.g., dairy products and alcoholic beverages) and during processing (e.g., deep-fat fried foods) and ripening (e.g., pears, bananas, peaches).

Lipids are not only important for flavor, they are essential in many product formulations because of their ability to tenderize, to aerate doughs or batters, to serve as heating and frying media, to act as separating agents, to emulsify, to control viscosity, smoothness, and texture, to stabilize foams, to provide structure, to improve moisture retention, and to act as carriers for pigments and vitamins. Bakery products, for example, require shortening for tenderness/flakiness, and whole eggs contribute to leavening in the creaming process. Replacements for shortening and eggs such as oil and egg whites and/or the addition of fiber must deliver comparable functional attributes in order for the products to perform under normal processing conditions and to guarantee a desirable end product. In each of these functional applications, the fat ingredient must also possess the proper chemical structure, ionization and solubility characteristics. In emulsions, hydrophilic and lipophilic compounds must be balanced to avoid separation of compounds within a food product. A systematic approach to fat-reduced product development was recently reported [13].

II. SUCROSE POLYESTERS

A. Definitions

Sucrose polyesters (SPEs) and sucrose esters (SEs) are synthesized by esterifying sucrose with long- and short-chain fatty acids from vegetable oil sources that may be saturated or unsaturated. As esterification proceeds from the mono- to an octaester form, the originally hydrophilic compound becomes increasingly lipophilic (Table 1). The nature of the polymer can be altered by changing the constituent fatty acids; the shorter and more unsaturated they are, the more hydrophilic the molecule becomes. These two variables—the degree of esterification and fatty acid type—provide SPEs with their different functionalities and physicochemical properties. Sucrose polyesters are not a completely new class of food additives since the lower esters (mono-, di-, and tri-) have been used in foods for some time as emulsifiers. However, use of the higher esters (hexa-, hepta-, and octa-) as fat substitutes in foods may prove to be the most versatile and significant application.

Table 1 Some Properties of Sucrose Polyesters Associated with Esterification Level

Sucrose	Esterification level							
	Mono	Di	Tri	Tetra	Penta	Hexa	Hepta	Octa
Hydrophilic	More hydrophilic → More lipophilic							→
	More sugarlike → More fatlike							→
Digestible	Digestible →						
	Not digestible or absorbable →						
Absorbable	Absorbable →						

Source: Ref. 21. By permission of American Association of Cereal Chemists, St. Paul, MN.

1. Sucrose

Sucrose itself is unique in its physical and chemical properties. It is a nonreducing disaccharide that is extremely stable except to hydrolysis at the glycoside linkage. The sucrose moiety, consisting of glucose and fructose (Fig. 1), can be esterified at eight positions giving ample opportunity for substitution. It is highly soluble in water, is the least expensive polyhydric alcohol readily available, and has the world's highest production of any single pure organic chemical [14]. Sucrose and its by-products have been used to make ethanol, butanol, and acetone by fermentation. Wallboard and paper come from sugarcane bagasse, which has also served as a raw material for furfural production [15]. Of the eight hydroxyl groups of sucrose, three are primary (C1', C6', C6) and five are secondary; the primary hydroxyl groups are about 10 times more reactive than the secondary hydroxyls [16] (see Figure 1).

Initially, the most reactive sites were determined to be the C6 position of glucose, with appreciable substitution at C4 of glucose and C1' of fructose [17]. However, more recent studies have concluded that C6, C6', and C1' are the most reactive sites with C1' of minor importance due to steric hindrance [18]. Research on the cyclic acetals of sucrose and their derivatives has allowed selective reactions with previously inaccessible hydroxyl groups, specifically at C2, C3, C3', and C4' [19].

2. Lower Esters

The lower esters are generally referred to as sucrose esters and are not fat substitutes since the mono-, di-, and triesters are digested by pancreatic li-

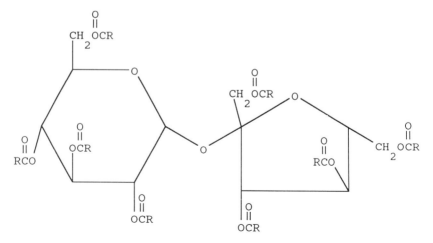

Figure 1 Sucrose moiety with all eight hydroxyl groups esterified.

pase and therefore absorbed. Due to their hydrophilic nature, SEs are used primarily as emulsifiers but are also used as lubricants for producing tablet candy in molds, as anticaking agents in dry soup mixes, as viscosity reducers in chocolate manufacturing, and as inhibitors of heat-resistant, spore-forming bacteria in hot canned drinks sold in vending machines [20]. The history and synthesis of SEs and SPEs occurred simultaneously, and even though this chapter focuses on fat substitutes, the lower esters will be included briefly for the sake of accuracy. Additional information on SEs can be obtained from a 1989 review by the authors [21].

3. Higher Esters

Olestra, a product developed by Procter & Gamble and formerly known as sucrose polyester, is the common name for the mixture of hexa-, hepta-, and octaesters formed by the esterification of sucrose with long-chain fatty acids derived from edible oils. Olestra is typically comprised of greater than

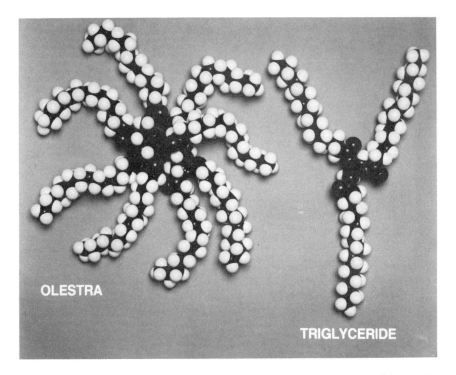

Figure 2 Molecular models of olestra and triglyceride. (Reproduced with permission of the Procter & Gamble Company.)

80% octaesters and less than 0.1% lower esters. Figure 2 illustrates the structure of a sucrose octaester (olestra) with all eight hydroxyl groups substituted by fatty acids and the structure of glycerol with three fatty acids (a traditional triglyceride). By way of clarification, in studies on sucrose polyesters cited in this chapter, the compounds are identified either as SPEs or olestra, depending on the name used by the investigators. Most of the work done on SPEs in the past 20 years has focused on olestra.

B. History

The concept of SE/SPE production in the United States was probably initiated in 1952 when Henry Hass, then president of the Sugar Research Foundation, urged Foster D. Snell to investigate the possibility of "hanging a fat tail" on sucrose to make detergents [22]. Due to the hydrophilic nature of sucrose and the lipophilic nature of fatty acids, the esterified derivatives could act as surfactants. It was hoped that the new product would be easily synthesized and purified, produced at a reasonable cost, and biodegradable under both aerobic and anaerobic conditions.

1. Sugar Research Foundation

The Sugar Research Foundation (SRF), established in the United States in 1954, made efforts to expand the applications of sucrose other than as a sweetener. Foster D. Snell initially responded to the inquiry of Henry Hass by interesterifying sucrose with methyl esters of fatty acids in the presence of an alkaline catalyst, using as the solvent dimethylformamide (DMF), in which both sucrose and fatty acids are sufficiently soluble. The Snell process was patented in 1959 [23] and assigned to the Sugar Research Foundation. A similar process for preparing fatty acid esters of nonreducing oligosaccharides was patented by Procter & Gamble Co. in 1958 [24–26]. Also in 1958, a chemist from Dainippon Sugar Mfg. Co. Ltd. (parent to the Ryoto Co. Ltd.) negotiated a license with SRF for the Snell process; SE was approved as a food additive in Japan in 1959.

It is interesting to note that industrialization of SEs has occurred in Japan, which is totally dependent on imports of the main raw materials, sugar and edible fats, and whose per capita consumption of emulsifiers is lower than that of Europe or of the United States [27]. Japan is the largest producer of SEs with 70% of the world's sales [28]. The Snell process was licensed in 20 foreign countries, including Germany, France, Italy, and Brazil, for the manufacture of surfactants [29] and sucroglycerides [30]. SEs were recommended for general admission within the "horizontal" European Economic Community in 1974; in 1980 FAO/WHO gave SEs permanent approval. In 1983,

FDA permitted the use of sucrose fatty acid (lower) esters as additives in the U.S. market.

2. Procter & Gamble

Fred Mattson and Robert Volpenhein, who had been conducting basic research on the absorption of fats since 1948 at Procter & Gamble, analyzed the ability of intestinal lipases (lipase and nonspecific lipase) to cleave fatty acid esters of various sugars. In 1968 they worked on the relative digestibility and absorbability of fats and related compounds for the purpose of developing formulas for premature infants. By altering the alcohol backbone instead of the fatty acid groups, they determined in vitro that the rate of lipase-catalyzed hydrolysis was dependent on the number of fatty acids. Hydrolysis increased as the oleic acid esterified polyol size increased from one (methanol) to three (glycerol), but hydrolysis dramatically decreased to almost zero as the polyol size increased from six (sorbitol) to eight (sucrose) [30]. Subsequent investigations with octa-esterified sucrose showed that it was not hydrolyzed by gastric or pancreatic lipases and that it was not absorbed from the intestinal tract [31,32]. The dual attributes of nonhydrolysis and nonabsorption paved the way for the noncaloric group of octaesters, later called olestra.

The original patent for "Low Calorie Fat-Containing Food Compositions" was granted to Procter & Gamble in 1971 [33] based on the work of Mattson and Volpenhein. After several decades of laboratory and clinical research on nonabsorbability, calorie and cholesterol reduction, physical and chemical properties, nutrient absorption, and other safety issues (all of which will be covered in this chapter), Procter & Gamble petitioned FDA in April 1987 to approve olestra as a food additive. The petition included 20,000 pages of data from more than 100 animal studies and more than 25 clinical trials. The original petition requested that olestra be used as a replacement for up to 35% of the fat in cooking oils and shortenings for home use and up to 75% of the fat used in commercial deep-fat fryers and in fried snack foods. In August 1990, Procter & Gamble narrowed its food additive petition to 100% olestra substitution for conventional fats (instead of 75%) in the preparation of savory snacks only, deferring the retail and food service use of shortenings and oils. In the petition, savory snacks include flavored and unflavored vegetable chips and crisps (e.g., corn, potatoes) and flavored and unflavored extruded snacks. Even though it is physically possible to incorporate olestra in a variety of foods such as margarine, ice cream, and cheese, these applications will require separate FDA approval.

Although Procter & Gamble's original SPE patent expired in 1988, attorneys for the company are seeking a 10-year extension on four individual patents for olestra, citing the precedent set by Congress in 1982 when it enacted a patent extension measure for aspartame [34]. Reasons for the patent extension include the diligent and lengthy petition review process and the importance of adequate testing for a substance that is more like a new drug than a food additive. The FDA has agreed that olestra is unique in that it is a macroingredient and also pointed out that the average time for approval of usual food additives is 5 years [34].

C. Industrial Production

SEs/SPEs can be synthesized in the laboratory by various means, but certain methodologies do not lend themselves to commercial production. Over time, the synthesis of SPEs has evolved from a solvent method to a solventless process. Purification procedures, quality and availability of raw materials, and projected costs are important aspects of delivering SPEs as fat substitutes to the marketplace. If and when FDA grants olestra clearance, public acceptance of the product will depend on such factors as palatability, safety, cost, and consumers' overwhelming desire to reduce fat intake.

1. Solvent Processes

The Snell process for nonionic surfactants [35,36], described earlier, was an interesterification reaction in a homogeneous system whereby the solvent (DMF) was mutual for both the sucrose and the fatty acids. However, DMF had an offensive odor and left a toxic nitrogen residue in the esters; as a result, FDA set a zero-tolerance level for DMF and did not permit SPE produced by the Snell process to be used in edible food products. In the 1960s, two significant process improvements were introduced: formation of a microemulsion and a heterogeneous reaction mixture, which favors one compound. The state of Nebraska cooperated with the laboratories of Foster D. Snell in an attempt to use surplus raw materials, particularly sugar beets and tallow. In the Nebraska-Snell process [37,38], sucrose was dissolved in a single solvent, propylene glycol, and methyl esters of selected fatty acids were added, with potassium carbonate as catalyst. A microemulsion was formed after the mixture was vigorously stirred, and as the propylene glycol was distilled off, complete conversion of the methyl esters occurred. This method was improved upon by a Japanese company that succeeded in industrializing it by using water instead of propylene glycol as the solvent [27].

2. Solventless Processes

In 1970, workers in the USDA Southern Regional Research Laboratory developed a solvent-free method [39,40] by interesterifying molten sucrose and methyl esters of fatty acids with the aid of potassium and sodium soaps as catalysts and solubilizers. The soaps and types of fatty acid esters used differed markedly in performance and yield of SPE. Rizzi and Taylor [41,42] refined the process further by employing a two-stage reaction sequence to improve the conversion level of sucrose. The first stage involves a 3:1 molar ratio of methyl esters to sucrose to form a one-phase melt containing lower esters of sucrose; in the second stage, additional methyl esters are added to produce SPEs with a distribution of 70% octaester, 25% heptaester, and 5% hexaester in yields up to 90% based on sucrose. In 1985, two more patents were issued to Procter & Gamble for work by Robert Volpenhein using potassium carbonate as a reaction catalyst [43] and for developing optimum soap to polyol ratios [44].

3. Purification

According to Spinner [45], the starting material for olestra will directly influence the efficiency of the reaction and will determine the extent of the post-process cleanup. High quality and fully refined sucrose and triglycerides are essential. The fatty acids are converted to methyl esters by reacting them with methanol using either sodium or potassium methoxide as a catalyst and the glycerol by-product is then removed by settling. The crude reaction products of olestra synthesis are purified before the material can be directly substituted for conventional oils. The standard edible oil refining process is employed. Olestra esterification specified 70–95% octaesters with a lower ester content of not more than 0.1%. Residual levels of starting material in the finished product are designated not to exceed 1000 ppm of methyl esters and 10 ppm of methanol, in addition to all the traditional impurity specifications for fats and oils.

4. Market Analysis

Salzman and Ostroff [46] estimated the size of the nonbeverage diet food market to be $750 million to $1 billion annually at retail, including snack foods, nutrient products, and frozen dinners. In a National Food Review study [47], the market potential for fat substitutes was determined by two factors: the size of the product markets in which fat substitutes are used and the fat content of the products. Figures based on 1987–88 data showed that baking/frying fats and salad/cooking oils accounted for 98% of the over 14 billion pounds of fats and oils produced annually. Most of this was used by cookie makers, snack food companies, and other food processors that make mayonnaise and dressings. Baking/frying fats and salad/cooking oils average 100% fat content and, when combined with mayonnaise at 80% fat content, represent a fat substitute market that could potentially replace over 13 billion pounds of traditional fats and oils used annually in these products. Annual production of selected dairy products totaled more than 12 billion pounds, with most of it at retail, and a total potential replacement market for fat substitutes of 2.8 billion pounds.

The ability of fat substitutes to replace existing low-fat items or to expand the popularity of low-fat foods depends on several factors—FDA approval, the substitutes' quality and versatility, marketing strategies, and the strength of consumer demand and willingness to pay for reduced-fat products. Estimates on the cost of fat substitutes by assessing their raw material and processing costs (excluding research and development) placed existing starch-based substitutes in the low-cost group at $1/lb or less, the undigestible fats at $1–2/lb, and Simplesse at $2–3/lb; by comparison refined soybean oil sells at 20–30 cents/lb and milk fat costs about $1.35 [47].

Even though Procter & Gamble has changed its initial food additive petition from partial substitution in cooking oils to total replacement in savory snacks, concerns voiced by the National Renderers Association [48] could become an issue if and when the original petition is resubmitted. The rendering industry collects and refines 2.5 billion pounds of spent oil annually from fast food restaurants, selling 95% of it as a high-calorie, low-cost feeding fat to the animal feed industry. But dilution with olestra reduces the caloric value of the rendered oil, which may eliminate it from feed formulations and consequently raise production costs in the feed industries as well as putting many renderers out of business. A quick assay for olestra content may be necessary and the cost of chemical separation could be prohibitive.

Possibly the largest concern is the disposal of spent oil if it is not collected by renderers, since currently there is no place to legally dispose of such large quantities. Could olestra be rejuvenated by a bleaching and/or deodorizing process and reused? The U.S. Environmental Protection Agency is examining the environmental impact aspects of introducing olestra into the food supply, since it is not clear how its presence in wastewater will influence sewage treatment processes; although olestra is excreted unmetabolized in the feces, it was reported to adsorb onto sewage sludge where it was degraded by aerobic bacteria [49].

D. Properties

1. Functionality

Since each SPE molecule has six to eight fatty acids, one would expect it to exhibit properties similar to traditional fats. By modifying the fatty acid chain length and degree of saturation, SPEs could conceivably be tailor-made to simulate fat in baked and fried foods, frozen products, cooking oils, margarine, shortening, and dairy foods. Functionally, they could be used in the same food applications as triglycerides to replace fat calories without sacrificing taste, texture, color, mouthfeel, satiety, shelf life, or convenience. However, the literature does not contain much information on the physical and chemical properties of SPEs.

The physical properties of nine sucrose octaesters of homogeneous fatty acid makeup were reported in 1978 [50] and included polymorphism, melting point, molecular weight, heat of fusion, refractive index, viscosity, density, and interfacial tension. Mattson and coworkers [51] reported that SPE was completely miscible with triglycerides and insoluble in water; mixtures of water, triglycerides, and SPEs separated into water and oil phases, the latter containing triglycerides and SPEs. In formulating SPE-vegetable oil blends for margarine, shortening, and cooking oils, Procter & Gamble claims that olestra is completely miscible with fats containing the same fatty acid side chains.

An early version of SPEs [52] contained some high-melting fatty acids from soybean oil. Subjects reported that many of the food items containing SPEs had a waxy or greasy feel or taste due to their semisolid consistency at room temperature. A reformulated SPE with safflower oil fatty acids remained liquid at room temperature and had the appearance and consistency of corn oil [53]. A mixture of this SPE (80%) and hydrogenated palm oil (20%), when included in a diet, was accepted better by human subjects.

For clinical studies conducted since then, SPEs were incorporated into margarinelike spreads, olestra-butter blends, and mayonnaiselike salad dressings with appearance and texture apparently identical to those made with traditional fats; subjects ingesting SPE blends and placebos were not able to distinguish between them. According to Procter & Gamble sensory data, the organoleptic qualities of fats and olestra substituted with the same fatty acids are virtually indistinguishable from one another, and by adjusting the fatty acid composition, olestras can be formulated for many different applications.

The rate of olestra and olestra-soybean oil polymerization under food service frying conditions was identical with that of triglycerides. Cross-linking at unsaturation points on the fatty acid side chains was identical, regardless of the backbone structure [54]. Linoleic acid appeared to be the major contributor in the polymerization process.

The similarity of physical properties between SPEs and traditional fats and oils ends in the digestive tract, which is why olestra and other fat substitutes as well as dietary fiber are such important compounds. SPEs are not enzymatically hydrolyzed in the lumen. When Mattson and Volpenhein [30] first discovered these compounds, they stated that it was tempting to invoke steric hindrance as an explanation for the inability of lipase to hydrolyze them.

Initial nondigestibility studies led researchers to investigate numerous related properties such as nonabsorbability, cholesterol lowering, calorie reduction, and bioavailability. Health and safety risk and benefits of these properties have been the focus of extensive investigations for years [55,56].

2. Nonabsorbability

The pioneering work of Mattson and Volpenhein [30,31] and Mattson and Nolen [32] provided evidence that enzyme-catalyzed hydrolysis was indeed the obligatory first step before absorption of lipid components could occur. The belief that some emulsified but unhydrolyzed triglyceride droplets could be absorbed from the intestine proved to be false when these workers discovered that the unhydrolyzed larger polyols were not absorbed. It is now generally agreed that absorption requires hydrolysis of fats by the action of lipases, producing fatty acids and monoglycerides which form mixed micelles with bile salts for transport to the intestinal cells.

Typically, intestinal emulsion after a meal contains lipid material dissolved as fat droplets in an oil phase and an aqueous phase containing bile salt micelles. The fat droplets combine with bile salts to become more soluble so that lipases can hydrolyze the triglycerides to fatty acids and monoglycerides. Ordinarily, as triglyceride hydrolysis proceeds, the oil phase disappears as these lipolytic end products are transported to the micellar aqueous phase and then absorbed. However, if the oil phase cannot be hydrolyzed and subsequently absorbed, it moves down the intestine and out of the body. This has been described as the "solvent effect" of SPE, a persistent oil phase that remains undydrolyzed and is excreted from the system intact. The solvent effect also inhibits intestinal absorption of other lipids such as cholesterol and fat-soluble vitamins; they will be discussed in the following sections.

Fatty acid absorption studies on SPEs using fat balance techniques in rats [32] showed that the compounds with one, two, or three ester groups hydrolyzed rapidly, those with four or five esters digested more slowly, and those with six or eight ester groups were not hydrolyzed. This experiment correlated well with the earlier in vitro hydrolysis study using preparations of pancreatic juice [30]. Since water-insoluble fatty acids enter the body by way of the thoracic duct, the appearance of these substances in the thoracic duct lymph afforded another technique by which the absorption of lipid-soluble material can be measured as a function of time. The cumulative recoveries in 24 hours of radiolabeled acids fed to rats as esters of various polyols were 88% from glycerol, 67% from erythritol, 24% from xylitol, and 2% from sucrose [31], all of which were in good agreement with the fat balance study. These two methods—fat balance and thoracic duct lymph—showed that compounds containing more than three ester groups were incompletely absorbed and that absorption continued to decrease as the number of ester groups increased.

Pancreatic amylase activity in rats consuming high levels of SPEs (16%) resembled that of rats eating a low-fat diet in which energy was derived from carbohydrate and protein, indicating that the pancreas responded to SPE as a nonnutritive ingredient rather than as a digestible lipid [57]. Olestra was also found not to be metabolized by colonic microflora under anaerobic conditions [58].

Cortot et al [59] demonstrated in human subjects that when ingested as part of an ordinary mixed meal, water and fat have different patterns of emptying, with water leaving the stomach first. A second study by the same workers [60] showed that the SPEs were emptied very rapidly and at about the same rate as water. These results implied that gastric emptying of the oil phase was controlled by receptors sensitive to the hydrolytic products of fat digestion (with SPEs and water there are none) and that the slow emptying of dietary fat was not simply due to its lower density.

3. Laxative Effect

One of the most publicized issues regarding olestra has been oil loss or anal leakage of SPEs at high dosage levels. Fifty grams of SPE, either substituted for the same amount of ordinary fat in the diet or added to the base diet, induced a laxative side effect in several subjects [52]. SPE was reformulated because research with rats had shown that oil loss could be prevented by using palmitic or longer chain saturated fatty acids introduced in a form that made the saturated acids unabsorbable [53]. Completely hydrogenated palm oil (HPO) fulfilled these requirements. When introduced into the diet as a portion of the SPE, as much as 50 g/day of SPE were consumed without leakage [53]. This formulation has been used in subsequent studies conducted by Procter & Gamble to provide stiffening of fecal fat and to control oil loss. A Procter & Gamble patent [61] for "Compositions for Treating Hypercholesterolemia" included the addition of saturated fatty acids to prevent a laxative side effect. SPE-containing saturated fatty acids would not appear to be in conflict with current health recommendations for lowering saturated fat intake, since SPEs are neither digested nor absorbed.

SPE/oil loss can also be viewed as an efective laxative. Subjects in several cholesterol studies who were previously constipated experienced temporary relief and/or more frequent bowel movements and loose stools. Procter & Gamble holds a patent on "Compositions for Inhibiting Absorption of Cholesterol" [62] relating to a stool-softening formula for use particularly by obese or hypercholesterolemic patients. The estimated size of the laxative market is approximately $500 million at retail [47], but Procter & Gamble has not submitted a new drug application to FDA for this use of SPE.

4. Cholesterol Reduction

Since the distribution coefficient of cholesterol between a micellar phase and an oil phase of either triglyceride or SPE was the same, and since these fats were alike in their capacity to dissolve cholesterol, it was reasoned that they had the same potential for influencing the absorption of cholesterol. Yet the two lipids were not alike in their abilities to contribute to the micellar phase because SPE did not supply monoglycerides and free fatty acids via hydrolysis for the formation of mixed micelles with bile salts. Because SPE was neither digested nor absorbed, Mattson and coworkers in 1975 hypothesized that its presence in the lumen of the intestinal tract acted as a persistent oil phase and therefore a portion of the luminal cholesterol should dissolve in SPE and not be absorbed.

Cholesterol-reduction studies involving analysis of both blood and feces have shown that dietary SPE inhibits or interferes with cholesterol absorption and enhances fecal excretion of neutral sterols [52,53,57,61–75]. Blood serum total and LDL cholesterol levels were reduced by up to 20% in either case when SPE was included in the diets. As a consequence, Procter & Gamble was issued several patents on the pharmaceutical use of SPE for cholesterol reduction [61,62] but has not submitted a new drug application for this use of SPE.

5. Calorie Reduction and Obesity

With the assurance that SPE was neither hydrolyzed nor absorbed but was excreted from the system intact, the possibility of SPE as a weight-reduction tool appeared promising. Glueck and coworkers [76] designed a study to determine whether SPE reduced total caloric intake when covertly substituted for traditional dietary fats under double-blind conditions of free food choice. In the SPE study period, 40 g of SPE replaced 40 g of traditional fat for every 1200 cal of mandatory intake, covertly deleting 30% of mealtime calories and allowing subjects to freely choose non-SPE food items at snacktime to compensate for the covert caloric dilution. The SPE was administered in three different forms—as an oil in salad dressings and other recipes, as a 54% SPE bread spread, and as an SPE emulsion milk-shake type beverage. The average daily weight loss was 0.18 kg, and mean total caloric intake (meal and snack) fell 23% during the SPE period. There was no difference in snack calorie intake between test periods and no significant increase in snack caloric density. The subjects failed to compensate for the dilution of fat calories, and the subjective hunger data revealed that they did not feel more hungry when consuming SPE. It was concluded that SPE, by providing the taste, bulk, and consistency of a high-fat, high-calorie diet without the calories, was promising as a dietary treatment of obesity but that long-term studies were necessary to determine the efficacy of SPE substitution.

Crouse and Grundy [63] examined the effects of SPE on saturation of gallbladder bile. Since previous work had shown that caloric restriction in obese subjects may enhance saturation of bile and consequently increase the risk of cholesterol gallstones, it was suggested that SPE might reduce saturation of gallbladder bile by decreasing cholesterol absorption because a potential source of biliary cholesterol is absorption from the intestine. Their results revealed that the mean saturation level of gallbladder bile decreased but not significantly, although a greater reduction might have been achieved with a higher cholesterol level in the basal diet. It appeared unlikely that the addition of SPE accentuated the risk of gallstones in patients already on reduced calorie diets. Procter & Gamble received a patent in 1981 for "Gallstone Dissolution Compositions and Methods" [77], which described various treatments of gallstones including surgical removal, bile acid therapy, and bile acid binding with chenodeoxycholic acid (CDCA) and ursodeoxycholic acid (UDCA).

6. Vitamin Availability

Many cholesterol-lowering studies also monitored fat-soluble vitamin losses [52,53,63,68,71–73]. The initial SPE cholesterol study in humans [52] reported the first signs of lowered plasma vitamin A and E levels due to the same mechanism that decreased the absorption of cholesterol and reduced the levels of plasma cholesterol—the solvent effect of SPE. Both the normolipidemic men and the hypercholesterolemic women in the study responded to the addition or substitution of SPE in their diets with significantly lowered levels of vitamin A (10%) and E (21%). In the six subjects studied for 10 days after cessation of SPE ingestion, plasma vitamin A and E levels returned to pre-SPE baseline levels. Subsequent investigations confirmed the SPE effect of lowering the levels of plasma vitamin A [53,68,71,72,78,79] and vitamin E [53,63,71–73,79] as well as those of vitamin D [71,73] and K [71]. Other studies showed little if any effect of dietary SPE on levels of plasma vitamin A [63,73], E [68], D [53,80], or K [72,73,81].

At the Calorie Control Council meeting in February 1990, a Procter & Gamble official reported on these vitamin studies by concluding that although olestra caused a slight reduction in absorption of vitamin D_2, it did not affect overall vitamin D status because that level was primarily determined by sunlight, with only 15% coming from the diet; additionally, other studies showed no effect on absorption of vitamin A or K. However, he stated that the fat substitute would be supplemented with one milligram of vitamin E per gram of olestra because a small decrease in vitamin E absorption occurred with olestra ingestion and because vitamin E is normally found in vegetable oils [82].

7. Effects on Other Lipophiles

Because lipid absorption is facilitated by transport in bile-salt micelles, removal of cholesterol and fat-soluble vitamins from the micellar phase by SPE inhibited the absorption of these compounds and increased their excretion. However, SPEs did not reduce the absorption of all lipophilic substances; as reported in several studies, the absorption of triglycerides and their lipolytic products—fatty acids and monoglycerides—were unchanged by SPE ingestion. But results using a representative halogenated hydrocarbon—DDT (dichlorodiphenyltricholorethane)—suggested that SPEs might reduce the absorption of undesirable dietary lipophiles such as halogenated herbicides and pesticides that are either chronically absorbed trace contaminants of foods or acutely ingested lipophilic poisons [83,84]. Intestinal excretion of DDT metabolites stored in body tissues was dramatically increased by a combination of food restriction and administration of SPE [85]. There were no significant differences observed in the absorption of five lipophilic drugs when administered with olestra, triglyceride oil, or water [86] and the effect of olestra on the absorption and efficacy of a highly lipophilic oral contraceptive indicated that there was little potential for olestra to reduce the absorption of oral drugs [87].

8. Toxicity and Safety

Because SPEs alter the intestinal environment due to the persistent oil phase, the effects of various levels of SPE on the reproductive characteristics of two generations of rats were studied. It was concluded that SPEs, even at a high dietary level of 10%, did not present any adverse reproductive or developmental effects in rats and, therefore, that SPEs would not pose a reproductive hazard for humans [88]. Since olestra is neither absorbed nor enzymatically broken down, the possibility of accumulation of intact olestra in body organs during chronic ingestion was evaluated for its genotoxic potential in the *Salmonella*/mammalian microsome test, the L5178Y thymidine kinase (TK $+/-$) mouse lymphoma assay, an unscheduled DNA synthesis assay in primary rat hepatocytes, and an in vitro cytogenetic assay in Chinese hamster ovary (CHO) cells [89]. From these studies it was concluded that olestra was nongenotoxic in short-term assays. A 91-day feeding study [90] in rats was conducted to assess the potential toxicity of heated olestra/vegetable oil blends (OA/VO). Although a number of statistically significant differences were observed in clinical chemistry and haematology determinations, each of the differences was considered to represent normal biological variation and not effects of treatment. This conclusion was supported by the observations that the alterations occurred sporadically across all groups, that there were no consistent significant differences noted between groups receiving heated OA/VO blends and the controls, and that there was no dose-response relationship for any observation.

Two 2-year feeding studies [91] in rats were conducted to evaluate the chronic toxicity and the carcinogenic potential of olestra. Isolated statistically significant differences in mortality, mononuclear cell leukemia, and pituitary adenomas were observed but were not considered to be related to olestra ingestion since they were not reproducible across the two studies, generally not dose-responsive, not consistent between sexes, and the incidences were within the ranges for historical and contemporary laboratory controls. It was concluded that olestra was not toxic or carcinogenic when fed to rats at up to 9% of the diet for 24 months.

Olestra accumulation of an ingested dose was measured in various organs in rats [92,93]; studies [94] using intravenously dosed olestra in monkeys verified that the liver was the primary target organ for olestra absorption and accumulation. Feeding studies showed that less than $2 \times 10^{-6}\%$ of the total amount of olestra (9%) eaten by rats over 24 months and less than $4 \times 10^{-5}\%$ of the amount (8%) eaten by monkeys over 29 months accumulated in their livers, indicating that olestra did not accumulate in the body following chronic ingestion [94].

E. Regulatory Implications

1. Testing Protocols

The potential for fat substitutes in the marketplace has created interesting scientific and legal issues, not the least of which are how to deal with the rearrangement of a traditionally GRAS food, and whether a rearranged food can be considered as safe as the food from which it was derived [95]. Initially, these concerns applied specifically to Simplesse, which has since been approved as GRAS. But F. E. Scarborough, Deputy Director of FDA's Office of Nutrition and Food Science, claimed that fat substitutes are different from other food additives because they could represent up to one-third of the calories consumed. If large amounts are eaten, it would be impossible to administer test dosages at exaggerated levels [95]. S. Miller, formerly Director of FDA's Center for Food Safety and Applied Nutrition, pointed out that FDA is likely to examine these substances more carefully because fat substitutes may be used by all sectors of the population at 30–40% levels, whereas other additives may make up only 1–2% of a food product. Furthermore, testing of fat substitutes creates scientific problems not normally found with more traditional food additives, and FDA may have to address them in a different way by establishing experimental food additive rules that would regulate clinical trials [95].

W. H. Glinsmann, Associate Director for Clinical Nutrition in FDA's Center for Food Safety and Applied Nutrition, made a similar suggestion about the increased need for human clinical testing prior to approval of new food additives such as nonabsorbable fat substitutes, where a no-effect level cannot be established and the agency cannot extrapolate fully what an effect will be, based on prior experience [96]. A "no-effect level" is the highest dose of a substance (mg/kg body weight/day) that does not adversely affect the test animal and is used to establish an acceptable daily intake by adding a margin of safety that may be 100–1000 times greater than the approved level. But how can a synthetic fat be tested at 100 times the normal rate of ingestion? Discussing safety issues of fat substitutes, Glinsmann [97] explained that FDA was concerned with characterization of exposure, extrapolation from animal to human data, validation of pharmacokinetic models, and the usefulness of pooled data from experiments, adding that clinical testing was needed but that current guidelines were not clearly defined.

2. Labeling Standards

FDA requires a food to be labeled as "imitation" if it resembles another food and can be substituted for it, yet is nutritionally inferior to the food it imitates. According to Scarborough [95], the term "imitation" revolves around vitamin and protein content; fat and calories are not considered in determining whether a food is nutritionally inferior to the original. If fat substitutes were included in reduced-calorie foods, they would not require "imitation" labeling and would simply be part of the ingredient listing. The criteria for determining nutritional inferiority are obviously not adequate when applied to fat substitutes or to the foods into which they are added.

Standards of identity present another labeling hazard because adding a fat substitute to a dairy product would prevent it from being called a dairy product. The label would have to clearly distinguish products containing the fat substitute from products covered by the standards by using either the word "imitation" or by developing a completely new name [95].

III. OTHER SYNTHETIC OIL COMPOUNDS

A. Trialkoxytricarballylate (TATCA)

In 1984, Hamm [98] reported on the preparation and evaluation of trialkoxytricarballylate (TATCA), trialkoxycitrate (TAC), trialkoxyglyceryl ether (TGE), SPE, and jojoba oil as low-calorie replacements for fats and oils. The compounds were tested as substitutes for fat in mayonnaise, margarine, egg frying, cake baking, and were tested for resistance to digestion by pancreatic lipase in vitro. TATCA proved to be the most versatile of the group due to its close structural resemblance to a triglyceride, and in 1985 a patent for its use was assigned to the Best Foods division of CPC International [99]. The patent describes low-calorie oil substitutes based on thermally stable polycarboxylic acids esterified with saturated or unsaturated alcohols that can be used in oil-based food compositions. The fatty alcohol analogs of similar fatty acids are esterified onto a polycarboxylic backbone, and because the ester units are reversed from the corresponding esters present in triglyceride oils, the esters in the low-calorie substitutes are not susceptible to enzymatic hydrolysis by lipases [5]. Results of feeding studies in rats of up to 9% TATCA over a 2-week period showed 97% recovery of excess fecal lipid, and the high pressure liquid chromatography (HPLC) fingerprint of the compound extracted from the fecal lipids was identical to that fed [100].

B. Dialkyl Dihexadicyclomalonate (DDM)

PepsiCo's Frito-Lay division was granted a patent [101] in 1986 for "dicarboxylic acid esters," which can be used in the preparation of fatty oil–containing food products or for use in frying foods. Fatty alcohol esters of malonic and alkylmalonic acids—dialkyl dihexadicyclomalonate (DDM)—are liquids or semi-liquids synthesized from diethyl malonate or malonyl dichloride and are suitable for high-temperature applications [102]. In vitro lipase assays used to determine DDM digestibility relative to triolein (100%) measured 4.7% for dialkyl malonate, 3.3% for dialkyl hexadecylmalonate, and 2.5% for DDM. Absorption was assessed by feeding trials in rats using oil recovery in feces and radio-labeled tissue distribution/balance studies; it was concluded that less than 0.1% ingested DDM was absorbed [100]. Subchronic feeding studies at low concentrations showed no toxic effects, but higher exposure rates produced oil leakage in rats. Other important assessments such as the impact of DDM on drug and vitamin absorption, the pharmacokinetics and disposition of DDM, and the effects of gut integrity on DDM absorption are being examined [103]. Sensory panels reported that a blend of DDM and soybean oil used for frying potato and tortilla chips resulted in products that were equally crisp but less oily than those fried in regular vegetable oils. The DDM-soybean oil blend provides a 33% reduction in calories and a 60% reduction in fat [104].

C. Esterified Propoxylated Glycerols (EPG)

Esterified propoxylated glycerols (EPG) are a new family of propylene oxide derivatives developed by ARCO Chemical Company with a structure similar to natural fats and oils. A glycerol backbone is reacted with propylene oxide to form a poly ether polyol which is then esterified with fatty acids to produce the modified triglyceride EPG. The compound is heat stable for baking and frying and can be used in applications such as salad dressing, mayonnaise, ice cream, toppings, and sauces. EPG functional properties can be tailored to the desired product application. Irritation and sensitization tests on laboratory animals have proved negative. Hydrolysis was not observed in EPG containing more than five oxypropylene units during in vitro digestion studies using pancreatic lipase and hydrochloric acid. When rats were fed diets containing 5% EPG, body organs and tissues were unaffected, but in another tolerance study, one version of EPG produced oil leakage in some animals at the 10% level [105]. Radio-labeled metabolism testing on different EPG versions resulted in low metabolism levels but much work remains before clinical trials can be conducted. A joint agreement signed in 1990 between CPC International and ARCO combines expertise in food technology and product development with chemical processing knowledge for the development of EPG and the eventual bid for FDA approval [106]. ARCO was issued a U.S. patent for EPG in 1989 [107] and a European patent in 1990 [108].

D. Raffinose Polyesters (RPEs), Alkyl Glycoside Fatty Acid Polyesters, and Methyl Glucoside Polyesters

Akoh and Swanson synthesized liquid polyesters of raffinose by a one-stage solvent-free interesterification of raffinose undecaacetate and fatty acid methyl esters of salad oils, long-chain fatty acids, and blends of both [109]; preparations of trehalose octaoleate and sorbitol hexaoleate were also interesterified by a one-stage solventless process [110]. Physical properties such as refractive index, specific gravity, and density were similar in those polymers to those exhibited by SPEs and commercial vegetable oils, and they were not susceptible to in vitro hydrolysis.

Synthesis and purification of RPEs and SPEs were optimized in another study [111] that measured the melting properties of both compounds. Subsequent work produced high yields of alkyl glycoside fatty acid polyesters and stachyose fatty acid polyesters with physical properties not unlike those of triglycerides. There was no evidence of in vitro hydrolysis in these compounds [112]. Preliminary feeding trials of 13% liquid raffinose polyesters or semi-solid methyl glucoside polyesters (MGPE) in mice resulted in fecal recovery of 98% and 60% of these compounds, respectively, with no oil leakage from either polyester [113]. U.S. patents for these compounds have been assigned to Curtice-Burns Foods [114,115].

E. Olestrin™ and Prolestra™

Reach Associates Inc. introduced a new fat replacer in 1988 [116] called olestrin, which combines dextrins and maltodextrins of high molecular weight (and less than 5 dextrose equivalents) with sucrose polyesters and triglycerides in a particle engineering process similar to that applied in microparticulated proteins. Olestrin delivers fewer than 3 cal/g; formulas can be tailored to provide the texture and mouthfeel of fat—the preferred composition includes 33% triglyceride oils (canola and olive oils), 33% dextrins (0.5–5.0 dextrose equivalents), and 33% SPE. Applications for olestrin cover most products that incorporate fat such as ice cream, frozen deserts, yogurt, salad oils, and baked goods. However, dextrins are destroyed by prolonged frying; therefore, incorporation into french fries is not included as an application. But heat-resistant formulas can be customized for frying and other cooking and baking applications. Reach projects olestrin could capture 500,000 tons of the 60 million ton world market for edible oils. Prolestra is another Reach product formula, which combines 30% or less SPE with a variety of animal and vegetable proteins for a maximum of 76% triglyceride substitution; the composition can be used in mayonnaise, spreads and sauces, ice cream, salad oil, and baked goods [117].

F. Caprocaprylobehenin (Caprenin)

Procter & Gamble is seeking regulatory approval of caprenin as a GRAS ingredient since it is a triglyceride made from fatty acids contained in common foods [118]. The caprenin molecule contains caprylic (C8), capric (C10), and behenic (C22) acids. It provides only five calories per gram instead of the usual nine because behenic acid is poorly absorbed in the intestinal tract. The two short-chain fatty acids have not been linked with increased blood cholesterol levels, and they impart a functionality similar to that of cocoa butter, making caprenin suitable as a fat replacer in soft candies and confectionary coatings. Three laboratory feeding studies have indicated that it is utilized in the body like other fats containing these fatty acids. Procter & Gamble commissioned a FASEB expanel to determine the safety of caprenin; they found no evidence of significant adverse health effects in the available information on caprenin at the estimated potential levels of consumption [119]. All data have been submitted to FDA in a final petition process.

Procter & Gamble sold the fat substitute to M&M Mars Co., which has formulated a Milky Way II candy bar with 25% fewer calories and half the percentage of calories from fat compared with the original [120].

REFERENCES

1. C. E. Morris, Focus on fat reduction, *Food Eng.*, *62*(6): 91 (1990).
2. A. E. Przybla, Formulating healthy foods, *Food Eng.*, *62*(2): 49 (1990).
3. C. M. Kroskey, Creating guilt-free bakery products, *Prep. Foods*, *159*(10): 76 (1990).

4. D. D. Duxbury and N. M. Meinhold, Dietary fats and oils: Continued controversy, new research findings, *Food Proc.*, *52*(3): 58 (1991).
5. B. F. Haumann, Getting the fat out—researchers seek substitutes for full-fat fat, *J. Am. Oil Chem. Soc.*, *63*: 278 (1986).
6. R. G. LaBarge, The search for a low-caloric oil, *Food Technol.* *42*(1): 84 (1988).
7. J. Probber, Future foods: What Americans will eat in the year 2000, *The New York Times*, Jan. 27 (1988).
8. R. Johnson, Nutritionists detect a dark side in new world of food substitutes, *The Wall Street Journal*, Feb. 3 (1988).
9. A. D. Campbell, M. P. Penfield, and R. M. Griswold, *The Experimental Study of Food*, Houghton Mifflin Co., Boston, MA, p. 247 (1979).
10. T. P. Coultate, *Food; The Chemistry of Its Components*, Royal Society of Chemistry, London, p. 51 (1989).
11. G. M. Wardlow and P. M. Insel, *Perspectives in Nutrition*, Times Mirror/Mosby College Publishing, St. Louis, MO, p. 133 (1990).
12. H. B. Heath and G. Reineccius, *Flavor Chemistry and Technology*, Van Nostrand Reinhold Co., New York, p. 44 (1986).
13. D. Best, Getting more for less: The challenges of fat substitution, *Prep. Foods*, *160*(6): 72 (1991).
14. K. J. Parker, K. James, and J. Hurford, Sucrose ester surfactants—a solventless process and the products thereof, *Sucrochemistry* (J. L. Hickson, ed.), American Chemical Society, Washington, D.C., p. 97 (1977).
15. H. B. Hass, The concept of sucrochemistry, *Sucrochemistry* (J. L. Hickson, ed.), American Chemical Society, Washington, D.C., p. 4 (1977).
16. S. P. Rowland, V. O. Cirino, and A. J. Bullock, Structural components in methyl vinyl sulfone modified cotton cellulose, *Can. J. Chem.* *44*: 1051 (1966).
17. M. Gee and H. G. Walker, Jr., Gas chromatographic analysis of sucrose monostearate, *Chem. Ind.*: 829 (July 1961).
18. H. Chung, P. A. Seib, K. F. Finney, and C. D. Magoffin, Sucrose monoesters and diesters in breadmaking, *Cereal Chem.*, *58*: 164 (1980).
19. R. Khan, Some fundamental aspects of the chemistry of sucrose, *Sucrochemistry* (J. L. Hickson, ed.), American Chemical Society, Washington, D.C., p. 40 (1977).
20. Sucrose polyester, *Food Eng.*, *59*(11): 49 (1987).
21. K. A. Harrigan and W. M. Breene, Fat substitutes: Sucrose esters and Simplesse, *Cereal Foods World*, *34*: 261 (1989).
22. H. B. Hass, Early history of sucrose esters, *Sugar Esters*, Noyes Development Corp., Park Ridge, NJ, p. 1 (1968).
23. H. B. Hass, F. D. Snell, W. C. York, and L. I. Osipow, Process for producing sugar esters, U.S. Patent 2,893,990 (1959).
24. N. B. Tucker and J. B. Martin, Method for producing fatty esters of nonreducing oligosaccharides in the presence of an amide, U.S. Patent 2,831,854 (1958).
25. N. B. Tucker and J. B. Martin, Method for producing fatty esters of nonreducing oligosaccharides in the presence of pyridine, U.S. Patent 2,831,855 (1958).
26. J. B. Martin, Method for producing fatty esters of nonreducing oligosaccharides in the presence of an amide, U.S. Patent 2,831,856 (1958).

27. T. Kosaka and T. Yamada, New plant and new applications of sucrose esters, *Sucrochemistry* (J. L. Hickson, ed.), American Chemical Society, Washington, D.C., p. 84 (1977).

28. N. Kawase, Sucrose ester and its application for sugar manufacturing, *Sugar y Azucar*, *76*(7): 29 (1981).

29. L. Bobichon, A sugar ester process and its applications in calf feeding and human food additives, *Sucrochemistry* (J. L. Hickson, ed.), American Chemical Society, Washington, D.C., p. 115 (1977).

30. F. H. Mattson and R. A. Volpenhein, Hydrolysis of fully esterified alcohols containing from one to eight hydroxyl groups by the lipolytic enzymes of rat pancreatic juice, *J. Lipid Res.*, *13*: 325 (1972).

31. F. H. Mattson and R. A. Volpenhein, Rate and extent of absorption of the fatty acids of fully esterified glycerol, erythritol, xylitol and sucrose as measured in thoracic duct cannulated rats, *J. Nutr.*, *102*: 1177 (1972).

32. F. H. Mattson and G. A. Nolen, Absorbability by rats of compounds containing from one to eight ester groups, *J. Nutr.*, *102*: 1171 (1972).

33. F. H. Mattson, and R. A. Volpenhein, Low calorie fat-containing food compositions, U.S. Patent 3,600,186 (1971).

34. P. B. Hutt urges patent extension provisions for additives, *Food Chem. News,* *33*(24): 37 (1991).

35. L. I. Osipow, F. D. Snell, W. C. York, and A. Finchler, Fatty acid esters of sucrose. Methods of preparation, *Ind. Eng. Chem.*, *48*: 1458 (1956).

36. L. I. Osipow, F. D. Snell, and A. Finchler, Sugar esters, *J. Am. Oil Chem. Soc.*, *34*: 185 (1957).

37. L. I. Osipow and W. Rosenblatt, Micro-emulsion process for the preparation of sucrose esters, *J. Am. Oil Chem. Soc. 44*: 307 (1967).

38. L. I. Osipow and W. Rosenblatt, Esterification of polyhydric compounds in the presence of transparent emulsifying agent, U.S. Patent 3,480,616 (1969).

39. R. O. Feuge, H. J. Zeringue, Jr., T. J. Weiss, and M. Brown. Preparation of sucrose esters by interesterification, *J. Am. Oil Chem. Soc.*, *47*: 56 (1970).

40. R. Feuge, T. Weiss, and H. Zeringue, Process for the production of sucrose esters of fatty acids, U.S. Patent 3,714,144 (1973).

41. G. P. Rizzi and H. M. Taylor, Synthesis of higher polyol fatty acid polyesters, U.S. Patent 3,963,699 (1976).

42. G. P. Rizzi and H. M. Taylor, A solvent-free synthesis of sucrose polyesters, *J. Am. Oil Chem. Soc.*, *55*: 398 (1978).

43. R. A. Volpenhein, Synthesis of higher polyol fatty acid polyesters, U.S. Patent 4,517,360 (1985).

44. R. A. Volpenhein, Synthesis of higher polyol fatty acid polyesters using high soap:polyol ratios, U.S. Patent 4,518,772 (1985).

45. J. Spinner, Olestra update, World Conference on Oleochemicals '90, American Oil Chemists' Society, Kuala Lampur, Thailand (1990).

46. J. L. Salzman and G. M. Ostroff, Sucrose polyester: An in depth study. Fat chance for Procter and Gamble, Goldman Sachs Investment Research, New York (1985).

47. R. M. Morrison, The market for fat substitutes, *National Food Review*, USDA, Econ. Res. Serv., *Apr/Jun 13*(2): 24 (1990).

48. Renderers hit potential impact of fat substitute approvals, *Food Chem. News, 31*(5): 23 (1989).

49. J. O'Brien, Olestra: Conference report of the 200th American Chemical Society national meeting, *Trends in Food Science and Technol., 1*(5): 123 (1990).

50. R. J. Jandacek and M. R. Webb, Physical properties of pure sucrose octaesters, *Chem. Phys. Lipids, 22*: 163 (1978).

51. F. H. Mattson, R. J. Jandacek, and M. R. Webb, The effect of a nonabsorbable lipid, sucrose polyester, on the absorption of dietary cholesterol by the rat, *J. Nutr., 106*: 747 (1976).

52. F. W. Fallat, C. J Glueck, R. Lutmer, and F. H. Mattson, Short-term study of sucrose polyester, a non-absorbable fat-like material, as a dietary agent for lowering plasma cholesterol, *Am. J. Clin. Nutr., 29*: 1204 (1976).

53. C. J. Glueck, F. H. Mattson, and R. J. Jandacek, The lowering of plasma cholesterol by sucrose polyester in subjects consuming diets with 800, 300, or less than 50 mg of cholesterol per day, *Am. J. Clin. Nutr., 32*: 1636 (1979).

54. D. R. Gardner and R. A. Sanders, Isolation and characterization of polymers in heated olestra and an olestra/triglyceride blend, *J. Am. Oil Chem. Soc., 67*: 788 (1990).

55. R. B. Toma, D. J. Curtis, and C. Sobotor, Sucrose polyester: Its metabolic role and possible future applications, *Food Technol. 42*(1): 93 (1988).

56. R. W. Boggs, Sucrose polyester (SPE)—a non-caloric fat, *Fette Seifen Anstrichmittel, 88*(4): 154 (1986).

57. M. H. Hager and B. O. Schneeman, Pancreatic enzyme and plasma cholesterol response to chronic ingestion of a nonabsorbable lipid in rats, *J. Nutr., 116*: 2372 (1986).

58. B. A. Nuck and T. W. Federle, Inability of the human colonic microflora to metabolize olestra, Abstracts of the Annual Meeting of the American Society for Microbiology, Washington, D.C., p. 275 (1990).

59. A. Cortot, S. F. Phillips, and J-R. Malagelada, Gastric emptying of liquids after ingestion of a solid-liquid meal in humans, *Gastroenterology, 80*: 922 (1981).

60. A. Cortot, S. F. Phillips, and J-R. Malagelada, Parallel gastric emptying of non-hydrolyzable fat and water after a solid liquid meal in humans, *Gastroenterology, 82*: 877 (1982).

61. R. J. Jandacek, Compositions for treating hypercholesterolemia; fatty acid esters of polyol, U.S. Patent 4,005,195 (1977).

62. F. H. Mattson, Compositions for inhibiting absorption of cholesterol; polyol fatty acid esters, fat soluble vitamins, U.S. Patent 4,034,083 (1977).

63. J. R. Crouse and S. M. Grundy, Effects of sucrose polyester on cholesterol metabolism in man, *Metabolism 28*(10): 994 (1979).

64. R. W. Fallat, C. J. Glueck, F. H. Mattson, T. T. Ishikawa, and J. Brazier, Sucrose polyester: Effects on fecal cholesterol, total neutral sterol and fatty acids, *Clin. Res., 24*: 360A (1976).

65. R. J. Jandacek, F. H. Mattson, S. McNeely, L. Gallon, R. Yunker, and C. J. Glueck, Effect of sucrose polyester on fecal steroid excretion by 24 normal men, *Am. J. Clin. Nutr., 33*(2): 251 (1980).

66. C. J. Glueck, R. J. Jandacek, M. T. R. Subbiah, L. Gallon, R. Yunker, C. Allen, E. Hogg, and P. M. Laskarzewski, Effect of sucrose polyester on fecal bile acid excretion and composition in normal men, *Am. J. Clin. Nutr.*, *33*(10): 2177 (1980).

67. F. H. Mattson and R. J. Jandacek, The effect of a non-absorbable fat on the turnover of plasma cholesterol in the rat, *Lipids*, *20*(5): 273 (1985).

68. C. J. Glueck, M. M. Hastings, C. Allen, E. Hogg, L. Baehler, P. S. Gartside, D. Phillips, M. Jones, E. J. Hollenbach, B. Braun, and J. V. Anastasia, Sucrose polyester and covert caloric dilution, *Am. J. Clin. Nutr.*, *35*: 1352 (1982).

69. M. R. Adams, M. R. McMahan, F. H. Mattson, and T. B. Clarkson, The long-term effects of dietary sucrose polyester on African green monkeys, *Proc. Soc. Exp. Biol. Med.*, *167*: 346 (1981).

70. R. W. St. Clair, L. L. Wood, and T. B. Clarkson, Effect of sucrose polyester on plasma lipids and cholesterol absorption in African green monkeys with variable hypercholesterolemic response to dietary cholesterol, *Metabolism*, *30*: 176 (1981).

71. M. J. Mellies, R. J. Jandacek, J. D. Taulbee, M. B. Tewksbury, G. Lamkin, L. Baehler, P. King, D. Boggs, S. Goldman, A. Gouge, R. Tsang, and C. J. Glueck, A double-blind, placebo-controlled study of sucrose polyester in hypercholesterolemic outpatients, *Am. J. Clin. Nutr.*, *37*: 339 (1983).

72. C. J. Glueck, R. Jandacek, E. Hogg, C. Allen, L. Baehler, and T. Tewksbury, Sucrose polyester: Substitution for dietary fats in hypocaloric diets in the treatment of familial hypercholesterolemia, *Am. J. Clin. Nutr.*, *37*: 347 (1983).

73. M. J. Mellies, C. Vitale, R. J. Jandacek, G. E. Lamkin, and C. J. Glueck, The substitution of sucrose polyester for dietary fat in obese, hypercholesterolenic outpatients, *Am. J. Clin. Nutr.*, *41*: 1 (1985).

74. S. M. Grundy, J. V. Anastasia, Y. A. Kesaniemi, and J. Abrams, Influence of sucrose polyester on plasma lipoproteins, and cholesterol metabolism in obese patients with and without diabetes mellitus, *Am. J. Clin. Nutr.*, *44*(5): 620 (1986).

75. R. J. Jandacek, M. M. Ramirez, and J. R. Crouse, Effects of partial replacement of dietary fat by olestra on dietary cholesterol absorption in man, *Metabolism*, *39*(8): 848 (1990).

76. C. J. Glueck, M. M. Hastings, C. Allen, E. Hogg, L. Baehler, P. S. Gartside, D. Phillips, M. Jones, E. J. Hollenbach, B. Braun, A. S. Anastasia, and J. V. Anastasia, Sucrose polyester and covert caloric dilution, *Am. J. Clin. Nutr.*, *35*: 1352 (1982).

77. R. J. Jandacek, Gallstone dissolution compositions and method; polyol-fatty acid esters and a lipophilic bile acid, U.S. Patent 4,264,583 (1981).

78. F. H. Mattson, E. J. Hollenbach, and C. M. Kuehlthau, The effect of a non-absorbable fat, sucrose polyester, on the metabolism of vitamin A by the rat, *J. Nutr.*, *109*: 1688 (1979).

79. M. Meydani, J. D. Ribaya-Mercado, J. K. Ellis, J. B. Macauley, J. McNamara, J. B. Blumberg, R. M. Russell, and E. J. Schaefer, Effects of sucrose polyester (SPE) on the absorption of dietary vitamins A and E, *Am. Soc. Clin. Nutr.*, Abstracts of Annual Meeting in Washington, D.C., p. 697 (1986).

80. D. Y. Jones, K. W. Miller, B. P. Koonsvitsky, M. L. Ebert, P. Y. T. Lin, M. B. Jones, and H. F. DeLuca, Serum 25-hydroxyvitamin D concentrations of free-living subjects consuming olestra, *Am. J. Clin. Nutr.*, *53*: 1281 (1991).

81. D. Y. Jones, B. P. Koonsvitsky, M. L. Ebert, M. B. Jones, P. Y. T. Lin, B. H. Will, and John W. Suttie, Vitamin K status of free-living subjects consuming olestra, *Am. J. Clin. Nutr.*, *53*: 943 (1991).

82. Reduced vitamin D, E absorption noted with olestra, *Food Chem. News*, *31* (52): 36 (1990).

83. R. A. Volpenhein, D. R. Webb, and R. J. Jandacek, Effect of a nonabsorbable lipid, sucrose polyester, on the absorption of DDT by the rat, *J. Toxicol. Environ. Health*, *6*: 679 (1980).

84. R. J. Jandacek, The effect of nonabsorbable lipids on the intestinal absorption of lipophiles, *Drug Metab. Rev.*, *13*(4): 695 (1982).

85. L. C. Mutter, R. V. Blanke, R. J. Jandacek, and P. S. Guzelian, Reduction in the body content of DDE in the Mongolian gerbil treated with sucrose polyester and caloric dilution, *Toxicol. Applied Pharm.*, *92*: 428 (1988).

86. R. J. Roberts and R. D. Leff, Influence of absorbable and nonabsorbable lipids and lipidlike substances on drug bioavailability, *Clin. Pharmacol. Ther.*, *45*(3): 299 (1989).

87. K. W. Miller, D. S. Williams, S. B. Carter, M. B. Jones, and D. R. Mishell, The effect of olestra on systemic levels of oral contraceptives, *Clin. Pharmacol. Ther.*, *48*(1): 34 (1990).

88. G. A. Nolen, F. E. Wood, and T. A. Dierckman, A two-generation reproductive and developmental toxicity study of sucrose polyester, *Food Chem. Toxicol.*, *25*(1): 1 (1987).

89. K. L. Skare, J. A. Skare, and E. D. Thompson, Evaluation of olestra in short-term genotoxicity assays, *Food Chem. Toxicol.*, *28*(2): 69 (1990).

90. K. W. Miller and P. H. Long, A 91-day feeding study in rats with heated olestra/vegetable oil blends, *Food Chem. Toxicol.*, *28*(5): 307 (1990).

91. F. E. Wood, W. J. Tierney, A. L. Knezevich, H. F. Bolte, J. K. Maurer, and R. D. Bruce, Chronic toxicity and carcinogenicity studies of olestra in Fischer 344 rats, *Food Chem. Toxicol.*, *29*: 223 (1991).

92. L. Aust, J. Bruckner, R. Noack, and G. Mieth, Accumulation of sucrose polyester in different organ lipids of rats, *Die Nährung*, *26*: K3 (1982).

93. L. Aust, G. Mieth, J. Bruckner, A. Weiss, and R. Noack, Accumulation of sucrose polyester in different organ lipids of rats in dependence on duration of application, *Die Nährung*, *30*: 453 (1986).

94. F. E. Wood, B. R. DeMark, E. J. Hollenbach, M. C. Sargent, and K. C. Triebwasser, Analysis of liver tissue for olestra following long-term feeding to rats and monkeys, *Food Chem. Toxicol.*, *29*: 231 (1991).

95. A. Gillis, Fat substitutes create new issues, *J. Am. Oil Chem. Soc.*, *65*(11): 1708 (1988).

96. Glinsmann sees need for clinical testing regs for food additives, *Food Chem. News*, *30*(38): 49 (1988).

97. Fat substitute approval process scored at NAS meeting, *Food Chem. News*, *32* (10): 51 (1990).

98. D. J. Hamm, Preparation and evaluation of trialkoxytricarballylate, trialkoxycitrate, trialkoxyglycerylether, jojoba oil, and sucrose polyester as low calories replacements of edible fats and oils, *J. Food Sci.*, *49*: 419 (1984).

99. D. J. Hamm, Low calorie edible oil substitutes, U.S. Patent 4,508,746 (1985).
100. M. Bieber, TATCA: results of a two-week dietary exposure study in rats, Annual Meeting Abstracts, *J. Am. Oil Chem. Soc.*, *66*(4): 480 (1989).
101. J. Fulcher, Fried food product fried in synthetic cooking oils containing dicarboxylic acid esters, U.S. Patent 4,508,746 (1986).
102. M. E. Spearman and J. G. Fulcher, Malonate esters: new synthetic fat substitutes for food use, Annual Meeting Abstracts, *J. Am. Oil Chem. Soc.*, *66* (4): 470 (1989).
103. Frito-Lay testing fat simulant for use in frying snack foods, *Food Chem. News*, *31*(13): 57 (1989).
104. Fat substitutes update, *Food Technol.*, *44*(3): 92 (1990).
105. T. A. Beck, EPG: A versatile fat substitute, Calorie Control Council Meeting, Washington, DC (1990).
106. Quest for fat substitutes taking many routes, *Inform, 2*(2): 115 (1990).
107. J. F. White and M. F. Pollard, Non-digestible fat substitutes of low-caloric value, U.S. Patent 4,861,613 (1989).
108. C. F. Cooper, Preparation of esterified propoxylated glycerin from free fatty acids, European Patent 356,255 (1990).
109. C. C. Akoh and B. G. Swanson, One-stage synthesis of raffinose fatty acid polyesters, *J. Food Sci.*, *52*: 1570 (1987).
110. C. C. Akoh and B. G. Swanson, Preparation of trehalose and sorbitol fatty acid polyesters by interesterification, *J. Am. Oil Chem. Soc.*, *66*: 1581 (1989).
111. C. C. Akoh and B. G. Swanson, Optimized synthesis of sucrose polyesters: Comparison of physical properties of sucrose polyesters, raffinose polyesters and salad oils. *J. Food Sci.*, *55*: 236 (1990).
112. C. C. Akoh and B. G. Swanson, Synthesis and properties of alkyl glycoside and stachyose fatty acid polyesters, *J. Am. Oil Chem. Soc.*, *66*(9): 1295 (1989).
113. C. C. Akoh and B. G. Swanson, Preliminary raffinose polyester and methyl glucoside polyester feeding trials with mice, *Nutr. Rep. Int.*, *39*(4): 659 (1989).
114. R. S. Meyer, J. M. Root, M. L. Campbell, and D. B. Winter, Low caloric alkyl glycoside fatty acid polyester fat substitutes, U.S. Patent 4,840,815 (1989).
115. R. S. Meyer, C. C. Akoh, B. G. Swanson, D. B. Winter, J. M. Root, and M. L. Campbell, Polysaccharide fatty acid polyester fat substitutes, U.S. Patent 4,973,489 (1990).
116. New entry in the fat-substitute sweepstakes; olestrin, *Food Eng.*, *60*(5): 60 (1988).
117. R. S. Aries, Prolestra—a new sucrose polyester and protein composition, Annual Meeting Abstracts, *J. Am. Oil Chem. Soc.*, *66*(4): 470 (1989).
118. D. D. Duxbury, New fat replacers sourced from GRAS ingredients, *Food Proc.*, *52*(9): 86 (1991).
119. FASEB panel finds new fat substitute GRAS, *Food Chem. News, 33*(49): 50 (1992).
120. Reduced-calorie candy bar, *Food Chem. News, 33*(47): 2 (1992).

11
Bulking Agents and Fat Substitutes

Amanda M. Frye and Carole S. Setser *Kansas State University*
Manhattan, Kansas

I. INTRODUCTION

Nutrition is driving consumer demands for less fat, sugar, and calories [1, 2]. In 1988, the Surgeon General recommended that food manufacturers could contribute to an improved American diet by increasing the availability of palatable, easily prepared food products that could help consumers follow dietary principles [3]. The food industry is challenged to redesign traditional foods for optimal nutritional value while making them taste the same or better [1,2]. New food-production technologies introduce new materials—both natural and synthetic—to use as ingredients in food products [4]. Bosselman et al. reported that flavor, texture, mouthfeel, and smell are critically important in the development of these new foods [5].

One way to achieve a healthful food product is to omit ingredients. However, in most foods the removal or reduction of ingredients causes readily detectable loss of appearance, texture, and mouthfeel. Carbohydrate and fat components provide the desirable bulk and mouthfeel in many food products. Ingredients that replace the bulk and functional properties of these usual carbohydrates or fats are called bulking agents [6].

Bulking agents aid formulation of food products with a reduction in fats or carbohydrates and calories [6]. The ideal bulking agent would contribute no calories, introduce no taste of its own, have good to excellent solubility, be compatible with a wide range of food materials, be near neutral pH, be tolerant to conventional processing technologies, and be void of any food safety issues [7]. Selection of a bulking agent requires an analysis of the food system for its intended use and determination of the factors of importance. Generally, a major factor is the caloric contribution, however, other factors need to be considered. These include sweetness, solubility (usually in water), retention (and release) of water, air incorporation in some products, ability to contribute viscosity, ability to alter gelatinization and coagulation temperatures in bakery products, ability to depress freezing point in frozen products, and control of crystal formation in confectionary products. However, no single alternative meets these criteria or fulfills all of the functional properties of sucrose or fats in all food products. Each bulking agent has unique properties that make its applications limited; frequently combinations are needed. The following is a discussion of bulking agents used to replace either the carbohydrate or fat components in foods. Some bulking agents can function as both fat and sugar replacements.

The two broad types of carbohydrate bulking agents are soluble and insoluble materials. Carbohydrate bulking agents can replace some of the non-sweet functional characteristics of sucrose [6]. Although some agents are sweet, none are as sweet as sucrose. These bulking agents can be grouped into three broad classifications: polyalcohols, carbohydrate polymers, and fibers or gums. In many instances, combinations of several bulking agents are needed to provide properties similar to the original sucrose-sweetened product.

Fats contribute the highest caloric value of any energy nutrient, 9 kilocalories/gram (kcal/g). Therefore, to achieve caloric reduction in fat-based foods, a reduction of the fat component is the simplest approach. The roles of fat in food products are numerous and give food unique identifiable characteristics. In many products some fat can be removed without a noticeable deviation from the original product. However, the replacement or total removal of the fat alters the flavor [9], texture, tenderness, body, and smoothness of a product. Fats also contribute moistness and a rich mouthfeel. Fats produce emulsions and aid in the incorporation of air in batters. The various fat replacers are novel for mimicking certain fat properties. However, the universal fat substitute does not exist. Thus, different fat replacers contribute distinct properties suitable to replicating a limited number of food products.

Specific products discussed in this review are intended as examples of types of bulking agents without any intended recommendations. All products that are discussed are not approved, as yet, for use in all types of food products in the United States, although some of them have been approved for use in other countries.

II. POLYALCOHOLS

The polyalcohols (see also Chapter 8) are bulk sweeteners related to sucrose and have many properties similar to monosaccharides and disaccharides [6,10]. Several of the polyalcohols are not low calorie. Sugar alcohols have laxative effects if consumed in excess; thus, daily intake should be limited to 60–80 g and below 20 g per single dose [11]. In general, all of the polyols are significantly less cariogenic than sucrose, and they can offer advantages for diabetics.

A. Sorbitol

Sorbitol is the oldest and the most thoroughly investigated polyalcohol. It was first isolated in 1872 from the mountain ash berry (*Sorbus aucuparia*) by the French chemist, Joseph Boussingault [11–13]. Later, sorbitol was discovered in varying levels in many plants. Today, sorbitol is produced by the catalytic hydrogenation of dextrose [11], sucrose, or starch. The syrup is refined and evaporated to a 70% dry substance [11]. Sorbitol cannot be crystallized directly from an aqueous solution except by special techniques, thus crystallization is completed after dehydration. Crystallized sorbitol is a polymorphous substance. Three crystalline forms exist, of which only the gamma form is stable under normal conditions. The other forms are converted to a less stable form, which results in caking or surface recrystallization [14].

Sorbitol is well utilized by the body and has an energy content of approximately 4 kcal/g for the solid [6,12,15] or 2.8 kcal/g for the 70% solution [12]. Sorbitol is highly palatable and odorless with a sweet, pleasant taste [12,16]. The crystalline form is a white powder or granule, whereas the syrup is clear.

B. Lactitol

Hydrogenation of the glucose moiety of lactose (milk sugar) yields a polyol with the systemic name of 4-β-D-galactopyranosyl-D-glucitol, or lactitol [17–19,20]. Lactitol is purified into a syrup, which can be crystallized into mono- or dihydrate forms depending on conditions [21]. Lactitol is more stable than the parent, lactose. Lactitol has an energy value of 2.0 kcal/g [19–21].

Lactitol hydrate is described as a white, odorless, crystalline, free-flowing powder without the sandy mouthfeel of lactose [19]. In general, lactitol has a clean, sweet taste with no aftertaste, closely resembling sucrose in character [17,20–22]. Compared to other polyols, lactitol is the lowest in sweetness [17,20,21]. A 10.0% lactitol solution can be made to equal a 10.0% sucrose solution with the addition of 0.033% aspartame or acesulfame-K or 0.013% sodium saccharin [20,21].

C. Isomalt (Palatinit®)

Isomalt is the generic name for Palatinit, named after the region in West Germany where it was discovered [23]. Isomalt is classified as a sugar alcohol derived from sucrose via a two-step process. The first step is the enzymatic rearrangement of the $1 \rightarrow 2$ glycosidic linkage of the glucose and fructose moieties. This rearrangement leads to the formation of the disaccharide isomaltose (Palatinose®). The enzyme used for this transformation is sucrose-glucosylfructose-mutase from *Protaminobacter rubrum*, which is a nonpathogenic organism found in beet sugar factories [23]. Isomaltose is purified through crystallization and then hydrogenated to yield isomalt, an equimolar mixture of α-glucopyranosyl-$1 \rightarrow 6$-sorbitol (GPS) and α-D-glucopyranosyl-$1 \rightarrow 1$-mannitol (GPM). It contains about 5% bound water as GPM, is crystallized with two molecules of water, and GPS forms anhydrous crystals [23–26].

Isomalt is a white, odorless, sweet-tasting crystal. The energy value is 2.0 kcal/g, half that of sucrose [27]. Different isomalt types are recommended depending on the food system or product. Isomalt has a sweet taste similar to sucrose without any aftertaste. In flavored foods, isomalt was reported to intensify aroma and flavor of products. Synergistic effects were reported if isomalt was combined with other sugar alcohols (sorbitol, Lycasin®, xylitol) or other potent sweetening agents (saccharin, cyclamate, aspartame). Isomalt can be substituted for traditional sweeteners in a ratio of 1:1 in some products compensating for its lower sweetness by changing the flavoring so that increasing the amount of isomalt is not necessary [24].

D. Xylitol

Xylitol is a naturally occurring, five-carbon sugar alcohol with the empirical formula of $C_5H_{12}O_5$ and a molecular weight of 152.15 [28]. It has a caloric value of 4 kcal/g. Because the human body produces xylitol naturally, it is fully metabolized. Xylitol is a constituent of many fruits and vegetables (such as raspberries, strawberries, yellow plums, lettuce, and cauliflower) as well as mushrooms, yeast, and seaweed [9,29]. In humans and animals, xylitol is an intermediate product of carbohydrate metabolism. Like many of the other polyols, it is a white, odorless, crystalline powder. Xylitol is manufactured by hydrolyzing natural sources of hemicellulose such as hardwoods; pecan, coconut, and almond shells; cane sugar bagasse; rice, cottonseed, and oat hulls; corncobs or cornstalks to D-xylose. The D-xylose then undergoes hydrogenation, purification, and crystallization to produce xylitol.

E. Maltitol

Maltitol (D-glycosyl-α(1 $\rightarrow$ 4)-D-glucitol) is a polyalcohol produced by the hydrogenation of maltose in the presence of a nickel catalyst [30,31]. Maltitol can exist in syrup or crystalline form. Different producers provide pure maltitol with purity of 99% or a mixture with < 90% maltitol and > 5% maltotritol Malbit®) [31]. Maltitol is a major component of the hydrogenated glucose syrup, Lycasin, discussed later.

F. Mannitol

Mannitol can be produced from seaweed or, preferably, invert sugar. Mannitol is produced by catalytic hydrogenation of glucose/fructose (invert sugar) mixtures resulting in 75% sorbitol and 25% mannitol [32], which is separated by crystallization or chromatography. Alternatively, mannitol is produced from mannitol/fructose yielding 62-66% mannitol [32], which is easily crystallized [30].

G. Hydrogenated Starch Hydrolysate Mixtures (Lycasin)

The composition and properties of hydrogenated starch hydrolysates differ depending upon the manufacturing process. Lycasin usually is derived from potato or corn starch [14]. The starch hydrolysis must be controlled carefully to achieve a syrup with a specified glucose and maltose content, which then determines the sorbitol and maltitol content after hydrogenation. Hydrolysis is accomplished by the use of acids or enzymes [30,33,34].

Lycasin 80/55, Lycasin 5/60, and Lycasin 80/33 are all hydrogenated glucose syrups. To avoid confusion among the various products, the manufacturer (Roquette Corporation) reserved the name Lycasin for Lycasin 80/55. Lycasin 5/60 and Lycasin 80/33 were renamed Polysorb® 5/60 and Polysorb® 80/33, respectively [14].

Lycasin 80/55 is the most fully developed syrup. The 80 represents the dry substance content, and the 55 refers to dextrose equivalent (DE) of the starch syrup prior to hydrogenation [33]. Lycasin is a mixture of sorbitol, maltitol, and various hydrogenated oligosaccharides and polysaccharides [35]. The overall composition is approximately 44% sorbitol (6-8% free sorbitol) and 66% dextrose (no free dextrose) [13,36]. Further discussions of Lycasin 80/55 will be referred to as Lycasin.

Lycasin was developed to be a noncariogenic replacer of corn syrup for the confectionery industry. It is a colorless, odorless, pleasant-tasting syrup that is sweeter than glucose or sorbitol [13,33,36], achieved by increasing the maltitol content. This is done by subjecting the corn starch hydrolysate to β-amylase enzyme to yield a high-maltose syrup [14,35]. Lycasin has been evaluated as 75% as sweet as an equivalent sucrose system [13,36]. It is also available as a hygroscopic powder [13,34].

III. CARBOHYDRATE POLYMERS

A. Polydextrose

Polydextrose is a low-calorie bulking agent that can replace some of the functions of sucrose or fat in food products. It is formed by the random polymerization of glucose, sorbitol, and citric acid in a ratio of 89:10:1 [37]. Small amounts of glucose, sorbitol, and citric acid are present in the polymer [38, 39]. Sorbitol helps to control the upper molecular weight limit and the formation of water-insoluble material during polymerization [38]. Trace amounts of $1 \rightarrow 6$ anhydro-D-glucose and 5-hydroxymethyl furfural are produced as by-products of glucose caramelization [40]. The polydextrose polymer contains all types of glycosidic bonds with the $1 \rightarrow 6$ bond predominating [38,39].

Polydextrose is available in four forms: polydextrose powder, polydextrose Type N (70% solution), polydextrose Type K (powder), and polydextrose Type F (powder, Litesse®, Pfizer Inc., Chemical Division, New York). Polydextrose powder is amorphous, white to light tan in color with a pH of 2.5-3.5 because of the residual acid content. The addition of a neutralizing buffering agent sometimes is needed [38]. The Type N polydextrose is a 70% solution neutralized with potassium hydroxide to a pH of 5.0-6.0. Type K polydextrose is the dry buffered form, neutralized with potassium bicarbonate to the same pH as the Type N solution [41]. Polydextrose has almost no sweetness. The sweetness of a product can be adjusted by the addition of a high-potency sweetener. A 10% weight/weight (w/w) aqueous solution of polydextrose has been described as slightly sweet-sour-bitter and Type N as slightly sweet-salty-bitter [39]. High levels have been found to increase bitterness in reduced-calorie bakery products [42], but reportedly Litesse reduces bitter notes in food products (F. Kopchik, personal communication) and is virtually tasteless [43].

Metabolic studies by Figdor and Bianchine [44] showed that the utilization of polydextrose in humans is 1 kcal/g, which confirmed earlier rat studies [45]. Therefore, polydextrose contributes 25% of the caloric value of sucrose or 11% of fat's energy. A laxative effect has been observed in some people who consumed high levels of polydextrose; thus, products containing more than 15 g polydextrose per serving must be labeled [43].

Polydextrose in the powdered form and in solution has high stability. The powder remained stable after storage for 90 days at temperatures of 25, 35, and 60 °C [38,40]. Color change in polydextrose-N was reported when the product was stored for 3 months, at elevated temperatures, or when heated to dryness at temperatures greater than 135 °C [38–40].

B. Sucrose Polyesters

Sucrose polyesters are noncaloric fat substitutes produced from soybean oil and sucrose [46–50]. These are described in detail in Chapter 10. Sucrose polyester is claimed to have excellent sensory characteristics as a fat substitute [51]. It has an appearance, flavor, heat stability, flash point, and shelf life similar to fats [47].

C. Maltodextrins and Starch Derivatives

Maltodextrins are partial hydrolysates of starch [31], defined by the Food and Drug Administration as follows:

> Maltodextrin [$(C_6H_{12}O_5)_nH_2O$] is a non-sweet saccharide polymer that consists of D-glucose units linked primarily by alpha 1-4 bonds and that has a D.E. (dextrose equivalent) less than 20. It is prepared as a white powder or concentrated solution by partial hydrolysis of corn starch with safe and suitable acids or enzymes [52].

They are described as filling the void between starch and sugar [53]; low DE products serve as fat and oil replacers. Maltodextrins substituted on an equal-weight basis provide 4 kcal/g [46]. However, when maltodextrins are used as fat replacers, they usually are dissolved in a water:maltodextrin ratio of 3:1, thus producing a sol or gel providing only 1 kcal/g. Maltodextrin uses are widespread in the food industry; a wide range of products are available in powdered and syrup forms. The functionality of each type varies with the extent of starch degradation. The varying properties are indicated by the DE and degree of polymerization (DP), which change with the degree of hydrolysis and enzymatic treatment [31,53]. DE is expressed as the percentage hydrolysis of the glycosidic bonds. It reflects the amount of reducing power and, therefore, indicates stability and functionality. Maltodextrins are metabolized similarly to starch, thus they can be used by diabetics [54]. Maltodextrins possess a low sweetness level with a bland, not starchy flavor that does not mask other flavors [53,54].

Maltodextrins perform multifaceted functions in food systems. Some characteristics include: (1) bulking, (2) resistance to caking, (3) bland taste, (4) texture and body, (5) film forming, (6) binding of flavor and fat, (7) high nutritive value, (8) oxygen barrier, (9) surface sheen, and (10) dispersibility and solubility. The varying DE and/or bulk density give maltodextrins their varying characteristics and functionality [54]. For example, the high DE maltodextrins have solubility, bulking, and bodying characteristics more similar to the corn syrup sweeteners. The low DE maltodextrins have binding properties of starch and can function more effectively as fat binders than high DE maltodextrins. The surface sheen and creaminess can be related to the concentration; higher concentrations tend to be more brittle and lower concentrations have a "slimy" rather than creamy character.

Several commercial products marketed as fat replacers include: Maltrin® M040 (Grain Processing Corporation, Muscatine, IA); Paselli SA2 (Avebe Americas Inc., Princeton, NJ); Sta-Slim® 143 and Star Dri® 1 and 5 (A.E. Staley, Decatur, IL); N-Oil®, Instant N-Oil®, Instant N-Oil® II, and N-Flate™ (National Starch and Chemical Corp., Bridgewater, NJ); Rice Trin™ (Zumbro, Inc., Hayfield, MN); and Amalean™ (American Maize Products, Hammond, IN). More are being developed. Characteristics of some of these products are described further to provide the reader an idea of the variety of maltodextrins used for these purposes.

Maltrin M040 is a white powder with a DE of 5 produced from corn starch. The powder is completely soluble in hot water. Solutions of 30–50% dry solids of the Maltrins produce thermoreversible gels with a bland flavor, smooth mouthfeel, and a texture similar to hydrogenated oils or butterfat [47,55,56].

Paselli SA2 is a maltodextrin enzymatically converted from potato starch [57]. It is a fully digestible off-white powder, which can replace more than 50% of the fat in many products [58,59]. It has a DE of less than 3 and a pH between 5.5 and 7.0 [57]. The bulk density is 400 kg/m³. Used at the appropriate level and temperature, it forms a shiny, white, thermoreversible gel with a smooth, fatlike texture and neutral taste that is also suited for acid formulations. Undiluted, it has a value of 3.8 kcal/g [59]. Thus a typical gel with 25% solids contains less than 1 kcal/g. Paselli SA2 should not be stored more than 1 year because of its hygroscopicity [57].

Paselli SA2 can be used in aqueous systems by homogenization or by heating and stirring. In dry systems, it should be mixed with other dry ingredients to avoid lumping [57]. A gel is formed with concentrations greater than 20% [59] 2–3 hours after hydration, which is stable with fat and oil products and is easily mixed with other ingredients. The final gel strength usually is reached within 24 hours. The gel strength increases with increasing concentration and is maximized in the pH range of 3.5–5 if the hydration occurs within the temperature range of 90–194 °C [59]. It will be higher if the maltodextrin is not held at temperatures over 100 °C for long time periods [57].

A tapioca maltodextrin, N-Oil contains 4 kcal/g, but like the other products, if used in a 25% solution the yield is 1 kcal/g [58]. An instant pregelatinized tapioca maltodextrin form (N-Oil II) is available to use as a fat enhancer. The instant, pregelatinized form is designed for use in foods that require little or no heat or high-temperature, short-time processing [60]. The white to off-white powder has a pH of 4 (pH 6 for the instant product). Stability to low temperature for long storage periods is possible [62]. It also is heat-stable and can withstand high temperatures, high shear, and acidic conditions. To produce a gel for fat replacement, the solution should be heated to 190 °F (88 °C). It is added directly to food products as a hot liquid or cooled before using, depending upon the product. Upon cooling, the solution will develop the texture of hydrogenated shortening. N-Flate, which contains a mixture of ingredients that includes a modified food starch, also is available as a fat replacement for bakery products, and is discussed later.

Amalean I is a modified high-amylose food starch, which can replace 100% of fat [63], achieved by using 8% solids yielding 0.32 kcal/g. This results in a caloric reduction of 96%. Amalean I can be dry blended or used as a precooked paste. A gel for fat replacement can be achieved by heating a paste or slurry to 195–200 °F (88–90 °C) for 3 minutes. For cold-processed foods, the gel should be cooled to room temperature before using [64]. Amalean I can be used in applications requiring clear pastes [65].

All of the Star-Dri maltodextrins are prepared from waxy corn starch; Sta-Slim® 143 is prepared from a modified potato starch. Sta-Slim 143 is used as a fat mimic in products low in natural fats and is said to increase the perception of "creaminess." Usually it is slurried in water at 3–20% solids and heated with agitation to 150–160 °F (65–71 °C) before blending hot with other ingredients. In contrast, with several other maltodextrins used as fat replacers, it usually is processed as a warm liquid in formulations [66].

Stellar™ (A.E. Staley, Decatur, IL) was introduced recently as a fat-mimicking microparticulate corn starch gel that restructures and immobilizes water uniquely [131]. The acid-hydrolyzed corn starch's submicron crystallites are hydrated and shear-processed to provide a large surface area for the immobilized water [132]. The tightly bound water does not migrate in bakery products, which apparently is responsible for slowing the staling process and retarding water migration from cakes to fillings and vice versa. Staling and toughening, normally noted with reheating of bakery products, are reduced because water binding inhibits the starch-protein and protein-protein interactions [133].

Maintaining small, intact swollen starch granules duplicates the mouth sensation of fat. The irregularly shaped particle aggregates are 3–5 μm in diameter, slightly larger than the protein-based fat replacers, but approximately the same size as the fat crystals that they replace [133]. Its short, pseudoplastic texture is attributed to the low degree of association among the aggregates of submicron particles (about 0.02 μm) as compared to continuous, polymer gel networks that many gums form. This system was likened to fat crystals in a continuous oil phase. The particulate gel was confirmed by transmission electron microscopy and small angle x-ray scattering data [134]. The particle gel character was maintained with multiple heating/cooling cycles within the temperature range of 0–70 °C. This gives the 20% solids creme a plastic character that readily deforms similarly to the fats. Heating the creme to temperatures greater than 105 °C solubilizes the starch and decreases its funtional properties [131].

Applications for this fat replacer include low-fat margarines, soups, salad dressings, confections, bakery goods, frostings, fillings, cheese, and dairy products, frozen dairy desserts, and meat products. A low-fat (2.2%) Danish pastry formulated with Stellar™ stayed soft for up to 35 days [133]. These and additional starch derivatives that are used as fat-replacing bulking agents are listed in Table 1.

D. Fibers

Fiber can fulfill some of the bulking properties of sucrose and fat. A partial replacement of flour can be another way to provide bulk and reduce calories. Fiber will imbibe large quantities of water, contribute no calories, and also has been indicated to have nutritional benefits. A wide array of fiber products are commercially available from numerous plant sources—cereals, fruits, legumes, nuts, and vegetables—and they differ depending on their components [67]. In this review, fiber includes the celluloses, hemi-celluloses, gums, pectins, beta glucans, and lignins.

Gums, also referred to as hydrophilic colloids or hydrocolloids, give a thickening or gelling effect. Frequently, gums do not serve as direct fat, sugar, or flour substitutes, but they are used at low levels (0.1–0.5%) to imbibe water and contribute viscosity [47]. One part gum, often guar, locust bean, or carboxymethyl cellulose (CMC), can replace 10 parts starch as a thickening agent to reduce calorie content in sauces or puddings. Gums also contribute viscosity in "lite" syrups when the sugar is removed [68]. Added to dry ingredients in bakery products, they increase the soluble dietary fiber content and increase water-holding capacity so that water serves as the bulking agent without altering the original identity of most products. Gums useful for these purposes include agar, alginate, arabic, carrageenan, konjac, guar gum, high-

and low methoxyl pectins, xanthan gum, and cellulose derivatives. Several hydrocolloids currently marketed as fat replacers are listed in Table 2. The low solubility of many fibers and some gums can make them difficult to incorporate and contributes "grittiness" to finished food products. Grittiness can be minimized by soaking the fiber in the formula water before it is added. Clumping can be prevented by mixing with a carrier such as the flour in the system.

Cellulose derivatives include α-cellulose, CMC, hydroxypropyl cellulose, microcrystalline cellulose (MCC), and methyl cellulose (MC). Cellulose contains zero calories and is white and flavorless [69]. Various grades of cellulose are available for different processes and products [69] with the average particle sizes ranging from 20 to 120 μm. The finer grades (20–60 μm) are more suitable for baking purposes [70]. Water absorption is a function of particle size; the coarse grades absorb more water because of a more open structure than the fine grades [70]. Colloidal grades give a gel network that functions as a fat substitute. Such a gel network will stabilize foams and emulsions, modify texture, improve cling, contribute viscosity, suspend particles, control syneresis, add dietary fiber, and control ice crystal growth in frozen products [69].

A MCC dispersion has many physical properties of an emulsion. The particle size of approximately 0.2 μm simulates the fat sensations of an oil-in-water emulsion. Cellulose gels can contribute body, stability, creaminess, mouthfeel, and the glossy appearance of high-fat emulsions [70]. This sensation has been said to result from the three-dimensional network that is formed with water, which is similar to the three-dimensional network of fat [70]. Thus the rheological properties of the colloidal dispersion are similar to fat [71].

Oatrim (U.S.D.A., Peoria, IL) is a cold-water-dispersible amylodextrin derived from whole oat or debranned whole oat flour and is an example of a fiber that is rich in β-glucans [72]. Oatrim can be used to form a gel (25% dry solids) and function as a fat replacer. Oatrim can also function as a flour replacer in bread [72].

IV. EMULSIFIERS

Emulsifiers can replace all or part of the fat in many food products. Some emulsifiers used include mono- and diglycerides, sucrose esters, propylene glycol monoesters, sorbitan fatty acid esters, polysorbates, and various combinations. They retain moisture, reduce fat content, reduce calories, match or reduce the cost of fats, aid aeration, increase volume, and soften the crumb if used in bakery products [73]. The mono- and diglyceride emulsifiers are produced from vegetable oils by completely replacing all of the triglycerides.

Table 1 Selected Commercially Marketed Fat Replacers Derived from Starches

Replacer	Trade name (developer)	Conc. used (% solids)	Special features
Corn starch	Steller™ (A.E. Staley)		Acid hydrolyzed; forms microparticulate gel; extends shelf life in laminated pastries up to 2 weeks
Corn maltodextrin	Maltrin® M040 Maltrin® M100 Maltrin® M520 (Grain Processing Co)	35	Used for dairy products, frozen foods, sauces, salad dressings, confectionery products, and dry mixes
Corn maltodextrin	Lycadex® 200 (Roquette Corp.)	10–20	Enzymatically hydrolyzed; nongelling for sauces, salad dressings
Modified high-amylose corn starch	Amalean I™ Amalean II™ (American Maize-Products Co)	I–8 II–25	Acid, heat, shear tolerant; Amalean II developed to aid batter aeration in bakery products
Modified potato starch	Sta-Slim™ 143 Sta-Slim™ 141 (A.E. Staley)	3–20	Suggested for use in salad dressings, cheese products, soups
Potato maltodextrin	Paselli SA2 (Avebe America Inc)	>20	Enzymatically hydrolyzed; used in dips, dressings, frozen desserts, frostings, and bakery products
Potato maltodextrin	Lycadex® 100 (Roquette Corp.)	25	Enzymatically hydrolyzed; forms gel after 12 hr for bakery products, frozen dairy desserts, spreads
Whole rice maltodextrin	Rice*Trin 3 Complete® (Zumbro/IFP)	>20	Hydrolyzed by α-amylase; contains 10% protein as 1–5 μm particles; used in frozen desserts, bakery products, salad dressings
Pregelatinized rice starch	Remyrise AP® (A&B Ingredients)		

Tapioca dextrin	N-Oil®, Instant N-Oil® (National Starch & Chemical)	20–35	Used for frozen desserts, salad dressings
Tapioca maltodextrin	Instant N-Oil® II (National Starch & Chemical)	30–40	
Modified tapioca starch	Slenderlean™ (National Starch & Chemical)	1	Holds up to 10% formula weight in water in sausages and ground beef
Modified tapioca starch	Sta-Slim™ 150, 151 (A.E. Staley)	4–10	Provide creamy texture for wide range of food products but particularly suited for salad dressings
Tapioca	Tapiocaline® (Tipiak Inc.)		Partially pregelatinized; 50% nonsoluble remains granular shaped
Modified starch	CrystaLean™ (Opta Food Ingredients Inc.)		High fiber; high levels can be used without grittiness
Modified starch	N-Lite™ D (National Starch & Chemical)	2–4	Used for dairy products if slight gelling is desirable, e.g., frozen desserts, yogurts, and sour cream
Agglomerated waxy corn maltodextrins	Star-Dri® (A.E. Staley) LoDex (American Maize Products Co.)		Available as DE 1, 5, 10, 15, or 20; high bulking ability
Modified waxy corn	N-Lite™ L N-Lite™ LP (National Starch & Chemical)	2–10	Used for soups, sandwich spreads, salad dressings, and dips
Waxy corn maltodextrin	N-Lite™ B (National Starch & Chemical)	25–30	Used as gel in laminated doughs; extends shelf life and replaces up to 100% shortening
Blend of hydrolyzed wheat, potato, corn, and tapioca starches	Colestra™ (Reach Associates)	25%	

Source: Ref. 139. Reprinted with permission from *CRC Critical Review in Food Science and Nutrition.* Copyright CRC Press, Inc. Boca Raton, FL.

Table 2 Selected Hydrocolloids (Nonstarchy) Used as Fat Replacers

Product components	Trade Name (Developer)	Special features
β-Glucan from yeast	Fibercel™ (Alpha-Beta Technology Inc.)	Non-gelling for use in liquids; microspherical
β-1→4-Glucan polymer	Solka Floc® (James River Corp.)	Various fiber lengths and bulk volumes available
β-Glucans (dextrins) from oat flour	Oatrim (UDSA NRRL, Peoria) marketed as TrimChoice (Con-Agra Specialty Grain Products Co.)	
Microcrystalline cellulose + carboxymethyl-cellulose gel	Avicel® (FMC Corp.)	Insoluble cellulose crystallites prehydrated prior to adding to formulations
Cellulose + maltodextrin + xanthan gum (75:25:5)	Avicel® RCN-30 (FMC Corp.)	
Cellulose + guar gum	Avicel® RCN-15 (85:15) Avicel® RCN-10 (85:10) (FMC Corp.)	
Gellan gum	Kelcogel BF (Kelco)	

Hemicelluloses	Fibrex® from sugar beets (Delta Fibre Foods) Fibrim® from soy (Protein Technologies International) AF Fiber® from almonds (ITD Corp.)	Fibrex® high in protein and contains 74% total dietary fiber, 24% soluble dietary fiber
Inulin	Raftiline® Raftincreaming® (Tiense Suikkerraffinaderij Services)	Extracted from chicory roots; also considered a sucrose replacer; used in Europe but not yet approved in U.S.
Konjac flour gel	Nutricol® (FMC Corp)	Hot, cold, acid, alkali stability
Golden pea fiber	Centu Tex (Woodstone Foods)	High water absorption; used in low-calorie icings
Microfibrillated cellulose	(ITT-Rayonnier)	3–5% levels suggested for use in icings and fillings
Mixture of gum arabic, modified starch, alginate	Pretested Colloid No Fat 102 (TIC Gums Inc.)	
Pectin gel	Slendid™ (Hercules Inc.)	Extracted from citrus peel; acid and heat stable; levels < 5% suggested for wide range of food products including salad dressings, soups, sauces, frozen desserts, bakery products

Source: **Ref.** 139. Reprinted with permission from *CRC Critical Review in Food Science and Nutrition.* Copyright CRC Press, Inc., Boca Raton, FL.

These emulsifiers tend to be low in alpha-monoglyceride content and high in diglycerides. Dur-Lo (Durkee Industrial Foods Corp., Lisle, IL) is one such example. Butylated hydroxytoluene (BHT) and citric acid usually are added to protect the flavor. They are plastic with an ivory color and have a shelf life of about 6 months when stored at 60–80 °C [74]. The calorie content is the same as fat, however, a reduction in calories is achieved by reducing (25–78%) the amount of emulsifier used to obtain similar characteristics.

N-Flate is a blend of mono- and diglyceride and polyglycerol monoester emulsifiers; modified, pregelatinized food starch; guar gum; and nonfat dry milk developed especially for use in cake mixes [75,76]. The dry, free-flowing powder increases whippability and air incorporation in a cake batter.

V. OTHER LIPIDS AND PROTEINS AS FAT SUBSTITUTES

A. Simplesse® and Other Protein-Based Substitutes

Simplesse (NutraSweet Company, Skokie, IL) is produced from milk and/or egg white proteins [46,47,77]. This development is described in Chapter 9.

Each gram of this fat substitute will contribute 1.3 kcal/g versus 9 kcal/g by fat. Thus, 1 gram of protein and 2 grams of water replace 3 grams of fat [46,47,58] to achieve significant calorie reduction in nonheated products. Simplesse contains egg protein, therefore, food products containing the fat substitute carry warning labels to alert individuals who are allergic to egg protein and who might react to Simplesse [78].

Three forms of Simplesse are now available. A new version, Simplesse 100, is a thixotropic fluid made from whey protein concentrate, which can be used in bakery products and soups as well as cheese, butter, sour cream, yogurt, and other products also made with the original Simplesse. Simplesse Dry 100 is a readily hydratable powder, and the Simplesse 300 is a mixture of egg white and milk proteins with pectin and sugar (135). The Simplesse 100 can be used in foods that require heating, but they are not usable in fried foods or as a frying medium.

Semi-solid foods containing microparticulated proteins were compared to those containing fat or products with gums or maltodextrins as replacements (136). The microparticulated proteins were said to result in products more similar to the full-fat products than if maltodextrins or gums were used. However, they gave a less oily, more cohesive consistency than the full-fat product. Commercial products that have been formulated with the egg white/milk protein include the frozen dairy dessert (Simple Pleasures®, The Simplesse Co.) with sugars and with aspartame. The sugar product contains 120–150 kcal/4-oz serving, depending upon the flavoring used, and the aspartame product contains 80–90 kcal/4 oz (137,138). Another fat-free product that has been developed as a vanilla frozen dessert sandwiched between two fat-free chocolate wafers (Fat Freedom™ Eskimo Pie® sandwich, Eskimo Pie Corp.) containing 130 kcal. The traditional counterpart contains 180 kcal.

Trailblazer® (Kraft General Foods, NY) and Finesse™ (Reach Associates, South Orange, NJ) are yet other egg albumin and milk protein fat substitutes but made by different processes. Other milk protein hydrolysates are being developed to provide creamy mouthfeel in dairy products [79], and examples of similar protein-based fat substitutes likely will increase rapidly.

B. Developmental Lipids

Dialkyl dihexadecyl malonate (DDM), prepared from malonate esters (Frito-Lay, Inc., Dallas, TX), esterified propoxylated glycerol (EPG, ARCO Chemical Co., Newtown Square, PA), trialkoxytricarballylate (TATCA, CPC International, Englewoods Cliffs, NJ), trialkoxyglycerylether, trialkoxycitrate, and refined jojoba oil are all examples of synthetic fat substitutes under development. Each is noncaloric, or nearly so, and expected to have good stability for baking and frying [47,58,61]. Other low-calorie carbohydrate-lipid combinations that have been developed include Prolestra™, Nutrifat™ (Reach Associates, South Orange, NJ), and Colestra™ (Food Ingredients and Innovations, Ashland, MA) [47]. However, the safety of these fat substitutes has not been established.

VI. PHYSICOCHEMICAL PROPERTIES RELATED TO FOOD FUNCTION

A. Maillard Browning and Caramelization

The carbonyl-amine (or Maillard) browning reaction involves the interaction of an amino acid and a reducing sugar. Caramelization of sugars occurs at elevated temperatures and is promoted by acidic and alkaline conditions. Either reaction can produce both desirable and undesirable aroma and flavor compounds. The food processor should know which bulking agents are susceptible to each of these reactions to maximize the desirable and minimize the undesirable effects.

Maltodextrins have the capacity to participate in Maillard reactions. The extent of the browning increases with increasing DE [53,54]. Low DE maltodextrins can be used as nonbrowning carriers for drying-sensitive products [81].

In contrast, sorbitol, lactitol, maltitol, or xylitol do not participate in Maillard reactions because they lack aldehyde groups. This also allows for the sorbitol and maltitol syrup to be concentrated to high dry substance levels without product discoloration [11]. The slight yellow color that occurs when sugar alcohols are heated above 150 °C results from the presence of low levels of impurities [80]. Furthermore, neither Lycasin nor isomalt participate in Maillard browning. Hydrogenation of the starch hydrolysis products of Lycasin leaves less than 0.2% free reducing sugars. During the production of Palatinit, the aldehyde group is hydrogenated; thus its reducing sugar content is only 0.8%.

Neither sorbitol, xylitol, maltitol, nor isomalt caramelize when crystalline or aqueous solutions are heated above their melting points. When exposed to conditions similar to those of baking or candy manufacturing (pH 3, 145 °C), lactitol content remains virtually unchanged [17,20]. Lactitol, maltitol, and Lycasin do not decompose at temperatures less than 200 °C [11,82]. The missing carbonyl group also makes lactitol more stable than lactose in alkaline mediums. In an acid medium, lactitol's glycosidic linkage stability is about the same as lactose [17,20]. Xylitol can polymerize slightly if heated at a temperature above 300 °C for a prolonged period [84]; sorbitol is thermally stable up to 250 °C without decomposition or caramelization in either acidic or alkaline conditions [11,12,85].

Food products made with isomalt experience little composition change, caramelization, discoloration, or dehydration during melting, extrusion, or baking [86,87]. Isomalt is stable in acid or alkaline media; it does not caramelize when crystalline substances or aqueous solutions are heated above its melting point, 200 °C or greater [24,26,87]. Its stability can be attributed to the $1 \rightarrow 6$ disaccharide linkage because it takes more energy to hydrolyze the $1 \rightarrow 6$ linkage compared to the $1 \rightarrow 2$ linkage found in sucrose. Complete hydrolysis requires 5 hours in 1.0% HC1 at 100 °C, whereas sucrose is completely hydrolyzed within a few minutes at the same HCl concentration and temperature [23,24]. No more than 10.0% hydrolysis should occur when isomalt is subjected to harsh conditions that might be found in food manufacturing, pH 2 and heating for 100 °C for more than 1 hour [24].

B. Crystallization

Polyols vary in crystallization ability. Lactitol has a crystallization pattern similar to sucrose [19]. Compared to other polyols, isomalt has a low solubility, thus a higher tendency toward crystallization [25]. Pure sorbitol solutions tend to crystallize at temperatures below 21–23 °C. To combat this crystallization problem, "noncrystallizing" grades containing oligosaccharides have been developed [13]. The texture of the xylitol-containing product differs from a product containing sucrose because of differences in crystallization and water-binding capacity; therefore, substitution of xylitol for sucrose in food products can require modification of the processing conditions [80]. In jams and jellies, xylitol at concentrations greater than 40% likely will crystallize during storage [80]. Even dust particles have been demonstrated to trigger crystallization of xylitol solutions [84]. With Lycasin, no sugar inversion takes place with acidic conditions during processing [13]. Crystallization does not occur at reduced temperatures or high concentrations. This property allows Lycasin to serve as an anticrystalline inhibitor in many confectionery products [13,36].

Low DE maltodextrins are effective in preventing formation of coarse crystals. The variety of sugar polymers in maltodextrins prevents formation of large, gritty crystals as sugar mixtures will not crystallize as readily as pure compounds [54]. And the fine particle size of maltodextrins contribute to a smooth, creamy, mouthfeel in many food products [88]. Polydextrose also does not crystallize [38].

C. Cooling Effects

Polyalcohols have cooling effects because of the negative heats of solution, which can be used advantageously to provide a clean, refreshing taste in products such as mints. The cooling effects of various polyalcohols are listed in Table 3.

D. Fermentation

Sorbitol, mannitol, and xylitol are nonfermentable by yeast and fairly resistant to bacterial growth [16,19,28]. Longer fermentation time is required to prepare yogurt with xylitol [28]. The osmotic pressure of a sorbitol solution (70%) is high enough to prevent microbial spoilage [12]. Lactitol is metabolized slowly by some yeasts. However, it is fairly resistant to bacterial growth [22].

Table 3 Cooling Effect of Selected Polyalcohols

Polyalcohol	Cooling effect (kcal/g at 25 °C)	Ref.
Isomalt	− 9.4	26
Lactitol		
Monohydrate	− 12.7	
Dihydrate	− 13.9	17,89
Mannitol	− 28.9	13
Sorbitol	− 26.5	11
Xylitol	− 34.8	28

Isomalt cannot be used as a substrate by microorganisms because the $1 \rightarrow 6$ linkage is resistant to microbial attack. Thus isomalt has high microbial stability in foods and beverages [23,26,87]. This ability to impair mold growth and microbial activity is the result of lowered water activity.

E. Hygroscopicity and Flowability

Hygroscopic properties influence moisture levels in food products. The rate of moisture change can be affected by the nature of the food, the formulation used, and the product packaging. Low moisture absorption is particularly important in crisp baked goods such as cookies. Various bulking agents can serve as humectants in many food products.

Polydextrose can serve as a humectant to slow moisture changes (either an increase or a decrease) in food. The powdered form absorbs moisture under normal, controlled atmospheric conditions until equilibrium is reached. Polydextrose can be used to improve the flowability of dry ingredients in a dry mix. It can serve as a formulation aid to assure uniform dispersions and help to prevent lumping of dry ingredients. At 52% relative humidity (RH) and 25 °C, polydextrose powder absorbs 10% moisture, whereas at 75% RH and 25 °C, it gains 25% water. Polydextrose-N loses water to attain the same equilibrium concentrations, approximately 80% w/w at 75% RH and 90% w/w at 52% RH [38–40]. When the equilibrium relative humidity (ERH) of different concentrations of polydextrose solutions is compared with sucrose and sorbitol solutions, polydextrose is similar to 50 and 60% sucrose equivalent weight solutions, but its ERH is higher than sorbitol's [38]. The hygroscopic properties necessitate polydextrose's storage in tightly sealed, moisture-proof containers.

The hygroscopicity of the maltodextrins increases with increasing DE [53,54]. Thus, their humectant properties vary inversely with DE; the lower the DE, the greater the flowability at higher ERH [56]. Maltrin 040 and Paselli SA2 are two examples of low-DE maltodextrins that have low humectant properties and remain free-flowing [56,81]. Such maltodextrins can be used in spray-drying hygroscopic materials.

Xylitol is among the most hygroscopic polyols, although less hygroscopic than sorbitol [90]. At 20 °C and 77% RH, crystalline or powdered xylitol has a moisture content of 0.5%, but at 85% RH xylitol absorbs enough water to nearly liquefy the crystals [28,84]. The moisture uptake accelerates rapidly above 85% RH. At higher temperatures the increase occurs at lower relative humidities. Xylitol may be unsuitable as a humectant at low temperature/humidity combinations. In most tropical regions, the storage of xylitol or xylitol products may present packaging problems [84].

Sorbitol often is regarded as a humectant. However, this is a misconception, because this is a property only of sorbitol solutions [13,14]. When sorbitol syrup is subjected to changes in ambient humidity, it is less prone to gain or lose water compared to other humectants such as glycerol, and the ERH also is reached more slowly [11]. The gamma crystalline form of sorbitol is only slightly hygroscopic, and it remains free-flowing during storage at cool temperatures [11,12]. The limiting relative humidity of the crystalline form is 70–73% at 20 °C compared to 80–84% for sucrose [13].

Isomalt's low hygroscopicity and low solubility are important properties in food applications. No moisture pickup was noted at 25 °C with up to 85% RH. At temperatures of 60 and 80 °C, water absorption commenced with 75 and 65% RH, respectively [25,26].

Lactitol's mono- and dihydrate forms and solutions are nonhygroscopic, although the anhydrous form is hygroscopic [17,18,20,22]. Lactitol monohydrate is less hygroscopic than sorbitol and xylitol, but at high relative humidities it is more hygroscopic than mannitol. Moisture is absorbed by lactitol at a relative humidity greater than 50% at 30 °C [17,20]. The low hygroscopic properties of lactitol monohydrate make it free-flowing, but do not allow it to be used to regulate water-binding properties. Its nonhygroscopic properties are desirable in crisp baked goods and coatings of moisture-sensitive sweets (e.g., jellies) where crystalline lactitol will protect against water absorption [19,22].

Mannitol and maltitol are much less hygroscopic than sorbitol [91]. Maltitol has a moisture content of 6% at 75% RH at 35 °C [83]. Lycasin syrup is only slightly hygroscopic. However, the powdered form is hygroscopic, and requires careful handling and holding before use [13]. A combination of isomalt and Lycasin in a ratio of 60:40 yields a product that is not hygroscopic or caramelized, and sweeter than each bulking agent if used separately because of synergism [24,26].

F. Melting

The melting points of some bulking agents are listed in Table 4. Paselli SA2 gels will melt when heated to 50–90 °C, yielding viscous solutions. However, the solutions will gel again when cooled and can be maintained several hours at room temperature [57]. Polydextrose is amorphous and melts above 130 °C. Upon cooling it produces a clear, brittle glass [38]. All commercially produced xylitol is of the stable *ortho*-rhombic form with a melting range of 92–96 °C [84].

G. Solubility

Aqueous solutions of polydextrose can be prepared with concentrations as high as 80% [39,92]. The rate of solution of the amorphous powder depends upon the equipment and the manner in which the powder is added to the

Table 4 Melting Points of Bulking Agents

Bulking agent	Melting point (°C)	Ref.
Isomalt	145–150	26
Lactitol monohydrate	95–97	17
Maltitol	130–142	83
Mannitol	165–168	30
Mono- and diglyceride emulsifiers	113–120	74
Maltodextrin (Paselli SA2)	50–90	57
Polydextrose	130	38
Sorbitol		
Gamma form	96	13,30
Anhydrous form	110–112	13
Xylitol		
Ortho-rhombic form	92–96	84
Metastable monoclinic	61	84

water [39,40]. Difficulties in dissolving polydextrose can be overcome by slowly dispersing polydextrose in hot water with sufficient mechanical agitation. Solubility also can be facilitated by blending dry polydextrose with a soluble diluent [38–40,93]. Polydextrose is insoluble in ethanol and only partially soluble in glycerin and propylene glycol [38].

All of the sugar alcohols are nonvolatile, completely miscible with each other and other sugars [17,18], only slightly soluble in the organic solvents, such as ethanol and methanol [13,28], and vary in their solubility in water. Sorbitol and xylitol are readily soluble in water and are similar to sucrose at temperatures between 10–30 °C. However, in higher temperatures (40–50 °C), their solubilities increase more rapidly than sucrose. At 25 °C, 235 g of sorbitol are soluble per 100 cc of water [35]; the concentration of a saturated solution (% w/w) is 72 g [13]. The solubility of xylitol is approximately 65g/100g solution at 30 °C [28,84].

Lactitol's solubility also increases linearly with increasing temperature. At 25 °C, 149–150 g lactitol monohydrate (or 140 g of dihydrate) will dissolve in 100 ml water with a dry solids content of 60.0% [19,20]. A wide solubility temperature range makes lactitol applicable to a variety of food products. However, products with a high dry solids content (67%) will crystallize [21]. Maltitol at 25 °C has a solubility of 100 g in 100 g water [83]. Mannitol has a solubility of 22 g in 100 g water at 25 °C. This low solubility may be a disadvantage, as it will prevent it from being used in many products [30].

Isomalt has limited solubility compared to sucrose. Increasing temperatures produce increased solubility [23,24]. In water, a maximum concentration of 25% solids at 20 °C, which is less than half the solubility of sucrose, can be achieved [86,87]. To prevent the recrystallization of α-D-glucopy-ranosido-1→6 mannitol, the total dry solids content must not exceed 46% [24]. Isomalt, too, is characterized as insoluble in ethanol [26]; however, in aqueous ethanol solutions, the solubility of isomalt increases linearly with increasing temperature and decreasing alcohol content [24]. Isomalt's solubility range is sufficient for most food products except fruit jams, marmalades, preserves, and jellies. In food systems with relatively high water content (e.g., jams, preserves, ice cream, and candies), the low solubility of isomalt can be counterbalanced by the addition of another sugar alcohol such as Lycasin or maltitol, to prevent recrystallization in products.

The solubilities of maltodextrins increase with increasing DE [53,54]. Some maltodextrins are cold water soluble. For example, the levels of Paselli SA2 used in food systems (less than 30% w/w) swell in cold water [57], and up to 40% Maltrin 040 dissolves in water [81]. They can produce a solution, which is clear or cloudy, depending upon specific properties [53]. Some forms of maltodextrins can be agglomerated for increased bulking, solubility, and dispersibility [54].

H. Texturizing and Bodying

Polydextrose can be used to control, modify, and improve texture in food products. It improves mouthfeel and viscosity in many products [39]. Polydextrose has been reported to mimic the effects of sucrose on starch gelatinization by increasing the temperature at which it occurs [95]. Therefore, it can be useful in bakery products.

Polydextrose solutions behave as typical Newtonian liquids that are slightly more viscous than equal concentrations of sucrose or sorbitol. Increasing temperatures decrease viscosity of polydextrose solutions. When comparing 70% solutions of polydextrose, sorbitol, and sucrose at 20°C, polydextrose is approximately 1000 centipoises (cps) more viscous than sucrose and 15000 cps more viscous than sorbitol [38,40]. Increasing concentrations of polydextrose gave rise to increased viscosities [38].

Sorbitol adds body to products such as pudding, jelly, and carbonated beverages [29]. The viscosity of sorbitol (70% dry substances) at 25°C is approximately 120 cps [14]. The noncrystallizing syrups are somewhat more viscous than the crystallizing syrup [11]. This viscosity is the same as fructose. Xylitol's substantially lower viscosity than sucrose is the result of its lower molecular weight. Xylitol, like all polyols, has a decreased viscosity at increased temperatures [13,28]. Xylitol has relatively poorer bodying effects because of its substantially lower viscosity. Therefore, it is necessary to modify standard procedures by increasing the proportion of high molecular weight components such as increasing the level of gelling agents in jellies [90]. Solutions of isomalt and lactitol have similar viscosities as equivalent sucrose solutions [20,24-26,29]. The viscosity of Palatinit solutions increases with dry solids content and decreases with increasing temperatures [26]. Lactitol solutions are less viscous than the parent lactose solutions. This decrease in viscosity can be attributed to the opening of the pyranose ring of the glucose moiety. Lactitol solutions are more viscous than similar sorbitol or xylitol solutions [18,19]. At 30°C with 60% dry solids, the viscosity is 47-50 cps [17,19]. A 70% maltitol solution at 40°C has a viscosity of 241 cps, higher than that of sorbitol [14].

The viscosity of Lycasin is higher than a comparable sucrose solution. At 25°C, its viscosity with 75% dry solids is 500 cps [13,14,36]. The high viscosity results from the presence of 23% hydrogenated polysaccharides in the range of trisaccharides to septasaccharides (DP3-DP7) and 18% hydrogenated higher polysaccharides (DP > 8) [36].

Maltodextrins help to control body or viscosity while giving a smooth and stable texture. Viscosity decreases with increasing temperature and DE [56]. A 25% w/w Paselli SA2/demineralized water system at 20°C yields a viscosity of 100 cps [27]. Paselli SA2 acts as a binding and filling agent, texturizing such products as powdered baby foods. Maltrin 040 retains its viscosity in solutions. Solutions using 20-40% dry solids are more viscous than high DE products of equal concentration [81]. At 80°C Maltrin 040 has a viscosity of 100 at 38% solids content. The viscosity of Amalean I increases with pH, concentration, and time [64].

Gums that have viscosity at low concentrations, such as guar, locust bean (carob), xanthan, MC, and CMC, are used to thicken syrups. They also are added to batters to allow for more even crumb expansion as the product bakes. Locust bean and xanthan gums, by increasing the viscosity of the water phase, also can enhance the foam stability of whipped products and cake batters.

VII. APPLICATIONS

A. Bakery Products

1. Replacing Sucrose

Polydextrose has been used in many bakery goods and mixes including biscuits, pound cake, yellow cake, angel food cakes, brownies, butter cookies, doughnuts, wafers, pastries, and pudding- and custard-filled pies [92,93]. As a bulking agent it contributes solids and improves textural qualities and palatability without contributing sweetness. Its low caloric content aids in the development of reduced- or low-calorie products. In bakery mixes, polydextrose can improve the flowability, assure uniform dispersion, and help to prevent lumping of dry ingredients.

The acidity of polydextrose can be adjusted by using a small quantity of sodium bicarbonate to a pH of 5.5 or higher or by using the buffered type K in the formulation [38,39]. Torres and Thomas [39] noted that leavening and batter absorption could need adjustment when substituting polydextrose for sucrose.

Several studies [42,92,93,96–100] report the use of a polydextrose/high-potency sweetener combination for the partial replacement of sucrose in layer cakes to achieve one-third or more calorie reductions. Kamel and Rasper [97] found adverse effects when polydextrose replaced 50% of the sucrose in a reduced-calorie cake system. These cakes were described as having a "heavy" texture, "syrupy" mouthfeel with a mild, detectable, bitter after-taste. A 70:30 sucrose:polydextrose combination, however, was found to have a volume similar to the sucrose control cake. For partial replacement of sucrose in reduced-calorie cake systems, an appropriate level and combination of emulsifiers was suggested as necessary [100]. Combinations of bulking agents/sweeteners were used with specially treated emulsifier systems to partially or completely replace sucrose and shortening in layer cakes [8,97, 98]. A sucrose/polydextrose and a sorbitol/polydextrose system did not differ from two commercial products in several sensory textural attributes.

Reduced-calorie cakes made by totally replacing the nonsweetening functions of sucrose with polydextrose (62.5–79.0% flour weight basis, fwb) or a polydextrose, sorbitol, and maltodextrin combination were reported by Neville and Setser [42] and Freeman [96], respectively. In the study by Neville and Setser [42], polydextrose had no influence on cell uniformity but inversely affected specific gravity, volume, and shrinkage. All cakes containing polydextrose were found to be "gummier" than a standard yellow layer cake. Bitterness and sweetness intensities were found to increase even though sweetener levels were held constant. These bitterness findings were confirmed in studies using polydextrose and high-potency sweeteners in a shortbread system [102].

Polydextrose in shortbread cookies, compared to the sucrose counterpart, was found to increase spread, hardness, and fracturability while decreasing cohesiveness of the mass [102]. Freeman totally replaced sucrose with polydextrose and fructose in a chocolate brownie. Hedonic tests indicated that the brownies as well as yellow and chocolate cakes with partial sucrose replacement by polydextrose had "good flavor, color, and symmetry and acceptable sweetness and eating characteristics" [92].

Freeman [96] also developed formulas using polydextrose to replace sucrose and cellulose to replace flour. Prepared cake and cookie mixes were reported to have good storage stability for 6 months at room temperature.

Powdered cellulose has been used in conjunction with polydextrose and other gums for up to 75% flour replacement [69]. Guar gum replaced up to 15% of the flour in several types of cakes [103], and Zabik and coworkers [104] reported that good quality cakes could be made with any of several cellulose fiber types substituting for 30% of the flour. Cakes can achieve 10–20% greater volume with 2% (dry ingredient weight) powdered α-cellulose [105]. The short-fibered grade replaces the bulk of the sugar and flour, and the long-fibered product is said to add structure, strength, and bite. "Light" breads also can be produced replacing part of the flour with cellulose [106]. However, gluten must be added to ensure proper dough structure [69], and water content must be increased. Polydextrose cannot be used in yeast-leavened breads if all fermentable sugars are replaced [39] unless enzymes or cereal malt to provide enzymes are added to break down the starch in flour to fermentable sugars [107].

Polyalcohols have been used in reduced-sugar bakery products for several years. Sorbitol has been the standard bulking agent for dietetic products [13,108]. Xylitol in bakery goods is feasible with no alterations in formulation. Fructose can be added to improve crust formation, caramelization, and nonenzymatic browning. However, products with polyalcohols likely will have a volume that is slightly smaller than that of similar sucrose products [28]. The low hygroscopicity of several polyalcohols lends itself to use in crisp baked goods [109]. Bollinger [26] reported that yeast dough can be made from isomalt without modifying traditional recipies even though it is not used as a substrate by yeast.

Lactitol is reported to totally or partially replace sucrose with relatively few formulation changes [17] producing cakes with similar specific volume, shelf life, texture, and eating qualities [17,20,21]. The low calorie content of lactitol lends its application to reduced-calorie products. Lactitol/sucrose combinations are also suggested [22]. Successful development of a "light biscuit-like product" (cookies) is reported with a total carbohydrate content of less than 10% and a sugar content below 4% using lactitol for the sweetener and calcium caseinate as a flour substitute [17,20,22].

Traditional bakery good formulations have been made with isomalt with few changes [26,110–112]. Sweetness was increased by the addition of high potency sweeteners [25,87] or the addition of fructose in an isomalt:fructose ratio of 85:15 to increase both sweetness and crust browning [23,26]. However, Brack et al. [110,111] found that 50:50 and 67:33 isomalt:fructose combinations produced unacceptable cake products with "poor form," a dark crumb, a dark and thick crust, and burnt notes. A high-protein flour and wheat starch were used to compensate for the low solubility properties of isomalt, which might have partially caused the unacceptable cakes. Johnson [8] found that thick, leathery crusts were associated with cakes containing high levels of a high-DE maltodextrin (Maltrin M180) or polydextrose and with combinations of the maltodextrin and polyols, including isomalt.

Cakes with isomalt as a complete sucrose replacement were found to have similar volume, shape, and color as sucrose cakes [110], but the cake crumb was reported to be soft and gluey. The crust was described as dull and shriveling, and crystallization occurred upon standing for more than 2 days. After 14 days of storage, the cake crumb was dry and crumbly with a stale flavor.

Crystallization on the cake surface and a dry crumb because of moisture migration from crumb to crust [26,110] also were reported in pound or madeira cakes, sponge flans, and sponge fingers. Increasing the moisture content increased number and size of white crystals that formed on the cake crust [110]. Bollinger suggested that sorbitol or fat level increases could decrease moisture migration [26]. Gums or glycerine could be added to decrease water activity and, therefore, help control moisture migration in bakery goods. Icing or glossing also can conceal this problem. The low hygroscopic properties of isomalt can be advantageous or detrimental in bakery products depending on the product characteristics. In short-pastry biscuits (cookies) low hygroscopicity improves shelf life. Short crust dough with isomalt hardens after processing. To keep dough pliable it is necessary to increase the water in formulations, but consistency corrections by the addition of water after mixing are not advised. To decrease the risk of short crust becoming tough, 10–30% of the flour can be replaced by starch, which can increase the risk of dough separation. The addition of small amounts of emulsifier reduced separation. Stiffening and toughness were reduced by replacing flour with some fiber. In hard cookie doughs, hardening still can be a problem when using isomalt and can be corrected by increasing the water content. Fructose/isomalt combinations in hard cookies usually are not recommended because excessive crumb darkening results. In gingerbread cookies, a suspension of isomalt, fructose, and water heated to 50 °C can be substituted for a standard invert sugar solution.

2. Replacing Fat

Various emulsifiers have been demonstrated to partially or totally replace fat in reduced-calorie cake products [96,98–101]. The emulsifiers promote increased aeration of the products. The substitution of emulsifiers can be in combination with carbohydrate bulking agents such as sorbitol, polydextrose, or combinations thereof [8,98–100].

Mono- and diglycerides replaced 50% of the fat in cookies, cakes, and cake mixes by using a 50:50 emulsifier:water ratio. The emulsifiers absorb water and maintain moisture in the bakery products [73]. Mixtures of sodium stearoyl lactylate, sorbitan monostearate, and polysorbate 60 at high hydration levels gave cakes of good quality with only 3–6% oil (flour weight basis) in cakes [100]. A hydrated blend of emulsifers developed specifically for use in reduced-calorie, flour-based bakery goods includes stearyl monoglyceridyl citrate, propylene glycol monostearate, and lactylated monoglycerides [113]. N-Flate replaced up to 50% of the shortening in cookies resulting in an increased volume, height, softer, more cakelike texture than the original cookie. N-Flate at the 6–8% level (of the total batter weight) can replace all 10–12% of the shortening in several bakery products [76]. Several studies used sucrose polyesters in low-calorie bakery goods [114–116].

Maltodextrins can be used in a gram-for-gram fat or sucrose replacement in bakery goods. Paselli SA2, for example, has been used as a fat replacer in cakes, muffins, and cookies [57], and Amalean I has been used in reduced-fat bakery products such as cake, muffins, and cheesecake [65].

Olestra can be used at high temperatures including baking and deep-fat frying applications. Since proteins are subject to heat denaturation, Simplesse's functionality likely is altered when exposed to heat [78]. Therefore, use of Simplesse as a substitute in food products that require baking or frying has been limited. Coagulation of proteins with heat likely would alter the mouthfeel [47].

B. Beverages

Sugar alcohols, including isomalt [24], add body to beverages such as low-alcohol beer. Sucrose polyesters are used in nonalcoholic beverages to incorporate aromatics [50,113–115]. Neither is fermentable, so they are effective in the low-alcohol beer application. The choice of sugar alcohol depends on the characteristics desired [14]. Sorbitol, lactitol, and Lycasin all have been suggested to add body to soft drinks [13,33,36,50], although high levels of the sugar alcohol are not recommended in soft drinks because of the laxative effects. Zimmerman states that the sweetening power of Lycasin is not sufficient for soft drinks. Acids (citric and lactic acid) are more detectable at this sweetness level; their addition in products should be reduced 20–30% [131]. An isosweet soft drink with fewer calories was produced by using xylitol in combination with high-potency sweeteners; it can be used in milk-based chocolate drinks to give similar physical properties as the sucrose-sweetened products [28].

Gums are added to sugar-free beverages to give viscosity similar to sugar-sweetened products. MCC, for example, was used to increase the concentration of fiber in high protein drinks while imparting a creamy mouthfeel [69].

C. Confectionery Products

Polydextrose can be used in both hard and soft candies and in frostings [92, 118] to partially replace either sugar, including corn syrup, or fat. It will produce a good-textured product without other bulking materials such as cellulose, and it is almost equivalent to invert sugar or corn syrup as a humectant [118]. Since polydextrose is acidic, sodium citrate must be added to optimize flavor and to reduce sugar inversion. Polydextrose produces a slightly lighter colored and less tacky product with reduced calories than is obtained with the sugars. In soft candy (toffees, caramel, gum drops), its humectant properties help to retain softness.

Polyalcohols are used widely in the confectionery industry because of their noncariogenic properties [119]. Lycasin was especially manufactured for the confectionery industry. When used in boiled confections, it produces hygroscopic sweets that will not crystallize on the surface if water is absorbed. Therefore, these products, as well as those prepared with any of the hygroscopic polyols, need to be packaged in hermetic materials to prevent stickiness [120].

Sorbitol is marketed in "sugar-free" candies where it serves as a total sucrose or glucose replacer. As a general rule the crystalline form will replace sucrose and the syrup will replace glucose syrups. The balance of components used depends on the product [14]. Sorbitol can be used in hard-pan coating, pressed tablets, chocolates, hard candies, or partially crystallized products such as fondants, chewy candies, and chewing gums. Hard candies, again, must be wrapped in moisture-proof material to prevent moisture absorption. Sorbitol can be used for the production of pastilles using a 50:50 gum arabic: sorbitol ratio. Gum pastilles made with maltitol syrups are less hygroscopic than those from sorbitol. Additions of mannitol will aid to prevent stickiness and glycerol improves plasticity in chewing gums. Chewing gum also can be made using sorbitol powder and maltitol syrup (85%) [11]. Appropriate granule size and temperatures less than 50 °C must be used to totally replace sucrose with sorbitol in chocolate.

Levels of 5–10% sorbitol will improve textural properties of conventional sweets [11]. An advantage of sorbitol in confectionery goods is that it does not cause the inversion of sucrose [13]. Isomalt also does not cause sugar inversion, and isomalt hard candies are less hygroscopic that traditional sugar/glucose sweets [26]. The low solubility and tendency to recrystallize requires usage of other sugar alcohols, such as Lycasin or maltitol, when using isomalt [23].

Xylitol's cooling effects can be exploited [80] in mints and chewing gums, and it can be substituted for sucrose on a 1:1 basis. Since xylitol is less viscous than sucrose, using gum arabic increases viscosity and helps to decrease mixing time in chewing gum. Kneading operations can be controlled by using an aqueous xylitol solution or adding glycerol as with sorbitol gums. Particle size of the xylitol should not exceed 50 μm and the temperature should be 10 °C less than for the sucrose/glucose gum. The addition of water should be kept at a minimum to avoid hardening [28]. If isomalt is used in chewing gums, temperatures need to exceed 50 °C to prevent loss of water with crystallization [26].

Xylitol can be used for tablet coatings, hard candies, and chocolate with certain deviations from conventional techniques. Xylitol chocolates were noted to have a coarse, sandy texture after storage in RH exceeding 85% [28]. Xylitol concentration in chocolate bars ranges from 17 to 42%. Chocolates might need additives to increase the viscosity [80]. In toffees and caramels, xylitol must be used with an agent, such as maltodextrins or Lycasin, to prevent hardening and crystallization. The absence of Maillard browning and caramelization requires the addition of coloring and flavoring agents. Toffees tend to have a short texture [28]. Modifications in procedures are needed to produce a hard candy from xylitol. If clear, hard-boiled sweets are desired, xylitol needs to be used in combination with natural polymers; however, nonclear products can be achieved without additives [80]. The use of glucose as a crystallization inhibitor reverses xylitol's noncariogenic benefit [28]. Xylitol candies crystallize during the cooling phase leaving brittle drops, but it has been used in combination with polydextrose and hydrogenated glucose syrups to provide a boiled hard candy that has a one-third calorie reduction.

Gum drops using xylitol plus gum arabic, pectin, or gelatin tend to harden during storage. Sorbitol or Lycasin helps to retard crystallization [13,14]. Pectin jellies with 75% xylitol will crystallize, but if xylitol is used in lower proportions, the pectin will no longer gel. This can be overcome with the addition of gelatin or agar.

Lactitol can be used in the production of chewing gum and hard candies with a 100% replacement of sucrose. Additional sweetness will need to be imparted with a high-potency sweetener. In chocolates, lactitol can replace sucrose in a ratio of 1:1. The lactitol is said to enhance the chocolate flavor [17]. Lactitol candies are not hygroscopic and are easy to wrap [20]. It should be used with another sugar alcohol in pastilles to prevent crystallization [21].

Sucrose polyesters can be used as lubricants for producing tablet candy in molds or as viscosity reducers in chocolate manufacturing [50]. Some gums and maltodextrin gels (e.g., MCC, Paselli SA2, Amalean I, and N-Oil) can be used in confections and frostings to add creaminess and replace fat [47, 57,58].

D. Dairy Products

Removal of conventional sweeteners from ice creams increases the freezing point; reversal of this effect is necessary for a bulking material to be used in non-sugar-sweetened, frozen desserts. Polyols used as bulk sweeteners in frozen desserts include sorbitol, lactitol, xylitol, and isomalt. Sorbitol will cause a slight depression of the freezing point in ice cream [11,13] and is effective in limiting the formation of ice crystals [14]. Lactitol can be used in ice cream in conjunction with a potent sweetener [20]. Its level in low-fat ice creams is about 14% [21].

Xylitol will alter melting properties of frozen products producing softer products at the same temperature. This condition can be improved with the addition of thickeners [80]. Frozen stability of xylitol ice cream is good during storage. Xylitol can be used in yogurt with no effect on pH when added after incubation. The viscosity of presweetened xylitol yogurt is lower than that of its sucrose counterpart [28].

Isomalt can be used in yogurt, ice cream, ice milk, pudding, and other milk-based desserts [23,26]. However, the Palatinit content cannot exceed 15% in ice cream products because it recrystallizes. If a higher dry substance content is desired, fructose or another sugar substitute should be added [26]. A novel approach to add "bulk" with the high-potency sweeteners is the use of increased nonfat milk solids with lactase to hydrolyze the lactose and prevent the grittiness that is usually associated with high lactose levels [121].

Milkfat content can be reduced in frozen dairy desserts using a variety of gums and maltodextrin gels. The ability to depress the freezing point by maltodextrins increases with increasing DE [53,54]. Low DE maltodextrins, such as Paselli SA2, can be used in cold-prepared, pasteurized foods including frozen desserts if they are soluble in cold water as well as thermostable and able to form stable mixtures with other food components. Gums, especially the cold water–soluble hydrocolloids, are used widely to imbibe water and control crystallization in cold-processed foods. The cold water–soluble gums, such as carrageenan, guar, CMC, and MCC, will replace either fat or sucrose in frozen dairy desserts. They help to control crystallization and meltdown in soft-serve products as well as to serve as heat shock stabilizers and to provide other benefits of the butterfat [69]. An oatrim frozen dessert with fewer than half the calories compared favorably with a premium ice cream on sensory evaluations of sweetness, vanilla flavor, and creamy taste [122]. A 35% solution of Maltrin 040 was used to replace the fat on a 1:1 basis [129], and a 25% solution of N-Oil was used in a 12% butterfat ice cream to replace 33, 50, or 100% of the fat. A 4% butterfat frozen dessert was prepared using 6% of the 25% gel to simulate a 10% fat product [62]. Paselli SA2 enhances creaminess in creamed fillings, frozen desserts, and toppings [57]. Specter [123] and others [92] found that polydextrose powder and polydextrose N (70% solution) totally replaced sugar and partially replaced the butter fat in frozen dairy desserts. Either Paselli SA2, N–Oil, or polydextrose could substitute for up to 67% of 12% butterfat in a frozen dessert [123]. Polydextrose will depress the freezing point and contribute creaminess and smoothness to the mouthfeel [92,123].

Simplesse, protein hydrolysates, Sta-Slim 143, or sucrose polyesters have been used as fat substitutes in dairy products such as yogurt, cheese spread, cream cheese, and sour cream as well as in frozen dairy desserts [47,117]. The milkfat impacts cheese firmness, adhesiveness, and mouthfeel, and these must be considered in the fat replacements for cheese. Aqueous dispersions of soluble hydrocolloids were used effectively to replace lipids in process cheese spreads [124]. The 25% fat level of the control cheese spread was reduced 40–50% by increasing the moisture and adding either 2.2% lambda-carrageenan, 1.7–2.2% pectin, or 1.7% low-viscosity guar gum. Various maltodextrins have been suggested to reduce the fat content in cheese products: Amalean I or Paselli SA2 in a cheese spread [64] and instant N–Oil in microwavable cheese sauce [47]. Reduced–fat sour creams with 50% of the fat of standard sour cream with acceptable flavor and texture have been made from MCC [70], Amalean I, and Maltrin M040, [47]. Polydextrose also has been used in yogurt products. The mouthfeel of noncarbohydrate sweetened yogurts was improved with an addition of 5–14% polydextrose [38].

Mono- and diglyceride emulsifiers can be used in dairy systems to achieve a 100% fat replacement. These products include vegetable protein cream cheese, spray–dried whipped toppings, frozen desserts, sour dressings, and sour cream dips. The emulsifiers absorb water and are easily mixed [74].

In both instant and regular puddings, xylitol or polydextrose can be used for sweetener bulk with no alteration in process [38,80]. The polydextrose contributes a creamy texture and aids in the uniform dispersion of cocoa and starch [92]. Maltodextrin gels also are effective as fat replacers in puddings [47].

E. Fruit Products (Including Gelatin Gels and Pectin Jams, Jellies, and Preserves)

In general, in products like jellies where the texture is given by gelatin, pectin, or gums, the high molecular weight polysaccharides limit setting. Xylitol can replace sucrose on a 1:1 basis [80], although in pectin jellies concentrations greater than 40% can result in xylitol crystallization during storage. An increase in the pectin or gelatin content can compensate for the lower viscosity and gel strength of xylitol products. Preservative agents are not needed with polyol gels because they have high osmotic pressure and are not fermented by yeast, molds, and bacteria. A 30% xylitol solution and a 70% sucrose solution have about the same osmotic pressure. Low-methoxyl pectin jellies benefitted by the addition of calcium salts [28].

Sorbitol, lactitol, or Lycasin can be used in jellies, jams, and preserves [11,13,17,33,36,117]. Typically, pectins with low methoxyl levels are used as gelling agents to prevent syneresis. Sorbitol jellies and jams are clear and do not mask fruit flavors [13].

Isomalt also can be used in jams and preserves, but because of its tendency to recrystallize, the level should not exceed 25% [26]. A change in procedures is needed to produce these products. Fructose is recommended to be used in conjunction with the isomalt because it will increase the dry substance content and sweetness and enhance fruit flavor [26].

Polydextrose or MCC can be used to achieve 90% or greater calorie reduction in gelatin-type desserts [92]. They are used in conjunction with high-potency sweeteners and usually with other hydrocolloids as well [69].

F. Margarine, Fats and Oils, and Salad Dressings

Olestra has been proposed as a partial fat substitute in shortening, margarines, and home cooking oils [113–115]. It could be used as a 35% (by weight) cooking oil substitute in foodservice applications or up to 75% substitute (by weight) in shortenings and deep fat trying oils [117].

Simplesse and the maltodextrins are used in margarine spreads [47]. Standard margarine contains approximately 7 kcal/g, and a typical Maltrin 040 reduced–calorie table spread contains 4.5 kcal/g. This spread has been reported to have the mouthfeel, flavor, and spreading properties of a soft margarine.

Salad dressings need to duplicate the viscosity, eating equality, shelf stability, and flavor release properties associated with traditional salad dressing emulsions. Gums widely used to add viscosity for reduced–calorie salad dressings include those stable at low pH such as xanthan gum, MCC, and gum tragacanth. Maltodextrins in salad dressings are reported to result in a product that is less stringy in texture than when gums are used for fat replacement [55]. Paselli SA2, N–Oil, and Instant N–Oil are applicable in dips, both spoonable and pourable salad dressings, and imitation mayonnaise. A low-calorie dressing with Maltrin 040 was reported to have a calorie content of 1.5 kcal/g [47]. A 25% maltodextrin solution can replace 30% and 50% of oil in a 30% oil spoonable salad dressing. Or the maltodextrin can be dry blended and added to the liquids in the paste portion of the formula [62]. Even lower concentrations of Amalean I can be used [64]. Sta–Slim 150 and 151 acid– and shear–stable tapioca starches are said to be particularly suited for salad dressings and mimic the "creamy" fatty texture of oils [125].

Simplesse and sucrose polyesters can be used in salad dressings and mayonnaise [47]. Polydextrose has been used to replace the vegetable oil in a nonstandard French-type dressing [40].

G. Meats, Gravy Mixes, Sauces, and Condiments

Paselli SA2 was used in meat products to decrease the fat levels [47], and in Europe, N–Oil has been used in breakfast sausage [74]. Several novel approaches have been developed to reduce fat levels in meat products. Hamburger with 9% fat content relied upon carrageenan and hydrolyzed vegetable protein to retain a moist texture and duplicate the sensory properties of the typical 15–20% fat product. In hot dogs, cellulose gum, alginate, and oat hull fiber were used to compensate for the texture, moisturizing, and lubricating properties of fat [126]. A thermally stable konjac gel is ground into macroscopic pieces and added to ground meat to simulate the fat properties of a hardened fat [127]. Even precooked rice has been reported to replace 60% of the fat in a conventional sausage providing the moist, fatlike character and structure of the product without diluting the flavor [128].

Maltodextrins can be used in soup and gravy mixes [81,129] to reduce the fat content [130]. The sensory characteristics of soft fats for reduced-fat condiments has been duplicated by hydrating konjac flour in the presence of 1–2% fat [127]. In marinades, sauces, and paste, xylitol can be substituted for sucrose in a 1:1 substitution with no problems. Browning and spoiling can be avoided by replacing sugar with xylitol [80].

REFERENCES

1. New foods for a new century, *Prep. Foods, 158*(2): 47 (1989).
2. M. E. Carter, Agricultural Research Service: Food research in the nineties, *Food Technol., 43*(12): 48 (1989).
3. Human Health Services, *The Surgeon General's Report on Nutrition and Health*, U.S. Department of Health and Human Services, U.S. Government Printing Office, Washington, D.C. (1988).
4. E. Sills-Levy, U.S. food trends leading to the year 2000, *Food Technol., 43*(4): 128 (1989).
5. R. H. Bosselman, F. P. Lattuca, and P. B. Manning, Food technology: In the 21st century, the science of food production will have significantly altered the available supply; The future of food service, *Restaurant Business, 86*(May): 166 (1987).
6. J. J. Beereboom, Low calorie bulking agents, *CRC Critical Rev. Food Sci. Nutr., 11*(4), 401 (1979).
7. R. McCormick, Considerations in selecting bulking agents or food ingredient carriers, *Prep. Foods, 156*(6): 131 (1987).

8. A. M. Johnson, *Sucrose replacement in reduced-calorie layer cakes using response surface methodology*, M.S. thesis, Kansas State University, Manhattan, KS (1990).

9. V. Young, Nutritional implications of microparticulated protein, Nutritional and functional qualities of microparticulated protein: A Symposium Summary, University of California, Berkeley, CA, p. 122 (1989).

10. J. D. Dziezak, Special report: Sweeteners and product development 2. Types and characteristics, *Food Technol.*, *40*(1): 114 (1986).

11. A. Rapaille, Application of hydrogenated products, *Starch*, *40*(9): 356 (1988).

12. T. M. Friedman, Sorbitol in bakery products, *Baker's Digest*, *52*(6): 10 (1978).

13. P. J. Sicard and P. Leroy, Mannitol, sorbitol and Lycasin: Properties and food applications, *Developments in Sweeteners-2* (T. H. Grenby, K. J. Parker, and M. G. Lindley, eds.), Elsevier Science Publ. Co. Inc., New York, p 1 (1983).

14. M. Serpelloni, The food applications of sorbitol-mannitol and hydrogenated glucose syrups, Roquette Corp., Gurnee, IL (undated).

15. A. H. Wick, M. C. Almen, and J. Lionel, The metabolism of sorbitol, *J. Am. Pharm. Assoc. 40*: 542 (1951).

16. C. A. M. Hough, Sweet polyhydric alcohols, *Developments in Sweeteners-1* (C. A. M. Hough, K. J. Parker, and A. J. Vlitos, eds.), Applied Science Publ. Ltd., Essex, England, p. 69 (1979).

17. J. A. van Velhuijsen, Food additives derived from lactose: Lactitol and lactitol palmitate, *J. Agric. Food Chem.*, *27*(4): 680 (1979).

18. P. Linko, Lactose and lactitol, *Nutritive Sweeteners* (G. G. Birch and K. J. Parker, eds.), Applied Science Publ. Ltd., Essex, England, p. 109 (1982).

19. C. J. Booy, Lactitol: A new food ingredient, *Bull. Int. Dairy Fed.*, *212*: 62 (1987).

20. C. H. den Uyl, Lactitol: A new reduced calorie sweetener, Presented at International Symposium on Polyols and Polydextrose, New Carbohydrate Ingredients for Food Industries, Paris, France (1985).

21. C. H. den Uyl, Technical and commercial aspects of the use of lactitol in foods as a reduced-calorie bulk sweetener, *Developments in Sweeteners-3* (T. H. Grenby, ed.), Elsevier Applied Science Publ. Co., Inc., New York, p. 65 (1987).

22. P. Linko, T. Saijonmaa, N. Heikonen, and N. Kreula, Lactitol, *Carbohydrate Sweeteners in Foods and Nutrition* (P. Koivistoinen and L. Hyvönen, eds.), Academic Press Inc., New York, p. 243 (1980).

23. W. E. Irwin, Palatinit-technological properties. An overview, Presented at International Conference on Sweeteners: Carbohydrate and Low Calorie, Agricultural and Food Chemistry Division, American Chemical Society, Los Angeles (1988).

24. H. Schiweck, Palatinit®-Preparation, technological properties and analysis of Palatinit containing foods, *Alimenta, 19*: 5 (1980).

25. P. J. Sträter, Palatinit: Technological and processing characteristics, *Alternative Sweeteners* (L. O'Brien Nabors and R. C. Gelardi, eds.), Marcel Dekker, Inc., New York, p. 217 (1986).

26. H. Bollinger, Palatinit® Info Pac, 2nd ed., Palatinit® Süssungsmittel GmbH, Germany (1987).

27. U. Grupp and G. Siebert, Metabolism of hydrogenated Palatinose, an equimolar mixture of α-D-glucopyranosido-1, 6-sorbitol and α-D-glucopyranosido-1,6-mannitol, *Res. Exp. Med. (Berlin)*, *173*: 261 (1978).

28. L. Hyvönen, P. Koivistoninen, and F. Voirol, Food technological evaluation of xylitol, *Advances in Food Research*, Vol. 28 (C. O. Chichester, E. M. Mark, and G. F. Stewart, eds.), Academic Press Inc., New York, (1982).

29. M. M. Bean and C. S. Setser, Polysaccharides, sugars and sweeteners, *Food Theory and Applications* (J. A. Bowers, ed.) Macmillan Publishers, New York (1991).

30. B. K. Dwivedi, Polyalcohols: Sorbitol, mannitol, maltitol, and hydrogenated starch hydrolysates, *Alternative Sweeteners* (L. O'Brien Nabors and R. C. Gelardi, eds.), Marcel Dekker Inc., New York, p. 165 (1986).

31. S. C. Ziesenitz and G. Siebert, The metabolism and utilization of polyols and other bulk sweeteners compared with sugar, *Developments in Sweeteners-3* (T. H. Grenby, ed.), Elsevier Applied Science Publ. Co. Inc., New York, p. 109 (1987).

32. H. Röper and H. Koch, New carbohydrate derivatives form biotechnical and chemical processes, *Starch, 40*(12): 453 (1988).

33. E. Rockström, Lycasin hydrogenated hydrolysates, *Carbohydrate Sweeteners in Foods and Nutrition* (P. Koivistoinen and L. Hyvönen, eds.), Academic Press, Inc., New York, p. 225 (1980).

34. R. Havenaar, Dental advantages of some bulk sweeteners in laboratory animal trials, *Developments in Sweeteners-3* (T. H. Grenby, ed.), Elsevier Science Publishing Co., Inc., New York, p. 189 (1987).

35. P. J. Sicard, Hydrogenated glucose syrups, sorbitol, mannitol and xylitol, *Nutritive Sweeteners* (G. G. Birch and K. J. Parker, eds.), Applied Science Publishers Ltd., Essex, England, p. 145 (1982).

36. D. A. Whitmore, Developments in the properties and applications of Lycasin and sorbitol, *Food Chem., 16*: 209 (1985).

37. R. P. Allingham, Polydextrose—a new food ingredient: Technical aspects, *Chemistry of Foods and Beverages:Recent Developments,* Academic Press, Inc., New York, p. 293 (1982).

38. P. R. Murray, Polydextrose, *Low Calorie Products* (G. G. Birch and M. G. Lindley, eds.), Elsevier Applied Science Co., Inc., New York, p. 83 (1988).

39. A. Torres and R. D. Thomas, Polydextrose . . . and its applications in foods, *Food Technol., 35*(7): 44 (1981).

40. R. E. Smiles, The functional aspects of polydextrose, *Chemistry of Foods and Beverages: Recent Developments*, Academic Press, Inc., New York, p. 305 (1982).

41. *Polydextrose*, Pfizer Chemical Division, New York, (1985).

42. N. Neville and C. Setser, Optimization of reduced calorie layer cake texture, *Cereal Foods World, 31*: 744 (1986).

43. S. Hegenbart, Formulating "lite" bakery foods with sweeteners, *Prep. Foods, 159*(7): 97 (1990).

44. S. K. Figdor and J. R. Bianchine, Caloric utilization and disposition of [^{14}C] polydextrose in man, *J. Agr. Food Chem., 31*(2): 389 (1983).

45. S. K. Figdor and H. H. Rennhard, Caloric utilization and disposition of [^{14}C] polydextrose in rat, *J. Agr. Food Chem., 29*(6): 1181 (1981).

46. A. M. Altschul, Low-calorie foods—a scientific status summary by the Institute of Food Technologists' expert panel on food safety and nutrition, *Food Technol.*, *43*(4): (1989).
47. Fat substitute update, *Food Technol.*, *44*(3): 92 (1990).
48. Community Nutrition Institute, Indigestible fat appears on U.S. food horizon, *Nut. Week, 17*(21): 6 (1987).
49. C. J. Glueck, R. Jandacek, E. Hogg, C. Allen, P. A. Baehler, and M. Tewksbury, Sucrose polyester: substitution for dietary fats in hypocaloric diets in the treatment of familial hypercholesterolemia, *Am. J. Clin. Nutr. 37*: 347 (1983).
50. K. A. Harrigan and W. M. Breene, Fat substitutes: Sucrose ester and Simplesse, *Cereal Foods World, 34*: 261 (1989).
51. R. W. Fallat, C. J. Glueck, F. Mattson and R. Lutmer, Sucrose polyester: A cholesterol lowering, noncaloric, unabsorbable, synthetic, fat food additive, *Clin. Res. 23*: 319A (1975).
52. Anonymous, Maltodextrin 184.1444. Code of Federal Regulations, 21 parts 170–199. p. 456. Office of the Federal Register National Archives and Records Administration (1989).
53. C. E. Morris, 1984. New applications for maltodextrin, *Food Eng. 56*(7): 48 (1984).
54. *Maltrin® Maltodextrins and Corn Syrup Solids: Brilliance in Food and Pharmaceutical Technology*, Bulletin 11005, Grain Processing Corp., Muscatine, IA (undated).
55. J. B. Klis, Ingredients round table, *Food Technol.*, *38*(11): 92 (1984).
56. *Maltodextrins—Corn Syrup Solids*, Bulletin 10003, Grain Processing Corp., Muscatine, IA (undated).
57. *Paselli SA2*, Avebe Product Information Ref. No. 05.12.31.167 EF, Veendam-Holland, (1988).
58. Calorie Control Council, Fat substitutes menu, *Calorie Control Comment., 12* (1): 5 (1990).
59. F. S. Kaper, and H. Gruppen, Replace oil and fat with potato-based ingredient, *Food Technol.*, *41*(3): 112 (1987).
60. J. D. Dziezak, Fats, oils, and fat substitutes, *Food Technol.*, *43*(7): 72 (1989).
61. D. J. Hamm, Preparation and evaluation of trialkoxytricarballylate, trialkoxycitrate, trialkoxyglycerylether, jojoba oil and sucrose polyester as low calories replacements of edible fats and oils, *J. Food Sci., 49*: 419 (1984).
62. R. G. LaBarge, The search for a low-calorie oil, *Food Technol., 42*(1): 84 (1988).
63. F. LaBell and D. Duxbury, Ingredient trends, concepts shown at 1990 IFT Food Expo, *Food Processing, 51*(8): 88 (1990).
64. *Fat/Oil Sparing Starch—Amalean I*, America Maize Products Company, Corn Processing Division, Hammond, IN (undated).
65. *Amalean I™ Product Data*, America Maize-Products Company, Corn Processing Division, Hammond, IN (undated).
66. *Technical Data Sheet 441*, Staley Industrial Products, A. E. Staley Manufacturing Co., Decatur, IL (undated).
67. B. O. Schneeman, Dietary fiber, *Food Technol., 43*(10): 133 (1989).

68. S. A. Andon, Applications of soluble dietary fiber, *Food Technol. 41*(1): 74 (1987).

69. *Avicel®* *in Low and Reduced Calorie Foods*, Bulletin C–53, FMC Corp., Philadelphia, PA (1987).

70. Lose the fat, retain the taste: Cellulose gel helps do both, *Prep. Foods, 159*(5): 157 (1990).

71. *Avicel®* *in Low/Nonfat Systems*, Bulletin C–96, FMC Corp., Philadelphia, PA (1989).

72. Fiber-based fat filler feels its oats, *Prep. Foods, 159*(7): 31 (1990).

73. C. M Kroskey, Creating guilt-free bakery foods, *Prep. Foods, 159*(11): 76 (1990).

74. D. D. Duxbury, Vegetable oil emulsifier replaces fat component in bakery and non-dairy foods. *Food Process., 51*(14): 37 (1990).

75. *N-Flate*, Bulletin No. 501, National Starch and Chemical Corp., Bridgewater, NJ (undated).

76. S. Waring, Shortening replacement in cakes, *Food Technol., 42*(3): 114 (1988).

77. H. Sampson, Microparticulation of protein and allergenicity, *Nutritional and Functional Qualities of Microparticulated Protein: A Symposium Summary*, University of California, Berkeley, p. 8 (1989).

78. T. T. Boutte, The present state of artificial fats, *Audits International/Monthly* (March–April, 1990).

79. F. LaBell, Milk hydrolysate enhances mouth feel in low-fat foods, *Food Process., 51*(7): 102 (1990).

80. A. Emodi, Xylitol—its properties and food applications, *Food Technol., 32*(1): 28 (1978).

81. *Maltrin®* *M040—Maltodextrin Product Data,* Ref. No. 0212387, Grain Processing Corp., Muscatine, IA (1989).

82. *Lycasin*, U.S. Department of Labor Occupational Safety and Health Administration Material Safety Data Sheet, Roquette Corporation, Gurnee, IL (1989).

83. *Crystalline Maltitol*, Technical Information #870601, Towa Chemical Industry Co., LTD., Tokyo, Japan (undated).

84. F. Voirol, Xylitol—its caries-preventive and technical properties and food applications, Presented at *Journées Internationales D'Information sur les Polyols et le Polydextrose 6 and 7 Mai*, Paris, France (1985).

85. G. Von Hertzen and C. Lindqvist, Comparative evaluation of carbohydrate sweeteners, *Carbohydrate Sorbitol in Foods and Nutrition* (P. Koivistoinen and L. Hyvönen, eds.), Academic Press, New York, p. 127 (1980).

86. Future ingredients—focus of OVIFT meeting, *Food Technol., 42*(1): 60 (1988).

87. P. J. Sträter, Palatinit® (isomalt) an energy-reduced bulk sweetener derived from saccharose. *Low Calorie Products* (G. G. Birch and M. G. Lindley, eds.), Elsevier Applied Science, New York, p. 63 (1988).

88. *Maltrin®* *Maltodextrin Product Data*, Grain Processing Corp., Muscatine, IA (1987).

89. *Lacty®* *A New Reduced Calorie Sweetener*, CCA biochem b.v., Purac Inc., Arlington Heights, IL (undated).

90. T. Pepper and P. M. Olinger, Xylitol in sugar-free confections, *Food Technol., 42*(10): 98 (1988).

91. S. Hegenbert, Critical factors in sweetener selection, *Prep. Foods*, *159*(10): 89 (1990).

92. T. M. Freeman, Polydextrose for reduced calorie foods, *Cereal Foods World*, *27*(10): 515 (1982).

93. N. Ernest, Low-calorie baked foods possible with polydextrose bulking agent, *Baker's J.*, *42*: 320 (1982).

94. J. D. Dziezak, Special report: Sweeteners and product development 4. Applications of polydextrose. *Food Technol.*, *43*(1): 129 (1986).

95. K-O. Kim, L. Hansen, and C. Setser, Phase transitions of wheat starch-water systems containing polydextrose, *J. Food Sci.*, *51*: 1095 (1986).

96. T. M. Freeman, Sweetening cakes and cake mixes with alitame, *Cereal Foods World*, *34*: 1013 (1989).

97. B. S. Kamel, and V. F. Rasper, Effects of emulsifiers, sorbitol, polydextrose, and crystalline cellulose on the texture of reduced-calorie cakes, *J. Texture Stud.*, *19*: 307 (1988).

98. A. Johnson and C. Setser, Sucrose replacement in reduced-calorie layer cakes, Abstract 160, American Association of Cereal Chemists Annual Meeting, Dallas, TX, (1990).

99. C. S. Setser, Low calorie chemically leavened cakes and surfactant systems therefor, Patent Application 7,821,319 (1992).

100. V. F. Rasper and B. S. Kamel, Emulsifier/oil system for reduced calorie cakes, *J. Am. Oil Chem. Soc.*, *66*: 537 (1989).

101. B. S. Kamel and S. Washnuik, Composition and sensory quality of shortening-free yellow cakes, *Cereal Foods World*, *28*: 731 (1983).

102. H. Lim, C. Setser, and S. Kim, Sensory studies of high potency multiple sweetener systems for shortbread cookies with and without polydextrose, *J. Food Sci.*, *54*: 625 (1989).

103. R. Dogra, M. A. Hill, and R. Strange, The acceptability of three cake types incorporating varying levels of guar gum, *Food Hydrocolloids*, *3*: 1 (1989).

104. M. E. Zabik, M. A. M. Shafer, and B. W. Kukorowski, Dietary fiber sources for baked products. Comparison of cellulose types and coated-cellulose products in layer cakes, *J. Food Sci.*, *42*: 1428 (1977).

105. J. F. Ang, W. B. Miller, and I. M. Blais, The chemical and functional properties of powdered cellulose as a low-calorie food ingredient, Presented at International Conference on Sweeteners: Carbohydrate and Low Calorie, Agricultural and Food Chemistry Division, American Chemical Society, Los Angeles, CA (1988).

106. W. B. Miller, Seeing the 'light'—cellulose in reduced-calorie baked goods, *Baker's Digest*, *60*(1): 18 (1986).

107. C. D. Magoffin, P. L. Finney, and K. F. Finney, Short-time baking systems. II. A 70-min sugar-free formula for conventional and high-protein breads, *Cereal Chem.*, *54*: 760 (1977).

108. E. C. Torr and W. W. O'Hara, Sorbitol-sweetened sugar-free mix makes cakes with "real cake" taste, *Baking Ind.*, (*Nov.*): 22 (1976).

109. A. Bär, Xylitol, *Alternative Sweeteners* (L. O'Brien Nabors and R. C. Gelardi, eds.), Marcel Dekker, Inc., New York, p. 185 (1986).

110. G. Brack, W. Seibel, and F. Bretschneider, Backtechnische Wirkung des Zuckeraustauschstoffes Palatinit (Isomalt) 3. Mitteilung: Massen mit Aufschlag, *Getreide Mehl und Brot*, *40*(10): 302 (1986).

111. G. Brack, W. Seibel, and F. Bretschneider, Backtechnische Wirkung des Zuckeraustauschstoffes Palatinit (Isomalt) 2. Mitteilung: Feinteige ohne Hefe, *Getreide Mehl und Brot*, *40*(9): 269 (1986).

112. W. Seibel, G. Brack, and F. Bretschneider, Backtechnische Wirkung des Zuckeraustauschstoffes Palatinit (Isomalt) 1. Mitteilung: Feinteige mit Hefe, *Getreide Mehl und Brot*, *40*(8): 239 (1986).

113. E. J. Hollenbach and N. B. Howard, Emulsion concentrate for palatable polyester beverage, U.S. Patent 4,368,213 (1983).

114. M. B. Robbins and S. S. Rodriguez, Low calorie baked products, U.S. Patent 4,461,782 (1984).

115. B. A. Roberts, Oleaginous compositions, U.S. Patent 4,446,165 (1984).

116. J. S. Wittman, III, Hydrated emulsifier for use in flour based baked goods, U.S. Patent 4,424,237 (1984).

117. R. McCormick, New ingredient developments augur lean times ahead, *Prep. Foods*, 157(4): 120 (1988).

118. C. D. Barnett, Try new polydextrose in low-calorie candies, *Candy Ind.*, (Feb): (1986).

119. A. G. Dodson and T. Pepper, Confectionery technology and the pros and cons of using non-sucrose sweeteners, *Food Chem.*, 16: 271 (1985).

120. *Lycasin®* *in Confections*, Roquette Corporation, Gurnee, IL (undated).

121. S. E. Keller, J. W. Fellows, T. C. Nash, and W. H. Shazer, Formulation of aspartame-sweetened frozen dairy dessert without bulking agents, *Food Technol.*, *45*(2): 102 (1991).

122. Anonymous. USDA's oatrim replaces fat in many food products, *Food Technol.*, *44*(10): 100 (1990).

123. S. Specter, *The effect of sucrose and milkfat substitution on sensory textural and physical properties in a frozen dessert system*, M. S. thesis, Kansas State University, Manhattan, KS (1988).

124. S. E. Brummel and K. Lee, Soluble hydrocolloids enable fat reduction in process cheese spreads, *J. Food Sci.*, 55: 1290 (1990).

125. Low-fat salad dressings demand a "total systems" solution, *Prep. Foods*, 160 (2): 73 (1991).

126. D. Best, Technology fights the fat factor, *Prep. Foods*, *160*(2): 48 (1991).

127. R. J. Tye, Konjac flour: Properties and applications, *Food Technol.* 45(3): 82 (1991).

128. Rice replaces fat in sausage, *Food Process.*, *51*(14): 116 (1990).

129. *Using Maltrin®* *Maltodextrine to Reduce or Replace the Fat in Food Formulations*, Technical Bulletin M-TB10-022390, Grain Processing Corp., Muscatine, IA (undated).

130. *Instant N-Oil®* *II*, Technical Service Bulletin 15889-238, National Starch and Chemical Division, Bridgewater, NJ (undated).

131. Pszczola, D. E. Carbohydrate-based ingredient performs like fat for use in a variety of food applications, *Food Technol.*, *45*(8): 262 (1991).

132. Technical Data TDS 513, A.E. Staley, Decatur, IL (1991).
133. Anti-staling fat mimetic: Too good to be true? *Prep. Foods*, *160*(9): 127 (1991).
134. Technical Data T1B 29, A.E. Staley, Decatur, IL (1991).
135. Pszczola, D. E., New ingredients and applications, *Food Technol. 46*(1): 129, (1992).
136. Civille, G. V., The sensory properties of products made with microparticulated protein, *J. Amer. Coll. Nutr. 9*: 427, (1990).
137. *Simplesse® All Natural Fat Substitute: A Scientific Overview*, 2nd ed., The Simplesse Company, Deerfield, II., (1991).
138. All-natural fat substitute cuts fat, not flavor, *Prepared Foods* 160 (6): 123, (1991).
139. Setser, C. and Racette, W., Macromolecule replacers in food products, *CRC Crit. Rev. in Food Sci. and Nutr.* (In Press).

12
Low-Fat Dairy Products

Charles H. White *Mississippi State University, Mississippi State, Mississippi*

I. INTRODUCTION

The consumption of low-fat foods certainly appears to be more than just a trend; it has become a way of life. This is certainly true with regard to dairy products, since low-fat products have been available for many years. Examples include low-fat milk, skim milk, ice milk (reduced-fat ice cream), and low-fat yogurts. Standard formulas have been available for most of these low-fat foods, but the emphasis on premium low-fat foods is a relatively recent concept. When dairy products are named, many items come to mind, but discussion in this chapter will include the following: fluid milk products, including flavored milks, cultured milk, (i.e., buttermilk, cream, and half and half); cheese, including both unripened and ripened; frozen dairy desserts; and other cultured or fermented dairy products, e.g., sour cream and regular yogurt.

The general trend for consumption of regular dairy products contrasted with that of low-fat dairy products may be seen in Table 1. With regard to

Table 1 Per Capita Sales of Selected Dairy Products

Year	Whole milk (lb)	Low-fat milk (lb)	Skim milk (lb)	Creamed cottage cheese (lb)	Low-fat cottage cheese (lb)	Ice cream (qt)	Ice milk (qt)
1975	168.0	53.2	11.5	4.0	0.6	15.53	5.55
1980	137.5	70.0	11.6	3.6	0.8	14.61	5.17
1985	116.7	83.3	12.6	3.0	1.0	15.16	5.07
1990	83.8	97.1	23.0	2.2	1.2	13.09	5.59

Source: Refs. 1, 2.

fluid milk products, one can easily observe the downward trend just in the past 15 years, with the consumption of whole milk dropping from 168 pounds per capita in 1975 to 83.8 pounds in 1990. The fat level for whole milk must be 3.25% or greater. The consumption of low-fat milk has likewise increased from 53.2 pounds in 1975 to 97.1 pounds in 1990. The year 1989 was significant to the dairy industry in that it was the first year that the consumption of low-fat milk surpassed that of whole milk. By definition, low-fat milk must contain between 0.5 and 2.0% fat. Skim milk, which must contain less than 0.5% fat, remained relatively constant until the last few years in which consumption has increased from 12.6 pounds per capita in 1985 to 23 pounds in 1990.

The consumption of creamed cottage cheese (minimum 4.0% milk fat) has decreased from 4.0 pounds per capita in 1975 to 2.2 pounds in 1990. While the consumption of low-fat cottage cheese (0.5-2.0% milk fat) has increased from 0.6 pound in 1975 to 1.2 pounds in 1990, this increase does not offset the decrease in consumption of creamed cottage cheese. Hence, the total per capita consumption of cottage cheese has decreased. This fact is particularly puzzling to most leaders of the dairy industry since cottage cheese is an excellent food from a nutritional standpoint and lends itself quite well to the diet of many weight-conscious Americans. A couple of reasons have been suggested, with one being the quality of the cottage cheese and the other being a lack of a concerted marketing push towards the consumption of this dairy product.

Finally, the consumption of ice cream has decreased from 15.53 quarts in 1975 to 13.09 quarts in 1990. The consumption of ice milk has remained relatively constant. It should be noted that the federal standard for ice cream is a minimum of 10.0% milk fat while that of ice milk is 2.0-7.0% fat. The figures shown for ice milk reflect both the production of soft-serve products as well as the hard frozen ice milk. In the past 3 or 4 years there has been a big increase in the production of premium hard frozen ice milk products.

Many of these products compare quite favorably to their whole fat counter-parts.

While not listed in Table 1, frozen yogurt should be mentioned due to the current interest in this product. For example, the International Ice Cream Association reports [1] the per capita consumption of frozen yogurt in 1989 to be 1.34 quarts, increasing to 1.90 quarts in 1990.

Many of the trends observed in the low-fat dairy food items have come about because of the major change in recommended eating habits. With the recommendation that no more than 30% of our calories come from fat, the emphasis has been placed on low-fat and nonfat items. The impact is especially profound with regard to dairy products since these products are considered to be nutritious and a necessary item in anyone's diet as well as being refreshing, good-tasting products. The dairy food industry has been faced with the option that many other segments of the food industry have, i.e., the simple removal of fat and/or the substitution of some other ingredient for the replaced milk fat.

II. EFFECT ON FORMULATION AND PROCESSING

Bannar [3] reported that a 1990 Gallup Survey found that 74% of consumers indicated that they were reducing fat in their diets, while a 1990 Harris Poll indicated that 48% of consumers canvassed had purchased a reduced-fat product within the last 30 days. He reported that Kraft General Foods has reduced the fat and cholesterol in products covering seven of the most popular food categories . Olson [4] reported that Chuck Haberstroh of *Food Engineering* indicated that about 232 "light" dairy products were introduced in 1990, accounting for 39% of all "light" introductions for the year. Most of these products were ice creams and other frozen desserts, but introductions of "light" cheeses, including 23 low-fat Cheddar-type cheeses, tripled. Olson stressed that problems would be encountered not only in making technological advances but also in marketing strategies of major companies as well as regulatory constraints. The Food and Drug Administration (FDA) is now developing regulations on the labeling of low-fat foods with these due to be completed in 1993.

Best [5] stressed that fat and calorie reduction remains the leading research and development priority slated for increased investment by 76% of the 352 food processors polled in the 1991 *Prepared Foods* Third Annual R&D Survey. Realizing that repeat sales depend on a product that tastes good, Best concluded that the challenge for food product developers lies in providing fat-reduced products that offer little or no sacrifice in quality or value to consumers. Duxbury and Meinhold [6] reported that FDA's surveys in 1983, 1986, and 1988 showed a dramatic increase in public perception of the health risks of dietary fat. Awareness almost doubled in the previous 5 years among college-educated adults, more than doubled with high school-educated adults, and almost tripled among grade school–educated adults. They cautioned that specific facts such as whether cholesterol-free foods were also low in saturated fats or whether one kind of fat was higher in calories were not known to American consumers.

III. DEVELOPMENT OF LOW-FAT FOODS

Olson [4] indicated that the development of low-fat foods has followed two approaches: elimination of all or part of the fat with concomitant increases in the remaining components of the product; and partial or total replacement of the fat with a substitute material. Fat replacers have been categorized into fat mimetics and fat substitutes.

Fat mimetics mimic the mouthfeel of fat but cannot completely substitute for it. They are not useable for frying because of the water content and heat sensitivity of some products. Fat mimetics are starch-, cellulose-, or protein-based. At least four starch-based products are being marketed, some being used in frozen desserts. Cellulose-based mimetics and a related oat-derived fiber are either noncaloric or low in calories. Starch- and cellulose-based mimetics are being used in fresh cheeses, like cream, cottage, and processed cheese products, all of which offer the most potential at present, according to Olson. He stated that protein-based mimetics have been evaluated in a wider range of cheeses.

Fat substitutes are compounds that resemble fat chemically to some extent and have chemical and physical properties that are similar to fat. Olestra (Procter & Gamble) was the first such product to be developed and has been tested primarily as a fat replacer in deep fat frying and in fried snack foods [4].

A. Milk Solids as an Ingredient

As fat is reduced and/or replaced in different dairy products, new ingredients may be added. The dairy processor is faced with many options and will be faced with many more. One very basic source of these ingredients is other milk solids. An example would be the whey protein concentrates (WPCs). Morr [7] indicated that although a number of protein fractionation processes have been considered, ultrafiltration (UF) has become the process of choice for making WPCs. He cautioned that one major disadvantage of this process is that it concentrates the lipids and lipoproteins along with the proteins. The U.S. Dairy Industry is currently producing approximately 150 million pounds of WPCs annually, with additional quantities being produced around the world. He reported that there was a consensus that the WPCs lacked consistency of composition and of sensory and functional properties. While not the only reason, he suggested that the primary reason was due to the different whey sources with resultant variation in composition, pretreatment, fractionation, and processing conditions. Morr added that the dairy industry has more recently produced and introduced whey protein isolates (WPIs), which are manufactured by an ion-exchange adsorption process. The protein content is higher, and it is essentially fat-free with excellent sensory and functional properties.

Mangino [8] indicated that the WPCs cost 3–15 times as much as dried whey on a solids basis. Hence, these higher-priced products must possess functionality that justifies the additional cost. This often means that the WPC will replace a higher-cost functional ingredient.

B. Fat Replacers

Four basic sources discuss fat replacers in foods, especially dairy products [6,9,10,11]. The fat replacers are classified as follows [9].

1. Protein-based mimetics
2. Synthetic compounds as substitutes
3. Carbohydrate or starch-based replacements
4. Combination products

1. Protein-Based Mimetics

Mixtures of protein and water are also used as partial fat replacements [6]. Most of the proteins used for fat mimetics may be found in eggs, milk, and other foods that have noted fatlike properties.

In the United States, Thomas J. Lipton, Inc. (Unilever) has test–marketed a lowfat "butter" made with a fat substitute that uses either gelatin or milk proteins and is reported [6] to be evaluating the results. The product can supposedly withstand some heat, which means that it can be used for baking and light frying and sauteing.

Another product in this category is Simplesse®, developed by the NutraSweet company (Skokie, IL). The proteins from milk or eggs are subjected to a patented heating and blending processes called "microparticulation." As the proteins are heated, they coagulate, forming large particles of gel. Further processing blends and shears the gel into spheroidal particles so small that the tongue perceives them as fluid rather than individual particles, approximating the richness and creaminess normally associated with fat [6,9]. This product was approved in February 1990 by FDA for use in frozen dairy desserts. Kraft General Foods developed a product, Trailblazer® , which is said to be similar to Simplesse but made by a different process. The product is based on egg albumin and milk protein.

2. Synthetic Compounds

These are fatlike substances that are resistant to hydrolysis by digestive enzymes and are being promoted as partial or complete replacers for fats and oils [6,9]. Olestra is the suggested name for this synthetic sucrose polyester (SPE) that can reportedly substitute for virtually any edible fat [6,9]. This is a nonabsorbable, synthetic fat produced by Procter & Gamble (Cincinnati, OH).

Another synthetic fat substitute is esterified propoxylated glycerol (EPG). This product is sold by the ARCO Chemical Company (Newtown Square, PA). The structure of EPG is similar to that of natural fat and, like olestra, is reported to be undigestable.

A third synthetic product is dialkyl dihexadecylmalonate (DDM). This is a fatty alcohol ester of malonic and alkyl-malonic acids. This product is being developed as a fat substitute for high-temperature applications by Frito-Lay, Inc. (Irving, TX). Another synthetic product is trialkoxytricarballate, a tricarballic acid esterified with fatty alcohols. This is being evaluated as an oil substitute by Best Foods (CPC International, Inc., Englewood Cliffs, NJ).

3. Carbohydrate-Based Replacements

Several carbohydrates are being promoted and effectively used as partial or total fat or oil replacements. These include:

1. Gums or hydrocolloids or long-chain, high molecular weight polymers that dissolve or disperse in water. Usage level is suggested at 0.1–0.5% [6].
2. Polydextrose, a polymer of dextrose with small amounts of sorbitol and citric acid (Pfizer Chemical Division, NY). While marketed primarily as a bulking agent, it may also be used as a partial replacement for fat. Litesse™ has been introduced by Pfizer to provide favorable fat-sparing properties while maintaining texture and mouthfeel.
3. Cornstarch maltodextrin [6] is produced by Grain Processing Corporation (Muscatine, IA) and is a nonsweet saccharide polymer produced by a limited hydrolysis of cornstarch. It consists primarily of alpha-1-4-linked dextrose units, which are capable of being inverted into maltose. The product is called Maltrin® M040 and is a white spray-dried powder having a dextrose equivalent (DE) of five. The DE of starch is 0, while the DE of dextrose is 100 [6].

4. Tapioca dextrins designated N-Oil® and a tapioca maltodextrin called instant N-Oil® II are marketed by the National Starch Chemical Corporation (Bridgewater, NJ). Both products are reported to be used to produce no-fat frozen desserts. The instant maltodextrin is also recommended for applications in the production of microwaveable cheese sauces [6]. The dextrin products are usually used at 20–35% aqueous solutions. Typically, one part of a 25% solution is considered the equivalent of one part of oil.

5. Potato starch maltodextrin, known as Paselli SA2, is produced by Avebe America Inc. (Princeton, NJ). The product may be used to replace fats or oils in many foods to include frozen desserts. The ingredient is reported to have a DE of less than 5.

6. Modified potato starch, in a product called Sta-Slim™ 143, may be used to partially replace fats and oils in a wide variety of food products, including imitation cream cheeses.

4. Combination Products

There are two basic products in this category [2]: Prolestra™ (Reach Associates, Inc., South Orange, NJ) and Colestra™ (Food Ingredients and Innovations, Ashland, MA).

IV. FUNCTIONAL ASPECTS OF FAT REDUCTION

Best [5] indicated that reduced-fat product development should begin by identifying how fat removal will affect a product's "key factors for success" (KFS). This term was coined by Kenichi Ohmae and means the manufacturing, consumer, and strategic variables that are critical to a product's mass marketplace success. For consumers, flavor is always a KFS, but appearance, storage stability, versatility, and ease of handling need also be considered. Specifically the functional aspects of fat reduction, as he identified them, are appearance, texture, flavor, mouthfeel, handling, processing and preparation, and storage stability. When all of these factors are considered, a reduced-fat product can be effectively produced.

Medcalf [12], discussing the functional role of fat in dairy products, indicated that fat contributes to the following:

1. Flavor, both as a carrier for flavor and also with regard to flavor stability
2. Texture, especially as related to meltability
3. Mouthfeel, particularly from the standpoint of the coating that the mouth is given

4. Structural stability

5. Actual appearance

While chemically some of the fat replacers are satisfactory, physiologically and from a regulatory standpoint many of these replacers are just not acceptable. Further, it is important to evaluate the functionality of fat in dairy products. This would emphasize the type of product being manufactured whether it happened to be a frozen dairy dessert, a processed cheese–type product, or a creamed cheese product. In addition, it is important to consider functionality of the fat replacer with respect to flavor, texture, appearance, and stability.

Altschul [13] indicated that reduced-fat or low-fat products offer more nutrients per 100-gram serving than do traditional products, for example, skim milk, which contains 43% fewer calories and 95% less fat (4.6% calories from fat), as well as more protein, vitamin A, riboflavin, and calcium than whole milk. Moreover, low-fat milk, which has a more acceptable flavor than skim milk to many individuals, contains 22% fewer calories and 48% less fat (35% of calories from fat), as well as more protein, vitamins, and calcium than whole milk. These same differences are observed for modified mozzarella and ricotta cheese and ice cream.

With a tremendous increase being predicted in the sale and consumption of low-fat foods in general, the future is very bright for those processors who venture into this area. Howard Dean, chairman and chief executive officer of Dean Foods Company, was quoted [14] as saying, "Lowfat, low cholesterol dairy products will bring the consumer away from soft drinks and beer and back to the dairy industry."

V. LOW-FAT/REDUCED-FAT CHEESES

Jameson [15] indicated that there are marketing opportunities for cheeses with lower fat contents, but to be successful, it is essential that such cheeses be organoleptically acceptable. Due to its minor role in most cheese classification schemes, fat content might be considered not to play a dominant role in determining the flavor and texture of cheese. Major reductions in fat content do, however, affect the sensory properties of cheese sufficiently to seriously impede attempts to manufacture attractive low-fat products.

A. Problems with Low-Fat Cheeses

The two primary complaints about low-fat cheeses in recent years have been (1) lack of flavor of the cheese variety [34], and (2) a body/texture that is hard and rubbery lacking the pliable characteristics of that specific variety of cheese. Olson [4] indicated that reduction of fat in semisoft and hard ripened cheeses has followed more traditional approaches. Lowering the fat content by one-third with simultaneous increases in water and protein has been partially successful. A critical factor in that process is adjusting the ratio of water to protein to obtain physical properties close to the traditional counterpart. Cheddar-type cheeses in which fat is reduced by one-third can simulate the texture of full-fat cheeses with proper compositional and manufacturing controls.

Johnson and Chen [16] listed three factors that are primarily responsible for the reduced quality of lowfat cheese relative to their higher-fat counterparts: (1) lack of flavor, (2) development of off-flavors, generally characterized as meaty-brothy, bitter, and unclean, and (3) body defects—too firm or too soft, weak and pasty. They indicated that lower quality may go hand in hand with prolonged shelf life requirements, in that the longer a high-moisture, low-salt cheese ages, the more its quality is likely to deteriorate. In experiments conducted in their laboratories, three manufacturing practices were found to substantially influence the quality of reduced-fat cheese: (1) starter selection, (2) moisture control, and (3) control of the level of lactic acid in the cheese.

These workers [16] and Olson [4] indicated that the proper choice of the lactic starter culture is important for all cheeses but especially for low-fat cheese. Apparently not all starters are suitable for manufacturing reduced-fat cheese. There is evidence that the slower acid-producing starters are more desirable in the manufacture of reduced-fat cheeses. However, the assumption could not be made that the use of any slow acid producer would result in higher-quality cheese while all fast acid producers would not. Research is needed in this area to further clarify the selection of starters. Moisture control and control of lactic acid in a higher-moisture cheese($>47\%$) were reported to develop undesirable flavors more readily than in lower-moisture cheeses (43–44%). Unless the lactic acid levels in high-moisture cheeses are reduced, the cheeses are very acid and the body may become weak and pasty with age [4].

Most, if not all, high-moisture cheeses are rinsed to remove lactose and lactic acid [16]. These "washed" cheeses may be more susceptible to off-flavor development. Also, the washed cheeses are less flavorful than unwashed cheeses regardless of fat content. Higher-moisture reduced-fat cheese has some advantages over lower-moisture reduced-fat cheese. Higher-moisture cheeses are more economically attractive, but their body and flavor qualities deteriorate rapidly with age. Lower-moisture cheeses require more ripening to develop desirable body characteristics but have a longer shelf life than their higher-moisture counterparts.

The increase in cheese yield on processing the reduced-fat hard or semi-hard cheeses ranges from 14 to 20% [17]. Simard adds that in processing milk of low fat content, a cheese yield advantage is also gained in terms of a higher recovery of milk fat in the curd as the casein-to-fat ratio is increased, the major advantage being the greater moisture content.

For low-fat cheese manufacture, Olson and Johnson [18] advocate the concept of moisture in the nonfat substance (MNFS). They indicate that the development of more objective methods for grading cheese has included this concept of using the MNFS [MNFS = %H_2O/(100 − %fat)]. This is essentially a ratio of water to protein. The theory is that adjusting the fat content of cheese within certain limits, while maintaining a constant MNFS, should yield cheeses with fairly uniform firmness. However, this cannot be extrapolated to cheese in which fat content has been reduced by more than 33%. Some of this work along with that of Emmons et al. [19] indicates that MNFS had to be priced higher than predicted in low-fat Cheddar cheese to attain firmness approximating that of Cheddar cheese. This was attributed to a greater amount of protein (30% more) per unit volume of low-fat cheese as compared to Cheddar cheese.

Certainly moisture is a key to the control of the body characteristics of low-fat cheeses. This MNFS or the ratio of moisture to fat-free substance (MFFS) as described by Jameson [15] can actually be a basis for cheese classification systems and is done so in various cheesemaking regions of the world. For example, Jameson [15] described the typical composition of Cheddar cheese in Australia as being 36% moisture, 33% fat, 52% fat on a dry matter (FDM) basis, and 54% MFFS. He concluded that it is now generally accepted that when low-fat versions of traditional cheese varieties are made, the preferred MFFS range to obtain optimum organoleptic properties will usually be slightly higher than that for the full-fat cheese. He reasoned that this overcomes the increased firmness and elasticity due to the partial replacement of fat by proteinaceous matrix [19] but may require the cheese to be manufactured at a composition outside the range specified for that variety in current food legislation.

Jameson [15] stated that an alternative approach to the problem of maintaining acceptable texture in lowfat cheese is to replace some of the fat with a filling material which does not contribute either to structure formation or undesirable flavor generation. Due to the regulatory constraints on acceptable materials for use in cheese manufacturing, the use of whey protein aggregates would probably be subject to fewer objections than non-dairy materials. An alternative approach would be to incorporate undenatured whey proteins through the use of ultrafiltration (UF)-based cheese making technology. Olson [4] revealed that higher pH values at whey drainage and at milling (salting) are preferable for lowfat Cheddar-type cheeses.

B. Functions of Milk Fat

Milk fat serves several functions in cheese. Olson and Johnson [18] describe these functions as follows.

1. Cheese Firmness

As indicated previously, MNFS is a key index in the manufacture of low-fat cheeses. Relative amounts of water, protein, and fat are dominant factors affecting the cheese firmness. Prentice [20] found that the firmness of cheese was also affected by the melting point of milk fat. An indirect linear relationship was observed between penetrometer readings of cheese and iodine number of milk fat, which is a measurement of saturation and an indication of meltability.

2. Elasticity

Masi and Addeo [21] observed a linear decrease in elasticity of mozzarella cheeses as the ratio of fat to solids-not-fat increased. Olson and Johnson [18] further state that the effect of milk fat on cheese elasticity may be related to the interaction between the fat globule surface membrane and the cheese protein matrix.

3. Adhesiveness

Low-fat cheeses exhibit stickiness when masticated. This is especially evident with cheeses with higher moisture content, with fat content of 15% or less, and after aging. Olson and Johnson [18] indicated that it has not been demonstrated whether removing a portion of the fat in cheese affects adhesiveness directly or indirectly because of the concomitant increase in the protein level.

4. Flavor

The principle attribute of milk fat is its unique flavor and high concentrations of short-chain fatty acids that are flavor active. Free fatty acids contribute substantially to the flavor of several varieties such as Romano, bleu, and feta cheeses, but do not seem to be very important and are detrimental at high concentrations in other varieties such as Cheddar and Gouda. Lack of flavor in low-fat cheeses should not be related to lack of triglycerides, since intense free fatty acid flavors can be produced in these cheeses with added lipases. Olson and Johnson [18] stress the need for a study of the fat-protein serum interface for effects on flavor development and structure of low-fat cheeses. Low-fat cheese would have fewer fat globules that were more widely dispersed; this would lessen the access of flavor compounds generated in the serum to the protective solvent, fat, in low-fat cheeses.

C. Manufacture of Low-Fat Cheeses

McGregor and White [22] used ultrafiltration (UF) to produce a high-quality, low-fat Cheddar cheese. Acidification to pH 6.2 by the addition of lactic acid and diafiltration by concentrating the UF milk to 65% original volume and then bringing the concentrate level back to its original volume with the addition of 50 °C water were performed during UF to optimize manufacturing conditions. Analyses showed significant reductions in lactose and calcium content of the retentate. Sensory evaluation of the low-fat Cheddar cheese manufactured from the acidified and diafiltered UF lowfat milk revealed a significant improvement in the flavor and body and texture of the cheese upon extended storage (12 months) at 8 °C when compared with that of UF low-fat Cheddar cheese made without these two steps. These same researchers in a related study [23] added a flavor-enhancing enzyme to UF low-fat milk as a means of improving the flavor and body/texture of the low-fat Cheddar cheese. The enzyme treatment did appear to stimulate the production of organic acids in low-fat Cheddar cheese by yielding higher mean levels of citric, orotic, pyruvic, acetic, and propionic acids. Neither UF nor enzyme treatment significantly improved the flavor or body and texture of the treated cheese types.

Olson and Johnson [18] emphasize that cooking temperatures typically are lower in the manufacture of low-fat cheeses. Selection of lactic bacteria strains that will not impart bitterness with the use of lower temperatures is important. Although the reasons are obscure, pH values at whey drainage and salting should be higher during manufacture of low-fat Cheddar-type cheese to obtain better quality. Higher pH values would result in lower retention of chymosin but more retention of the milk proteinase plasmin. It is advisable to use lower levels of milk-clotting enzymes. Washing low-fat cheese curd or partially diluting whey with water may be necessary to control the pH of the cheese. This would be more critical in cheese of higher moisture content and consequently higher lactose concentrations.

These researchers also compared the economics of low-fat cheese manufacture with that of regular Cheddar cheese. A calculated net return in manufacturing Cheddar cheese (38% moisture, 33.5% fat) was $2.33 per 100 pounds of whole milk. The net return from the same 100 pounds of milk that had been standardized by removing cream and converted into low-fat cheese (47% moisture, 19.5% fat) was only $1.84. Manufacturing low-fat cheese (19.5% fat) priced at $1.45 per pound and containing 43% moisture from this standardized milk yielded a net return of only $0.66. Standardizing the milk with nonfat dry milk (NDM) or skim milk is attractive for low-fat cheese containing 47% moisture. Other alternatives for standardization exist, such as skim milk, condensed skim milk, and UF retentate, and the latter (UF retentate) may be attractive since less lactose would be added to the standardized milk.

Groves [24] indicated in an editorial comment that some of the new reduced-fat cheese on the market established two facts:

1. It is an inaccurate overgeneralization to assert that less fat means less cheese flavor or inferior cheese texture.
2. Typical flavor and texture associated with each cheese variety are recognized and identifiable.

Moreover, the recognizable flavor and texture can be achieved in a reduced-fat cheese. Therefore, the typical flavor and texture should be expected and required with respect to each reduced-fat cheese described through reference to product meeting the Cheddar standard.

VI. LOW-FAT FROZEN DAIRY DESSERTS

The International Ice Cream Association has proposed new standards of identity for ice cream–related products to FDA as follows:

Product	Proposed fat content
Ice cream	10%
Reduced fat or "light"	2–7%
Low-fat	0.5–2%
Nonfat	<0.05%

According to Marshall [25], the United Dairy Industry Association's 1990 Attitudes and Usage Trend Study showed that 25% of those surveyed had cut down on dairy products and that the majority were actively trying to consume less fat. Only 39% considered ice cream to be a healthy food. Recent legislative and regulatory developments are creating opportunities to market to those health-conscious consumers and perhaps to regain lost sales.

Marshall further stated that the emphasis for product development is coming not only from the proposed standards (mentioned above) but also from new ingredient, processing, and equipment technology. he listed four promising categories:

1. Reduced fat, low-fat, and nonfat
2. Modified fat

3. Lactose modified
4. Protein-modified, frozen desserts

With regard to reduced fat, low-fat, and nonfat ice cream–related products, the major challenges are:

1. Building body
2. Minimizing ice crystal size
3. Providing creaminess
4. Finding the best stabilizing formula
5. Finding the best flavoring system
6. Preventing shrinkage
7. Slowing textural change

Marshall [25] states that the industry's resources for producing these products depend on "fake fats" and bulking agents, as described earlier (see Sec. III.C). He concludes that high-quality ice creams most likely will contain fat for many years to come and stresses the need for more research to create a more desirable fatty acid profile, such as by removing saturated fat and increasing the percentage of unsaturated fat.

Tharp and Gottemoller [26] indicate that frozen dairy desserts differ from other dairy products in three major ways:

1. They are intended to be consumed in the frozen state.
2. Substantial volume is made up of an ingredient—air—which contributes absolutely no calories.
3. The levels of fat and total solids vary over a broad range.

Even if the fat is completely removed, the calorie level at conventional overruns is borderline for reduced-calorie status. Reduction of fat level also invokes additional challenges in replacing its contribution to the flavor and richness that the consumer has come to expect in frozen desserts similar to ice cream.

These workers [26] conducted a "functionality appraisal" of supplemental ingredients that might be included in low-fat frozen dairy desserts. Each of the ingredients was rated based on its effect on functionality over factors such as bulking, freezing point depression, water control, sweetness, and fat substitution. These are summarized in Table 2. The drastic compositional changes required to achieve reduced-calorie status create special problems in achieving acceptable flavor, body/texture, and heat-shock protection. Identifying the problems to be overcome and understanding the role of available ingredients in surmounting those problems are key steps in that process.

Lee and White [27] used UF retentates and whey protein concentrates to replace different levels of solids-not-fat (SNF) in vanilla ice cream at 25, 50, or 75% and 25, 50, 75, or 100%, respectively. Sensory evaluation showed

Table 2 Functionality Appraisal of Supplemental Ingredients Studied

Ingredient	Bulking	Freezing-point depression	Water control	Sweetness	Fat substitution
Polydextrose	3	2	1	0	0
Maltodextrin	3	0	2	0	2
Glycerine	1	3	0	0	0
Propylene glycol	1	3	0	0	0
Pure crystalline fructose	2	3	0	3	0
Sorbitol	2	3	0	2	0
Emulsifier	0	0	1	0	2
Conventional stabilizer	0	0	3	0	1
Microcrystalline cellulose	1	0	3	0	3
Aspartame	0	0	0	3	0

Source: Ref. 26.
0 = negligible, 1 = slight, 2 = moderate, 3 = strong.

that ice cream made with substitution of SNF with UF retentate had higher flavor and body texture scores than that made with whey protein concentrate. Substitution with 25% UF retentate produced the highest mean flavor score of any of the ice creams tested. This work encourages the use of UF retentates in reduced-fat/low-fat frozen dairy desserts. Several bulking agents are now on the market, as described previously.

According to Rogers [28], production history and industry estimates point to increases in ice milk, frozen yogurt, and other frozen dairy desserts at the cost of ice cream. The predictions are that the super premium segment should continue to increase. The key for all frozen dairy desserts, he described, is that of quality. He stated that quality, many believe, is what is causing many consumers to rediscover or increase their consumption of ice cream. At any rate, the producers of lowfat and nonfat frozen dairy desserts must keep the issue of taste and mouthfeel foremost in their mind in order to retain a significant segment of the market.

VII. LOW-FAT/NONFAT YOGURT PRODUCTS

As much or more so than any other dairy product, yogurt has been the vehicle for the ideal low-fat, low-calorie food. Most yogurts on the market today are low-fat, and some are nonfat. In addition, many of the yogurts are sweetened with aspartame and advertise the fact that they contain fewer than 100 calories per unit serving. This trend will continue as long as the quality of these products are maintained.

In two related studies, McGregor and White [29,30] evaluated the effect of sweeteners on the quality and acceptability of yogurt. They specifically looked at sucrose and the high-fructose corn syrups. High-quality yogurts, both plain and fruit-flavored, were effectively made with both corn syrup and high-fructose corn syrups. In fact, there appeared to be a preference for yogurt made with 90% high-fructose corn syrup especially in the strawberry yogurt. Most panelists preferred the level of 4% added sweetener. It was noted that as the amount of sweetener increased, the time required to get to the breaking pH of 4.4 increased. The 42% high-fructose corn syrup was significantly less sweet than the other sweeteners evaluated. Acetaldehyde decreased significantly during storage, whereas diacetyl increased significantly.

In a subsequent study, Keating and White [31] evaluated plain, strawberry, and cherry swiss-style yogurts utilizing alternative sweetening agents. The sweeteners studied were sucrose (control), aspartame, calcium and sodium saccharin, sorbitol, high-fructose corn syrup, high-fructose corn syrup plus monoammonium glycyrrhizinate, sucrose plus monoammonium glycyrrhizinate, acesulfame-K, and dihydrochalcone. For each flavor and over all storage periods (up to 42 days), yogurts sweetened with sorbitol or aspartame were among those consistently favored. Fructose samples had a significantly higher viscosity. Both time and sweetener type significantly affected the growth of the microorganisms.

VIII. FLUID MILK

As already mentioned, fluid milk has offered the consumer low-fat and non-fat options for many years. An increase in consumption of skim milk during the past several years has substantially altered the marketing strategy of many dairy companies. A major regulatory and legislative decision will soon be made regarding the requirement of adding nonfat solids to fluid milk. While this will increase the viscosity of the milk, there is a legitimate question as to whether or not this improves the quality of the milk as perceived and actually received by the consumer.

Skim milk sales rose from 5.7% of total fluid milk sales in the United States in 1987 to 10.3% in 1990 [2]. Skim milk and low-fat milk (both 1% and 2%) represent 55.6% of total fluid milk sales, while plain whole milk represented only 33.9% in 1990.

In conjunction with the low-fat and nonfat fluid milk products, there is also the question of cholesterol-reduced milk fat in fluid milks. Kosikowski

[32] reported that the cholesterol content of fat in milk and milk products varies widely. The fat of whole milk averages 4 mg of cholesterol per gram, whereas fat from ripened cheese contains about 3 mg per gram and that from skim milk about 16 mg per gram. These concentrations reflect differences in fat globule size and effects of manufacturing steps, product fermentation, and ripening. Further, the labeling proposals of the FDA define cholesterol labeling and establish new serving sizes for many foods, and a new classification was introduced specifically concerning foods processed or formulated to lower cholesterol concentration or density. This category is entitled "reduced cholesterol" and applies to foods that have a reduction of at least 75%. The cost of producing cholesterol-free milk and milk products is yet to be fully documented. These foods will apparently cost considerably more than standard milk and its products. Also, when the FDA labeling proposals of 1990 are implemented, these may exert a restraining force on future research in cholesterol removal from dairy foods due to an inability of the food to meet the qualifier requirements. However, cholesterol-removal processes have the ability to convert many dairy foods to "reduced-cholesterol" status and potentially to cholesterol levels below 2 mg per serving. Furthermore, the opportunity allowed in these new proposals to list a value of less than 2 mg per serving on the food carton as "0 cholesterol" could prove advantageous enough to stimulate continued research activity.

Schroder and Baer [33] used steam-stripping to reduce the cholesterol content in fluid milks, and they reported the following results:

1. Cholesterol-reduced milk fat (CRMF) milk can be processed using typical milk-processing equipment.
2. Low cholesterol fluid milks can be produced.
3. CRMF fluid milks can be acceptable to consumers.

Since their work was done on a pilot plant scale, they recommended the following:

1. CRMF milks should be evaluated at a commercial fluid milk plant.
2. A regional market test of 1 and 2% CRMF milks should be undertaken.
3. Further testing should be conducted with CRMF in flavored milks.

Thus, cholesterol reduction does appear to go hand in hand with the emphasis on low-fat and nonfat fluid milk products.

IX. COMMENTS ON PRICE STRUCTURE

Currently, milk is paid for based on fat content and total quantity (weight). Thus, the higher the fat content of the product, the higher the price. However, as consumers become more and more concerned about their nutritional well-being, the price of a food item becomes less critical as to whether or not the food will be purchased. As a consequence, low-fat dairy products can cost even more than their whole-fat counterparts. If the basis for payment of milk shifts to a total solids or protein content rather than fat, the price structure can be changed even more dramatically. Premiums are already being paid to dairy farmers meeting certain protein standards. Therefore, the dairy food processor should be able to receive top dollar when distributing and marketing premium low-fat/nonfat dairy products.

REFERENCES

1. The latest scoop, International Ice Cream Association, p. 4 (August 1991).
2. Milk facts, Milk Industry Foundation, p. 14 (August 1991).
3. R. J. Bannar, Free food: Fat-free, that is, *Dairy Frozen Foods, 2*: 43 (1991).
4. N. F. Olson, A report from the conference on fat and cholesterol reduced foods, *Dairy Field, 174*: 34 (1991).
5. D. Best, The challenges of fat substitution, *Prep. Foods, 159*: 72 (1991).
6. D. D. Duxbury and N. M. Meinhold, Fat replacers—key ingredients in new product R & D efforts, *Food Process. 61*: 58 (1991).
7. C. V. Morr, Whey protein functionality: current status and the need for improved quality and functionality, Presented at the Dairy Products Technical Conference, ADPI, CDR, Chicago, April 25–26 (1990).
8. M. E. Mangino, Functionality of whey protein concentrates, Presented at Dairy Products Technical Conference, ADPI, CDR, Chicago, April 25–26 (1990).
9. Fat substitute update, *Food Technol., 44*: 92 (1990).
10. R. M. Morrison, The market for fat substitutes, *Natl. Food Rev., 13*: 24 (1990).
11. B. Salvage, Cutting fat, building profits, *Dairy Field, 174*: 48 (1991).
12. D. G. Medcalf, The use of fat substitutes in dairy products, Presented at Fat and Cholesterol Reduced Foods Conference, New Orleans, March 22–24 (1990).
13. A. M. Altschul, Low-calorie foods, *Food Technol., 43*: 113 (1989).
14. E. Dexheimer, Straight talk, *Dairy Foods, 91*: 13 (1990).
15. G. W. Jameson, Cheese with less fat, *Aust. J. Dairy Technol., Nov.*: 93 (1990).
16. M. E. Johnson and C. Chen, Making quality reduced-fat 1991 cheese, Proceedings of the Cheese Research and Technology Conference, Madison, WI, p. 35, March 6–7 (1991).
17. R. E. Simard, Evaluation of lowfat cheese problems, Proceedings of the Cheese Research and Technology Conference, CDR, Madison, WI, p. 37, March 6–7 (1991).
18. N. F. Olson and M. E. Johnson, Light cheese products: Characteristics and economics, *Food Technol., 44*: 93 (1990).
19. D. B. Emmons, M. Kalab, and E. Larmond, Milk gel structure. X. Texture and microstructure in Cheddar cheese made from whole milk and from homogenized lowfat milk, *J. Texture Stud., 11*:15 (1980).

20. J. Prentice, Cheese rheology, *Cheese: Chemistry, Physics, and Microbiology* (P. F. Fox, ed.), Elsevier Appl. Sci., New York, p. 299 (1987).
21. P. Masi and Addeo, An examination of some mechanical properties of a group of Italian cheeses and their relation to structure and conditions of manufacture, *J. Food Eng., 5*: 217 (1986).
22. J. U. McGregor and C. H. White, Optimizing ultrafiltration parameters for the development of a lowfat Cheddar cheese, *J. Dairy Sci., 73*: 314 (1990).
23. J. U. McGregor and C. H. White, Effect of enzyme treatment and ultrafiltration on the quality of lowfat Cheddar cheese, *J. Dairy Sci., 73*: 571 (1990).
24. D. Groves, Standards not taken lightly, *The Cheese Reporter, 116*(2): 4 (1991).
25. R. T. Marshall, Fat in ice cream: Can we live with it? *Dairy Field, 174*: 35 (1991).
26. B. W. Tharp and T. V. Gottemoller, Light frozen dairy desserts: Effect of compositional changes on processing and sensory characteristics, *Food Technol., 4*: 86 (1990).
27. F. Y. Lee and C. H. White, Effect of ultrafiltration retentates and whey protein concentrates on ice cream quality during storage, *J. Dairy Sci., 74*: 1170(1991).
28. P. Rogers, Split decision, *Dairy Foods, 92*: 46 (1991).
29. J. U. McGregor and C. H. White, Effect of sweeteners on the quality and acceptability of yogurt, *J. Dairy Sci., 69*: 698 (1986).
30. J. U. McGregor and C. H. White, Effect of sweeteners on major volatile compounds and flavor of yogurt, *J. Dairy Sci., 70*: 1828 (1987).
31. K. R. Keating and C. H. White, Effect of alternative sweeteners in plain and fruit-flavored yogurts, *J. Dairy Sci., 73*: 54 (1990).
32. F. V. Kosikowski, "Cholesterol-free" milk and milk products: Limitations in production and labeling, *Food Technol., 44*: 130 (1990).
33. B. G. Schroder and R. J. Baer, Utilization of cholesterol-reduced milk fat in fluid milks, *Food Technol., 44*: 145 (1990).
34. S. Newton, Facing the consequences. *Dairy Foods. 92*: 69 (1991).

13
Low-Calorie Bakery Foods

James L. Vetter *American Institute of Baking, Manhattan, Kansas*

I. INTRODUCTION

A. "Healthful" Bakery Foods

A walk through the supermarket aisles will quickly convince the observer that there has been a flurry of activity in the development, production, and marketing of "healthful" foods. This is as true for bakery products as it is for other categories of food. The word "healthful" is put in quotes, because some would argue that snack cakes, pies, cookies, and pastries are not really "healthful" foods even if calorie content has been reduced or fat and cholesterol have been removed. Perhaps a better term would be "more healthful" since some of the objectional components have been reduced or eliminated. Nevertheless, these nutritionally modified foods are considered more healthful than their normal counterparts by many consumers.

Although many of the "healthful" bakery foods are relatively new, some have been on the market for some time. High-fiber, reduced-calorie breads have been marketed since the mid-1970s and have become a mainstay of sales of the baking industry.

B. Modifying Nutritional Characteristics

These new "healthful" bakery foods represent a variety of approaches to modifying nutritional characteristics. Calorie reduction varies from a relatively low level (on a per-gram basis, but augmented by a reduction in serving size) to as much as one-third fewer calories than an equivalent serving of a normal counterpart product. Fat may be reduced to a few percent or, in many cases, to zero. Sodium content is often reduced, and cholesterol is reduced or eliminated. In some products, fiber is increased to add another reason for consumer purchase. Nutritionally modified bakery foods include saltines, breads, muffins, cakes, Danish, pies, cookies, and the possibility of fried foods such as doughnuts.

At the time of this writing, most low- or reduced-calorie bakery foods are based on the reduction or elimination of fat. In time, high-intensity sweeteners, when they are approved for use in bakery foods, will also be used to reduce calories. Suitable low-calorie ingredients will be used to replace the bulk of the sugar replaced by the high-intensity sweetener.

This chapter will review the rationale for modifying the nutritional characteristics of bakery foods, the technology currently available to achieve this modification, examples of products on the consumer market, and the outlook for the future.

II. ROLE OF BAKERY FOODS IN THE DIET

A. Consumption of Fat in Grain-Based Foods

Bakery foods are generally included in the category of grain products in many surveys of dietary patterns and food consumption trends. As a group, grain products contribute only 1.3% of total dietary fat [1], but this low level can be quite misleading because of the wide variety of foods that are considered "grain" products. Pastas and rice are quite low in fat, but are included in the grain products category. Grain-based snacks (most of which are relatively high in fat) are also part of this grouping. Some bakery foods are quite low in fat, while others contain significant amounts of shortening, frying fat, etc. Therefore, it is necessary to look beyond the 1.3% of total dietary fat contributed by grain products to understand the rationale and marketing opportunities behind the development, production, and sale of reduced-fat and other nutritionally modified bakery foods.

B. Fat Content of Bakery Foods

The range in fat content of selected bakery foods is illustrated by the data in Table 1. Yeast-leavened breads are quite low in fat, containing only 1–3%.

Table 1 Typical Fat Content of Bakery Foods

Product type	Typical fat content (%)	Approx. kcal/100 g	Approx. % kcal from fat
Yeast-leavened breads	1.0–3.0	250	3.6–10.8
Muffins	9–10	285	28–32
Cakes/Cupcakes	10–20	370	24–48
Danish pastry	23–25	425	49–53
Chocolate chip cookies	20–30	495	36–54
Yeast-leavened doughnuts	25–30	420	54–64

Source: Ref. 2.

In fact some breads (French, for example) contain essentially no fat. Yeast-leavened doughnuts are fried in fat or oil and contain much higher levels of fat. Doughnuts contain as much as 58% of their calories from fat, whereas most breads contain only about 10% of fat calories.

C. Consumption of Bakery Foods

In addition to considering the amount of fat in a product, consumption patterns are also important in judging the need for—or opportunity to market—reduced-fat bakery products.

The data in Table 2 illustrate the importance of considering patterns with a few selected bakery foods as examples. Note that for all age groups white bread is consumed at least once every 3 days by over 70% of the population. The percent of the population eating whole or cracked wheat bread at least once in 3 days is considerably less (10–28%), and for high-fiber, wheat germ, multigrain, and similar breads it is even lower at 0.8–3.4%. However, the amount of bread consumed per day is virtually the same (about 20–60 grams) regardless of the type chosen by individual consumers. This has led marketers to target a specific segment of consumers with nutritionally modified bakery foods.

D. Segmenting the Market

Although a whole wheat bread reduced in calories or fat may have little effect on the total calorie and fat consumption for the population as a whole, it could make quite a significant difference for that segment of the population that eats whole wheat bread. Although fewer adults than children eat chocolate cake or cookies, a product with fewer calories or less fat could be im-

Table 2 Consumption Data for Various Baked Foods

Product type	Age group (yr)	% Consuming	g/day consumed
White breads	1–8	76–87	27–40
	9–18	80–86	40–61
	19 +	70–77	38–59
Whole and cracked wheat bread	1–8	13–14	21–29
	9–18	10–12	29–50
	19 +	19–28	31–49
High-fiber, wheat germ, multigrain bread	1–8	0.8–1.0	15–25
	9–18	0.7–1.0	23–55
	19 +	1.4–3.4	31–59
Chocolate cake and cupcakes	1–8	6–16	22–29
	9–18	10–15	32–46
	19 +	4–9	27–51
Chocolate chip cookies	1–8	16–18	9–12
	9–18	12–14	11–16
	19 +	3–6	7–16

Source: Ref. 3.

portant to parents who are concerned about calorie or fat consumption by their children and to the fewer adults who continue to enjoy these products.

Food marketers also believe that consumption of many products that adults tend to avoid as they get older could be increased if a more healthful (fewer calories, less fat, no cholesterol, etc.) alternative were available. Thus, a variety of nutritionally modified bakery foods were developed and marketed. Most are targeted to a segment of the population: those who consume, but might consume more, and those who don't consume, but might begin, if reasons for not consuming or restricting consumption are reduced or eliminated.

III. FUNCTIONALITY OF FAT IN BAKERY FOODS

Fats and oils (or shortenings) have a number of important functions in bakery foods. These functions must be considered when reducing or eliminating shortenings from bakery products. In some cases, it is possible to achieve the desired functionality or, at least, end result with other ingredients or changes in processing conditions. In other cases, it may be necessary to accept a slight change in the quality characteristics of the finished product as a trade-off for reducing or eliminating fat. A good general discussion of the chemical, physical, and functional properties of fats and oils in bakery foods is given by Pyler [4].

A. Aeration

Shortenings are used to incorporate air during mixing of doughs or batters. This air or leavening gas from either chemical leavening systems or yeast activity is released into the cell nuclei generated during mixing and, in some cases, is entrapped by beta prime crystals of fat. Proper mixing and mixer design will break entrapped gas into small nuclei, which expand during baking and contribute to volume and grain of the final baked product. Grain, in this instance, refers to the visual characteristics of cell size and shape and cell wall thickness. This function of fats can often be simulated in reduced or fat-free products by gums, starches, or emulsifiers.

B. Lubrication

Shortenings, usually the liquid oil portion, provide important "lubrication" properties to doughs, batters, and the product during and after baking. This lubrication helps prevent sticking of the baked product to surfaces during baking. These surfaces may be pans for bread, cakes, muffins, etc. or the baking surface itself in the case of cookies or crackers that are baked directly on a traveling band or mesh. Lubrication is also important in slicing bread on high-speed, continuous slicing machines. Without proper lubrication from fat, oil, or substitute, there will be excessive "crumbing" (referred to as "snow" in the industry) on the slicing equipment creating an undesirable sanitation condition and poor appearance to the slice of bread. The lubrication function of oils may be achieved through the use of emulsifiers.

C. Texture

Texture refers to physical properties of toughness, tenderness, or "shortening" characteristics. Fats and oils obviously affect texture of baked products. Shortbread cookies owe their short, tender texture to the large amount of butter or other fat used in preparation. Fats and oils affect the eating characteristics of most baked foods in a similar manner. When fats or oils are reduced or eliminated, it is often very difficult to achieve the same texture with other ingredients or technology currently available.

D. Organoleptic Properties

Finally, fats and oils contribute to a variety of organoleptic characteristics of baked foods. These include "richness" (a term used to describe many high-fat baked products), flavor (as in butter cookies), flakiness (croissants, pie crust, etc.), and visual appeal such as an attractive shine on a snack cracker that has been sprayed with oil following baking. In many cases, a basic change in organoleptic characteristics must be accepted as a trade-off for reducing or removing fats and oils.

Continued work by ingredient suppliers and the baking industry itself will surely lead to even better ways to achieve the functionality of fats and oils with substitute ingredients or new processing technology.

IV. MARKETS AND MARKETING

A. A Multifaceted Market

There is no single market for bakery foods with reduced fat content. It is a multifaceted market, multifaceted because different consumers are looking for different things; some consumers will accept some trade-offs in product quality characteristics that other consumers will not accept.

1. Controlled Calories

Some manufacturers have targeted their products to those consumers who are more interested in controlled calories than in fat or cholesterol reduction. These products may have some adjustments in fat content and serving size in order to achieve a level of calories per serving that these consumers will accept. In general, these products have quality characteristics most similar to normal, counterpart products.

2. Fat and Cholesterol Removal

Some bakers have been able to achieve desired quality characteristics even when removing all fat- and cholesterol-containing ingredients, and their products appeal to those consumers who want it all or nothing. In some cases, a sacrifice in quality is accepted in return for a fat- and cholesterol-free product.

3. Reduced Fat

If a manufacturer cannot produce a fat-free product with a minimum level of quality considered necessary for the intended market segment, some fat may be included and the products marketed as "reduced fat" or "95% fat free."

B. Selecting a Segment of the Market

The market is varied and each manufacturer determines which segment to target. This selection may depend to some extent on the technical expertise of the baker, but more than likely is based on deliberate marketing decisions concerning estimates of size of various segments of the market and image the company wants to project for its product line to the consumer.

C. Market Size

It is virtually impossible to estimate the size of the current market or predict the size of the potential market for reduced-fat bakery foods. The market is so new that good data on market size have not yet been generated. The market is so dynamic that projections are almost meaningless. One thing appears certain, however. A growing number of consumers are concerned about diet and health, and a viable market exists for products designed for these consumers. The major unknown in the equation is whether or not the nature and quality of nutritionally modified bakery foods possible with today's technology meet the ever-changing needs of the consumer.

Furthermore, the need and desirability for most consumers to reduce fat and calorie intake from current levels is undoubtedly permanent; it will not change as a result of additional research on the relationship between diet and health. This same conclusion may not apply to other, more controversial issues concerning healthy eating practices.

V. INGREDIENTS FOR REDUCING CALORIES AND FAT

A. Introduction

1. Available Options

The new product formulator has a number of options available to reduce fat and/or calories in bakery products, and most are being used in commercial products today. These options will certainly be expanded in the future as the allied industry continues to develop new ingredients and technology to help the baking industry meet the needs of the consuming public.

In most cases, no one ingredient alone will provide all the quality characteristics desired. A combination of ingredients or other formula and processing modifications is usually required to meet both label claims and quality parameters.

2. Moisture and Weight Changes

In addition to ingredient changes to modify nutrient content, it is, of course, possible to reduce calories, fat, and other nutrients by increasing the moisture content of the final product or decreasing serving size. Both of these practices are being used in the production of reduced-calorie or reduced-fat bakery foods. They are often combined with ingredient substitution in order to achieve further reduction in calories and fat.

B. Ingredient Substitutions

The following is a discussion of the application of ingredient substitutions in the production of reduced-calorie or reduced-fat bakery foods with emphasis on special considerations or limitations in bakery applications.

1. Fiber Ingredients

High-fiber ingredients with low calorie content may be used as bulking agents to replace ingredients with higher calorie contents (see Chapter 11). These high-fiber ingredients are usually nonfunctional or "dead weight"; other formula modifications are necessary to minimize adverse effects on finished product quality. For example, when high-fiber ingredients are used to replace flour in the production of calorie-reduced bread, it is necessary to add vital wheat gluten to replace the gluten that has been removed with the flour and to "carry" the fiber ingredient.

In general, the amount of flour that can be replaced by fiber ingredients decreases in proportion to the final moisture content of the baked food because of adverse effects on textural characteristic in low-moisture products. The wide variety of available high-fiber ingredients vary in fiber content, color, flavor, particle size, and, of course, price. The new product formulator must choose the product or combination of products that provides the desired end product within well-defined parameters of cost and marketing objectives.

2. Starch-Based Fat Replacers

A number of starch-based products are being used as fat replacers (see Chapter 11). These products are generally low-DE (dextrose equivalent) maltodextrins manufactured by mild hydrolysis of starch resulting in relatively low levels of dextrose—the building block of the starch molecule. Solutions of about 25% solids of these low-DE maltodextrins have a short texture, which gives a fatlike sensation in the mouth. Starting formulas using this type of product are given in Tables 3–6.

Table 3 Starting Formula for 95% Fat-Free Cake Mix

Ingredient	Total mix (%)	Flour basis (%)
Cake flour	37.14	100.0
Sucrose	28.38	76.4
Krystar 300 fructose	15.57	42.7
Dur-Lo (Van Den Bergh)	4.03	10.8
Nonfat dry milk	3.56	9.6
Ultra-bake NF	2.99	8.0
Dried egg whites	1.79	4.8
Sta-slim 150 (Staley)	1.67	4.5
Salt	1.41	3.8
Baking soda	0.95	2.6
Stable 9 (Monsanto)	0.51	1.4
Panalite (Monsanto)	0.48	1.3
Creamy vanilla (Universal 464174)	0.48	1.3
Lecithin (Lucas Meyer MCP)	0.32	0.9
Butter vanilla (Fries & Fries)	0.32	0.9
Gatodan 415 (Grindsted)	0.10	0.3
(390 g water to 630 g dry mix)		

Source: A. E. Staley Mfg. Co., Decatur, IL.

Table 4 Starting Formula for Fat-Free Muffins

Ingredient	Flour basis (%)
Water	165.6
Cake flour	100.0
Granulated sugar	96.7
Dried fruit (Sun Diamond)	33.3
Brown sugar	32.2
Oat bran	27.8
Maltrin M100 (GPC)	13.9
Nonfat dry milk	12.2
Baking powder (ADM 112713)	8.9
Dried egg whites	6.7
Emulsifier (Dur-Lo, Van Den Bergh)	3.3
Salt	2.8
Vanilla	2.7
SSL (Emplex, Amer. Ingred.)	1.7
Xanthan	0.6
Guar	0.6
Cinnamon	0.6
Allspice	0.1

Source: Grain Processing Corporation, Muscatine, IA.

Table 5 Starting Formula for 75% Fat-Reduced Yellow Cake

Ingredient	Total mix (%)	Flour basis (%)
Flour	24.03	100.0
Sugar	28.41	118.3
Water	24.70	102.8
Whole eggs	11.90	49.5
Shortening	2.70	11.2
Nonfat dry milk	2.24	9.3
Baking powder	1.70	7.1
Salt	0.96	4.0
Vanilla extract	0.24	1.0
Emplex	0.12	0.5
Paselli SA2	3.00	12.5

Source: AVEBE America, Inc.

These starch-based fat replacers require moisture for their functionality and are most suitable for application in baked foods such as cakes, which contain a relatively high moisture content in the finished product. They are unsuitable for replacing fat in low-moisture products such as crisp cookies or crackers.

3. Polydextrose

Although polydextrose (see Chapter 11) is not a "fiber" in the usual sense of the word, its characteristics are fiberlike in many applications in bakery

Table 6 Starting Formula for 75% Fat-Reduced Cookie

Ingredient	Total mix (%)	Flour basis (%)
Flour	24.60	100.0
Chocolate chips	24.60	100.0
Shortening	4.12	16.7
Sugar	16.45	66.9
Whole eggs	8.20	33.3
Brown sugar	4.15	16.9
Water	3.81	15.5
Salt	0.50	2.0
Baking soda	0.50	2.0
Vanilla extract	0.50	2.0
Emplex	0.12	0.5
Paselli SA2 (20% gel)	12.45	50.6

Source: AVEBE America, Inc.

Table 6 Starting Formula for 75% Fat-Reduced Cookie

Ingredient	Total mix (%)	Flour basis (%)
Flour	24.60	100.0
Chocolate chips	24.60	100.0
Shortening	4.12	16.7
Sugar	16.45	66.9
Whole eggs	8.20	33.3
Brown sugar	4.15	16.9
Water	3.81	15.5
Salt	0.50	2.0
Baking soda	0.50	2.0
Vanilla extract	0.50	2.0
Emplex	0.12	0.5
Paselli SA2 (20% gel)	12.45	50.6

Source: AVEBE America, Inc.

foods. It is considered a low-calorie bulking agent and is most commonly used to replace sugar in formulating nutritionally modified bakery foods.

Polydextrose also has fat-sparing properties and may be used to reduce fat content in some bakery foods. It alone, however, cannot be used to replace all of the fat in these products; polydextrose is usually used in combination with other fat-sparing ingredients.

4. Beta-Glucan Fiber

Beta-glucan fiber derived from yeast is a new development that may have application in reduced-calorie and reduced-fat bakery foods. It is the major structural component of the yeast cell wall; a product with 86% fiber (all of which is beta-glucan) has been produced. Although originally developed for its cholesterol-lowering properties, reports from limited test results indicate that the beta-glucan may have functionality as a fat replacer [5].

5. Microparticulate Protein

Microparticulate protein (see Chapter 9) may be used to replace fat in some bakery applications. Although there have been concerns about the heat stability of microparticulate proteins during baking applications, these have been shown to be largely unfounded. Microparticulate proteins are being used in bakery products. However, the fatlike characteristics are achieved by hydrating the protein with about two times its weight of water. This amount of water would prevent the use of microparticulate proteins in products such as cookie sandwich cremes where the water would migrate to—and soften the texture of—the cookie base cake.

Nevertheless, it is anticipated that microparticulate proteins will find application in some components of bakery products such as icings and water-based creme fillings.

6. Fat Replacers

Whereas a number of nonfatty ingredients have been proposed and are being used as partial or complete replacements for fats and oils in bakery foods, a variety of fatlike materials that look, feel, and act like fat but do not provide the calories of fat are under development (see Chapter 10). None of these materials is commercially available at the present time because they have not yet been approved by the Food and Drug Administration (FDA) as food additives or accepted as generally recognized as safe (GRAS) substances.

It is difficult to say when any of these "synthetic" fats will be approved and available for use in bakery foods, but it is almost certain that this type of material will be part of the formulator's resources in new product development at some time in the future. Manufacturers of these materials must include bakery foods in their petitions for approval by FDA.

7. Emulsifiers and Blends

Emulsifiers have been proposed—and are being used—to replace fat in bakery foods. These products function by (1) making the fat go farther (fat-sparing actions), simulating the sensory characteristics of higher levels of fat, or (2) using a reduced-calorie, fatty-based substitute in place of the fat (see Chapter 11).

Mono- and diglycerides are, perhaps, the most common emulsifiers used to replace fat in bakery foods. Products relatively high in diglyceride content seem to be preferred. Although they are used at lower levels than the fat that they replace because of fat-sparing activity, there may be a question about whether or not the final baked product is indeed "fat-free." Other emulsifiers that may be used as fat replacers in bakery foods include sodium stearoyl lactylate, sorbitan monostearate, diacetyl tartaric acid esters (DATEMS), sucrose esters, and polysorbate 60.

Blends of emulsifiers are also available as fat-sparing agents. One commercial product is a blend of propylene glycol mono- and diesters of fats and fatty acids, mono- and diglycerides, partially hydrogenated soybean oil with lecithin, and butylated hydroxyanisole (BHA) and citric acid to help protect flavor. Another is a blend of emulsifiers, modified food starch, and guar gum on a nonfat dry milk base.

Whereas carbohydrate-based fat substitutes are used primarily in bakery foods with intermediate- or high-moisture contents, emulsifiers appear to function reasonably well in low-moisture products such as cookies. Blended products also work well in these low-moisture applications.

8. Gums

A variety of gums (see Chapter 11) may be found in reduced-fat or fat-free bakery foods. The most common are guar and xanthan. There is essentially no literature nor company technical data on the function of gums in this application. However, it can be speculated that gums increase viscosity of batter systems and assist in providing aeration during mixing, which would tend to improve baked volume and grain. Additional research on the functionality of gums in reduced-fat bakery foods should lead to further application in this area.

9. High-Intensity Sweeteners

Three high-intensity sweeteners (Sucralose, Alitame, and Sunette) are under review by FDA for approval to use in bakery foods. Small amounts of these sweeteners can provide the sweet taste of substantially larger amounts of sugar and other sweetening ingredients. However, sugar and other "traditional" sweeteners have functional properties other than just adding sweet flabor to bakery foods. These properties include fermentability, color development, and textural characteristics. Low-calorie bulking agents must be added to replace the weight of sugar and other ingredients replaced by small amounts of high-intensity sweeteners. These bulking agents themselves, or in combination with other ingredients, must simulate the nonflavor functional properties of the sweeteners they replace. The development of suitable low-calorie bulking agents to be used in conjunction with high-intensity sweeteners is needed, and work in this area is continuing.

VI. A LOOK AT THE MARKETPLACE

A. An Overview

The following discussion is intended to provide an overview of the wide variety of calorie- or fat-reduced bakery foods on the market today and to illustrate various approaches being taken to achieve labeling claims and the desired quality characteristics. Table 7 lists calorie characteristics of selected commercial bakery foods being marketed as reduced- or fat-free products. The data are taken from the nutrition labels of these products and are approximate to the extent that rounding off is used in developing the nutrition label

Table 7   Calorie Content and Percent Calories from Fat for Selected Commercial Bakery Products Marketed as Reduced-Fat or Fat-Free

Product	Serving size (oz)	kcal/g	Calories per serving	%Calories from fat
Fat-free saltines	0.5	3.5	50	0
Snack cakes				
Product				
A	1.5	3.0	130	7
B	1.5	3.0	130	7
C	1.5	3.0	130	14
D	1.2	2.6	90	10
E	1.25	3.1	110	16
Muffins				
Product				
A	2.25	2.0	130	7
B	2.25	1.9	120	0
Cakes, layer				
Product				
A	1.7	2.3	10	0
B	1.0	2.5	70	0
Cakes, loaf				
Product				
A	1.0	2.5	70	0
B	1.0	2.8	80	0
C	1.0	2.1	60	0
D	1.0	2.5	70	0
E	1.0	2.1	60	0
Cakes, coffee				
Product				
A	1.1	2.8	80	0
B	2.0	2.3	130	0
Cookies	0.8	3.5	80	0
Frozen dessert, Pie	2.25	1.9	120	0

declarations. Note the dramatic reduction in fat content compared to "normal" products described in Table 1.

There is, of course, a wide range in serving size: 0.5–2.25 ounces; lower-moisture products (crackers and cookies) have lower serving sizes. Calories per serving range from a low of 50 for fat-free saltines to a high of 130 for a number of reduced-fat and for one fat-free product. This range is a result of variations in serving size and the number of calories per gram of product. Many products being produced and marketed are fat-free. Although not shown in Table 7, most products are formulated to be free of cholesterol.

The data in Table 7 illustrate the need to read label information carefully and select products based on objective in modifying diet: controlling calories, minimizing fat, reducing calories from fat, etc.

B. No-Cholesterol Products

Many bakery foods are promoted as having "no cholesterol." This has been achieved by replacing animal fats with vegetable fats or oils and by eliminating whole eggs or replacing whole eggs with egg whites or an egg substitute. This is a rather straightforward and simple technology.

C. Reduced-Calorie Breads

A number of calorie-reduced breads are on the market, and these are also lower in fat. The fat content of normal bread is already quite low at 1–3%, but eliminating even this low level contributes to achieving the calorie reduction needed for reduced-calorie claims. The technology for producing reduced-calorie breads is relatively simple, although it has become that way only after some 15 years of experience! Nevertheless, it still requires manufacturing skills to produce quality products with minimum scrap on high speed, automated production equipment in the modern bakery. Reduced-calorie breads are made by replacing 25 to 30 percent of the flour with a high fiber ingredient, eliminating the fat, adding emulsifier and vital wheat gluten, and baking to a higher moisture content. In some cases, the size of the slice is also reduced slightly and adjustments are made in minor ingredients to optimize quality and to facilitate processing.

D. Far-Free Cookies and Crackers

A number of fat-free cookies and crackers are on the market. A fat-free saltine has about 17% fewer calories than its normal, fat-containing counterpart. It is produced by simply removing fat; the finished product has a slightly harder texture as would be expected in a fat-free cracker.

Fat-free cookies are generally intermediate-moisture, chewy types of products in contrast to the low-moisture, crisp cookies that constitute the largest share of the market. Fat (including butter, if used), eggs, and other fat-containing ingredients are removed and replaced with a starch-based fat replacer (maltodextrin), gums (guar and xanthan), and emulsifiers (lecithin and polysorbate 60).

E. Cake Products

A variety of calorie- and fat-modified cake and snack cake products are being produced. These range from calorie-controlled servings to reduced-calorie (one-third fewer calories) versions of "normal" products. In between these two extremes are less-fat and no-fat products. In some cases, products are baked to a slightly higher moisture content in order to reduce calories. Maltodextrins, gums, and emulsifiers are used to replace the functionality of fat and simulate the organoleptic properties of fat-containing products. The quality of these products varies, and, in some cases, there appears to have been a trade-off between quality and label claims. Some of the products, however, are quite good even with no fat and a high reduction in calories.

F. Other Bakery Foods

Increased final product moisture, smaller serving size, maltodextrin, gums, and emulsifiers are all used in varying combinations to achieve the properties needed to meet marketing objectives and labeling claims. Quality characteristics also vary. Some muffins have a tendency to stick to baking surfaces because of a loss of lubricity when fat is removed. Danish has less richness and a firmer texture due to loss of flakiness by eliminating dough laminations and the shortening than is normally incorporated between the layers of dough. Nevertheless, quality is generally acceptable or could be with more experience with the technology available to produce calorie- or fat-modified versions of these types of bakery products.

G. Applying the Technology

The technology for producing a variety of bakery foods with reduced, low, or no fat or cholesterol and fewer calories appears to be available. The application of this technology in producing good-quality, consumer-acceptable products appears to vary within the industry. This variation may well be due to the "newness" of the technology and will probably be minimized as bakers become more experienced in using the new tools available to them for formulating nutritionally modified bakery foods.

1. Eliminating Cholesterol

The reduction or elimination of cholesterol is relatively simple in many bakery foods since it requires the replacement of animal fat with vegetable products and the reduction or elimination of whole eggs. Both of these changes can usually be made without serious adverse effects on processing or quality characteristics of the finished product.

2. Reducing or Eliminating Fat

The reduction or elimination of fat is somewhat more difficult. However, a number of rather traditional ingredients have been shown to have fat-sparing or fatlike properties. The replacement of the sensory properties of fat is more difficult in low-moisture bakery foods such as cookies and may explain why few, if any, fat-modified, low-moisture cookies are being marketed.

3. Reducing Calories

The production of reduced-calorie versions of many bakery foods is quite difficult, unless the "normal" product is very rich and high in fat and calories, in which case a large part of the caloric reduction needed can be obtained by eliminating fat and the remainder can be obtained by other means. Hopefully, the development of suitable low-calorie bulking agents and calorie-free fat substitutes will some day make it possible to produce and market a broad line of high-quality reduced-calorie bakery products.

H. Consumer Prices

A very limited survey of pricing of regular and nutritionally modified bakery foods at the retail level was conducted in order to determing the extent to which a difference exists in the consumer prices for these products. The results are summarized in Table 8.

Table 8 Differential in Retail Cost per Ounce for Nutritionally Modified Bakery Products Compared to Similar Regular Products

Product	Differential for modified product (%)
"Pound" cake A	+7
"Pound" cake B	+20
Layer cake A	+64
Layer cake B	+72
Coffee cake A	+17
Coffee cake B	-21
Blueberry muffins	+32
Cookies	-9
White bread A	+72
White bread B	+34
White bread C	+47

Source: Based on limited retail market survey.

It was not always possible to find the exact normal counterpart of a nutritionally modified product; in these cases, a similar product, with perhaps a different characterizing ingredient, was chosen for comparison. The data in Table 8 should be viewed as approximate, but the conclusion that nutritionally modified bakery foods are more expensive than regular products appears to be justified with a few exceptions. The increase in cost per ounce of product may be as much as 75% based on this limited survey. The amount of increase varies from one manufacturer to another. It should be noted, however, that in some cases the cost of a nutritionally modified product is actually lower than the cost of a similar unmodified counterpart.

With the exception of reduced-calorie breads, fat-, cholesterol-, and calorie-modified bakery foods are relatively new on the marketplace. Current pricing may not necessarily be indicative of future pricing. Manufacturing experience and eventual sales volumes may dictate higher or lower prices for these products.

VII. REGULATORY CONSIDERATIONS

A number of regulatory issues, although they apply to all nutritionally modified foods, have special applications to bakery foods.

A. Nutritional Equivalence

According to federal regulations, reduced-calorie foods must contain one-third fewer calories than an equivalent serving of its normal counterpart and must be nutritionally equivalent except for calories. In some bakery foods nutritional equivalence will require the addition of vitamins and/or minerals to compensate for those lost in reformulation. For example, if a baker normally purchases enriched flour and then replaces 25–30% of it in producing high-fiber, reduced-calorie bread, additional quantities of enrichment nutrients must be added in order to achieve nutritional equivalency in the modified bread. A significant increase in moisture content of the finished product could also require the addition of nutrients so as to maintain nutritional equivalency.

B. Descriptors

Special consideration must be given to the use of descriptors such as "low," "free," and "light" or "lite." These terms will be defined by regulation for a number of nutrients and components of foods. What has been acceptable prior to formal definition may not be acceptable when new regulations are promulgated and become effective.

C. Analytical Methodology

Current regulations for labeling the fat content of a food product describe the analytical method to be used to determine fat content. FDA acknowledges [6] that this method does not pick up mono- and diglycerides, thus leading to a potential underreporting of fat content. FDA has suggested that if an analytical method underreports the content of a nutrient by 10% or more, another, more suitable method must be used.

These are current issues. Others will surely develop as the baking industry continues its efforts to meet the needs of the health-conscious consumer and Congress and/or FDA set appropriate parameters to prevent false and misleading claims.

REFERENCES

1. N. Raper and R. Marston, *Nutrient Content of the U.S. Food Supply*, Adm. Rep. No. 229-21, Human Nutrition Information Service, United States Department of Agriculture, (August 1988).
2. *Composition of Foods, Agriculture Handbook No. 8*, Agricultural Research Service, United States Department of Agriculture (1975).
3. E. M. Pao, K. H. Fleming, P. M. Guenther, and S. J. Mickle, *Foods Commonly Eaten by Individuals: Amount per Day and per Eating Occasion*, Home Economics Research Report No. 44, Human Nutrition Information Service, United States Department of Agriculture (1982).
4. E. J. Pyler, *Baking Science and Technology*, Vol. 2, Sosland Publishing Co., Kansas City, MO, pp. 443–487 (1988).
5. Yeast-derived beta glucan fiber shows cholesterol-reducing properties, *Food Process. (Dec.)*: 40 (1990).
6. Food labeling; mandatory status of nutrition labeling and nutrient content revision, *Fed. Reg., 55*(139): 29503 (1990).

14
Low-Calorie Foods: General Category

Lee Ann Quesada and Walter L. Clark *Chapman University, Orange, California*

I. INTRODUCTION

This chapter describes the following food categories:

Reduced-calorie margarines and spreads
Mayonnaise and salad dressings
Frozen entrees
Seafood
Salty or savory snacks
Egg substitutes

Margarines and spreads are water-in-oil emulsions. The viscous types of margarines and reduced- or low-calorie spreads differ primarily by the proportions of oil to water and the degree to which the products are hardened (hydrogenated).

The first portion of the mayonnaise and salad dressing section covers viscous, reduced-calorie, and nonfat dressings; the last portion covers pourable dressings. Nonfat dressings now exist that simulate mayonnaise and salad dressings.

Pourable dressing production as published by the U.S. Department of Agriculture (USDA) in 1990 is approximately 1.16 billion pounds per year in contrast to 1.71 billion pounds of mayonnaise per year followed by salad dressing and sandwich spreads at 0.91 billion pounds.

The category of health-oriented frozen entrees includes breakfast foods, single dishes, and dinners. They are formulated for lower calorie control, but also offer decreases in fat, cholesterol, and sodium content. Since these products are marketed as "lite, low calorie, or lower in calories" as compared to regular standard products, nutritional labeling is automatically required. As a whole these lower-calorie products are more expensive than their regular counterparts. The health-oriented entrees are the fastest growing segment of the frozen foods industry.

Seafoods are naturally low in fat and cholesterol. These include saltwater fish, some freshwater fish, and saltwater crustaceans and shellfish. Canned fish includes tuna, salmon, sardines, and herring. The per capita consumption of seafoods is low compared to other protein meat sources, tuna being the highest at 3.9 pounds per person per year.

Surimi is a term commonly used to describe shellfish analogs, crab being the dominant product with 90% of the analog sales. The reason surimi is included as a low-calorie food is that it contains less than one gram of fat per 3-ounce serving.

The category of salty or savory snacks includes, potato, corn, and tortilla chips; extruded snacks; pretzels; popcorn; and rice cakes. Low-calorie chips have one third fewer calories and have only recently come on to the market. Pretzels are inherently a low-fat and low-calorie snack; item sales have increased due to consumer awareness of these latter characteristics. Popcorn without butter or flavored oils is also a low-calorie food and has received the greatest application for home microwave use.

Light snacks in 1990 accounted for less than 3% of the potato and tortilla chip volume, but comprised 26% of the microwavable popcorn volume. Light snacks consumption was 145 million pounds in 1990.

Six egg substitute products are compared with whole egg and egg whites in the last section.

The number of low-calorie foods in this category is growing rapidly, and they are constantly undergoing change. This is a dynamic field. Consequently, it is impossible to be comprehensive or completely up to date. The examples cited do not exhaust the entire list of foods, rather they are representative of what is now available.

An effort has been made to compare costs of the regular versions and the low-calorie counterparts. Here, too, the marketing situation is in flux.

More time will be required to establish a stable pattern. Hence the comments on cost are, at most, tentative but important because the present cost structure may reflect long-term trends.

II. REDUCED-CALORIE MARGARINES AND SPREADS

A. Description

Margarine and spreads are made by emulsifying oil and water to form water-in-oil emulsions. In the United States, all of the major branded margarines and spreads are sold as all-vegetable oil products. However, lard and marine oils are available in some countries as relatively cheap fatty raw materials [1].

The various types of margarines and reduced- or low-calorie spreads differ primarily by the proportions of oil to water and the degree to which the products are hardened. To be labeled margarine in the United States, the product must have 80% fat by weight. Margarine, traditionally in stick form, is used for baking and cooking. It is hardened or hydrogenated more than margarine in tubs or squeeze bottles. Whipped and liquid margarines must contain 80% fat; however, whipped margarine has fewer calories per serving because the product is aerated. Liquid margarine has the same number of calories as solid margarine, but it has an increased amount of liquid vegetable oil to replace the hydrogenated oil on a weight-to-weight basis. All, however, contain 80% fat [2].

Lower-calorie, margarine-type products contain less than 80% fat by weight, and some may be as low as 20%. These include products called "light, diet, and reduced-calorie" margarines and spreads.

All products essentially contain the same ingredients. These include oils, salt, and vegetable-derived mono- and diglycerides and lecithin. These latter components act as emulsifiers and stabilizers. Sodium benzoate and potassium sorbate are used as preservatives with citric acid and calcium disodium EDTA added as antioxidants. Beta carotene and vitamin A palmitate are used to color margarine and to provide vitamin A. Milk products such as whey and flavorants such as diacetyl are added to give dairy notes. Lower fat products may contain gelatin to compensate for reduced oil content [2].

B. Typical Examples

Examples of reduced-calorie margarines or spreads are shown in Table 1. None of them meet the strict definition of low calorie (see Sec. II.C). However, Heart Beat Spread has half the calories of the other spreads. All of these examples claim zero milligrams of cholesterol per serving.

Table 1 Examples of Reduced-Calorie
Margarines/Spreads[a]

Brand	kcal	Fat (g)
Mazola Margarine[b]	**100**	**11**
Fleishmann's Light Spread[c]	80	8
Blue Bonnet Spread[c]	60	7
Mazola Light Spread[b]	50	6
Heart Beat Spread[d]	25	3

[a]Nutrition information provided on label based on
1 tbsp (14 g) serving. Regular counterpart is in bold
letters.
[b]CPC International, Inc., Englewood Cliffs, NJ
07632.
[c]Nabisco Brands, Inc., East Hanover, NJ 07936.
[d]GFA Brands Inc., Cresskill, NJ 07626.

C. Regulatory Status

In the United States, margarine is governed by the Code of Federal Regulations 1991 [3]. This sets forth a Standard of Identity for margarine specifying the minimum fat level at 80% and listing approved ingredients and their respective usage levels. Further, requirements also exist for the low- and reduced-calorie versions. For a food to be labeled as "low-calorie," it must provide 40 kcal/serving and 0.4 kcal/g as consumed. The requirements for a food to be labeled "reduced calorie" or "reduced in calories" requires one third fewer calories than in the regular or nonreduced counterpart [4]. There are no "low-calorie" margarines; however, several reduced-calorie margarines are available (see also Chapter 7).

D. Taste and Acceptability Compared to Common Counterpart

Taste panelists rated reduced-fat spreads as being "watery" or deficient in other areas compared to regular margarine [5]. In addition, these products cannot be used in baking applications as a direct substitute for margarine, as is noted on the packaging, since the fat level is reduced. Typically, low-fat spread emulsions are not stable at room temperature and may become watery. Further, due to the high water content they are not suitable for frying.

On the other hand, these spreads do provide an opportunity for calorie reduction and, as evidenced by continued sales, meet with consumer appeal.

Table 2 Percent Cost Differential of Reduced-
Calorie Margarine vs. Regular Margarine in the
Retail Market

Product	Store[a]		
	A	B	C
Fleischmann's 4 oz sticks (light spread/margarine)	0	0	0
Fleischmann's 2 8–oz tubs (extra light spread/ margarine)	0	NA	0
Imperial 2 8–oz tubs (diet, reduced-calorie/ margarine)	− 20	− 16	− 21
Blue Bonnet 16 oz tub/ 4 oz sticks (spread/margarine)	+ 16	+ 24	− 14

[a]Per ounce. Store A—Lucky; B—Stater Bros; C—Vons. Based on a
one-time survey (July 1991).
[b]NA = Not available at markets surveyed.

E. Sales

The U.S. retail sales of margarine and margarine-type spreads totaled over
1.9 billion pounds during 1988, a 5.2% increase over the previous year [2].
The annual per capita consumption of margarine was 10.1 pounds in 1989
[6]. Of the total retail margarine products manufactured in 1990, 41% were
diet or reduced-calorie versions with less than 52% fat [7].

F. Cost

As shown in Table 2, there is no uniform relationship in cost between regular
and reduced-calorie margarine.

III. MAYONNAISE AND SALAD DRESSINGS

A. Mayonnaise

1. Description

Mayonnaise is an emulsified semi-solid, viscous food prepared from edible
vegetable oil(s), acetic and citric acid, and egg yolk. Optional ingredients
permitted include salt, nutritive carbohydrate sweeteners, spices or spice oils,

monosodium glutamate, various harmless flavoring ingredients from natural sources, heavy metal sequestrants, and fatty crystal inhibitors [8].

Commercial mayonnaise generally contains 77–82% oil, usually unhydrogenated soybean oil because of its low cost. Other oils include winterized cottonseed, hydrogenated and winterized soybean, sunflower, safflower, corn, olive, and, most recently, canola (rapeseed with only a minor amount of erucic acid) oil. An oil that solidifies at refrigerator temperature is undesirable as the mayonnaise emulsion breaks as soon as the oil crystallizes; this emulsion also breaks upon freezing [9].

In mayonnaise, there is more oil than aqueous phase. Nevertheless, it is an oil-in-water emulsion where droplets of oil are dispersed in a continuous aqueous phase. Such an emulsion has a characteristic viscosity, mouthfeel, and taste due to its rigidity, which depends partly on the size of the oil droplets and how tightly they are packed. The more oil that is dispersed in the emulsion, the stiffer it will be.

Table 3 Examples of Viscous, Reduced-Calorie, and Nonfat Dressings[a]

Brand	kcal	Fat (g)	Calories from fat (%)	Cost differential over regular (%)
Hellmann's Real Mayonnaise[b]	**100**	**11**	**99**	
Miracle Whip Salad Dressing[c]	**70**	**7**	**90**	
Hellmann's Light Mayonnaise[b]	50	5	91	−8 to +4
Miracle Whip Light Salad Dressing[c]	45	4	80	−30 to −38
Heartbeat Reduced-Calorie Mayonnaise[d]	40	4	85	
Miracle Whip Free Nonfat Dressing[c]	20	0	0	+12 to +25
Kraft Free Nonfat Mayonnaise Dressing[c]	12	0	0	+5 to +39

[a]Nutrition information provided on label based on 1 tbsp (14–16 g) serving. Survey taken July 1991. The regular counterpart is shown in bold letters.
[b]CPC International Inc., Englewood Cliffs, NJ 07632.
[c]Kraft General Foods, Glenview, IL 60025.
[d]GFA Brands Inc., Cresskill, NJ 07626.

2. Typical Examples

Table 3 shows viscous mayonnaise and salad dressings in bold letters as references for comparative purposes to reduced-calorie and nonfat products. Reduced-calorie products usually contain half the calories per serving of regular products, though the percent calories from fat will range from 79 to 91 in contrast to 90–99% calories from fat for standard mayonnaise and salad dressing. The total fat content, however, is generally less than half that of regular mayonnaise (i.e., 4–6 grams per serving versus 11–12 grams for mayonnaise). The standard products contain greater amounts of poly-, mono-, and saturated fats than the reduced-calorie versions, as would be expected. Some reduced-calorie mayonnaise products (e.g., canola oil and corn oil Heartbeat mayonnaise products) claim on their labels to be free of saturated fat.

Cost range at the supermarket level was observed for several of the products in Table 3. Hellmann's Light Reduced-Calorie Mayonnaise showed a slight positive as well as a negative percentage change from their standard products, depending upon the jar size and the store. Two nonfat mayonnaise and salad dressings produced by Kraft General Foods are shown. The cost/serving compared to the regular counterpart increased from +5% to +39% for the first product and from +12% to 25% for the second product, respectively. Miracle Whip Light Reduced-Calorie Salad Dressing was 28–30% less costly than its counterpart Miracle Whip Salad Dressing.

3. Regulatory Status

This covers mayonnaise and salad dressing. Mayonnaise is defined by the Code of Federal Regulations 1991 [8] as a product in which the oil content is not less than 65% by weight. This standard specifies that the product contain edible vegetable oil, acetic or citric acid (2.5%), and egg yolk.

Standard salad dressing, also an emulsified semi-solid, is described in similar terms to those used for mayonnaise. This type of salad dressing is known as spoonable or viscous to distinguish it from pourable dressings, described later. Salad dressing under the standards resembles mayonnaise in that it is an emulsion of oil in vinegar using egg as an emulsifier. It differs from mayonnaise in that it also contains starch paste as a thickener [8]. There is no limitation on the level of total acid in vinegar or citrus juices. Salad dressing may also contain stabilizers and thickeners such as edible gums at not more than 0.7% by weight of the product. Gums are not permitted in mayonnaise. Salad dressing standards require not less than 30% vegetable oil nor less than 4% liquid egg yolk by weight. Salad dressings can be made with less than 30% oil and less than 4% egg yolk.

Polysorbate 60 is permitted at 0.3% maximum in eggless salad dressing [10]. Such dressings are nonstandard and are usually formulated as dietetic foods, either as "eggless" or "low-calorie" types. It was previously mentioned that for a food to be labeled as "low calorie," it must provide 40 kcal/serving and 0.4 kcal/g as consumed [4]. Likewise, for a food to be labeled "reduced calorie" or "reduced in calories," it must have one third fewer calories than the regular product.

Thus, strictly speaking, only the Heartbeat products along with Kraft General Foods nonfat dressings are "low-calorie" products. The other examples in Table 3 are "reduced-calorie" products.

Rules regulating the descriptions for "fat-free" products are being formulated by the FDA [11]. For example, a tablespoon of Kraft Free salad dressing qualifies as "fat-free" under current guidelines, but a larger serving does not. Consumers are surprised to see soybean oil listed in the ingredient statement of a "fat-free" product like Kraft Free.

5. Sales

There is still a difference of opinion as to whether fat-free products will replace existing lines or simply enhance them. According to Arbitron/SAMI figures [12], Kraft General Foods Kraft Free line of nonfat dressings, introduced in the spring of 1990, has resulted in sales of $33.9 million. This is 12.7% of the $268.2 million reduced-calorie segment for the year ended August 10, 1990. Clorox Company's Take Heart low-fat salad dressing registered $16.5 million in sales in the first 3 months it was on the market for a 6.2% share.

B. Pourable Dressings

1. Description

Pourable salad dressings contain oil, vinegar, spices, and other ingredients. They may be fully emulsified or may readily separate into oil and aqueous layers. They commonly are shaken and mixed well before use. Emulsifiers vary and include numerous gums and egg yolk.

In the United States, French dressing composition is covered by a Standard of Identity [11] that requires a minimum oil content of 35%, although higher levels of oil are common. The separating types of pourables are well mixed but need not be emulsified prior to bottling.

Kraft General Foods classifies these dressings as pourable (50–90 kcal/tbsp), reduced-calorie pourable (16–50 kcal/tbsp), and nonfat pourable (no fat, 4–20 kcal/tbsp) [13].

2. Typical Examples

a. Reduced Calorie. Examples of reduced-calorie, pourable dressings are listed in Table 4. Total fat controls, for the most part, the calories per serving and, hence, is listed along with the calories. When the fat content is 1 gram or less, the kcal/serving are 20. For 20–30 kcal/serving the fat increases from 2 to 3 grams. Likewise, 4 grams of fat yield 40–45 kcal/serving and, similarly, 5 and 6 grams of fat provide 50 and 60 kcal/serving, depending upon the calories derived from other components of the reduce-calorie, pourable dressings. Saturated fat is usually shown as zero and never more than one gram per serving. Polyunsaturated fats are still predominant.

Cost data were obtained from three different supermarket chains in August 1991. The reduced-calorie products providing 14–30 kcal/serving cost from 0–22% more than the regular products.

b. Nonfat. Examples of nonfat, pourable dressings can be found in Table 5. Active companies in this category include Kraft General Foods, Hidden Valley, Herb Magic, and Wish Bone; the latter, in the market since the mid-1970s, has just begun to advertise low-calorie products [14]. The products provide not more than 20 kcal/serving (with several below 10) and no fat whatsoever.

Table 4 Examples of Reduced-Calorie Pourable Dressings[a]

Brand	kcal	Fat (g)	Calories from fat (%)	Cost differential over regular (%)
Cheese Fantastic[b]	**50**	**6**	**100**	
Viva Red Wine,[c] Reduced-Calorie	40	4	90	0
Classic Lite Caeser Calorie-Reduced[d]	30	2	60	+15
Red Wine Vinaigrette[d]	20	1	45	0 to +22
Light Fantastic Cheese Fantastico Reduced-Calorie[b]	14	<1	45	0 to +22

[a]Nutrition information based on 1 tbsp (15 g) serving. Survey taken August 1991. The regular counterpart is shown in bold letters.
[b]Nalley's Fine Foods, Division of Curtice-Burns, Inc., Tacoma, WA 98411.
[c]Seven Seas Foods Inc., Glenview, IL 60025.
[d]Thomas J. Lipton, Inc., Englewood Cliffs, NJ 07632.

Table 5 Examples of Nonfat
Pourable Dressings[a]

Brand	kcal	Cost differential over regular (%)
Regular dressings	**40–90**	
Kraft Free Blue Cheese[b]	20	+ 18 to + 34
Seven Seas Ranch[c]	16	− 5 to − 12
Take Heart Blue Cheese, Reduced-Calorie[d]	12	− 2 to − 16
Wish Bone Lite Italian[e]	6	− 7 to + 44

[a]Nutrition information based on 1 tbsp (15 g) serving. Survey taken August 1991. The regular counterpart is shown in bold letters.
[b]Kraft General Foods, Glenview, IL 60025.
[c]Seven Seas Foods, Glenview, IL 60025.
[d]The Hidden Valley Ranch Co., Oakland, CA 94612.
[e]Thomas J. Lipton, Inc., Englewood Cliffs, NJ 07632.

Kraft General Foods and Lipton call their products "fat-free," while Clorox calls its Take Heart brand "low fat." Actually, Kraft Free and several of the Wish Bone and Take Heart flavors contain a small amount of fat, under 3%, but the FDA nutritional labeling guidelines allow these low levels of fat to be rounded down to zero grams. Take Heart Ranch flavor, with one gram of fat per serving or 9%, does not qualify as fat-free under the guidelines [14].

4. Sales and Cost

The production volume of pourable dressings, as reported by the U.S. Department of Agriculture [15], was 1.16 billion pounds in 1988, of which 45% went to retail and 55% went to food service. The average fat content as percent of calories was 36%. Any pourable dressing in Table 4 with ≤2 grams of fat per serving contains ≤25% of its calories as fat.

The Kraft General Foods products in this category cost 3–34% more than their regular counterpart dressings, having 50–90 kcal /serving. On the other hand, the Seven Seas series of products, now owned by Kraft General Foods, cost 5–12% less than the Seven Seas regular standard dressings. Thus, nonfat pourable dressings can in several instances be more economical for the consumer.

Are consumers willing to pay more for low-fat products? According to scanner checkout data, reduced-calorie liquid salad dressing sold today in food stores average about 10 cents more per pound than regular salad dressings [15]. The data in Table 5 indicate that in several instances, the cost differential over regular is as high as 34–44%.

Whether products containing new fat substitutes will replace existing or available low-fat products in the market place or even perhaps expand the availability of low-fat foods depends on several factors. These include, in order of priority, (1) FDA approval (2) the substitutes' quality and versatility, (3) strength of consumer demand and willingness to pay for reduced-fat products, and (4) marketing strategies. For new fat substitutes to be accepted by manufacturers and consumers and expand the low-fat market, they must be technically superior to existing substitutes and products and offer better taste and acceptability. Unlike today's fat replacements, true fat substitutes must mimic the taste, texture, and functions of fat. They may face real difficulty competing with highly flavored fats, such as milk fat and olive oil [15].

In 1990, *Gorman's New Product News* tracked 10,301 new food products in the marketplace, of which greater than 10% carried low/reduced-fat or reduced-calorie claims. For the 201 salad dressings introduced in 1990, this figure climbed to 24% [16].

The R. E. Staley Manufacturing Company (Decatur, IL) has developed a multifunctional, "total systems" approach for low-fat salad dressings as well as for other low-fat foods. The cornerstone for their low-fat ingredient systems is their line of Sta-Slim starches, which function as the primary fat mimetic [16]. Pfizer, Inc. has developed an improved polydextrose, Litesse, that can be used for the same purposes.

The low-calorie/reduced-fat products are now positioned with the regular, standard products in the stores. Producers and supermarkets have improved the image of the new nontraditional, modified, low-calorie products. These low-calorie/reduced-fat products are recognized not as diet products but as nutritious, lower-calorie, good-tasting counterparts. This has resulted in broader appeal than if they were positioned in the diet section of a supermarket [17].

In 1990, reduced-calorie salad dressings accounted for nearly one-quarter of the low-calorie foods (right behind diet soft drinks at 30%) [15] and led the new product introductions of low-calorie foods; sales should continue to increase, and eventually these may become the predominant category for salad dressings.

IV. FROZEN ENTREES

A. Description

Health-oriented frozen foods include breakfast foods, single dishes, and dinners. These products are formulated to help control intake of calories, fat, sodium, and cholesterol. While some products are promoted only on the basis of calorie reduction, most also offer decreases in content of fat, cholesterol, and sodium.

In the breakfast line, brands with items identified as health-oriented include Healthy Choice, Great Starts, Downyflake, Pillsbury, Aunt Jemima, and Krusteaz. Brands in single dishes and frozen dinners include Weight Watchers, Lean Cuisine, Budget Gourmet Light, Healthy Choice, Right Course, Le Menu Lightstyle, Le Menu Healthy, Ultra Slim Fast, Eating Right, and Tyson.

Since nutritional claims are made, nutritional labeling is required as regulated by the Code of Federal Regulations, Part 101.9 [18]. All products in this category are governed by regulations of the Food and Drug Administration (FDA). Those products containing meat or poultry also fall under USDA regulatory control and inspection.

B. Typical Examples

Tables 6 and 7 give examples of retail brands of frozen food entrees and frozen breakfasts. A regular counterpart is shown, wherever possible, for comparison. Several points are noteworthy. Notice the wide range in food energy per serving among the items listed. More pronounced is the range in fat content from 0% of the calories to 46%. The items presented as health-related generally have less fat and fewer calories per serving than the others. Reduction in caloric content is achieved in two ways: reduction in the portion size and in fat content. The former was the primary practice until recently when more manufacturers become sensitive to the public's interest in eating less fat.

Today, frozen entrees are being marketed as "lite, low-calorie, or lower in calorie" as compared with regular entrees. Achievement of calorie reduction is not always easy for this class of products because companies are limited in their formulation options. Several methods may be used to reduce calorie content. The standard main portion may be replaced with a lower-in-calorie substitute, such as replacing beef with a reduced-fat turkey roll or using lean cuts of meat. Further, the main portion can be replaced with an analog, such as a soy-based meat analog, which is lower in fat and calories. Fats inherent in sauces and gravies can be reduced or eliminated by using fat replacers such as starches or gums.

Depending upon an individual's dietary goal, emphasis can be on the total calories per serving regardless of the fat content or on reducing fat as the primary objective. A compromise may be achieved by considering the frozen dish that approaches both goals. Beef pepper steak (Healthy Choice) is among those foods in Table 6 that approach both goals.

Table 6 Comparison of Light or Health-Oriented
Retail Frozen Entrees

Product	Serving size (oz)	kcal	Fat (g)	Calories from fat (%)
Oriental				
Pepper steak[b]	**10**	**320**	**9**	**25**
Teriyaki chicken breast[c]	11	270	6	19
Beef pepper steak[d]	7.50	200	3	14
Sweet and sour chicken[b]	**10**	**340**	**5**	**13**
Sweet and sour chicken[d]	11.50	280	2	6
Poultry				
Roast turkey breast[e]	**7.88**	**300**	**13**	**39**
Baked chicken breast[e]	**7.38**	**190**	**6**	**28**
Herb roasted chicken[f]	9.25	240	7	26
Sliced turkey[f]	10	210	5	21
Glazed chicken breast[g]	10	240	4	15
Mesquite chicken[h]	12	360	1	3

[a]Nutritional information as given on the label, except percentage of
calories as fat which was calculated. Regular counterpart in bold letters.
[b]The Budget Gourmet, The All American Gourmet Co., Orange, CA
92913.
[c]The Budget Gourmet Light and Healthy.
[d]Healthy Choice, ConAgra Frozen Foods, Omaha, NE 68102.
[e]Stouffer's, Stouffer Foods, Solon, OH 44139.
[f]Le Menu Light Style/Le Menu Healthy Brands, Campbell Soup Company, Camden, NJ 08103.
[g]Eating Right, Kraft General Foods, Glenview, IL 60025.
[h]Ultra Slim Fast, ConAgra Frozen Foods, New York, NY 10150.

Table 7 Comparison of Light or Health-Oriented
Retail Frozen Breakfast Foods[a]

Product	Serving size (oz)	kcal	Fat (g)	Calories from fat (%)
Muffin[b]	4.25	200	3	14
Muffin[c]	**4.10**	**290**	**15**	**46**
Pancakes[d]	5.50	350	16	41
Pancakes[e]	**6.00**	**460**	**22**	**43**
Waffles[f]	1 waffle	80	3	34
Waffles[g]	1	80	0	0
Waffles[h]	**1**	**120**	**5**	**38**

[a]Nutritional information given on the label except percent of calories as fat, which was calculated. Regular counterpart in bold letters.
[b]Cholesterol-free egg, turkey, ham, and cheese. Healthy Choice, Con Agra Frozen Foods, Omaha, NE 68102.
[c]Egg, Canadian-style bacon, and cheese. Swanson, Campbell Soup Company, Camden, NJ 08103.
[d]Whole wheat with lite links. Great Starts, Harvest Grain, Swanson.
[e]With sausage. Great Starts.
[f]Oat bran. Belgian Chef. Chef America. Division of IEI, Chatsworth, CA 91311.
[g]Kellog's Special K, Eggo, Kellogg Co., Battle Creek, MI 49016.
[h]Homestyle. Eggo.

Overall, the health-oriented brands are more expensive than their regular counterparts. Table 8 lists frozen products from each category and their prices compared with regular counterparts.

C. Percentage of Market Share Compared with Regular Counterpart

Health-oriented frozen foods are the fastest-growing segment of that industry and have already reached significant proportions of the business in each category. For the 52-week period ending Sept. 7, 1990, health-oriented products accounted for 29.8% of the frozen single dishes and 20.8% of the basic dinner sales. Health-oriented oriental dishes were the most popular, accounting for 54% of the market share for single dishes and 81% for basic dinners in 1990 [19]. The health-oriented frozen market expanded to the area of children's meals with the introduction of Snoopy's Choice by ConAgra in late 1990 [20].

With respect to the future, it can be noted that ConAgra has taken the concept of the Healthy Choice frozen entree into a shelf-stable line called Healthy Choice Cans & Cups. Further, The Dial Corporation (Phoenix, AZ)

Table 8 Percent Cost Differential of Health-Oriented Frozen Foods vs. Regular Counterpart in Retail Market

Product	Per entree[a]			Per ounce		
	A	B	C	A	B	C
Sweet and sour chicken (Healthy Choice/The Budget Gourmet)	+29	+40	N.A.[b]	+16	+30	N.A.
Turkey (Le Menu Light-style/Swanson)	N.A.	+41	+47	N.A.	+50	+55
Chicken (Tyson/ Stouffer's)	N.A.	N.A.	+13	N.A.	N.A.	+8
Breakfast muffin (Healthy Choice/ Swanson)	+16	N.A.	+16	+12	N.A.	+14
Waffles (Special K/ Homestyle)	+17	+25	+19	+33	+39	+40

[a]Store: A—Lucky; B—Stater Bros; C—Vons. Based on a one-time survey, July 1991.
[b]Product(s) not available at markets surveyed.

launched Light Balance Microwave Meals (<220 calories) and Kraft General Foods lightened up a previous shelf-stable line and reintroduced it as Kraft Microwave Entrees in late 1990 [21].

V. SEAFOODS

A. General

1. Description

With relatively few exceptions, seafoods are naturally low in fat and cholesterol. The principal seafoods are saltwater fish, some freshwater fish, and saltwater crustaceans and shellfish such as shrimp, lobster, crab, and oysters [22]. The canned fish category includes tuna, salmon, sardines, and herring. The varieties of tuna available include white and light tuna packed in spring water or in oil.

2. Typical Examples

Tables 9 and 10 give the calorie and fat content of several of the seafood products mentioned above. As with any inherently low-calorie food, the method of preparation or cooking will alter its caloric density. Hence the products prepared by frying have much more fat than the original raw ma-

Table 9 Comparison of Haddock Using Different
Methods of Preparation[a,b]

Preparation	Serving size (oz)	kcal	Fat (g)	Calories as fat (%)
Raw	3	74	0.60	7
Smoked	3	99	0.80	7
Cooked, dry heat	3	95	0.80	8
Frozen, batter dipped, Van de Kamps[c]	4 2 (pieces)	240	10	38
Breaded, fried	3.5	206	10.60	46
Frozen, breaded, Van de Kamps[c]	5 oz piece	300	20	60
Frozen fillet, "Light & Crispy" Van de Kamps[c]	2 oz piece	180	15	75

[a]From A. D. Bowes and H. N. Church, *Food Values of Portions Commonly Used*, 15th ed., Harper & Row Publishers, New York, 1989. Percent calories as fat calculated from information provided.
[b]From Esha Research, *The Food Processor II Nutrition and Diet Analysis System Software Version 3.0*, Salem, OR 97309, 1990.
[c]Pet Incorporated, St. Louis, MO 63102.

terial or the canned, cooked, or smoked product. For example, breaded and fried haddock has 46% of the calories as fat compared with cooked haddock with 8% of the calories as fat.

Table 11 gives calorie and fat comparisons for the common packs of tuna. The differences between tuna packed in water and oil are dramatic: 13% compared with 78% of calories as fat in the latter. The caloric content of the water-packed product is 50% or less than that of the oil-packed counterpart.

3. Regulatory Status

Currently, seafoods fall under the jurisdiction of the FDA. Several bills are pending before the U.S. Congress to provide for a federally mandated fish inspection program. One bill, favored by the seafood industry, would allow the USDA to regulate seafood. This bill would require Hazard Analysis Critical Control Point monitoring [23].

4. Consumption

Seafood consumption is on the rise. According to sources at the National Fisheries Institute (NFI), seafood consumption reached a record high of 15.9 pounds per capita in 1989. NFI is anticipating that consumption will rise to

Table 10 Comparison of Shellfish Using Different
Methods of Preparation

Preparation of Seafood	Serving size (oz)	kcal	Fat (g)	Calories as fat (%)
Clams				
Raw	3 (4 large or 9 small)	63	0.80	11
Breaded, fried	3	171	9.50	50
Canned	3	126	1.70	12
Cooked by moist heat	3	126	1.70	12
Shrimp				
Raw	3 (12 large)	90	1.50	15
Breaded, fried	3 (11 large)	206	10.40	45
Canned	3	102	1.70	15
Cooked by moist heat	3 (15.5 large)	84	0.90	10
Frozen, breaded, raw	3.5	139	0.70	5
Imitation made from surimi	3	86	1.30	14

Data from A. D. Bowes and H. N. Church, *Food Values of Portions Commonly Used* 15th Edition, Harper & Row Publishers, New York, 1989. Percent calories as fat calculated from information provided. Also Esha Research, *The Food Processor II Nutrition and Diet Analysis System Software Version 3.0*, Salem, OR 97309, 1990.

more than 20 pounds per capita by the year 2000 (A. Wheeler, NFI, personal communication). This number is still far less than the consumption of meat, poultry, and dairy products. In 1989, per capita consumption of meat and poultry was 111.3 and 60.5 pounds, respectively [24].

Americans' favorite seafoods of 1989, in order of amount consumed, are shown in Table 12 [25]. Catfish is the fifth most popular fish, yet most of its production is by aquaculture, which is making an important impact in the seafood industry [23,45]. Aside from harvesting fish in locations where they are usually not found, the raw material is more uniform in size and quality. This allows for mechanization of processing and consistently high quality [26]. In the case of catfish, the product is less expensive than other seafood products.

5. Innovations That Could Improve Appeal to Consumers

According to figures published in 1989, 45% of all supermarkets had fresh fish/seafood departments. Typically, 85% of all fish comes into the store

Table 11 Calorie Comparison of Canned Tuna (2-oz serving)

Type	kcal	Fat (g)	Calories as fat (%)
Solid white in spring water	70	1	13
Solid white in vegetable oil	140	10	64
Solid light in spring water	60	<1	15
Solid light in vegetable oil	150	13	78
Chunk light in spring water	60	<1	15
Chunk light in vegetable oil	150	13	78

Nutritional information provided by Starkist Seafood Company, Heinz Nutrition Products, Inc., Pittsburgh, PA 15230. Percent calories as fat calculated from calorie and fat information.

Table 12 1989 Per Capita Consumption of Seafoods

Species	Pounds
Tuna	3.9
Shrimp	2.3
Cod	1.7
Alaskan pollock	1.4
Catfish	0.7
Clams	0.6
Flounder/Sole	0.6
Salmon	0.5
Scallops	0.3
Crabmeat	0.3

Source: Ref. 26.

precut and portioned (either fresh or frozen); the rest is as whole fish. Yet, less than 5% of store patrons purchase from the fresh fish section [27]. Apparently, despite encouragement from health-care professionals to eat more fish, consumers have not incorporated more seafood in their diets. They may not have sufficient comfort level with seafood preparation, may consider it too expensive, or may feel uneasy about the safety of fresh seafood [27].

Continued efforts by the food industry to develop low-calorie prepared seafood products and seafood entrees could influence further purchases. Also, continued efforts by NFI and the food retailers to educate consumers about the variety of ways of preparing seafood will improve appeal to consumers.

B. Surimi

1. Introduction

Surimi is the term most commonly used to describe shellfish analogs. The surimi process was developed centuries ago by Japanese fisherman as a means of preserving fish. Although the process has evolved further, it is essentially the same today. Surimi is processed from white fish; Alaskan pollock is most commonly used in the United States. The fish is deboned, then washed to remove undesirable flavor and color components, and, finally, minced into a paste that is shaped into blocks and frozen. These frozen blocks are shipped to food processors for the production of seafood analogs such as imitation crab or lobster. Surimi is marketed and sold as an alternative to more costly shellfish and is recommended in recipes as a direct substitute. It is convenient, reasonably priced, and nutritious, with a very low fat content.

Typical ingredients for a seafood analog might be as follows: pollock; water; sorbitol and/or sugar, sodium tripolyphosphate (these act primarily as cryoprotectants, but with the former, also impart a mild sweet flavor); starch and/or egg whites (these function as stabilizers and binders to achieve desired textural qualities). Salt, flavors, and colors are added to give characteristic flavor and appearance to the finished seafood products.

2. Description

While other seafood analogs are available, such as lobster, scallops, and shrimp, imitation crab remains the dominant product, comprising 90% of the analog sales (A. Wheeler, NFI, personal communication).

Surimi seafood is available at the supermarket at the seafood counter, the deli counter, or in the seafood section of the meat department. It can be bought by the supermarket frozen in large quantities, thawed as needed, and

Table 13 Composition of Surimi Products (3-oz Serving)

Nutrient	Imitation crab		Surimi[a]	King crab meat[a]
	Crab Delights[b]	Captain JAC[c]		
Calories (kcal)	81	70	87	82
Protein (g)	9.5	9	10.2	16.5
Carbohydrate (g)	9.9	9	8.7	0
Cholesterol (mg)	13.5	15	17	45
Fat (g)	<1	<1	1.1	1.3

[a]A. D. Bowes and H. N. Church, *Food Values of Portions Commonly Used*, 15th ed., Harper and Row, New York, 1989.
[b]Louis Kemp Seafood Co., Oscar Mayer Foods Corporation, Madison, WI 53707.
[c]SeaFest/JAC Creative Foods, Los Angeles, CA 90023.

repacked in smaller units for consumers to purchase. Also, surimi can be sold in packages labeled with one of several brand names. Usually these are available in the refrigerated seafood section. Surimi can be sold frozen to allow the consumer to thaw and use as desired [27,28].

Although the most common use for surimi is in seafood analogs, it has been used for hot dogs, sausages, and luncheon meats. Further, a number of products made from surimi or minced fish meat, including canned, frozen, and breaded items have been developed, consumer tested, test marketed, and even sold on a commercial basis [29]. Surimi, by itself, has no color, taste, or odor. It is, however, functional and adaptable in terms of texture, shape, and flavor. These characteristics have been the basis for analog production [30,31]. The finished product can be either refrigerated or frozen. Production of surimi seafood has increased nearly 450%, from 67 million pounds in 1987 to over 300 million pounds in 1989 (A. Wheeler, personal communication).

Table 13 gives the fat and calorie profiles of three surimi analogs compared to crabmeat. The fat content is very low. Surimi, therefore, is a good candidate for inclusion in a low-fat and low-calorie diet.

3. Labeling and Regulatory Status

No specific labeling laws for surimi exist. Companies presently selling seafood analogs label them as "Imitation Crab" or "Imitation . . . ," whatever the case may be, in accordance with 21 CFR 101.3 [32]. There is controversy concerning which agency will police this product. Typically, seafood is governed by the National Marine Fisheries Institute of the Department of Commerce, but in direct conjunction with the FDA.

4. *Status of Technology*

There is continued testing and evaluating of other underutilized species for use in the manufacture of surimi [31]. The process of surimi production provides the potential for introducing fish protein products in the form of intermediates for use as ingredients in other foods. From a functional standpoint, in ingredient technology, the future of surimi could be developed further. Based on its superior gelling properties, it could have application in food systems where previously fish protein would never have been considered [33]. Fish protein products can be added to meat and poultry products to improve binding properties, improve nutritional composition, change flavor and color, and reduce costs [34].

VI. SALTY OR SAVORY SNACKS

A. Description

The category of salty or savory snacks includes chips (potato, corn, and tortilla), extruded snacks, pretzels, popcorn, and nuts. It is difficult for an individual to restrain consumption of snack foods, once started. Seldom can we just eat one, a few, or a handful, but rather one bite leads to another. The snack food market in the United States continues to grow, with 1990 dollar sales at $12.67 billion and pound volume at 4.72 billion, an increase over 1989 of 6.2% and 3.5%, respectively [35].

Low-calorie options in the chip category became available for potato and tortilla chips with the 1990 roll-out of Ruffles Light and Doritos Light by Frito-Lay. These products offer a one-third reduction of calories compared to their regular counterpart. Cheetos Light cheese puffs were a part of this roll-out as well [35]. Thompson Kitchens (Springfield, IL) introduced corn chips made without oil, a first in the industry [36].

Pretzels are unique to this group of snacks since pretzels are baked, eliminating the oil used for the processing of the other items. This makes pretzels an inherently low-fat and low-calorie snack.

Popcorn is available in a variety of forms. It can be purchased as kernels to be popped by frying or in a hot-air popper. Prepopped popcorn is available with cheese or savory seasoning added or unflavored with oil and salt added. Light microwave popcorn is usually available as regular or butter flavored. Brands available in this category include Orville Redenbacher, Jolly Time, and Act II. By itself, popcorn is a very low-calorie food. The addition of butter, margarines or spreads, and oil contributes calories to this otherwise low-calorie snack.

314

Quesada and Clark

The oil content of nuts may represent as much as 50–70% of the total weight, making them inherently high in calories [37]. In order to lower the calorie content, these snacks are processed by dry-roasting methods. However, nuts still remain high in caloric density, even when dry-roasted.

In addition to salty snacks, rice cakes can be considered. Rice cakes can be made without added fat.

Labeling for any food claiming to be reduced or low calorie falls in the jurisdiction of the FDA Code Of Federal Regulations Section 21 Part 105.66. This states that for a food to be labeled as "light" it must provide at least a one-third reduction in calories over its regular counterpart [4].

B. Typical Examples/Range of Composition

Tables 14 through 16 show examples of "light" or reduced-calorie snacks and comparisons to their regular counterparts for calorie and fat content.

Table 14 Comparison of Low-Calorie Chips/Cheese/Pretzel Snacks[a]

Product/Brand	Serving size (oz)	kcal	Fat (g)	Calories as fat (%)
Ruffles Light Potato Chips[b]	0.9 (18 chips)	120	6	45
Ruffles Potato Chips[b]	**1 (18 chips)**	**150**	**10**	**60**
Pringles Light Potato Crisps[c]	0.9 (14 crisps)	130	6	42
Pringles Original Potato Crisps[c]	**1 (14 crisps)**	**160**	**11**	**62**
Doritos Light Tortilla Chips[b]	1 (16 chips)	130	4	28
Doritos Tortilla Chips[b]	**1 (16 chips)**	**140**	**7**	**45**
Cheetos Light Cheese Flavored Snacks[b]	0.9 (34 snacks)	120	6	45
Cheetos Cheese-Flavored Snacks[b]	**1**	**150**	**9**	**54**
Rold Gold[b] Thin Twists	1	110	1	8

[a]Nutritional information provided on label. Regular counterpart in bold.
[b]Frito-Lay, Inc., Dallas, TX 75235–5224.
[c]Procter & Gamble Co., Cincinnati, OH 45202.

Table 15 Comparison of Low-Calorie Popcorn Snacks[a]

Product	Serving size (cup)	kcal	Fat (g)	Calories as fat (%)
Popcorn kernels				
Air-popped[b]	3	40	< 1	< 23
Popped in pan with oil[c]	3	90	6	60
Microwave popcorn				
Orville Reden-bacher's Gourmet	3	80	5	56
Orville Reden-bacher's Gour-met light	3	50	1	18
Pop Secret[d]	3	100	8	72
Pop Secret, light[d]	3	70	3	39

[a]Nutritional information provided on label. Regular counterpart in bold letters.
[b]Orville Redenbacher's Gourmet Original, popping corn plain, Hunt-Wesson Inc., Fullerton, CA 93633.
[c]Orville Redenbacher's Gourmet Original, popping corn with oil.
[d]General Mills, Inc., Minneapolis, MN 55440.

Table 16 Comparison of Low-Calorie Rice/Popcorn Cakes[a]

Product/Brand	Serving size (cake)	kcal	Fat (g)	Calories as fat (%)
Chico San Popcorn Cake (lightly salted)[b]	1	40	0	0
Pritikin Rice Cakes (plain)[c]	1	35	0	0
Quaker Popped Corn Cakes (lightly salted white cheddar)[d]	1	40	0	0

[a]Nutritional information provided on label.
[b]Chico San, Pittsburgh, PA 15212.
[c]Pritikin Systems, Inc., Chicago, IL 60644-9003.
[d]The Quaker Oats Co., Chicago, IL 60644-9003.

Notice the wide range in fat content of the snacks listed as low-calorie or light. Only two among the chips listed have fewer than 40% of calories as fat. More lower-fat examples are found among the popcorn and pretzel products. The rice and popcorn cakes are truly low-fat foods. Since light snacks are relatively new on the market, a comparative cost survey is not possible at this time.

C. Production

Chips, as an entire category, derive their calorie content from the oil used in processing. There are several ways to lower calories in potato chip production. Selection of potato varieties that are high in solids is very important. Since moisture is driven off during the frying operation, a potato chip with high solids will have a lower moisture level requiring less frying time. For any frying operation, reducing the frying time results in less oil absorption and a product with fewer calories. Further, to reduce moisture level and subsequent frying time, the potato slices can be dried or partially dried before frying (W. Gould, Snack Food Association, personal communication).

In order to control oil absorption in the frying operation itself, the temperature of the oil is critical. Chips must be fried at the highest temperature possible to reduce cooking time and thereby reduce the amount of oil absorbed. In addition, the greater the surface area of the chip, the more oil will be absorbed. Consequently, thicker slices will have lower oil content.

After the frying operation the slices can be put through a superheated tunnel to force oil out of the chips. Supercritical carbon dioxide extraction also may be employed to remove excess oil after frying. The resultant chips have 75% less fat and 40% fewer calories than conventional chips yet retain the same flavor [38]. Tortilla chips and cheese puffs are baked rather than fried to reduce fat content [39]. Some or all of the above methods are currently employed by chip manufacturers to produce the "light" chips (W. Gould, Snack Food Association, personal communication).

Microwave popcorn achieves calorie reduction by decreasing the oil content used in each individual bag. Unflavored prepopped popcorn controls calories by the same means; the amount of oil used in popping is set at the minimum level is required for flavor and processing. The same principal applies at home. Popping in a hot-air popper and adding a reduced calorie spread in a controlled amount will provide fewer caloriess than popping in a pan with butter or oil.

D. Percentage of Market Share Compared with Common Counterparts

In 1990, light snacks comprised less than 3% of the total potato and tortilla chip volume, but 26.1% of microwavable popcorn volume. This represents an 800% increase in sales of low-oil microwave popcorn over 1989. Some ready-to-eat or prepopped popcorn products and Cheetos Light extruded snacks also contribute to light snack sales. Overall, 145 million pounds of light snacks were consumed in 1990 [35].

Pretzel sales increased dramatically in 1989 by 12.8%, and again in 1990 by 5.7%. This represents a significant turnaround for this category after a 2.8% decrease of sales in 1988 [35]. This can be attributed to increased consumer concern for fat and calorie consumption.

E. Status of Technology

The control of calories for all chip snacks covered in this section is contingent upon their oil content, which in turn depends upon absorption during processing. Hence, future developments in the area of fat substitutes have application to the further evolution of low-fat snacks. The Procter & Gamble Company has a Food Additive Petition under review by FDA for use of olestra, their zero-calorie fat replacement, in savory snacks. This includes snacks made from sliced vegetables, such as potatoes, and mixtures consisting predominately of dried potatoes or corn meal, including flavored and unflavored extruded snacks. These fat-free snacks would be prepared by frying in 100% olestra (C. M. Bergholz, Procter and Gamble, personal communication).

VII. EGG SUBSTITUTES

Egg substitutes make it possible to enjoy some of the taste of eggs without the cholesterol. Designed primarily for dietary control of cholesterol consumption, some of them are also low-fat foods compared to the eggs themselves. Hence, they are included in this chapter. Table 17 gives the composition of some of the available products showing how they compare to eggs.

VIII. COMMENTS AND NOTES

Prepared soups should be mentioned. They are advantageous in two ways: they provide for portion control and are available in low-calorie versions. Canned soups vary widely in caloric density, ranging from 0.12 to 0.88 kcal/g [40]. Their fat contents range from 22 to 50% of total calories. Soups prepared with milk are higher in caloric density than those prepared with water, such as bouillon or vegetable soups. Soups prepared from dry mixes usually contain less fat (10–20% of calories from fat).

It is reasonably accurate to conclude that many food manufacturers are expending much effort in satisfying America's pursuit of health and fitness

Table 17 Egg Substitutes

Brand	Calories from fat (%)	kcal	Cholesterol (mg)	Sodium (mg)	Form
Egg (one whole)	64%	79	204	69	Fresh
Scramblers[a] (Morning Star Farms)	45%	60	0	130	Frozen
Egg Beaters[a] with Cheese (Fleischmann's)	42%	65	2.5	210	Frozen
Second Nature[a] Refrigerated (Avoset Food Corp.)	30%	60	0	90	
Healthy Choice[a] (ConAgra)	<27%	30	0	90	Frozen
Egg white (two)	0	32	0	100	Fresh
Egg Beaters[a] (Fleischmann's)	0	25	0	80	Frozen
Egg Beaters[a] with Vegetables (Fleischmann's)	0	27	0	97	Frozen

[a]1/4 cup = 1 egg.
Source: *Cooking Light* Magazine. Copyright July/August 1991. Reprinted with permission.

with a wide assortment of lower-calorie food products as reported in this chapter and elsewhere in the book. The volume of low-cholesterol and low-fat foods is estimated by a New York market research firm (FIND/SVP) to climb from $25 billion at the end of 1990 to $33 billion at the end of 1993 [41]. The Calorie Control Council has reported that two out of three adult Americans consume "light" products an average of nearly four times per week [41].

The approach by the major food brand companies to expand their respective businesses rests not only on their respective reputations but also on their overall promise to the consumer. Friedman [41] refers to this concept as "the cross-category label," meaning that the same brand name appears on a variety of products (Kraft Free, Heinz Weight Watchers, ConAgra Healthy Choice, Ultra Slim-Fast, etc.). In most cases, the cross-category label promises nutritional benefit for the consumer.

Heinz Weight Watchers was the first major cross-category label to enjoy sales success. Using its lower-calorie and diet reputation concept, some 60 dry grocery products have been grouped into a single store-within-a-store section. This company has recently introduced the "Grand Collection," which includes a line of fat-free frozen deserts, ultra-pasteurized nonfat milk, an extensive breakfast foods line, and a line of 97–98% of fat-free luncheon meats [41].

ConAgra's Healthy Choice has created the most marketplace excitement in the last 2 years with its cross-category label, which promises low fat/low cholesterol, with secondary emphasis on sodium and calorie reduction. Healthy Choice, beginning with a very successful line of frozen dinners and entrees ($200 million annual sales), is running across new categories as fast as they can develop co-packers. This brand now has a frozen egg substitute and shelf-stable versions of Healthy Choice frozen dinners, entrees, breakfast items, and frozen dairy desserts [41].

Thompson Medical's Ultra Slim-Fast brand is the latest newcomer to cross-category labeling. Besides its shake drinks, Slim-Fast has introduced snack bars in several flavors, along with cheese curls and popcorn. In addition, they market hot cocoa mix, frozen desserts, shelf-stable puddings, and shelf-stable entrees. Their frozen line of Slim-Fast entrees is produced by ConAgra.

The expansion of the cross-category label strategy must be pursued with care. Friedman [41] concludes that Sara Lee and Pepperidge Farm Ice Cream are among a number of cross-category failures because they lacked the consumer benefit that characterizes the "new healthy choice" successful products in the market.

REFERENCES

1. R. E. Morse and W. L. Clark, The potential for modification in fats and oils, *The Role of Food Product Development in Implementing Dietary Guidelines* (G. E. Livingston, R. J. Moshey, and C. M. Chang, eds.), Food and Nutrition Press, Inc., Westport, CT, p. 106 (1982).
2. B. F. Haumann, New ideas for margarine, *INFORM.*, *1*: 174 (1990).
3. CFR, Margarine, *Code of Federal Regulations*, Title 21, Sect. 166.110, U.S. Government Printing Office, Washington, DC (1991).
4. CFR, Label statements, *Code of Federal Regulations*, Title 21, Sect. 105.66. Relating to usefulness in reducing or maintaining caloric intake or body weight, U.S. Government Printing Office, Washington, DC (1991).
5. New generation of foods with reduced fat, *Food Eng.*, *2*: 23 (1990).
6. United States Department of Agriculture, Per capita consumption of major food commodities (Table 41), *Agricultural Outlook, AO-168(10)*: 62 (1990).
7. National Association of Margarine Manufacturers, *Margarine Statistical Report*, Margarine production, January–December 1990, Washington, DC (March 1991).
8. CFR, Mayonnaise. *Code of Federal Regulations*, Title 21, Sect. 169.140, U.S. Government Printing Office, Washington, DC (1991).

9. T. J. Weiss, Mayonnaise and salad dressing, *Food Oils and Their Uses*, 2nd ed., AVI Publishing Company, Inc., Westport, CT, p. 211 (1983).
10. CFR, Salad Dressings. *Code of Federal Regulations*, Title 21, Sect. 169.150, U.S. Government Printing Office, Washington, DC (1991).
11. CFR, French dressing, *Code of Federal Regulations*, Title 21, Sect. 169.115, U.S. Government Printing Office, Washington, DC (1991).
12. J. Liesse Fat-free: Fad or food of the future? *Advertising Age* (9): 6 (1990).
13. Nutrition and Health Information, Kraft General Foods, Inc., Technology Center, 801 Waukegan Road, Glenview, IL 60025.
14. Low-fat dressings pour it on, *Grocery Supermarket News* (June 17, 1991).
15. R. M. Morrison, The market for fat substitutes, *National Food Review*, U.S. Department of Agriculture, Economic Research Service, pp. 24–30 (April-June 1990).
16. Low-fat salad dressings demand a "total systems" solutions, *Prep. Foods, 160* (2): 73 (1991).
17. F. T. Orthoefer, Update: Reduced-fat margarines and dressings. *J. Am. Oil Chem. 65*(4): 574 (1988).
18. CFR, Nutrition labeling of food. *Code of Federal Regulations*, Title 21, Sect. 101.9, U.S. Government Printing Office, Washington, DC (1991).
19. Trend holds momentum as health-oriented prepareds top $1.5 billion, *Frozen Food Age., 39(11)*: 14 (1990).
20. A. P. Wilkes, Frozen and shelf stable meals, *Food Eng., 63*(1): 69 (1991).
21. S. Davis, Healthy fare leads dinner parade, *Prep. Foods New Prod. Annu.:* 103 (1991).
22. N. N. Potter, Seafoods, *Food Science* (N. N. Potter, ed.), The AVI Publishing Company, Inc., Westport, CT, p. 424 (1986).
23. S. Montero, Seafood consumer expenditure study, *Super. Bus., 45*(9): 131 (1990).
24. United States Department of Agriculture, Per capita consumption of major food commodities (Table 41), *Agricultural Outlook, AO–168*(10): 62 (1990).
25. Anonymous, American's favorite seafoods of 1989 announced, *Frozen Food Digest., 6*: 58 (1990).
26. F. W. Wheaton and T. B. Lawson, Waste production and management, *Processing Aquatic Food Products.*, John Wiley & Sons, Inc., New York, p. 349 (1985).
27. Fresh fish and seafood 1989 department operations review, *Super. Bus., 44*(11): 31 (1989).
28. Surimi Seafood Education Center, National Fisheries Institute, The many styles of surimi seafood, Release #90-37.
29. J. Vondruska, Market trends and outlook for surimi-based foods, *Engineered Seafood Including Surimi* (R. E. Martin and R. L. Collette, eds.), Noyes Data Corporation, Park Ridge, NJ, p. 321 (1990).
30. C. M. Lee, Surimi process technology, *Food Technol., 38*(11): 69 (1984).
31. C. M. Lee, Surimi manufacturing and fabrication of surimi-based products, *Food Technol., 40*(3): 115 (1986).
32. CFR, Identity labeling of food in packaged form, *Code of Federal Regulations*, Title 21, Sect. 101.3 U.S. Government Printing Office, Washington, DC (1991).

33. T. C. Lanier, Functional properties of surimi, *Food Technol.*, *40*(3): 107 (1986).

34. W. H. Doyle and J. R. Brooker, Megatrends in seafood marketing, *Engineered Seafood Including Surimi* (R. E. Martin and R. L. Collette, eds.), Noyes Data Corporation, Park Ridge, NJ, p. 402 (1990).

35. A. Rickard and B. Levy, *1991 Snack Food Association State-of-the-Industry Report*, Snack Food Association, Alexandria, VA 22314.

36. D. Crawford, Snacks span the spectrum of tastes, *Prep. Foods New Prod. Annu.*: 103 (1991).

37. J. I. Duffy, Nuts and legumes, *Snack Food Technology Recent Developments* (J. I. Duffy, ed.), Noyes Data Corporation, Park Ridge, NJ, p. 121 (1981).

38. Anonymous, SCE produces low-fat potato chips, *Food Eng.* (7): 82 (1990).

39. P. M. Dillon, Let the chips fall where they may, *Food Eng.* (7): 72 (1990).

40. A. M. Altschul, Low-calorie foods, *Food Technol.*, *43*(4): 113 (1989).

41. M. Friedman, Healthy foods and cross-category niches, *Prep. Foods* (10): 61 (1991).

42. R. T. Lovell, Foods from aquaculture, *Food Technol.*, *45*(9): 87 (1991).

15
Artificially Sweetened Beverages

William T. Miller *The Beverage Research Center, Inc.,*
Columbus, Georgia

I. INTRODUCTION

Artificially sweetened beverages first appeared in the early 1950s. They grew from a tiny 1.5% of the market in 1958 to 29.4% of the much bigger market in 1990—an estimated total of 2330.5 million cases of 24–12-oz containers, equal to 5,243,625 gallons.

This chapter will discuss why these drinks came into being, the improvements necessary before they could gain wide acceptance, and the resistance by the industry, states, and federal government. This is a thrilling and exciting story.

The banning of cyclamate on October 18, 1969, led to financial losses of some half-billion dollars. Then there was the proposed banning of saccharin and a stay of the ban by Congress. The sales of artifically sweetened beverages continue to grow some 40 years later. Sucralose, a new sweetener that may soon be approved, may offer another big boost to artificially sweetened beverages.

Has the consumption of caloric sweeteners (sugar and high-fructose corn syrup) decreased or increased because of artificial sweeteners? Are artificially sweetened beverages displacing water? An effort will be made to answer these questions.

II. THE BEGINNING OF ARTIFICIALLY SWEETENED DRINKS

A. Diabetic Population

During the 1950s food manufacturers became more conscious of diabetics and their needs. Stores had diabetic sections with a variety of foods especially prepared for the diabetic.

B. Reduced Need for Calories

Men and women no longer spend long hours in manual labor. Since 1850 the output per man-hours has increased fivefold. Whereas in 1850 machines did 6% of the work, in 1960, machines did better than 94% of the work. The hand pump, scrub board, flatirons, wash tubs, ice boxes, coal stoves, and food pedal machines were all replaced, resulting in greatly reduced physical activity. Food energy intake needed downward adjusting to match the reduced energy output; otherwise, there would be energy imbalance and general weight gain above normal (see Chapter 2).

C. Health Concerns Regarding Sugar

The health concerns regarding sugar are reflected in a 1950 study on consumer attitudes toward soft drinks, which revealed that 49% of those surveyed thought soft drinks were harmful or somewhat harmful to the teeth since they contained so much sugar. Eighteen percent said they were too filling and spoil their appetite; 14% thought the sugar content was excessive; 13% showed concern over the fattening qualities. In total, 38.7% of the people surveyed expressed an objection to sugar in soft drinks (Life Magazine Marketing Laboratory, personal communication).

III. IMPROVEMENTS

Artificially sweetened soft drinks in the early years were restrained from broad acceptance by taste characteristics. A typical early descriptions was that they tasted like a motorman's glove. These offtastes were the result of flavor technologists' inexperience in working with artificial sweeteners, impurities in the sweeteners, and inherent taste characteristics of the sweeteners.

The earliest artificially sweetened beverages were sweetened only with saccharin. In 1949, the Food and Drug Administration (FDA) approved cyclamate. It was discovered that a mixture of 10 parts cyclamate with one part saccharin produced the most satisfactory combination and the most desirable sweetness. The use of this combination greatly improved the taste and acceptability of these beverages.

The next step was to improve the purity of the sweeteners. As more and more artificial sweeteners were used, greater efforts were made to remove impurities. Abbott Laboratories made several improvements in cyclamate in reducing the cyclohexylamine level. Monsanto reduced levels of orthotoluenesulfonamide and other impurities in saccharin.

Saccharin produced by the Maumee process from anthranilic acid was considered to have less impurities and less aftertaste than that from Remsen-Fahlberg process. The combination of these purifications with improved efforts by the favor technologists resulted in continued improvement in taste.

IV. RESISTANCE

A. States

In the 1950s and 1960s, when artificially sweetened beverages were being introduced, many states had laws preventing the use of saccharin in soft drinks. These laws had been sponsored by bottlers to prevent economic adulteration. When bottlers began to market artificially sweetened beverages, it became necessary to have these laws repealed.

The mid-continental group of states consisting of Kansas, Arkansas, Missouri, Oklahoma, and Mississippi met in August 1955 to consider their objections to artificially sweetened, carbonated beverages. At this meeting objections were raised concerning various statements on the label. A statement by the National Reseach Council, which cast doubt on the advisability of general distributions of artificially sweetened foods, was emphasized. A lawsuit was threatened by one of the states to declare the trademark "Diet-Rite" misleading, forcing the use of a different brand name in these states for a short time. The state of Connecticut required a label with white letters on a royal blue background. Today, all artificially sweetened carbonated beverages have the word "diet" in their name.

B. Federal

New federal regulations were enacted requiring a cola to be called a cola-flavored beverage. The words "special dietary" or "dietetic" were required to appear prominently on the container along with the words "artificially sweetened carbonated beverage."

Federal regulation number 125.7 provided for a statement: "Contains saccharin, a non-nutritive artificial sweetener which should be used only by persons who must restrict their intake of ordinary sweets" [1].

C. Industry

Until 1960, artificially sweetened carbonated beverages were maverick products. The leaders in the industry would not produce them. One large soft drink company wrote its bottlers that it would never produce one.

V. TRANSFORMATION OF THE SOFT DRINK INDUSTRY

The Royal Crown Cola Company decided, in 1961, to market artificially sweetened drinks in returnable glass bottles at regular prices. Within 90 days an average of 30% was added to this bottlers' volume. America's bulging waistlines and middle-age spread connected with the idea of artificially sweetened drink to transform soft drinks into a $2 billion industry within the space of 2 years.

Pepsi entered the market with Patio Cola in February 1963, and Coke with Tab in May 1963. The May 1963 issue of the *Atlanta Magazine* contains a special report by Bill Diehl, "A Behind the Scene Story of How Tab Was Born." This article describes the Coca-Cola Company's decision to produce an artificially sweetened beverage and how they went about developing the product and a package.

VI. CYCLAMATE DECLINE

In 1966, Kojima and Ichibagase discovered that cyclohexylamine was a metabolite of sodium cyclamate [2]. In 1963, Leahy et al. found cyclohexylamine excretors among human volunteers given cyclamate [3]. In 1969, Bajusz observed calcification of the myocardium after feeding calcium cyclamate to the Syrian hamster [4]. On June 5, 1969, a preliminary verbal report was given to Abbott Laboratories at the University of Wisconsin stating that a significant incidence of tumors had been found in the urinary bladder of mice that had been surgically implanted with pellets containing four parts of cholesterol and one part of sodium cyclamate.

On September 14, 1969, Dr. Marvin Legator made a public statement concerning a technical report published in *Science* stating that chromosome breaks were produced in both bone marrow cells and reproductive cells of male rats receiving injections of cyclohexylamine [5].

On October 1, 1969, a local news program on WNB-TV in Washington, D.C., carried a taped interview with FDA scientist Dr. Jacqueline Verrett. She described a photograph of deformed chicken embryos and stated that "cyclamates are more dangerous than Thalidomide."

On October 8, 1969, Abbott Laboratories was notified of bladder tumors found in rats fed a cyclamate/saccharin mixture in a study conducted at the Food and Drug Research Laboratories [6]. On October 18, producers of cyclamate products were called to Washington, D.C., where Robert H. Finch, the Secretary of Health, Education and Welfare, announced, "My order requires the use of cyclamate in the production of general purposes foods and beverages be discontinued forthwith."

VII. PRODUCT REFORMULATION

A. 1970–1973: Saccharin and Sugar

The industry was back on the market with reformulated products in record time. The saccharin ban was announced on Friday afternoon and Royal Crown Cola Company had a reformulated product by the following Monday. Pepsi, Seven–Up, and Coke followed shortly thereafter. Most of these products contained 3–6 calories of sugar per fluid ounce, with the exception of Fresca, which contained 0.04% saccharin.

B. 1973–1983: Saccharin

By 1973, sugar had been deleted. The consumers sacrificed taste characteristics to obtain fewer calories.

In 1974 a report of a saccharin feeding study conducted by the Wisconsin Alumni Research Foundation stated that bladder tumors were found in second-generation male rats [7]. In 1977, after a Canadian feeding study also found bladder tumors in second-generation male rats, FDA proposed a saccharin ban. The public outcry caused the Congress to delay the ban, but required a statement on the containers that "This product contains saccharin which is known to cause cancer in laboratory animals."

C. 1983–1985: Saccharin and Aspartame

On July 8, 1983, aspartame was approved for use in carbonated beverages. A mixture of aspartame and saccharin was used in artificially sweetened drinks until 1985 when the industry switched to 100% aspartame.

Table 1 Growth of Market for Artificially Sweetened Beverages During Different Periods of Product Formulation

Dates	Product Contained	Market (%)	Growth (millions)	Average annual growth (millions)
1952–1953	Saccharin and cyclamate product being improved	0–5	0–70.8	7.8
1963–1967	Saccharin and cyclamate (cyclamate banned 1969)	5.9–11.2	70.8–184	28.2
1970–1973	Saccharin and sugar (1st reformulation)	7–9	144–226	27.3
1973–1983	Saccharin only (2nd reformulation)	9–20	226–782	55.6
1983–1985	Saccharin and aspartame (3rd reformulation)	20–23.1	782–1000	109
1985–1989	Aspartame only (4th reformulation)	23–27.9	1000–1426	106.5

Source: National Soft Drink Association, personal communication.

D. 1985–Present: Aspartame

Major brands of diet soft drinks, bottled or canned, now contain 15–17.5 mg of aspartame per fluid ounce (507–592 ppm). Fountain syrups are sweetened with a blend of saccharin/aspartame with 8 mg saccharin and 3 mg aspartame per fluid ounce (National Soft Drink Association, personal communication) Table 1 shows the growth of artificially sweetened beverages during the various stages of product formulation.

VIII. EFFECT ON SUGAR CONSUMPTION

While consumption of artificially sweetened soft drinks has grown from nothing in 1952 to 1560 million 288-oz cases in 1989, consumption of regular sugar-sweetened soft drinks grew from 755 million cases in 1952 to 4073 million cases in 1989, an increase of 3318 million cases. This increase is more than double the increase in artificially sweetened soft drinks.

One must conclude that artificially sweetened soft drinks are not replacing sugar-sweetened soft drinks. This increase must be coming at the expense of other liquids. In 1986 Americans, for the first time, drank more soft drinks than water. Water, beer, and coffee are declining in per capita consumption, while soft drinks, both sugar- and artificially sweetened, continue to grow.

In 1989 per capita consumption of soft drinks was 46.6 gallons; tap water, 37.3 gallons; coffee, 24.7 gallons; beer, 23.3 gallons; milk, 20.9 gallons; and tea, 7.3 gallons [8].

From 1980 to 1988, total sweetener consumption grew by 26%. Caloric sweeteners grew by 17% and artificial sweeteners by 181%. In 1988 per capita sweetener consumption reached a record high of 154 equivalent pounds of sugar [9].

IX. COST

The relative higher price of artificial sweeteners does not affect the retail price of artificially sweetened soft drinks. The cost of 12 ounces of artificially sweetened soft drink is approximately one cent more than the regular soft drink. At retail, the prices are usually the same, the manufacturer preferring average pricing rather than a higher price for the artificially sweetened product.

REFERENCES

1. 57,707, Label statements relating to nonnutritive constituents, *Food Drug Cosmetic Law Reports, 21 CFR 125.7*, Commerce Clearing House, Inc., p. 36,505 (1963).
2. S. Kojima and H. Ichibagase, Studies on synthetic sweetening agents. VII Cyclohexylamine, a metabolite of sodium cyclamate, *Chem. Pharm. Bull., Tokyo, 14*: 971 (1966).
3. J. S. Leahy, M. Wakefield, and T. Taylor, Cyclohexylamine excretors among human volunteers given cyclamate, *Fd. Cosmet. Toxicol., 5*: 595 (1967).
4. E. Bajusz, Myocardial lesions: A reassessment of the toxicology of calcium cyclamate. *Nature, ii, 223*: 406 (1969).
5. M. S. Legator, K. A. Palmer, S. Green, and K. W. Peterson, Cytogenic studies in rats of cyclohexylamine, a metabolite of cyclamate, *Science, 165*: 1139 (1969).
6. J. M. Price, C. G. Biava, B. L. Oser, E. E. Vogin, J. Steinfeld, and H. C. Ley, Bladder tumors in rats fed cyclohexylamine or high doses of a mixture of cyclamate and saccharin, *Science, 167*: 1131 (1970).
7. Subcommittee on Nonnutritive Sweeteners, Committee on Food Protection, *Safety of Saccharin and Sodium Saccharin in the Human Diet*, National Academy of Sciences–National Research Council, Washington, DC, p. 63 (1974).
8. *90–91 Annual Manual*, Beverage Industry, 7500 Old Oak Blvd., Cleveland, OH 44130, p. 8 (1991).
9. U.S. Department of Agriculture, *Sugar and Sweetener Situation and Outlook Report*, March 1989, p. 62 and June 1988, p. 56.

16
Artificially Sweetened Low-Calorie Foods Other than Drinks

Basant K. Dwivedi   *NuGen Foods, Ltd., Paterson, New Jersey*

I. INTRODUCTION

The need for sweeteners in our diet has been a subject of relentless debate. We are constantly reminded that nutritive sweeteners, such as corn syrups and sugars, are not only unnecessary but undesirable components of our food intake because they do not provide essential nutrients other than calories, and thus may be responsible for America's ever-widening girth. Why then do we continue to ingest sweetened foods in ever-increasing quantities? Two million years ago or so, when the human species evolved on earth, primitive humans sought out fruits, nuts, and berries along with animal prey for survival. For more than 99% of human history, our diet has remained the same, slowly adapting to animal products, fruits, nuts, and vegetables. During the last 5000 years, however, technological changes have been so rapid that there has not been enough time for genetic selection and adaptation to our changing environment. It should be noted that the sweetness of sugar does not reside within the sugar molecule. Rather, sweetness is our brain's

Table 1 Saccharin Production
in Germany

Year	kg × 1000
1894	30
1922 (World War I)	300
1931	96
1944 (World War II)	500
1965	27

Source: Ref. 10.

interpretation of electrical signals produced by taste buds in response to sugar. David Barash, a well-known sociobiologist, explained our craving for sugar as follows: [1]

> Our primate ancestors probably ate a great deal of fruit, which is more nutritious when it is ripe and rich with sugars. We were, therefore, selected for responding positively to the taste of those chemicals that categorized ripe fruit. Accordingly, sugar tastes sweet to us. An articulate giant panda would probably say the same about bamboo shoots.

Our adaptive liking for sugar has become a major problem. Barash goes on: "Through culture, we provide ourselves with essential non-nutritive cakes, cookies, chocolates, and essential effluvia of the sweet tooth industry. We know it is not good for us, but we are still biological creatures and cannot easily resist our fondness for sugars."

Some evidence supports this position. For example, let's take a look at the impact of two world wars on saccharin production in Germany (Table 1). These data show that when the supply of sugar was cut off because of war, saccharin was used as a substitute. The data also show that the German government, when faced with the shortage of sugar, recognized the need for a sugar substitute and allocated resources for the production and distribution of saccharin in order to satisfy the German sweet tooth.

In 1977, when the U.S. Food and Drug Administration (FDA) announced its intention to ban saccharin from foods and beverages, our legislators received almost one million letters of protest—more mail than was received on any single issue since the Vietnam war [2].

II. ARTIFICIAL SWEETENERS AND WEIGHT LOSS

Do artificial sweeteners help us in controlling our food intake? Scientific literature provides conflicting data on this subject. Some studies support the view that caloric dilution achieved by the substitution of artificial sweeteners for sucrose may facilitate compliance to a hypocaloric diet [3]. Other studies show that artificial sweetener users tend to gain more weight than nonusers, irrespective of initial relative weight [4].

A. Effect on Insulin Release

Stimulation of sweet taste by artificial sweeteners may promote insulin release in some way, leading to hypoglycemia in normal individuals and so perhaps fostering appetite. Additionally, hyperinsulinemia itself can stimulate hunger, increase the palatability of sucrose, and increase food intake [5]. Liang and associates have reported that acesulfame-K in high doses stimulated insulin release in rats, although it did not lead to hypoglycemia [6].

B. Effect on Weight Loss

There is no scientific documentation showing long-term weight loss in response to the use of artificial sweeteners. However, most nutritionists agree that calories do count and that excess caloric consumption inevitably causes weight gain. Also, there is some proof that low-calorie foods and beverages sweetened with artificial sweeteners permit people to consume fewer calories. For example, studies have shown that covert substitution of aspartame-sweetened products for their sucrose counterparts resulted in an immediate reduction in spontaneous caloric intake of approximately 25% [7]. It should be noted that subjects maintained on a low-calorie diet for a prolonged period do compensate for missing calories by increasing their food intake to some extent, but generally they continue to consume fewer calories (i.e., in a long-term study by Porikos et al. [8], the subjects consumed approximately 85% of normal intake).

C. Consumer Response

How is the consumer responding to the availability of artificially sweetened foods? Growth of low-calorie products, documented in Table 2, shows that in 1989 about 93 million consumers used low-calorie, artificially sweetened products, as compared to 78 million consumers only 3 years earlier. The market share of artificially sweetened products continues to grow at a very rapid rate, as shown in Table 3.

Because of increased consumer interest in artificially sweetened products, per capita consumption of artificial sweeteners has increased sharply within the last two decades (Table 4). Comparative costs for various commercial sweeteners (Table 5) show that artificial sweeteners, with the exception of

Table 2 Low-Calorie Artificially Sweetened Foods:
Trend in Use by Product Category

Product	Millions of Users 1986	1989
All products	78	93
Sugar-free carbonated beverages	60	69
Sugar substitutes	43	53
Sugar-free gum/candy	39	48
Sugar-free pudding, gelatin	28	33
Sugar-free frozen desserts	NA	25
Sugar-free powder drink mixes	27	21
Sugar-free cakes/cookies	7	13
Other foods/beverages Containing low-calorie sweeteners	24	24
Other low-calorie "light" Foods and beverages	34	40

Source: Calorie Control Council Focus, Calorie Control Council,
Atlanta, GA, Sept. 6, 1989.

Table 3 Artificially Sweetened Foods: Trend in Sales in
Millions of Dollars

Product	1982 Total	Artificially sweetened	1987 Total	Artificially sweetened
Powdered soft drinks	700	30	740	300
Hot cocoa mix	196	23	217	75
Gelatin mixes	226	14	234	60
Pudding mixes	231	6	254	50
Table-top sweeteners	115	115 (saccharin)	236	110 (saccharin) 126 (aspartame)

Source: Private communication, NutraSweet Company, Skokie, IL (1989).

Table 4 Artificial Sweetener Consumption (Sucrose Equivalent Sweetness per Capita per Day)

Year	Usage (g)	
1909–13	0.6	
1976	7.6	
1979	9.2	
1983	23.4	
	Aspartame	16.2
	Saccharin	6.8
	Other	0.4

Source: Adapted from G. T. Molitor, Directions in international sweetener regulation, Calorie Control Council, Annual Meeting, Scottsdale, AZ, Oct. 26, 1987.

Table 5 Comparative Cost of Sweeteners (Sucrose Sweetness Equivalent)

Sweetener	Cost/lb (cents)
Saccharin	1
Acesulfame-K	15–16
Aspartame	30–50
Sugar	32
High-fructose corn syrup	20

Source: Adapted from G. T. Molitor, Directions in international sweetener regulation, Calorie Control Council, Annual Meeting, Scottsdale, AZ, Oct. 26, 1987.

aspartame, cost less than sucrose on a sweetening equivalent basis. This permits food manufacturers to offer these products at prices comparable to sugar-sweetened products. This may explain, in part, several hundred new product introductions each year with low-calorie and reduced-/low-sugar claims.

III. ARTIFICIALLY SWEETENED FOODS

Each sweetener has a distinct flavor/taste profile, and a judicious selection of ingredients is of prime importance in product development when using artificial sweeteners. Aspartame displays a slow onset of sweetness coupled with lingering sweet taste, as compared to quick onset and sharp cut-off of sweetness from sucrose. Onset of acesulfame-K sweetness is rapid, without unpleasant delay. It decreases slowly, without unacceptable lingering taste. The sweetness, however, does persist longer than sucrose. Acesulfame-K has a slightly better taste profile than saccharin. However, the quality of sweetness is less desirable than aspartame. The sweetness quality of acesulfame-K can be improved by combining it with nutritive sweeteners (i.e., sucrose, sorbitol, fructose, etc). Also, acesulfame-K produces a strong synergistic effect with aspartame and sodium cyclamate, but shows a less pronounced effect in mixtures with saccharin. For these reasons artificial sweeteners cannot be substituted for sucrose on a sweetness basis alone. Also, since artificial sweeteners are needed in small quantities because of high sweetness potency, a need for low-calorie, inert bulking agents is created. Water, polydextrose, starch and starch derivatives, pectins, vegetable gums, and agar are often used alone or in combination as bulking agents in artificially sweetened, low-calorie products. For example, in reduced-calorie baked goods, bulking agents like polydextrose, when substituted for sugar and flour, would permit lower usage of fat.

A. Table-Top Sweeteners

Low-calorie, readily soluble, low hygroscopic sweetening compositions are produced by preparing solutions of approved sweeteners—aspartame, saccharin, and acesulfame-K—with various low-dextrose-equivalent starch hydrolyzates and spray drying them. Food-grade acids are often added to improve solubility of the finished product. In sweetness tablets, lactose is often used as a filler; bicarbonate and acidulant provide effervescence, and L-leucine in an amount not to exceed 3.5% may be added as a lubricant to release the tablet from the press. In the sachet, lactose and dextrose act as fillers.

Table 6 Consumer Usage Patterns of Saccharin-Based Table-Top Sweeteners in Homes Where Table-Top Sweeteners Are Used

	Average usage (%)	
Usage category	Packet	Bulk
Hot beverages (coffee, tea, cocoa)	44.2	33.1
Cold beverage	0.7	1.1
Cereal	11.4	9.1
Other additive usage (Sprinkled)	5.7	8.0
Ingredient in baking	1.2	3.3
Ingredient in stovetop cooking	0.9	2.8
Miscellaneous	36.0	42.7
Total	100.0	100.0

Source: Ref. 9.

About 15 years ago, G.D. Searle & Co. conducted a survey to determine usage patterns of saccharin-based table-top sweeteners in homes where artificial sweeteners are regularly used [9]. The data presented in Table 6 showed that about 40% of the table-top sweeteners were used in hot beverages; about 10% were used on a breakfast cereal. Other applications were quite diverse. Although the data are old, it is likely that the usage patterns today are similar to 1976 when the study was conducted.

B. Dry Mix Products

A wide variety of low-calorie mixes have been formulated with artificial sweeteners. These include

Cold beverage mixes
Gelatin dessert mixes
Pudding and pie filling mix
Hot cocoa mix
Whipped topping mix
Meal replacements
Salad dressing mix
Dip mix
Instant presweetened tea

From a formulation and processing point of view, artificially sweetened mixes are relatively simple. Because these products require dry blending of individual ingredients, loss of sweetness during processing is not a problem.

However, because of intense sweetness of sugar substitutes, bulk characteristics of sugar must be duplicated by other means. In addition, sugar acts as a processing aid. Also, due to its granular nature, it provides a subtle flavor-masking affect and adds mouthfeel to the product.

Polydextrose, vegetable gums, and maltodextrins alone or in combination are used in dry mixes to mimic the sensory properties of sugar besides sweetness. The selection of ingredients and usage level are determined primarily by the critical functionality desired (i.e., mouthfeel, taste, flow properties, dispersability, etc). Typical prototype formulations of artificially sweetened mixes using aspartame are given in Tables 7 through 9. Formulations using saccharin and acesulfame-K may be developed using the following sweetness values for the sweeteners (sugar = 1):

Aspartame	160
Saccharin	300
Acesulfame-K	130

Table 7 Formulation for
Aspartame-Sweetened Lemonade[a]

Ingredients	%
Citric acid	55.95
Maltodextrin	20.27
(e.g., Maltrin 010)	
Sodium citrate	8.60
Aspartame	5.84
Tricalcium phosphate	4.29
Ascorbic acid	3.11
Clouding agent	1.94
(e.g., Beatrice #3545)	
Flavor	to suit
Color	to suit

[a]Provides 4 kcal/serving. Equivalent sugar-sweetened products provide 90 kcal/serving.

Processing Steps:
1. Preblend 3 or 4 parts maltodextrin with 1 part aspartame.
2. Mix the preblend with all remaining ingredients.
3. For finished product, 16 grams of mix are dissolved in 2 quarts of cold water.

Table 8 Formulation for Aspartame-
Sweetened Gelatin Mix[a]

Ingredients	%
Gelatin (225 bloom)	70.4
Adipic acid	17.6
Fumaric acid	1.5
Sodium citrate	6.6
Aspartame	3.9
Flavor	to suit
Color	to suit

[a]If greater body is desired, maltodextrin or polydextrose may be used with aspartame. Calories are 12–
13% of the sugar-sweetened product if formula is used
without maltodextrin or polydextrose.

Processing Steps:
1. Preblend fumaric acid, sodium citrate, flavor, and
   color.
2. Mix together gelatin, adipic acid (maltodextrin or
   polydextrose, if used), and aspartame. Blend 3–7
   minutes or until uniform.
3. Add preblend from step 1 to dry mix from step 2.
   Blend 8–10 minutes or until uniformly mixed. All
   mixing should be done in a controlled atmosphere
   that is cool and dry (25 °C and 50% RH).
4. For finished product, dissolve 12 grams of mix in
   one cup of hot water. Stir in one cup cold water.
   Pour into dessert cups and chill until set.

C. Canned Fruits, Jams, Jellies, and Preserves

Because of low caloric density, canned fruits may be desirable in a weight-
loss program. However, loss of sweetness and off-taste development during
retorting is a serious problem. Aseptic processing of artificially sweetened
fruits offers a significant advantage over retorting and may lead to commercial application with highly acceptable products.

Artificially sweetened jams, jellies, and preserves are a viable category
of products offering up to 75% reduction in calories. Aspartame-sweetened
preserves offer an acceptable alternative to regular jams and jellies because
of clean sweet taste. Jelly formulation using aspartame at 0.12% level, with
carrageenan and pectin added for body, may be used as a prototype. Since
sugar plays a role in the setting of certain types of pectins and also has a preservative action by its osmotic effect, other ingredients must provide these
functions [9].

Table 9 Formulation for Aspartame-
Sweetened Hot Chocolate Mix[a]

Ingredients	%
Nonfat dry milk solids (NFDM)[b]	75.5
Cocoa (lecithinated)	23.2
Gum (guar or xanthan)	0.3
Flavoring (vanilla and/or vanillin)	to suit
Aspartame	1.0

[a]This product sweetened with aspartame contains only
55% of the calories found in an equivalent sugar-sweetened
product.
[b]NFDM solids may also be formulated as a dairy blend
to include sweet whey, sodium caseinate, and other diary
ingredients.

Processing Steps:
1. Blend aspartame with nondairy milk solids and mix
   for 5 minutes or until uniform.
2. Add cocoa and flavor components and mix for an additional 8–10 minutes or until mixture is uniform in appearance.
3. Processes other than dry blending—such as agglomera-
   tion—may also be used to provide a more uniform mixture with possible improvement in final product solubility.
4. Finished beverage would be 8.3% dry mix in water.

Prototype formulations of jams and jellies with acesulfame-K as a sweetener have been prepared with sorbitol as a bulking agent. Other sugar alcohols
and polydextrose have proved to be suitable too.

D. Frozen Desserts and Dairy Products

The typical calorie content of sugar-sweetened frozen desserts range from
90 to 250 calories per 4-fluid-ounce serving. A major portion of the calories
in these products comes from the sweetener used. By replacing carbohydrate sweeteners with artificial sweeteners, a 30–70% reduction in calories
may be realized. Low-fat systems (i.e., ice milk, sherbert, sorbet, mellorine,
and frozen yogurt) can be products with the caloric reduction towards the
upper range, whereas ice cream with 4% or higher butterfat would only permit about a 50% or less reduction in calories. Bulking agents, such as poly-
destrose with 1 kcal/g, impart the desired mouthfeel in frozen desserts with
only one-fourth the calories of sugar.

A combination of two or more bulking agents is often required to duplicate the functional properties of sugar such as freeze-point depression, ice crystal control, and structure/bulk contribution. For example, a low molecular weight substance such as sorbitol is a better freeze-point depressant than a high molecular weight substance such as maltodextrin. On the other hand, water binding capacity may be better accomplished by large molecules such as maltodextrin than by small molecules such as sugar alcohols.

Frozen dessert processing using aspartame as a sweetener is basically the same as for sugar-sweetened products. However, the use of batch pasteurization should be avoided for aspartame-sweetened products. Exposure of aspartame to prolonged heating at neutral pH results in unnecessary aspartame degradation. Acesulfame-K-sweetened products can be pasteurized by batch processing because of their good heat and shelf life stability.

IV. CONCLUSIONS

Because of high consumer demand and acceptance of low-calorie products, artificially sweetened foods will continue to grow rapidly. FDA, having adopted a multiple sweetener approach in order to limit average daily intake of any one sweetener, will help food scientists and technologists in developing low-calorie products with optimum sensory properties and satisfactory shelf life. Artificial sweeteners that may gain FDA approval within the near future include Sucralose (McNeal Laboratories) and Alitame (Pfizer). These sweeteners offer some functional benefits that are lacking in currently available artificial sweeteners, such as stability at high temperatures and a broader pH range. If FDA grants approval of a suitable fat replacer such as olestra brand sucrose polyesters from Procter & Gamble, we may see a day when one may indulge in food of all types without worrying about calories and weight gain.

REFERENCES

1. D. P. Barash, *Sociobiology and Behavior*, Elsevier, North Holland, Inc., New York (1977).
2. W. Bennett, The taste that failed, *American Health*: 22 (July/August 1983).
3. B. S. Kanders, P. T. Lavin, M. B. Kowalchuk, I. Greenberg, and G. L. Blackburn, An evaluation of the effect of aspartame on weight loss, *Appetite, 11*(Suppl.): 73 (1988).
4. S. D. Stellman and L. Garfinkel, Artificial sweetener use and one year weight change among women, *Preventive Med.*, 15: 195 (1986).

5. J. Rodin, J. Wack, E. Ferrannini, and R. A. DeFronzo, Effect of insulin and glucose on feeding behavior, *Metabolism, 34*: 826 (1985).
6. Y. Liang, V. Maier, G. Steinbach, L. Lalic, and E. F. Pfeiffer, The effect of artificial sweeteners on insulin secretion. The effect of acesulfame-K on insulin secretion in the rat (studied in vitro), *Horm. Metab. Res. 19*: 233 (1986).
7. K. P. Porikos and T. B. Van Itallie, Efficacy of low calorie sweeteners in reducing food intake: Studies with aspartame, *Aspartame—Physiology and Biochemistry* (L. D. Stegrik and L. J. Filler, Jr., eds.), Marcel Dekker, Inc., New York (1984).
8. K. P. Porikos, M. F. Hesser, and T. B. Van Itallie, Caloric regulation in normal weight men maintained on a palatable diet of conventional foods, *Physiol. Behav. 29*: 293 (1982).
9. C. I. Beck, Application potential for aspartame in low calorie and dietetic foods, in *Low Calorie and Special Dietary Foods* (B. K. Dwivedi, ed.) CRC Press, West Palm Beach, FL (1978).
10. R. F. Crampton, The question of benefits and risks, *Sweeteners—Issues and Uncertainties*, Academy Forum, Fourth of a Series, National Academy of Sciences, Washington, DC (1975).

17
Meat Products in a Low-Fat Diet

Floyd Michael Byers, Nancy D. Turner, and H. Russell Cross* *Texas A&M University, College Station, Texas*

I. INTRODUCTION

Americans are nearly overwhelmed by the choices of food products available to them today. You can easily see the dilemma experienced by most people in stores as they carefully choose which product they want and then have to decide which package or brand of the product to buy. This is not the case in some countries where availability of any food is limited and, when food is available, no one is choosy.

When given the ultimate choice, most people will pick a product that is pleasing to the eye, nose, and palate. When presented with a no-cost or no-risk decision, we seldom choose a product that is fat-free, sugar-free, bland, and generally unappealing. It is only when we weigh the desirability of one product that is considered healthy with that of another product that has some (at least perceived) risks that we will logically decide to purchase the product that is "good for us."

Current affiliation: U.S. Department of Agriculture, Washington, D.C.

The 1990s have become the decade of food safety and environmental awareness. The entire social contract between consumers, food producers, and provisioners is in transition. From a consumer's perspective, safety, healthfulness, and the environmental aspects of food are interrelated and inseparable. The dramatic success of agricultural biotechnology has led to expectations and demands for products with desirable composition and food value that are safe and wholesome and a food supply that is bountiful, appealing, nutritious, healthful, economical, convenient, and safe.

In addition, as the American consumer has become more weight- and health-conscious, food is expected to impart health benefits that extend beyond mere nutritive value. Consumers recognize weight gain and its associated effects on health as a national health problem. The Institute of Food Technologists (IFT) recently estimated that more than 34 million people in the United States are overweight—13% are described as severely obese. The population has evolved into a "lean conscious society" where a high priority is placed on ways to get and stay trimmer. People are more concerned about exercise, diet choices, and food quality assisting in this change in lifestyle. This consciousness is evident in the desire for leaner animal products with less fat and cholesterol than found in traditional animal products.

Over the last 20 years we have been told by everyone from the American Heart Association, the American Medical Association, to the guy next door that we are going to die if we eat meat, especially red meat. In a sense they are correct, we are all going to die. However, when intelligent choices are made concerning what products to consume, how best to prepare the products, and, quite possibly the most important choice, how much of the product to consume, then meat can easily be part of a balanced, low-fat diet that will fulfill the dietary requirements of most anyone.

This chapter will describe some of the characteristics of meat and how it can be produced or processed to reduce its inherent fat content. Another point presented will be the cost factors involved in producing low-fat meat. Meat encompasses a huge spectrum of possibilities, and our discussion will focus primarily on beef and chicken. These two meat sources are chosen because historically they have represented the perceived two extremes of "good" and "bad" sources of meat. Therefore, any information concerning these two products should permit anyone to make intelligent choices concerning most other meat products.

A. Fat Content of Meat Products

1. Change in Meat Fat Content over Time

Early beef production in the United States was based on Longhorn-type cattle, which were very lean when compared to the European breeds that are used as a genetic base in today's production systems. Over time, changes in trans-portation availability and the demand for higher-quality beef caused pro-ducers to shift to Angus and Hereford cattle that, when finished for slaughter, were excessively fat. Costs of producing these overly fat carcasses increased, and consumer awareness of the need for reduced fat consumption combined with cost-awareness to cause producers to develop and use better breeding, feeding, growth regulation, and management practices, which resulted in leaner carcasses during the last two decades.

Poultry production was historically based on animals scavenging for feed or consumption of human food waste. When the time for Sunday dinner arrived, the next available chicken became the main entree. Need was the main criterion for harvesting an animal to convert it to food. As America became urbanized, the family chicken coop became a thing of the past. Pro-duction of poultry products also became a modernized process. Animals were confined, provided with an adequate quantity of a nutritionally com-plete diet, and soon fat poultry products were appearing in the local grocery store. Modification of production practices and breeding has occurred at a much faster rate in poultry than in beef operations because of the short life span and the ease of integration in poultry-production systems. It is because of these attributes that poultry producers were able to more rapidly respond to consumer demands for leaner products.

2. Current Fat Content

a. Beef. The composition of beef, whether fresh or cooked, depends on cut, grade, cooking method, and whether fat is trimmed prior to or after cooking. Most consumers do not eat the separable fat in cuts of beef; it is trimmed off the carcass before cooking and at the time of eating (as plate waste).

Over all grades of beef, the separable fat (which is usually not eaten) constitutes an average of 26.7% of the raw edible portion of retail cuts [1]. After cooking, separable fat averages 27.7% of the edible portion for all grades of beef retail cuts. The fat content in 100 grams of edible beef from a composite of trimmed retail cuts is dependent on quality grade. Quality grades reflect fat in the muscle, called marbling, with Prime having the most, Choice an intermediate amount, and Select having the least marbling of the three most common grades. As a result, there is more fat in Prime beef (30.3%), while Choice (23.8%) and Select (21.9%) have less fat. Therefore, when using a typically fat cut of beef (e.g., a chuck blade), choosing the Select grade provides a product with only 13.7% fat, one third less than would be found in the same cut of Prime grade. Conversely, in top round, typically a lean cut, where even a Prime cut has less than 9% fat, the Select grade also has approximately half as much fat (5.4%).

All of these grades of beef are available to consumers in grocery stores, with Choice and Select being the most common. Prime beef is available as a gourmet item and is featured in finer restaurants. Of the fed beef marketed in the United States [1], Prime, Choice, and Select represent 6.0, 66.7, and 27.3%, respectively. Statistics on carcasses marketed demonstrate that, although fat content of meat has decreased since 1986, quality has increased (2.1% Prime, 82.4% Choice, and 15.4% Select).

Cooking of the three grades can increase fat content to 33.8, 27.1, and 25.1% for Prime, Choice, and Select, respectively. Fat content may increase with cooking because certain techniques result in a larger percentage of water than fat being released as drippings or evaporated (Table 1). The cut of meat being cooked also has an effect on whether fat content will increase or decrease during cooking. Further, whether the cut is trimmed prior to or after cooking also affects fat content.

Meat cuts are obtained from different muscle groups, and, therefore, individual cut composition (Table 2) will vary [2]. Therefore, careful selection by the consumer can reduce the fat available for consumption in the beef cut chosen.

Table 1 Effect of Cooking Technique on Fat Content of Selected Choice and Select Retail Cuts of Beef[a]

Retail cut	Broiled	Braised	Roasted	Fried
Choice				
Rib, whole	26.1		27.6	
Ribeye, large end	28.2		25.9	
Ribeye, small end	21.6		25.7	
Top round	7.7			14.5
Flank	13.9	13.2		
Tenderloin	15.1		19.2	
Select				
Rib, whole	23.3		24.9	
Ribeye, large end	25.1		24.5	
Ribeye, small end	19.4		22.3	
Top round	7.1			
Tenderloin	13.4		17.3	
Ground, lean	15.7			16.2

[a]Quantity is grams in an 85-gram (3-ounce) edible portion composed of separable lean and fat.
Source: Ref. 1.

Table 2 Fat Content of Selected Retail Cuts of Beef[a]

Retail cut	Raw	Cooked
Brisket, whole	28.2	32.4
Chuck		
Arm pot roast	19.8	26.0
Blade roast	23.6	30.4
Flank	12.6	15.5
Rib		
Whole	29.1	30.0
Eye, small end	19.3	20.6
Large end	31.4	32.3
Small end	26.0	24.8
Short ribs	36.2	42.0
Round		
Full cut	17.5	18.2
Bottom round	15.6	14.8
Eye of round	12.6	14.2
Tip round	13.8	15.3
Top round	8.8	8.8
Short Loin		
Porterhouse	23.3	21.2
T-bone	26.1	24.6
Tenderloin	18.0	17.2
Top loin	22.8	18.8
Wedge-bone sirloin	20.2	18.0
Ground beef[b]		
Extra lean	17.1	16.3
Lean	20.7	18.5
Regular	26.6	20.7
Liver	3.8	4.9

[a]Quantity (grams) in 100 g of edible portion (all grades) composed of separable lean and fat.
[b]Broiled, medium.
Source: Ref. 1.

While these data indicate the quantity of fat in the edible portion of a cut, as stated before, most consumers do not actually eat all of the fat in an edible portion, but trim the waste from meat they consume. So-called plate waste contains a large fraction of the subcutaneous, seam, and other large, extractable parts of fat from most beef cuts. Separable fat that would be removed from the purchased beef cut prior to cooking or eating ranges from 33% for a whole brisket to 5% for a flank steak. Therefore, evaluation of beef, as consumed, with separable fat removed, instead of as available, should be the point of reference for analysis of fat in all meat products.

Composition of beef cuts based on separable lean is indicated in Table 3. When the basis for comparison is the meat actually consumed, the fat content of a broiled chuck roast is 10.3%, a large end rib that has been roasted has 14.4% fat, a broiled top round steak has 6.5% fat, and a broiled T-bone steak contains 10.4% fat [3]. Comparisons of several cuts with different cooking methods (Table 3) indicate the range of fat, its composition, and calorie contribution in typical (100 g) portions of lean with separable fat removed. A recent survey [4] found that beef marketed today contains approximately 27% less separable fat than reported by the USDA [1].

One commonly asked question is: How much fat is enough? This depends on the type of product and the way in which it will be prepared, among other factors, such as taste preference, texture, and appearance. For eating quality comparisons, a window of acceptability (Fig. 1) developed at Texas A&M [5] indicates a range of fatness in which cuts from the rib and loin are acceptable in palatability and contribution of fat to the diet. A minimum of 3% fat is needed for acceptable palatability, a desirable characteristic that continues to increase (slowly) with additional fat. Fat improves palatability by increasing tenderness and juiciness. Beef cuts from low Select to high Choice fit this window. The 3% cutoff is a minimal level, and cuts in the 5 and 7% range may be more appropriate for some products and usages. Relationships of fat to palatability are less clear for other cuts, reflecting the way they are cooked and consumer expectations of these products [5].

Ground beef is a major component of beef consumption and presents some interesting challenges for the food industry and consumers alike. This product is available in grocery stores at several fat levels typically referred to as regular, lean, and extra lean. Composition of ground beef with these descriptions (see Table 3) indicates some reduction in fat in leaner products as expected, along with fewer calories. A recent survey conducted in 12 cities across the United States [4] found that ground beef being currently marketed by retailers contains 10% less fat than reported in the current USDA Agriculture Handbook [1]. New products recently introduced and in development with less than 10% fat promise to yield real options to reduce fat delivered to consumers through ground beef.

Table 3 Nutrient Composition of Beef (100 g, separable lean only, edible portion)

Cut and grade	kcal	Protein (g)	Total fat (g)	SFA[a] (g)	Stearic acid[b] (g)	MFA[c] (g)	PUFA[d] (g)	Cholesterol (mg)
Bottom round, braised								
Prime	249	31.59	12.65	4.49	1.24	5.78	0.52	96
Choice	225	31.59	9.96	3.54	0.98	4.55	0.41	96
Select	214	31.59	8.77	3.11	0.86	4.01	0.36	96
Chuck arm, braised								
Prime	261	33.02	13.36	5.07	1.58	5.82	0.54	101
Choice	234	33.02	10.32	3.92	1.22	4.50	0.42	101
Select	222	33.02	8.97	3.40	1.06	3.91	0.36	101
Chuck blade, braised								
Prime	318	31.06	20.53	8.37	2.68	9.18	0.69	106
Choice	275	31.06	15.80	6.44	2.06	7.06	0.53	106
Select	256	31.06	13.69	5.58	1.78	6.12	0.46	106
Eye of round, roasted								
Prime	198	28.99	8.25	3.16	0.91	3.63	0.29	69
Choice	184	28.99	6.69	2.56	0.74	2.94	0.23	69
Select	178	28.99	5.99	2.29	0.66	2.63	0.21	69
Ground beef, well done, broiled								
Regular	292	27.20	19.46	7.65	2.30	8.52	0.73	101
Lean	280	28.20	17.64	6.93	2.08	7.72	0.66	101
Extra Lean	265	28.58	15.80	6.21	1.86	6.92	0.59	99

Table 3 Continued

Cut and grade	kcal	Protein (g)	Total fat (g)	SFA[a] (g)	Stearic acid[b] (g)	MFA[c] (g)	PUFA[d] (g)	Cholesterol (mg)
Rib (6–12), broiled								
Prime	280	26.03	18.70	7.97	2.51	8.25	0.56	82
Choice	233	26.03	13.55	5.70	1.79	5.90	0.40	82
Select	213	26.03	11.27	4.80	1.51	4.97	0.34	82
Tenderloin, broiled								
Prime	232	28.25	12.36	4.83	1.62	4.81	0.49	84
Choice	207	28.25	9.59	3.74	1.26	3.73	0.38	84
Select	196	28.25	8.35	3.26	1.09	3.25	0.33	84
Tip round, roasted								
Prime	213	28.71	10.06	3.69	1.15	4.14	0.41	81
Choice	193	28.71	7.75	2.84	0.89	3.19	0.32	81
Select	183	28.71	6.72	2.46	0.77	2.77	0.27	81
Top round, broiled								
Prime	215	31.69	8.87	3.10	0.96	3.47	0.42	84
Choice	194	31.69	6.45	2.26	0.70	2.53	0.30	84
Select	184	31.69	5.38	1.88	0.58	2.11	0.25	84

Beef has no carbohydrates. USDA Prime, Choice, and Select grades of beef are from animals less than 42 months of age. The grades differ by the amount of fat within muscle tissue (marbling). Prime grade contains a slightly abundant, moderately abundant, or abundant amount of marbling. Choice grade contains a small, modest, or moderate amount of marbling. Select contains a slight amount of marbling.
[a]Saturated fatty acids.
[b]Stearic acid ($C_{18:0}$) is a saturated fatty acid that, unlike other saturated fatty acids, does not raise the plasma cholesterol level.
[c]Monounsaturated fatty acids.
[d]Polyunsaturated fatty acids.
Source: Ref. 9.

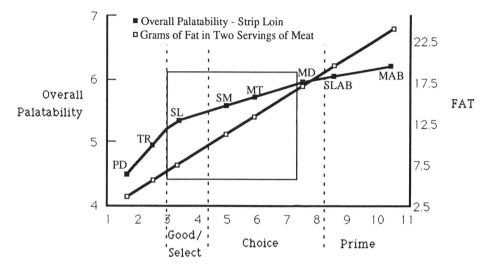

PERCENT OF FAT AND GRADE

Figure 1 Window of consumer acceptability of meat containing variable amounts of fat. PD = practically devoid; TR = traces; SL = slight; SM = small; MT = modest; MD = moderate; SLAB = slightly abundant; MAB = moderately abundant. Adapted from Savell and Cross [5]. Reprinted with permission from *Designing Foods,* © 1988 by the National Academy of Sciences. Published by National Academy Press, Washington, D.C.

Leaner beef products are also more valuable in contributions of other key nutrients: riboflavin, iron, niacin, phosphorus, pyridoxine, zinc, and vitamin B_{12} are important nutrients in beef whose contents increase in leaner products.

b. Pork. Pork has become leaner over the past 30 years, with substantial reductions in external fat. Selection for leaner types of pigs and emphasis on indices of lean along with improved feeding and management systems have dramatically altered the average fat content of pork (Table 4). As evident, the fat in the listed cuts dropped by 2–4 percentage units in two decades. In addition to genetic changes, improved protein nutrition and attention to caloric intake also contribute to this improvement in leanness.

Composition of pork reflects the type of muscle and product merchandized. For example, bacon is nearly half fat, while ham may be only one-tenth as fat. The fat content of cuts in Table 5 suggests the opportunity to reduce fat by one half and still have acceptable palatability. As for beef, a 3% fat level in pork loin muscle is probably a lower limit [5]; early research suggests a

Table 4 Comparison of Nutrient Composition of 1963 and 1983 Market Hogs

Cut	Year	kcal/100 g	Nutrient composition (%) Protein	Fat
Boston, blade	1963	180	18.0	11.4
	1983	165	19.0	9.3
Ham	1963	152	19.8	7.5
	1983	136	20.5	5.4
Loin, whole	1963	189	20.1	11.4
	1983	156	20.7	7.5
Picnic	1963	150	19.2	7.5
	1983	140	19.8	6.2

The 1963 data are based on an assumed distribution of 34, 40, and 25% of thin, medium, and fat pig types, respectively. For the 1983 data, 71.7% of the retail cuts were from U.S. Grade No. 1 carcasses; 24.2% from No. 2; and 3.7% from No. 3.
Source: Refs. 35–38.

3.5–4.5% fat level as adequate for acceptable palatability [6]. Unlike beef, the pork-grading system is not used on packaging to identify product fat content so that consumers could discriminate between low-fat and high-fat products. Grades of U.S. 1, 2, 3, 4, and U.S. utility are used to differentiate between carcasses. The numbers represent the degree of fat in the carcass, with a lower grade number indicating a carcass with less fat [7]. Although the official grades are usually not on packages, product labeling by retailers provides some options for selection when percentage fat appears on the label.

Although the pork industry has made significant strides to reduce the fat content of their products, the per capita consumption of pork has remained relatively constant since 1970 [7]. Further efforts to improve quality, to reduce fat, and to inform consumers about the merits of pork will be necessary if the quantity of pork purchased by consumers is to change.

c. Lamb. We consume very little lamb in the United States; current consumption averages just 1.1 pounds per capita annually. Therefore, it contributes very little to our diet. Lamb suffers, like other meats, from excess fat production through current production systems. On the basis of separable lean, lamb cuts range from 5.6 to 15.2% fat, depending on the cut and type of feeding system (Table 6). Lamb is one of the few meats where fat content has actually increased over the last two decades [7]. Technology is needed to reduce fat in lamb, both trim fat and in separable lean, to produce products consistent with needs of fat- and calorie-conscious consumers. If the

Table 5 Nutrient Composition of Pork (100 g, separable lean only, edible portion)

Cut	kcal	Protein (g)	Total fat (g)	SFA[a] (g)	Stearic acid[b] (g)	MFA[c] (g)	PUFA[d] (g)	Cholesterol (mg)
Bacon, Canadian, grilled	185	24.24	8.44	2.84	0.88	4.04	0.81	58
Bacon, fried	576	30.45	49.24	17.42	5.67	23.69	5.81	85
Ham, cured, roasted (11% fat)	178	22.62	9.02	3.12	1.05	4.44	1.41	59
Ham, extra lean, roasted (5% fat)	145	20.93	5.53	1.81	0.57	2.62	0.54	53
Leg, whole roasted	220	28.32	11.03	3.80	1.22	4.96	1.34	94
Rump	221	29.14	10.66	3.67	1.18	4.79	1.29	96
Shank	215	28.21	10.50	3.62	1.16	4.72	1.27	92
Loin, blade, roasted	279	24.68	19.30	6.65	2.13	8.68	2.34	89
Center, broiled	231	32.00	10.48	3.61	1.16	4.71	1.27	98
Center rib, broiled	258	28.82	14.94	5.15	1.65	6.71	1.81	94
Sirloin, roasted	236	27.49	13.17	4.54	1.45	5.92	1.60	90
Tenderloin, roasted	166	28.79	4.81	1.66	0.53	2.16	0.58	93
Whole, broiled	257	27.84	15.29	5.27	1.68	6.87	1.86	95
Shoulder, whole, roasted	244	25.38	14.99	5.17	1.65	6.74	1.82	97
Boston, blade, roasted	256	24.36	16.84	5.80	1.86	7.57	2.04	98
Picnic arm, braised	248	32.26	12.21	4.21	1.35	5.49	1.48	114

Pork products in this table have no carbohydrates.
[a]Saturated fatty acids.
[b]Stearic acid ($C_{18:0}$) is a saturated fatty acid that, unlike other saturated fatty acids, does not raise the plasma cholesterol level.
[c]Monounsaturated fatty acids.
[d]Polyunsaturated fatty acids.
Source: Ref. 38.

Table 6 Nutritional Composition of Cooked Lamb (100 g, separable lean only, edible portion)

Cut	Age group[a]	kcal	Protein (g)	Total fat (g)	Cholesterol (mg)
Arm chop, braised	A	227	35.97	13.81	119
	B	280	35.18	14.36	124
Blade chop, roasted	A	229	26.71	12.79	96
	B	197	25.79	9.65	86
Foreshank, braised	A	198	32.61	6.47	106
	B	176	29.42	5.57	102
Leg—shank, roasted	A	184	28.42	7.00	95
	B	176	27.84	6.35	79
Leg—sirloin, roasted	A	221	29.96	10.29	100
	B	187	27.00	8.05	84
Loin chop, broiled	A	221	29.77	10.42	97
	B	211	30.20	8.92	92
Rib roast, roasted	A	248	25.96	15.16	92
	B	217	26.36	11.57	83

[a]A animals were 4–4.5 months of age at slaughter and raised on shelled corn and mineral-vitamin pellets. B animals were 8–9 months of age at slaughter and raised on pasture supplemented with shelled corn and mineral-vitamin pellets. Most retail lamb in the United States is type B.
Source: Ref. 39.

fat content is not reduced, the already low level of consumption is sure to decline.

d. Veal.   Like lamb, veal is consumed in small amounts annually with a per capita consumption of 1.5 pounds in the United States. Several types of veal are marketed depending on age and nutritional program employed. Veal may be produced with calves receiving only milk for a month or a liquid diet with deficient or adequate iron to produce pale or pink meat products. Veal is normally a lean product, with between 3 and 10% fat in separable lean depending on cut of meat and feeding system (Table 7).

e. Poultry.   Poultry makes up a substantial fraction of meat consumed in the United States. The entire edible portion of a chicken, including skin, giblets, and neck, contains 14.8% fat when raw [8]. The content of fat in chicken changes dramatically depending on how it is prepared. When the whole chicken is batter dipped and fried, it will contain 17.5 g of fat in a 100-g edible portion. When it is flour coated and fried it will contain 15.3 g of fat. Roasting the same chicken would result in 13.3 g of fat per 100 g of edible meat, whereas if the chicken were stewed it would contain only 12.4 g of fat in the edible tissue.

Table 7 Nutritional Composition of Cooked Veal (100 g, separable lean only, edible portion)

Cut	Type of veal[a]	kcal	Protein (g)	Total fat (g)	Cholesterol (mg)
Arm steak, braised	B	173	33.9	3.09	174
	SFV	206	36.1	5.73	152
Blade steak, braised	B	163	31.4	3.15	182
	SFV	204	32.9	7.06	154
Cutlet, pan fried	B	178	32.7	4.24	154
	SFV	184	33.3	4.69	120
Loin chop, braised	B	188	31.7	5.82	192
	SFV	233	33.9	9.74	148
Rib roast, roasted	B	134	25.0	2.98	142
	SFV	185	25.9	8.23	128
Sirloin chop, braised	B	178	32.8	4.16	186
	SFV	208	34.1	6.93	133

[a]B = Bob veal, which is from animals raised on maternal milk and slaughtered at less than 4 weeks of age (predominantly grade USDA Select). SFV = special-fed veal, which is from animals fed a special formulated liquid diet and slaughtered at about 16 weeks of age (predominantly grade USDA Choice). USDA Choice and Select grades of beef are from animals less than 42 months of age.
Source: Ref. 40.

As specific cuts of the chicken are prepared differently, with or without the skin, fat content changes in a manner reflecting method of preparation, where on the carcass the cut is taken from, and the type of muscle tissue contained in that area. Table 8 illustrates selected cuts of chicken prepared in different ways, with and without the skin. Because chicken without skin tends to lose more moisture than chicken with the skin, the normal cooking techniques for skinless and skin-covered meat are different. While light meat without skin can be low in fat, most poultry is consumed with preparation methods that result in a much higher-fat product as consumed. Batter-fried chicken can have twice the fat as roasted chicken. Composition of fat in batter-fried chicken, therefore, reflects the composition of fat added in cooking, as well as fat in the fresh meat.

Dark meats also have more fat than light meats in both chicken and turkey, as noted in Table 9. Also, comparisons of chicken to other poultry products indicate a wide range in percentage fat in the edible portion from 3.2% in light meat from turkey to over 28% in duck.

f. Fish. A variety of fish and fish products are consumed in the United States, and their composition for comparison to animal products is indicated

Table 8 Effect of Cooking Technique on Fat Content of Selected Retail Cuts of Chicken[a]

With skin	Batter-dipped and fried	Flour-coated and fried	Roasted	Stewed
Light meat	15.4	12.1	10.9	10.0
Dark meat	18.6	16.9	15.8	14.7
Specific cuts				
Breast	13.2	8.9	7.8	7.4
Drumstick	15.8	13.7	11.2	10.6
Leg	16.2	14.4	13.5	12.9
Thigh	16.5	15.0	15.5	14.7
Wing	21.8	22.2	19.5	16.8
Without skin	Fried		Roasted	Stewed
Light meat	5.5		4.5	4.0
Dark meat	11.6		9.7	9.0
Specific cuts				
Breast	4.7		3.6	3.0
Drumstick	8.1		5.7	5.7
Leg	9.3		8.4	8.1
Thigh	10.3		10.9	9.8
Wing	9.2		8.1	7.2

[a]Quantity is grams in a 100-gram edible portion of broiler or fryer chicken.
Source: Ref. 8.

in Table 10. As with other meats, method of preparation has a major impact on composition of the product as consumed. As evident, steamed fish products tend to be very low in fat, while commonly consumed breaded forms have 10–12.6% fat. Thus, fish as commonly consumed in a breaded form, has more fat than commonly prepared beef and pork cuts as consumed.

B. Consumption of Meat and Poultry

In the years between 1965 and 1985, per capita disappearance of beef increased by about 7%. The annual disappearance of red meats had actually fallen to only 74.4 pounds, which is more than 16% less than it was for the all-time high of 89.0 pounds in 1976. During that time, however, the disappearance of chicken increased 72% [9]. The shift in consumer preference for poultry over beef has been in part a result of the change in consumer perceptions of what healthful foods are.

Table 9 Nutrient Composition of Poultry (100 g, edible portion)

Part	kcal	Protein (g)	Carbohydrate (g)	Total fat (g)	SFA[a] (g)	Stearic acid[b] (g)	MFA[c] (g)	PUFA[d] (g)	Cholesterol (mg)
Chicken, without skin									
Dark meat, roasted	205	27.37	0	9.73	2.66	0.63	3.56	2.26	93
Light meat, roasted	173	30.91	0	4.51	1.27	0.32	1.54	0.98	85
Chicken, with skin									
Breast									
Fried, batter-dipped	260	24.84	8.99	13.20	3.52	1.04	5.46	3.08	85
Fried, flour-coated	222	31.84	1.64	8.87	2.45	0.58	3.50	1.96	89
Roasted	197	29.80	0	7.78	2.19	0.45	3.03	1.66	84
Stewed	184	27.39	0	7.42	2.08	0.42	2.90	1.58	75
Leg									
Fried, batter-dipped	273	21.77	8.72	16.17	4.28	1.25	6.58	3.85	90
Fried, flour-coated	254	26.84	2.50	14.43	3.90	0.95	5.68	3.33	94
Duck, roasted									
Meat only	201	23.48	0	11.20	4.17	1.27	3.70	1.43	89
Meat with skin	337	18.99	0	28.35	9.67	2.43	12.90	3.65	84
Turkey, roasted									
Dark meat only	187	28.57	0	7.22	2.42	0.72	1.64	2.16	85
Dark meat with skin	221	27.49	0	11.54	3.49	0.90	3.65	3.09	89
Light meat only	157	29.90	0	3.22	1.03	0.31	0.56	0.86	69
Light meat with skin	197	28.57	0	8.33	2.34	0.55	2.84	2.01	76

[a]Saturated fatty acids.
[b]Stearic acid ($C_{18:0}$) is a saturated fatty acid that, unlike other saturated fatty acids, does not raise the plasma cholesterol level.
[c]Monounsaturated fatty acids.
[d]Polyunsaturated fatty acids.
Source: Ref. 8.

Table 10 Nutrient Composition of Fish (100 g, separable lean only, edible portion)

Product	kcal	Protein (g)	Carbohydrate (g)	Total fat (g)	SFA[a] (g)	Stearic acid[b] (g)	MFA[c] (g)	PUFA[d] (g)	Cholesterol (mg)
Crab, blue									
Crab cake	155	20.2	0.5	7.5	1.48	0.49	2.82	2.27	150
Steamed	102	20.2	0.0	1.8	0.23	0.06	0.28	0.68	100
Haddock									
Breaded-fried	205	19.2	7.5	10.4	2.60	1.04	4.38	2.71	80
Broiled	112	24.2	0.0	0.9	0.17	0.04	0.15	0.31	74
Halibut									
Breaded-fried	226	21.0	7.5	11.9	2.78	1.05	4.96	3.16	57
Broiled	140	26.7	0.0	2.9	0.42	0.06	0.97	0.94	41
Oyster, eastern									
Breaded-fried	197	8.8	11.6	12.6	3.20	1.11	4.70	3.31	81
Canned	69	7.1	3.9	2.5	0.63	0.06	0.25	0.74	55
Scallop									
Breaded-fried	215	18.1	10.1	10.9	2.67	1.06	4.50	2.86	61
Steamed	112	21.2	3.0	1.0	0.10	0.01	0.05	0.33	42
Shrimp									
Breaded-fried	242	21.4	11.5	12.3	2.09	0.54	3.81	5.09	177
Steamed	99	20.9	0.0	1.1	0.29	0.10	0.20	0.44	195
Surimi	99	15.2	6.9	0.9	0.18	0.03	0.14	0.46	30
Tuna									
Light, oil pack	199	29.1	0.0	8.2	1.53	0.09	2.95	2.89	65
White, water pack	136	26.7	0.0	2.5	0.65	0.10	0.65	0.92	56

[a]Saturated fatty acids.
[b]Stearic acid ($C_{18:0}$) is a saturated fatty acid that, unlike other saturated fatty acids, does not raise the plasma cholesterol level.
[c]Monounsaturated fatty acids.
[d]Polyunsaturated fatty acids.
Source: Human Nutrition Information Service, USDA, unpublished data, 1987.

The other and perhaps primary impetus for change in consumption patterns is relative cost. Overall, beef prices have fallen by nearly one third from the 1979 all-time high to 1989 prices. Poultry prices fell at the same time; however, their decline was more rapid, which resulted in a ratio of beef to broiler prices of 2.9 [10]. The combination of health concerns and price have primarily controlled most American's meat eating patterns. Some would argue that the beef:poultry price ratio needs to be 2:1 or less.

Concern over fat, saturated fat, and cholesterol content has caused many consumers to modify their intake of beef and chicken. In the 1930s fat intake was about 34% of energy intake. It rose to 40–42% in the 1950s and 1960s. Since that time fat intake has fallen to 36% [11]. Currently, 36% of the total calories in the food supply are from animal products. Of these calories, ~15% are from red meat, ~4% from animal fats, and ~3.5% from poultry. Of the fat available for consumption, approximately 57% is from animal products. However, as stated before, it is important to remember that a large percentage, ranging from 6 to 33% of the fat available, will be removed prior to cooking or as table waste and is never eaten. Animal fat's contribution to total fat intake has decreased from 70% in 1957–1959 to 58% in 1984 [9].

Because of the differences in distribution of fatty acids (saturated, monounsaturated, and polyunsaturated) between animal and plant tissues, it is normal for consumers to expect to alter their intake of fatty acids by modifying their diets. Of the total fatty acids in beef, 50.6% are saturated fatty acids. However, about one third of the saturated fat in beef is stearic acid, which may actually reduce cholesterol when fed in diets for humans, and cannot be considered as a health risk. Saturated fatty acids from chicken make up 31.1% of the total fatty acids. Further, it is important to remember that meats are trimmed of external fat prior to cooking and eating. Animals tend to deposit more saturated fatty acids in internal organ fat areas and in deposits with large fat cells than in fat found in marbling as intramuscular fat, which lends desirable flavor and textural characteristics.

Vegetable oils are one of the primary sources of saturated fatty acids in our diet. In 1985 the per capita disappearance of vegetable fat was 51.2 pounds, as compared to only 12.8 pounds of animal fat. Palm oil, palm kernel oil, and coconut oil have 51.2, 84.2, and 91% saturated fatty acids. Corn oil and olive oil fatty acids are less saturated (14.4 and 16.2%, respectively). However, because these oils are used in so many products and because of the large volume of them that are consumed, they contribute a significant amount of the total intake of saturated fatty acids for most diets [9].

C. Need to Modify Current Meat Composition

Current production practices, although better than those historically used for lean meat production, still result in approximately 6 billion pounds of waste and trim fat from beef alone [12]. Fat is not only expensive to produce and remove (about $2 billion each year) [13], but also poses a health threat to American consumers who consume between 29 and 35% of their dietary caloric intake as fat [14]. Any attempt to reduce fat intake would require that consumers purchase only those cuts of meat that already contain lower amounts of fat. However, if strategies were developed that would produce meat products that are inherently low in fat, consumers could easily have a wide array of choices made available to them.

According to the Surgeon General, dietary excesses or imbalances are the basis for 5 of the 10 leading causes of death in the United States [15]. Death is usually the result of prolonged exposure to such risks as high blood pressure, obesity, or carcinogens. The 1987 data report that 1.25 million heart attacks occur in the United States, causing more than 510,000 deaths. Cancers, some of which are diet related, cause more than 476,000 consumers to die each year. Nearly 2 million people suffer from stroke-related problems, with more than 148,000 dying as a result of strokes each year. The Surgeon General recommends choosing foods that are low in fat and cholesterol and using food-preparation methods that do not contribute additional fat to the foods to reduce the incidence of diet-related diseases. Foods that can be consumed without elevating fat intake include poultry and lean meats [15].

Cholesterol content of foods and dietary cholesterol intake is a perceived concern of many people, even though most circulating cholesterol comes from body synthesis and not the diet. Most individuals, not at risk because of genetic disease states, respond to increased dietary cholesterol by reducing absorption. Therefore, the contribution of dietary cholesterol to serum cholesterol is less than that of saturated fat [16]. Figure 2 indicates the relative cholesterol levels in a variety of foods consumed. It is apparent that those foods often considered by consumers to be low in cholesterol are actually quite high, and that beef, often considered as having the highest amount of cholesterol per serving, is quite similar to chicken or fish. Reiser and Shorland [17] have concluded, based on the results of several studies, that meat fats do not increase blood cholesterol when they are included in a balanced diet. They therefore concluded that all fat, in moderation, is safe for consumption.

It does not take much consideration to realize that the American diet could be causing a great deal of the discomfort, distress, and emotional or economic losses in the United States. Granted, everyone will die of some disease eventually and correlations between diet and cause of death are not cause-and-effect statements; it still becomes obvious that Americans (especially those at risk) should modify their diets to reduce total caloric intake. Reducing intake of fats, regardless of source, would be of assistance in reducing caloric intake because of the high energy density of fat and the lower desirability and, therefore, lower consumption of diets lower in fat.

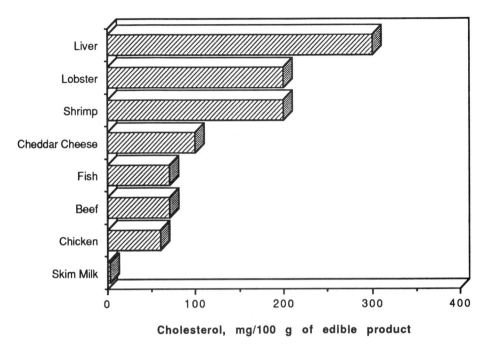

Figure 2 Cholesterol content of animal protein sources. (From Ref. 41.)

II. OPTIONS FOR MODIFYING CONTENT AND COMPOSITION OF ANIMAL PRODUCTS

A. What Needs to Be Modified in Animal Food Products?

Food products suitable for biotechnological modification include meat, milk, and eggs. Many animal products currently produced may need to be modified to provide foods more closely aligned with contemporary nutrient needs and food choices of specific consumers. For many reasons, the amount of fat, specifically those fatty acids known to elevate cholesterol production (e.g., 16:0, palmitic acid [42]) or those known to enhance tumor growth, may need to be reduced in the diets of some individuals. Hence, appropriate changes in both fat content of foods and composition of fat present (fatty acids) may be desirable. Cholesterol levels in foods per se are not as important, because only a small fraction of this cholesterol is absorbed—therefore diet contributes only a very small fraction of the overall daily cholesterol production in humans. Nevertheless, consumer perceptions indicate that a reduction in cholesterol levels in animal foods would also be desirable.

Other modifications could also be useful. For example, the amount and type of protein present in foods is also important, and changes in animal function to produce consumer-desired types of protein (e.g., white vs. red meat, fiber size, etc.) would be useful.

B. Mechanisms to Modify Animal Products

Animal food products represent an integration of events ranging from initiation to harvest, and from postharvest processing to produce, preserve, and deliver foods to consumers. In turn, biotechnological options to modify animal products exist in all segments of production. Some key options include modification of substrates used, modification of growth and systemic production processes, and postharvest product processing. These are accomplished in several ways and can be categorized as follows:

1. Genetic control of growth
2. Feedstuff selection and processing
3. Digestive tract processing physiology
4. Physiological repartitioning
5. Tissue-specific modification

Repartitioning of growth and the consequent modification of animal products has received major attention in recent years. Repartitioning clearly provides the most direct and efficacious mechanism for changing the protein and fat content of animal tissues. The objective is to repartition the growth patterns in animals to produce leaner animal products and less fat from all animals. While repartitioning is the eventual goal of many genetic engineering initiatives, systems employing these concepts such as transgenic animals are not likely to surface any time soon. A number of options are feasible in developing systems employing growth-regulating biotechnology in several forms to produce leaner animal products, including the following:

Genetics
Endogenous regulation
    Intact animals
    Castrated/spayed
    Autoimmunization
Exogenous regulation
    Repartitioning agents
        Estrogens
        Zeranol
        Androgens (e.g., teststerone benzoate)
        Growth hormone
        Beta agonists
        Growth hormone–releasing factor

Mechanisms of regulation include priorities for protein versus fat, redirection of nutrients, tissue mobilization, and limits for daily deposition.

All options listed above have been investigated to varying degrees across animal species in developing targeted growth-management systems to most efficiently produce desired leaner animal products. While genetic directives provide general targets for body and carcass composition, other factors really determine the extent to which these theoretical limits will actually be reached or how patterns and priorities for growth will be followed or translated into and realized as growth. In all animal types, the energy available translates genetic directives through tissue regulation into patterns of growth.

Carcass animal products reflect accumulative growth from birth to slaughter. As a consequence, use of growth-regulation biotechnologies from birth to slaughter provides lifetime growth regulation and provides the maximal redirection of nutrients from fat to protein and lean tissue production. The longer growth regulators are provided, the greater the increase in total lean animal product with a simultaneous reduction in fat.

While several options exist for producing leaner animal products, the product must be acceptable, even desirable, in the marketplace. Thus, the degree to which these production strategies impact the production of lean animal products must be assessed in terms of product acceptability. For example, forage-fed beef, because of its darker and softer lean, will not have the retail case shelf life equal to that of grain-fed beef. This presents a serious problem from the consumer acceptance standpoint. Meat from these carcasses is also borderline in taste acceptability.

1. Genetic Control Over Composition

One of today's easiest methods of controlling body composition is to use breeds of livestock that, because of genetically determined base patterns of metabolism or priorities for specific tissue growth, deposit less fat and more lean meat [18]. In general, typically lean, later-maturing animals have a greater capacity to deposit protein on a daily basis and will deposit more lean at any rate of gain. Therefore, when attempting to alter carcass composition, the genetic makeup of the animal, along with the rate of growth, must be considered because they are interrelated.

Although the route of genetic selection to decrease fat in the carcass is easy in concept, it is actually very difficult to achieve. Because of consumer preferences for products that meet certain desirability characteristics, animals that produce higher quantities of lean are not as acceptable. Fat contributes to taste, texture, and flavor of meats, and therefore, when it is drastically altered, consumer acceptance is also affected [5]. Therefore, animals that are extremely lean would not generate an acceptable carcass without using excessively long feeding periods to increase the quantity of intramuscular fat, if possible even then. This would also result in much larger-sized cuts of meat because of the larger mature size of these animals—a problem because beef carcasses are already often larger than desired and are discounted.

For example, the traditional method to increase the production of lean beef is by feeding larger mature-size cattle. However, an increase in mature size requires a larger mature-size cow, which also has greater requirements per unit of weight, greatly increasing maintenance energy committed to beef production. An example of this would be Chianina cattle, which can produce large, lean carcasses that concomitantly require more feed energy for maintenance due to their larger mature size. Large mature-size cows commonly require more feed resources, especially energy, than most range resources will support, requiring supplementation for much of the production cycle. Therefore, a more effective approach would be to modify the patterns of growth in cattle to produce more lean beef from all cattle produced. Similar concerns exist for other species but to differing degrees.

However, when growth is regulated in animals that typically produce a higher amount of fat, carcass fat content is reduced and the amount of edible lean tissue is increased. Regulation of growth and carcass composition can be achieved by several mechanisms aside from genetic factors, such as shortening the feeding period, feeding a calorically less dense diet, adjusting diet protein levels and fatty acid composition of the diet, and using exogenous growth regulators. These will be now discussed in detail.

2. Feeding Strategies to Modify Composition

a. Feedstuff Selection and Processing. Although this is an area that has received substantial attention, especially in recent years, feedstuff selection and processing is not a new phenomenon. For quite some time, mechanisms that modify the fatty acid composition of animal products have been established, particularly in animals, with minimal microbial modification of feeds prior to absorption. For example, the fatty acid composition of pork and poultry products largely reflects dietary fatty acid composition. As a consequence, composition of fat within some limits can be modified easily in meat products from these species through the selection of feed ingredients. Once a desirable combination of fatty acids for human needs is clearly established, feeding/management systems can be developed to produce products that better reflect these needs.

Further opportunities to modify the fatty acid composition of products such as meat and milk from cattle and sheep are limited currently and will require development of a novel biotechnology to make substantial progress. Selection and processing of feedstuffs to limit microbial access to, and modification of, fatty acids represents an area of current interest and considerable challenge. Some progress with calcium and other salts of fatty acids (i.e., fatty acid soaps) has been demonstrated, and products are currently being marketed for dairy cattle, primarily to increase energy intake and milk fat production with lesser emphasis on modification of milk fat composition. Further development of related biotechnology will be required to produce significant modification of fatty acid composition of beef or lamb products.

b. Digestive Tract Physiology. Much research has been conducted on digestive physiology in order to understand the absorption mechanisms for various nutrients and substrates for metabolism. Biotechnological applications in two major areas may be important. First, options that alter the distribution or function of specific microbes in the fermentative compartments of the digestive tract of ruminants may in turn alter the substrates delivered for use to the animal tissues. Possible modifications include volatile fatty acids and long-chain fatty acid modification and synthesis, resulting in altered composition of fat in animal food products produced. Second, modification of the digestive tract conditions and processing through pH, enzyme activity, flow rates, passage, retention time, and absorptive mechanisms, among others, will allow altered substrate delivery to animal tissues to modify growth and composition.

c. Feeding Systems Management. Meat production obviously starts with the young animal (Fig. 3). Therefore, it is not a surprise that the young animal is the logical starting point for altering nutritional management to effectively produce more lean, less fat, and fat of modified composition. Some of the possible management practices for preweaning cattle include reducing milk production of dams, not providing supplemental creep feeds, not castrating bulls, and providing an implant containing anabolic compounds [18].

Once the calf has been weaned and placed on a stocker or backgrounding program, it is important to manage stocking rates to control availability of supplements and high-quality forages to achieve desired growth rates and defer growth as needed [18]. Supplements should be limited to those key nutrients limiting in the primary feeds and forages. Growth-regulating implants should also be used in this phase.

The feedlot phase represents an opportunity for controlled feeding in production of beef. Animals are confined to an area and receive only the feed provided. This leaves the feeder in a position where the period length and level of nutrient availability can be closely controlled. For example, using shorter feeding periods to limit fat accretion, grouping cattle according to feeding period length, or slaughtering individual animals as they reach an established endpoint would reduce excess fat. Animals in feedlots should also receive exogenous growth-regulating agents to maximize protein gain and further control fat gain.

Animals, like humans, are the net result of what has happened to them and what they have consumed throughout their lives. Therefore, these strategies should be designed for each animal type and adhered to throughout

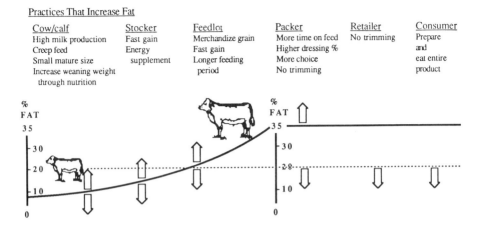

Practices That Increase Fat

Cow/calf	Stocker	Feedlot	Packer	Retailer	Consumer
High milk production	Fast gain	Merchandize grain	More time on feed	No trimming	Prepare
Creep feed	Energy	Fast gain	Higher dressing %		and
Small mature size	supplement	Longer feeding	More choice		eat entire
Increase weaning weight through nutrition		period	No trimming		product

Practices That Increase Lean or Reduce Fat

Lower milk production	Deferred growth	Shorter feeding period	Trim fat	Trim retail cuts	Trim products
No supplement	Implant hormones	Continuous implant	to 1/4"	to 1/4" or less	Discard plate
Implant hormones		of hormones	Yield grade	Boneless trimmed	waste
Bulls			specifications	products	Discard fat drippings

Figure 3 Practices that can be applied throughout the lifetime of an animal that affect the fat content of beef. Adapted from Byers et al., [18]. Reprinted with permission from *Designing Foods,* © 1988 by the National Academy of Sciences. Published by National Academy Press, Washington, D.C.

the animal's life (see Fig. 3) if the desired product is to be produced by the most efficient means.

3. Current Status of Composition Modifiers

Current technologies used in animal production modify growth, resulting in leaner products with less fat. For example, beef production incorporates anabolic implants, which produce a leaner product. Emerging technologies promise similar options for pork and poultry, with applications for fish as well. It would be unfortunate if safe, efficacious technologies for producing safer and healthier consumer-desired animal products were rejected by consumers on the basis of misinformation through special interest (i.e., vegetarian, animal rights) groups with unpublished agendas. In assessing options for the use of biotechnologies, those that enhance real and/or perceived product quality or safety and the quality of life of the consumer are most readily accepted. Unfortunately, the value of these technologies has not been communicated to consumers with the same message penetration as the emotional appeal for "natural" food-production systems.

Products approved for use in the United States to modify animal growth and body composition include zeranol, a combination of estradiol-17β and progesterone (for steers), and a combination of testosterone and progesterone (for heifers). These three products are used routinely in operations, primarily at the feedlot level. As one progresses further and further back in the life of an animal, fewer of these products are used. This is primarily because many cow/calf operators have only a few animals and are not prepared to use these technologies.

These compounds are estrogenic agents, in that their mechanism(s) of action closely resemble the response of an animal to estrogen. All three cause an increase in rate of gain. The amount of response will depend on animal size, availability of nutrients, and other production practices. An increase in the quantity of protein deposited is also achieved with these products at any rate of gain. Therefore, the animals are producing more protein at a constant rate of gain or are producing even more protein as the rate of gain increases with product usage [18].

As mentioned before, fat is essential for certain quality characteristics of meat. The estrogenic agents are capable of reducing the quantity of undesirable fat depot sites, such as internal fat, seam fat, and subcutaneous fat, while not significantly reducing the quantity of intramuscular fat [18]. Intramuscular fat, commonly called marbling, is primarily responsible for meat flavor, juiciness, and textural characteristics. Therefore, estrogenic agents are capable of inhibiting deposition of fat that is not essential for product quality without altering deposition of fat responsible for the attributes that make meat a desirable food item.

a. Safety Background. Growth regulators currently approved for use with beef cattle are either endogenous compounds already present in humans and animals (e.g., estrogen, testosterone, or progesterone), or are compounds developed through biotechnology to mimic these endogenous substances (e.g., zeranol or trenbolone acetate). None of these compounds are ever fed to animals in the United States. Instead, they are placed in the ear, which does not normally enter the food chain. When used in cattle, production residues in meat are extremely low and lower than naturally occurring levels in meat from cows and bulls. Levels of hormones produced in people every day are many thousands to millions times greater than present in meat either naturally or as a result of use of a growth regulator in cattle. Also, other foods, especially vegetables, salad oil, etc., provide thousands of times more estrogen than meat from cattle [43], whether receiving growth regulators or not, and less than 10% of what is consumed is absorbed by humans—so the contribution from beef is truly negligible.

Growth regulators in development, including growth hormone, beta agonists, growth hormone releasing factor, and immunization will be equally safe but also subject to public perception.

b. European Economic Community Safety Issues.   The European Economic Community (EEC) imposed a ban on beef imports from the United States and other countries using anabolic growth regulators commonly referred to as "hormones." The ban was originally launched under the guise of "safety" issues. The directive for the ban has been adopted by the EEC, although all safety issues were dismissed long ago by the EEC's own commission, "The Lamming Commission," and by the United States' own regulatory agencies, the Food Safety and Inspection Service (FSIS) branch of USDA and FDA.

In contrast to the United States, where biotechnology is tightly and efficiently regulated such that no violative residues were found in the past 4 years of the USDA-FSIS National Residue Program, as much as one fourth of the beef produced in the EEC contains unacceptable residues of compounds never cleared for use in cattle. Some of these compounds are known carcinogens such as diethylstylbesterol. A safety issue exists with EEC beef because of the use of unapproved "cocktails" of many potent drugs directly injected into the muscle of growing cattle on EEC farms, which came about as a result of bans on the use of approved products started in the late 1980s.

c. Animal Growth Regulators.   Some of the proposed new products for modifying animal growth and composition include growth hormone, growth hormone releasing factor, beta-adrenergic agonists, and immunization strategies for endogenous factors that limit growth or modify tissue deposition. Growth hormone, administered itself or via increased secretion caused by administering its releasing factor, causes increased rates of gain and an increase in the quantity of protein in gain [18]. Growth hormone also decreases the utilization of glucose for fat synthesis [19]. The combined effect of increasing rate of protein gain, rate of gain, and reduced fat deposition causes animals that have elevated levels of growth hormone to have larger carcasses that contain more lean retail product and less excess fat.

Beta-adrenergic agonists block beta-adrenergic receptors on the surface of adipocytes and skeletal muscles. Fat accretion in a carcass is the result of lipid synthesis, reesterification, and lipolysis. Beta-adrenergic agents stimulate lipolysis and inhibit lipogenesis [20]. As the quantity of nutrients used for lipogenesis is reduced and the quantity released by lipolysis is increased, nutrients are effectively shifted away from deposition of fat and are made available to support both maintenance energy needs and to support deposition of protein.

The net effect of growth is regulated by stimulators and inhibitors. One of the principal inhibitors of growth is somatostatin. Somatostatin inhibits the release of growth hormone and functions to regulate the growth of peripheral tissues in this manner. Therefore, by immunizing an animal against somatostatin, at least part of the normally circulating somatostatin would be bound to antibodies and be incapable of affecting growth hormone release. Research has indicated that this approach is capable of producing a short-term increase in the rate of growth in rats and steers [21]. Studies conducted by Spencer [22] indicated that although rate of gain was increased in lambs immunized against somatostatin, body composition was not changed. However, if one assumes that a standard size is preferable for most meat cuts, immunized animals would be slaughtered earlier than controls. Normal biological growth results in an increasing amount of fat being deposited as body size increases. Therefore, immunized lambs would have less fat at a given body weight [21].

4. Postharvest Mechanisms

a. Trimming.   Once the carcass is obtained, extensive trimming occurs to remove external and internal fat. The carcass is chilled and then processed into subprimal and primal cuts. At that point, further trimming of excess fat occurs. The primal cuts are prepared for boxed beef or shipped to retail distributors, at which point the meat is further trimmed in preparation for retail display. Currently, most large food chains adhere to a fat cover of 0.25 inch or less [9]. This alone has contributed greatly to the quantity of available fat presented to the consumer. However, further steps need to be taken. Some of the alternatives include use of injectors for delivery of tenderizers that might convert very lean meat sources into a more palatable product [23].

b. Processed Products.   One of the possibilities in generating a low-fat diet containing meat is to process prepared foods using lower-fat meats. However, depending on the product and the type of lower-fat meats used, consumer acceptability can be reduced [24]. Overall, if the product contains less than about 15% fat, acceptability is reduced. Achieving this fat level for most intact cuts of beef requires use of the growth regulators, integrated management systems, and extensive trimming after slaughter. However, these levels can be achieved in processed products.

Processed products include such foods as sausages, ground meat, frankfurters, and deli-style meat loaves. Research has centered on addition of products as a substitution for fat to reduce the overall fat content. In 1988 USDA changed its regulations to allow the substitution of water for fat in cooked sausages such as frankfurters, bologna, etc. [25]. Some of the other compounds used to dilute fat content are whey protein [26], soy flour [27], corn starch [28], and tofu [29]. These have met with moderate success depending on the product type developed and its preparation for consumption. Some of the research on various processing techniques have incorporated carrageenan [30], polydextrose or maltodextrins [31], methylcellulose [30,32], and synthetic products such as olestra into low-fat meat emulsions. Products (e.g., McDonald's McLean Deluxe) containing carrageenan, soy flours, wheat glutens, etc. are currently being marketed to fill consumer desires for lower-fat, lower-calorie ground beef products. Several other products are being tested, however, FDA approval for their use in nonexperimental foods has yet to be received [33].

5. Technologies, Management Strategies and Cost

The cost of beef from a Choice carcass is higher than that from a Select. Essentially, premiums are paid for Choice carcasses, whereas both Prime and Select carcasses are penalized. The actual price differential varies according to the area where the meat is produced and the local demand for certain types of products. However, certain cost factors are known to exist for producing established trim levels in carcasses of each grade (Table 11). For instance, to produce retail packages from 100 pounds of top round from a Select carcass of yield grade 2.5 would require 16–18 minutes, depending on the level of trim on the original material [34]. However, to produce the same product from a Choice carcass of yield grade 2.5 would require 18–20 minutes. This comparison points out the increased labor costs associated with producing a product with a desirable level of fat. Therefore, not only are the costs associated with producing an animal with a desirable carcass included in the cost of production, but so also are the extensive amount of labor required to achieve the desired level of fat in the marketed product. That is why use of technologies and management strategies to reduce fat content of meat will reduce final product cost.

Unique challenges face the animal industry in the design and development of new technologies that will allow production of lean animal products rather than require extensive trimming to make them lean. This will require development of greater lean tissue deposition throughout the life cycle and extensive redirection of feed energy from fat to protein growth through all phases of growth.

While the need to produce leaner, health-promoting animal products is clear, the segmentation of the industry, and its divergent goals, objectives, and profit centers, has resulted in mixed signals at best. In typical scenarios, incentives to produce fatter animal products often prevail. Incentives for producing leaner animal products must be established in all segments of the industry to assure coordination of growth toward optimal market endpoints.

Table 11 Time Required to Fabricate Selected Beef Cuts from Select or Choice Grade Carcasses[a]

Cut, initial trim	Retail trim	Select	Choice
Top round			
One inch	Quarter inch	17.09	19.16
	Eighth inch	17.26	19.32
	Total	15.91	17.97
Half inch	Quarter inch	18.16	20.22
	Eighth inch	18.02	20.08
	Total	16.81	18.87
Quarter inch	Quarter inch	15.85	17.91
	Eighth inch	16.03	18.09
	Total	16.56	18.62
Bottom sirloin			
One inch	Quarter inch	25.51	27.59
	Eighth inch	27.50	29.58
	Total	25.30	27.38
Half inch	Quarter inch	33.14	35.22
	Eighth inch	32.23	34.31
	Total	33.35	35.43
Quarter inch	Quarter inch	30.58	32.66
	Eighth inch	28.58	30.66
	Total	28.81	30.89
Rib			
One inch	Quarter inch	25.02	27.88
	Eighth inch	22.16	25.03
	Total	23.47	26.34
Half inch	Quarter inch	29.02	31.89
	Eighth inch	26.35	29.21
	Total	30.75	33.61
Quarter inch	Quarter inch	29.90	32.77
	Eighth inch	25.55	28.42
	Total	27.40	30.26

[a]All numbers are for yield-grade 2.5 carcasses. Time is in minutes.
Source: Ref. 34.

A primary challenge is to develop systems employing current and new biotechnologies that will allow us to produce specific uniform products from diverse animal production systems in a range of designer foods. Most important, we must (1) clearly define needed consumer attributes of specific products and then (2) derive targeted-integrated, biotechnology-based production systems to efficiently produce these products in order to (3) develop more desirable products than currently exist in the animal products industry. The food-production system from conception to consumption must be consumer driven and must focus on the final target product as biotechnology/production/management/marketing options are selected. Concurrently, all technology implemented in the production system must eventually be marketed to the final consumer as well; currently this is seldom accomplished. There will be increasingly limited opportunities to use technologies inconsistent with quality of life of consumers, and in the future, both the product as well as the system used to produce it will need to be consistent with consumer needs and attitudes.

The successful development and implementation of animal products will depend on consumer desires and demands. While animal-product biotechnologies have the potential to provide seemingly desirable products more efficiently than current systems, their introduction and development relies ultimately on consumer acceptance.

III. ROLE OF MEAT IN A LOW-FAT DIET

The information reviewed in this chapter has covered the basic level of fats in beef, pork, lamb, veal, chicken, and fish and how these levels are affected by the cut chosen, carcass grade, preparation, and cooking techniques. Also, we have presented information on why it is important to modify the current fat content of meat. Information concerning currently available techniques for modifying animal composition and developing techniques to reduce fat in meat in both the animal and product stages have been presented.

In concert with consumer desires to be, think, and eat "leaner," there is also an interest in reducing fat consumption (particularly saturated fat) and cholesterol levels—both dietary and circulating. The most common concerns are that animal products are high in calories, saturated fat, and cholesterol.

An average 3-oz serving of cooked lean beef, for example, provides only 73 mg of cholesterol, which is less than 25% of the American Heart Association's recommendation of less than 300 mg per day. This average 3-oz portion of cooked lean beef provides only 192 kilocalories of energy, less that 10% of a 2000-kilocalorie diet. Less than half of this energy (85 kcal) comes from fat, and the saturated fat component contributes only half of that. As is evident, lean animal products fit well within dietary guidelines; the challenge from the production perspective is to produce inherently lean animal products that do not require extensive trimming along the retail chain. Opportunities for reduction in fat and fatty acid modification will further advance the potential to deliver consumer-tailored, safe, and healthful animal products.

With this information as a base it is obvious that meat can be an integral part of a low-fat diet. The important criteria are an understanding of which cuts of meat to select, what the quality grades mean relative to fat content, and how to prepare the particular cut. Processed products are being developed that will further reduce fat content to the 5–9% level. Therefore, when part of a complete, varied diet, meat is easily included in a low-fat diet.

REFERENCES

1. USDA, *Composition of Foods: Beef Products,* Agriculture Handbook Number 8-13, U.S. Government Printing Office, Washington, DC (1986).
2. C. L. Davey and R. J. Winger, Muscle to meat (biochemical aspects), *Meat Science, Milk Science and Technology* (H. R. Cross and A. J. Overby, eds.), World Animal Science Series B, Elsevier Science Publishers, B.V., Amsterdam, pp. 3–31 (1988).
3. USDA, *Provisional Table on the Content of Stearic Acid, Total Fat and Other Fatty Acids in Selected Foods,* Human Nutrition Information Service Bulletin HNIS/PT-107 (1988).
4. J. W. Savell, J. J. Harris, H. R. Cross, D. S. Hale, and L. C. Beasley, National Beef Market Basket Survey, *J. Anim. Sci., 69*: 2883 (1991).
5. J. W. Savell and H. R. Cross, The role of fat in the palatability of beef, pork, and lamb, *Designing Foods: Animal Product Options in the Marketplace*, National Academy Press, Washington, DC, pp. 345–355 (1988).
6. G. C. Smith and Z. L. Carpenter, Eating quality of meat animal products and their fat content, *The Fat Content and Composition of Animal Products,* National Research Council, National Academy of Sciences, Washington, DC, p. 183 (1976).
7. H. R. Cross, K. E. Belk, and R. P. Garrett, *Pork and Lamb Quality*, A report submitted to the Task Force on Food Quality, L. Hill, Chairman, University of Illinois, (1991).
8. USDA, *Composition of Foods: Poultry Products*, Agriculture Handbook Number 8-5, U.S. Government Printing Office, Washington, DC (1979).
9. NAS/NRC, *Designing Foods: Animal Product Options in the Marketplace*, National Academy Press, Washington, DC (1988).
10. W. Kester, At the crossroads. Can the industry lower costs and satisfy customers?, *Beef, 27*: 6 (1991).

11. A. M. Stephen and N. J. Wald, Trends in individual consumption of dietary fat in the United States, 1920-1984, *Am. J. Clin. Nutr., 52*: 457 (1990).

12. F. M. Byers, Biotechnologically modified animal products, *Agricultural Biotechnology, Food Safety and Nutritional Quality for the Consumer* (J. F. McDonald, ed.), Union Press, Binghampton, NY, pp. 131-144 (1990).

13. Value Based Marketing Task Force, *The War on Fat!* National Cattlemen's Association and National Live Stock and Meat Board (1990).

14. W. C. Miller, A. K. Lindeman, J. Wallace, and M. Niederpruem, Diet composition, energy intake, and exercise in relation to body fat in men and women. *Am. J. Clin. Nutr., 52*: 426 (1990).

15. J. M. McGinnis and M. Nestle, The Surgeon General's report on nutrition and health: Policy implications and implementation strategies. *Am. J. Clin. Nutr., 49*: 23 (1989).

16. A. M. Gotto, Cholesterol intake and serum cholesterol, *N. Engl. J. Med., 324*: 912 (1991).

17. R. Reiser and F. B. Shorland, Meat fats and fatty acids, *Meat and Health: Advances in Meat Research*, Vol. 6 (A. M. Pearson and T. R. Dutson, eds.) Elsevier Applied Science, London, pp. 21-62 (1990).

18. F. M. Byers, H. R. Cross, and G. T. Schelling, Integrated nutrition, genetics, and growth management programs for lean beef production, *Designing Foods: Animal Product Options in the Marketplace*, National Academy Press, Washington, DC, pp. 283-291 (1988).

19. H. M. Goodman, The role of growth hormone in fat mobilization, *Designing Foods: Animal Product Options in the Marketplace*, National Academy Press, Washington, DC, pp. 163-172 (1988).

20. L. A. Muir, Effects of beta-adrenergic agonists on growth and carcass characteristics of animals, *Designing Foods: Animal Product Options in the Marketplace*, National Academy Press, Washington, DC, pp. 184-193 (1988).

21. G. T. Schelling and F. M. Byers. 1988. Immunization of beef cattle against somatostatin, *Designing Foods: Animal Product Options in the Marketplace*, National Academy Press, Washington, DC, pp. 200-207 (1988).

22. G. S. G. Spencer, Immuno-neutralization of somatostatin and its effects on animals production, *Domest. Anim. Endocr., 3*: 55 (1986).

23. P. J. Shand and G. R. Schmidt, New technology for low-fat meat products, *Proceedings of Reciprocal Meat Conference, 43*: 37 (1990).

24. A. M. Pearson, A. Asghar, J. I. Gray, and A. M. Booren, Impact of fat reduction on palatability and consumer acceptance of processed meat, *Proceedings of Reciprocal Meat Conference, 40*: 105 (1987).

25. USDA, Standard for frankfurters and similar cooked sausages, *Fed. Reg., 53*: 8425 (1988).

26. S. A. Ensor, R. W. Mandigo, C. R. Calkins, and L. N. Quint, Comparative evaluation of whey protein concentrate, soy protein isolate and calcium-reduced nonfat dry milk as binders in an emulsion-type sausage, *J. Food Sci., 52*: 1155 (1987).

27. R. K. Rockower, J. C. Deng, W. S. Otwell, and J. A. Cornell, Effect of soy flour, soy protein concentrate and sodium alginate on the textural attributes of minced fish patties, *J. Food Sci.*, *48*: 1048 (1983).

28. G. S. Mittal and W. R. Usborne, Meat emulsion functionality related to fat-protein ratio and selected dairy and cereal products, *Meat Sci.*, *18*: 1 (1986).

29. C.-Y. Jeng, H. W. Ockerman, V. R. Cahill, and A. C. Peng, Influence of substituting two levels of tofu for fat in a cooked comminuted meat-type product, *J. Food Sci.*, *53*: 97 (1988).

30. E. A. Foegeding and S. R. Ramsey. Effect of gums on low-fat meat batters, *J. Food Sci.*, *51*: 33 (1986).

31. B. F. Haumann, Getting the fat out. Researchers seek substitutes for full-fat fat, *J. Am. Oil Chem. Soc.*, *63*: 278 (1986).

32. S. E. Hill and K. J. Prusa, Physical and sensory properties of lean ground beef patties containing methylcellulose and hydroxypropylmethylcellulose, *J. Food Qual.*, *11*: 331 (1988).

33. J. T. Keeton, Fat substitutes and fat modification in processing, *Proceedings of Reciprocal Meat Conference*, *44*: (1991).

34. R. P. Garrett, R. W. Theis, J. P. Walter, D. B. Griffin, J. W. Savell, H. K. Johnson, T. Dockerty, J. W. Allen, and T. R. Pierson, *Communicating Cutability to the Retailer*, Final report to the Beef Industry Council of the National Live Stock and Meat Board (1991).

35. USDA, *Composition of Foods: Raw, Processed, and Prepared*, Agriculture Handbook No. 8, U.S. Government Printing Office, Washington, DC (1963).

36. USDA, *Marketing Research Report No. 849*, Economic Research Service, U.S. Department of Agriculture, Washington, DC (1969).

37. USDA, *ERS-675*, Economic Research Service, U.S. Department of Agriculture, Washington, DC (1982).

38. USDA, *Composition of Foods: Pork Products*, Agriculture Handbook No. 8-10, U.S. Government Printing Office, Washington, DC (1983).

39. K. Ono, B. W. Berry, H. K. Johnson, E. Russek, C. F. Parker, V. R. Cahill, and P. G. Althouse, Tables 2 and 5 in nutrient composition of lamb of two age groups, *J. Food Sci.*, *49*: 1233 (1984).

40. K. Ono, B. W. Berry, and L. W. Douglass, Table 2 in nutrient composition of some fresh and cooked retail cuts of veal, *J. Food Sci.*, *51*: 1352 (1986).

41. B. Simonsen, R. Hamm, and B. Rogowski, Meat as food, *Meat Science, Milk Science and Technology* (H. R. Cross, and A. J. Overby, eds.), World Animal Science Series B, Elsevier Science Publishers, B. V., Amsterdam, pp. 115–139 (1988).

42. A. Bonanome and S. M. Grundy, Effects of dietary stearic acid on plasma cholesterol and lipoprotein levels, *N. Engl. J. Med.*, *318*: 1244 (1988).

43. W. Velle, The use of hormones in animal production. FAO Animal Production and Health Paper, 31, Presented to Joint FAO/WHO Expert Committee on Food Additives, Geneva, 23 March–1 April, 1981, Food and Agriculture Organization of the United Nations, Rome (1982).

18
Impact of Low-Calorie Foods on Food Marketing

Robert C. Gatty *Gatty Communications, Inc., Columbia, Maryland*

This chapter describes the reaction of food retailers to the increased public interest in the role of diet in health and to the proliferation of new foods that seek to satisfy and capture this interest.

I. SURVEY OF SHOPPERS: NUTRITION SELLS

Food manufacturers and retailers operate by one simple rule: make and stock what sells. And today, what sells is food perceived as nutritious—that is, foods that are lower in fat, calories, cholesterol, and salt, and higher in fiber.

The 1990 annual survey of shoppers conducted by the Food Marketing Institute (FMI), a nonprofit research and education association for the retail grocery industry, found that 90% of shoppers pay at least some attention to the nutritional content of the food they eat [1]. More than half, 55%, are very concerned about nutritional content. At the same time, nearly two-thirds say that there is room for improvement in their diets. Shoppers say that they are eating more fruits and vegetables (57%); less red meat (34%), fats (27%), and sugar (19%); and more chicken (19%), fish (18%), and fiber (16%). Lower fat content in food emerged as the primary nutritional concern of shoppers, listed by 46% of those surveyed compared to 29% the previous year. Cholesterol, salt, and low calories also remained a concern.

But while interest in nutrition grows, retailers warn that taste remains the primary criterion in food selection. If something doesn't taste good, shoppers won't buy it, no matter how low in fat, sugar, or calories.

II. EFFECT OF NUTRITIONAL MESSAGE ON FOOD MARKETERS

A. More Nutritious Foods

Americans have grown used to a diet rich in salt, sugar, and fat. Until recently, food processors commonly added these ingredients to enhance flavor. The snack food craze further added to this dietary pattern.

The coming of age of the role of good nutrition in the healthy lifestyle has revolutionized food marketing. Foods in virtually every product category, from the most basic food staples like milk and bread to multicourse frozen dinners, are being produced and marketed in new forms perceived as being more nutritious. Old, familiar products are being cast in a new light. Best Foods is marketing its Karo corn syrup as a "user-friendly" way to bake without fat. Even pet foods are being touted as "lite" or "less fat."

B. Space and Presentation

A trip through a modern supermarket illustrates the impact of the heightened interest in healthier eating. Typically, the produce section is larger and offers a wide assortment of fruits and vegetables, all attractively displayed. Canned vegetables come in a low-sodium variety, and whole canned fruits may rest in natural juices as well as heavy or light syrup. An increased number of salad dressings are lower in calories or contain reduced amounts of oil.

Meat cases devote space to leaner cuts, while the amount of fat trimmed from all cuts have increased. The dairy category has exploded with more nutritious versions of traditional products. Lower-fat milk now outsells whole milk. Cheeses are made from a higher percentage of low-fat ingredients than in the past. Ice milk, frozen yogurt, and other frozen desserts elbow aside traditional ice cream in refrigerated cases. Low- or no-fat baked goods became an instant hit once consumers discovered taste had not been sacrificed for nutrition. There is still plenty of white bread, but whole grain breads and other varieties perceived as more nutritious are often featured more prominently.

C. Fish and Seafood

Americans have increased their consumption of fresh fish over the past few decades. Over half of the new stores studied in a 1989 FMI survey featured service seafood departments [2]. Store remodeling often includes the addition of a seafood department. Stores see this department as both a means of increasing traffic and as a profit center.

D. Convenience Foods

The busy lifestyle of many consumers has fueled the demand for convenience in the foods they choose. Ready-to-eat and heat-and-serve prepared foods have become a staple of today's supermarkets. Microwaveable products are big sellers in the frozen food aisles. Recognizing this trend, food manufacturers are developing products that offer both convenience and less of nutrient and calorie excesses. Healthy Choice® frozen dinners, for example, gained quick popularity as consumers sought to "eat the right thing"— quickly and easily. Introduced in 1990, Healthy Choice captured 37% of the frozen dinner market in slightly over a year [3].

Both food manufacturers and retail stores offering their own prepared foods are heeding consumer demands for nutritious foods. An FMI survey found that 69.6% of companies changed menus, 33.7% switching to lower salt, 31.5% to lower fat, and 28.1% to lower cholesterol [4].

E. Shelf Space and Position

In food marketing, store shelf space and position are critical factors in determining sales. The proliferation of lower-calorie foods has touched off a battle within the food distribution chain as new products vie with old ones for the best places.

Although shoppers have their own food preferences, most can be subtly influenced by product presentation. Shoppers tend to buy what is popular, and they make that determination, in part, by what they see. For that reason, food brokers and manufacturers scramble to get the most "facings"— horizontal shelf inches such as two of the same cereal boxes side by side. They also prefer shelf placement at eye level. Increasingly, "healthier" foods are claiming the better positions.

With a finite amount of space, stores are having to be more creative in their efforts to offer customers as many products as possible. New shelving designs have provided some extra space. In some cases, retailers have opted to maintain as many products and brands as possible, but carry less of them or limit the selection. A manufacturer may offer 12 flavors of yogurt, but the store will only carry seven of them. In other cases, store buyers may simply drop slow sellers. These days, in many cases, it's the products perceived as more healthy that are beating out the others.

F. Consumer Assistance

Food retailers are also capitalizing on the public's interest in nutrition to sell themselves as well as their products. Stores have adopted a number of ways to aid consumers to their search for more healthful foods.

With the use of simple symbols, shelf labels tell shoppers whether a product is higher/lower in sodium, fat, or fiber. Larger food chains have extensive consumer affairs departments, which produce materials targeting a health-conscious public. Low-calorie recipes for dieters, tips on food preparation, and manuals listing where specific products fall in fat, sodium, cholesterol, and calorie range are some of the most popular forms of outreach. Several retail chains have joined with recognized health groups such as the American Cancer Society or the American Hearth Association in promotional campaigns designed to encourage Americans to adopt a more healthy diet.

III. HEALTHY FOODS IN THE INNER CITY

While the hottest trend in food retailing is toward more nutritious products, actual stocking of such foods varies from store to store and area to area. The most striking difference is between a typical suburban supermarket and the smaller grocery stores in the inner city, where healthful foods tend to be the exception rather than the rule. A 1990 survey by Cornell University's Cooperative Extension Department found that only 25 of the 149 small grocers in New York City's poorer Bedford Stuyvesant section carried low-fat milk [5].

Inner city residents seeking nutritious foods face not only limited selections but also higher prices. Prices at smaller stores in these areas often run 10–20% higher than in the larger, suburban retail supermarkets. In late 1990, a box of Kellogg's Heartwise cereal sold for $3.39 in a Harlem store compared with $2.59 for General Mills's Kabboom. The owner of a Harlem food market said in the *Wall Street Journal*: "Healthy eating doesn't sell" [5].

IV. LABELS

While stores may put out shelf labels or put out flyers, it is the food label that is the primary source of nutritional information for consumers. Shoppers may want to eat foods lower in fat, salt, cholesterol, or calories, but only the food label can tell them how much of these components the product contains. More than 89% of shoppers in the 1990 FMI survey reported reading the label for ingredient or nutrition information. That figure rose to nearly 90% for first-time purchases only [1].

Consumer groups complained that labels often were misleading. Because there were no standardized definitions for most terms, terms such as "lite" of "lean" were generally meaningless. While a product may be touted as low in cholesterol and, therefore, helpful in reducing risk of heart disease, no mention is made of the fact that the product might be higher in fat, thus increasing the risk for the same disease. Or the new product might be lower in both fat and cholesterol but higher in sodium content. The FMI survey showed that 60% of shoppers found health claims at least somewhat believable, while 73% reported that the claims at least somewhat influenced their decisions to purchase the product [1].

Nutrition labeling was required only when a product made a nutrition-related claim, so some product labels contained no nutrition information. Some consumers also complained that the nutrition information provided was inadequate or hard to read.

Both the U.S. Food and Drug Administration (FDA) and the U.S. Congress began looking for ways to improve food labels to better serve consumers. The result was a new labeling law passed in 1990 that requires nutrition labeling on nearly all food products. At a minimum, labels must include amounts of total fat, saturated fat, cholesterol, sodium, total carbohydrates, complex carbohydrates, sugar, dietary fiber, and protein. The law requires standardization of descriptive terms and limits health claims to six well-documented relationships between a food component and a particular disease (see Chapter 7 for details). While applauding the new requirements, food retailers continue to urge manufacturers to include as much nutrition information as possible on the label.

V. NEW PRODUCTS

As more was being learned about the relationship between excesses of certain food components and disease, the public began to demand foods lower in those components. Products lower in sodium were among the first to meet this demand. The plethora of new low-calorie and low-fat ingredients and foods produced in response to this demand are described in Chapters 8–17.

Successful marketing of foods containing substitutes for familiar ingredients depends mainly on two factors—winning FDA approval and winning public acceptance. The former is a time-consuming process made even more difficult by existing standards of identity—requirements of what a product must contain in order to be called by a particular name. Food processors complain that these standards of identity are keeping otherwise more healthful products off the market. Acceptance, as mentioned earlier, depends on taste. Consumers will not accept a new product, no matter how well it is presented as providing good nutrition, unless the taste is acceptable.

Food processors continue to pursue new product development with an eye toward better nutrition. In its annual R&D survey of investment objectives, *Prepared Foods Magazine* found that 76% of the 352 food processors surveyed planned to increase development of reduced-calorie, reduced-fat, or diet food products [6]. A significant number (46%) were interested in developing all-natural, pesticide- and preservative-free products.

New product introduction continued unabated in 1990 despite the economic recession. According to *New Product News*, new product introductions arose 12%, with more than 10% of the food products touted as reduced-fat or reduced-calorie [6]. Introduction of new no- or low-cholesterol products rose 78%, low- or reduced-sugar products 76%, and natural food products 175%. Dairy and processed meat and poultry products led the way in the so-called "lite" foods.

VI. GRADING

Names can make a huge difference in food marketing. When the U.S. Department of Agriculture changed its meat standards to allow certain leaner cuts to be labeled "select" rather than "good," consumption rose by 17% [6]. Few people, argue food processors, are likely to rush out and buy a product labeled "meat substitute" even though it may taste the same and be more healthy. FDA is being pressured to change its standards of identity to allow more healthful alternatives to recognized products.

VII. CONCLUSION

Nutrition does sell, but, ultimately, it is taste that makes the difference in public acceptance. Americans want to eat better but they won't give up taste to do it.

The revolution in food marketing created by the public's desire for a slimmer, trimmer, more healthful self shows every sign of continuing. Food manufacturers and retailers are working together to give the public what they believe it wants. New products are hitting grocery shelves and the stores are doing their best to see that the shopper knows that they are there.

REFERENCES

1. *Trends: Consumer Attitudes and the Supermarket*, The Food Marketing Institute, Washington, DC, p. 50 (1991).
2. *Facts About Store Development*, The Food Marketing Institute, Washington, DC, p. 15 (1990).
3. A. Meyer, Healthy Choice transforms the freezer, *Prepared Foods New Products Annual, 1991*, Gorman Publishing, Chicago, IL, p. 34 (1991).
4. *FMI Speaks*, The Food Marketing Institute, Washington, DC, p. 10 (1991).
5. A. J. Freedman, Poor selection, *The Wall Street Journal*, Dec. 10 (1990).
6. K. Hochberg, Health claims shift into high gear, *Prepared Foods New Products Annual, 1991*, Gorman Publishing, Chicago, IL, p. 42 (1991).
7. *Meat Facts, 1989*, American Meat Institute, Arlington, VA, p. 22 (August 1990).

19
Impact of Low-Calorie Foods
on Nutrition Education

Janet K. Grommet   *Columbia University Teachers College, New York,
New York*

Janet Majewski Jemmott   *Cortlandt Group, Inc., Ossining, New York*

I. NUTRITION CONSENSUS REPORTS

Several reports released in recent years by expert committees provide dietary recommendations aimed at improving the health status of Americans [1–12]. Reports issued by government and government-related bodies have been particularly well publicized, for example, the U.S. Department of Health and Human Services' *Surgeon General's Report on Nutrition and Health*, the National Academy of Science's *Diet and Health*, and the U.S. Department of Agriculture and Department of Health and Human Services' revised *Dietary Guidelines for Americans.*

The reports are individually noteworthy since each represents the consensus of an expert committee. When viewed as a whole, the reports are remarkable for the consistency in recommendations from report to report (Table 1), which suggests a maturing scientific base underpinning these recom-

Table 1 Dietary Guidance for the Healthy U.S. Population

Title and organization	Type of guidance (general or specific)	Achieve and maintain desirable body weight	Fats (% kcal)		
			Total: limit or reduce	Saturated: reduce	Polyunsaturated: limit or reduce
Federal Government Agencies					
Nutrition and Your Health: Dietary Guidelines for Americans	General	Yes	Avoid too much	Avoid too much	[a]
U.S. Dept. Agriculture and Dept. Health and Human Services, 1990					
NCI Dietary Guidelines: Rationale	Cancer	Avoid obesity	To ≤ 30%	[a]	[a]
National Cancer Institute, 1988					
The Surgeon General's Report on Nutrition and Health	General	Yes	Yes	Yes	[a]
U.S. Department of Health and Human Services, 1988					
Report of the Expert Panel on Population Strategies for Blood Cholesterol Reduction (population panel)	Heart disease	Yes	≤ 30%	< 10%	[a]
National Cholesterol Education Program, USDHHS, PHS, NIH, NHLBI, 1990					
Other Scientific Groups					
Diet, Nutrition and Cancer	Cancer	[a]	30%	Yes	Reduce
Committee on Diet, Nutrition and Cancer, National Research Council, National Academy of Sciences, 1982					

| Cholesterol: limit or reduce | Carbohydrates | | | Sodium: limit or reduce | Alcohol:in moderation if at all |
	Complex: increase	Fiber: increase	Refined sugar:limit or reduce		
Avoid too much	Eat foods with adequate starch	Eat foods with adequate fiber	Avoid too much	Avoid too much	Yes
a	a	To 20-30 g/day, with an upper limit of 35 g	a	a	Yes
Yes	Consume more foods high in complex carbohydrates	Consume more foods high in fiber	Yes, especially children	Yes	Yes
< 300 mg/day	a	a	a	a	a
a	a	a	a	a	Yes

Table 1   Continued

Title and organization	Type of guidance (general or specific)	Achieve and maintain desirable body weight	Fats (% kcal)		
			Total limit or reduce	Saturated reduce	Polyunsaturated limit or reduce
Diet and Health: Implications for Reducing Chronic Disease Risk FNB/NRC/NAS, 1989	General	Yes	≤ 30%	< 10%	≤ 10%
Recommended Dietary Allowances Committee on Dietary Allowances FNB/NRC/NAS, 1989	General	Yes	≤ 30%	< 10%	≤ 10%
Health Organizations					
Nutrition Recommendations for Women American Dietetic Association, 1986	Healthy women	Yes	To <33% total kcal	Select a variety of fat sources	
Prudent Lifestyle for Children: Dietary Fat and Cholesterol American Academy of Pediatrics, 1986	Healthy children/heart disease	Yes; detect obesity by measuring height and weight	Optimal total fat intake is unknown, but 30-40% seems sensible for adequate growth and development; changes in current dietary practices for the first two decades of life are not recommended. Follow the current trends in the U.S.-decreased consumption of saturated fats, cholestrol, and salt and increased intake of polyunsaturated fats in moderation.		
Dietary Guidelines for Healthy American Adults American Heart Association, 1988	Heart disease	Yes	< 30%	< 10%	< 10%
The Healthy American Diet American Heart Association, 1990	General	Yes	Yes, especially saturated fat and cholesterol		

| Cholesterol limit or reduce | Carbohydrates | | Refined sugar limit or reduce | Sodium limit or reduce | Alcohol in moderation if at all |
	Complex increase	Fiber increase			
< 300 mg/day	≥ 55% of calories with ≥ 6 servings grains and legumes and ≥ 5 servings fruits and vegetables/day		Do not increase	2.4 g or 6 g salt/day or less	Does not recommend. If consumed, limit to less than 1 ounce/day
< 300 mg/day	Yes	Eat fiber-containing foods	Yes	Minimum of 0.5 g/day	
[a]	Consume at least 50% daily kcal from carbohydrates, select complex carbohydrates		Yes		Limit to 1 or 2 drinks/day
	[a]	[a]	[a]		[a]
< 300 mg/day	50-55% of calories with emphasis on complex carbohydrates		[a]	Limit to 3 g/day	Not to exceed 1-2 ounces of ethanol/day
	Yes	Yes	Yes, especially children	Yes	Yes. Children, adolescents and pregnant women should abstain

Table 1   Continued

Title and organization	Type of guidance (general or specific)	Achieve and maintain desirable body weight	Fats (% kcal)		
			Total limit or reduce	Saturated reduce	Polyunsaturated limit or reduce
American Cancer Society Dietary Guidelines	Cancer	Yes Avoid obesity	Yes. To 30% or less	a	a
American Cancer Society, 1990					

[a]No specific dietary advice given.
Source: National Dairy Council, *Dairy Counc. Dig.*, *61*(5): 27 (1990).

mendations for healthy eating. Any number of reports, for instance, recommends maintaining desirable (or healthy) body weight since excess weight is either an independent or a collaborating risk factor for chronic diseases such as diabetes, cardiovascular disease, and hypertension. Additionally, many of the reports recommend decreased consumption of fat, sugar, and salt and increased consumption of complex carbohydrates including dietary fiber. Thus, these reports infer that many Americans need to control the *quantity* of calories consumed while concurrently improving the *quality* of caloric intake.

II. LOW-CALORIE PRODUCT PROLIFERATION

The food industry, cognizant of the growing consensus regarding dietary recommendations plus consumers' increasing interest in healthful foods, responded by developing new product lines. In fact, a major technological change in food products in recent years has been the development of low-calorie foods and beverages. These products are achieved technically by one of several means: the addition of water or other ingredients such as polydextrose to dilute the caloric density of a product such as low-calorie salad dressing; the removal of fats and sugars in a product such as low-fat milk or low-calorie jam; the addition of noncaloric or low-calorie fat and sugar substitutes such as no-fat frozen dairy desserts or diet soft drinks [13].

Currently hundreds of low-calorie products are being produced annually in the United States that are reduced in fat or sugar compared to the standard counterpart. One prediction is that low-fat products alone will account for the introduction of over 2000 *new* products over the next several years [14]. This is in the context of a marketplace in which a total of over 12,000 new food products were introduced this year, continuing the steady growth trend

	Carbohydrates				
Cholesterol limit or reduce	Complex increase	Fiber increase	Refined sugar limit or reduce	Sodium limit or reduce	Alcohol in moderation if at all
[a]	[a]	Eat more high fiber foods such as whole grain cereals, vegetables and fruits	[a]	[a]	Yes

in annual product development [15]. The availability of low-calorie foods is intended to encourage healthful eating. Modifying traditional foods and producing low-calorie analogs theoretically remove barriers, thus simplifying food selections to achieve the goals of healthful eating.

Excessive proliferation of new products, however, runs the risk of being counterproductive for consumers by introducing too many confusing choices [16]. Additional choices force consumers to attempt to understand product difference to make intelligent decisions. At some threshold the number of choices adds such a burden that additional time spent studying the alternatives is more burdensome than the potential gain of choosing among the known choices. In this environment of an excessive number of choices the benefits of new and possibly healthier products can be lost.

Compounding the problem are inconsistencies in food labeling. Low-calorie foods as defined by the Food and Drug Administration (FDA) contain fewer than 40 calories per serving and less than 0.4 calorie per gram, whereas reduced-calorie foods contain at least 33% fewer calories than a conventional counter part [17]. The U.S. Department of Agriculture (USDA), which has jurisdiction over the labeling of meat and poultry products, however, defines low/reduced products as those containing at least 25% fewer calories. Similar discrepancies exist between the FDA and USDA's definitions of low fat.

Other descriptive terms lack legal definition. "Lite" or "light" can refer to fewer calories, less fat, lower cholesterol, reduced sodium, lighter color, lighter taste or texture. Thus, a product can be labeled "light" but not necessarily be low in fat content. Recent food label regulations proposed by FDA standardize definitions for "free," "less," "low," "reduced," "more," "fresh," "light," "high," and "source of" and will hopefully aid the consumer [18]. Until these regulations are enacted, food labels may function more to sell products than to educate consumers (see also Chapter 7).

III. IMPACT OF LOW-CALORIE FOODS
IN HEALTHY EATING

Although the recent nutrition consensus reports provide a context for formulating public policy, planning community interventions, or adjusting individual dietary habits, the recommendations of the reports are essentially endpoints. For instance, the majority of the recent reports recommends limiting fat intake. Limiting fat intake is *what* is to be achieved but does not encompass *how* to achieve this goal. The process of how to limit fat intake instead reflects various food behaviors. Numerous choices could be involved in the process of achieving this goal, which underscores that there is not one pathway to healthful eating.

The work of Kristal et al. takes a look at food behaviors that facilitate low-fat eating [19]. Their empirical study of food behaviors generated four dimensions of dietary behavior that facilitate low-fat eating: (1) *excluding* high-fat ingredients and preparation techniques, (2) *modifying* high-fat foods, (3) *replacing* high-fat foods with low-fat alternatives, and (4) *substituting* specially manufactured low-fat foods for the higher-fat counterparts.

The exclusion dimension includes eliminating certain classes of food items or preparation techniques to reduce caloric intake, specifically fat intake. This might include, for example, eliminating meat by having a vegetarian meal, eating breads without butter, eating potatoes without added butter or sour cream, or eating steamed vegetables without butter or cheese sauce, or excluding frying in food preparation.

The modification dimension includes altering commonly available foods to reduce fat content. This would include, for example, removing skin from chicken, trimming visible fat from meat, skimming congealed fat from a sauce, or modifying portion size, thus eating a smaller amount. The replacement dimension describes making deliberate changes in food choices in order to lower fat intake. This would include, for example, using lemon juice and herbs instead of salad dressing, using yogurt instead of sour cream, or eating fresh fruit instead of high-fat, baked products. Finally, the substitution dimension suggests maintaining the usual dietary pattern but using specially manufactured products that might include, for example, low-fat mayonnaise, low-calorie salad dressing, low-fat cheeses, or no-fat frozen dairy desserts.

Delineating dietary behaviors into these components highlights the variety of personal choices that can be exercised to lower fat intake. In mixing tuna salad, for example, low-fat mayonnaise could be *substituted* for regular mayonnaise to reduce the fat content. Alternatively, mayonnaise could be *replaced* with a spicy mustard in mixing the tuna salad. This would further reduce the fat content but, admittedly, deviates from the original concept of a mayonnaise-based spread. Another possibility is that the preparation could be *modified* by using a smaller portion of mayonnaise just to moisten the tuna. Or the mayonnaise could be *excluded* by serving the tuna flaked perhaps as an open-faced sandwich with a vegetable garnish.

Ironically, low-calorie foods that have proliferated in recent years tend to represent but one dimension of dietary behavior, i.e., substitution. Thus, although the vast array of new and changing low-calorie foods may overwhelm consumers, these products, when viewed from a behavioral perspective, are limited in scope.

Kristal et al.'s original dimensions of modification and substitution might be revised to take better account of low-calorie food technology. For example, low-calorie products based on the removal of fats and sugars, such as low-fat cheese or low-calorie pancake syrup, would be classified as modified products. The original description of modification focused on modifying foods during home preparation such as removing skin from chicken to lower fat content. The proposed revision broadens this dimension to include commercial, low-calorie modifications based on decreasing or diluting the traditional fat or sugar content of a food product.

The substitution dimension as originally described by Kristal et al. included all specially manufactured low-fat foods, but as revised would be limited to the array of food products that involve the use of fat and sugar substitutes, namely, the ingredients sucrose polyester (olestra) and microparticulated milk and egg proteins (Simplesse or Trailblazer) and nonnutritive sweeteners including saccharin, aspartame, and acesulfame-K.

The revised interpretation of modification and substitution dimensions is proposed because consumers may indeed have a different perception of food products that are low in calories as a result of decreasing or diluting traditional fat and sugar content as opposed to food products that are calorically reduced as a result of using fat and sugar substitutes. Heasman, for example, alludes to this when he writes, "Fat replacers are likely to provide an area of future interest as long as concerns about the mass marketing of synthetic foods do not dampen the market" [20]. But regardless of consumers' perceptions of low-calorie foods based on modifications versus ingredient substitutions, these food products, despite their large numbers, represent only a portion of the behaviors that an individual can invoke to limit fat/calorie intake.

Also, there is the realization that low-calorie foods tend to reinforce the existing food pattern since they require no change in food patterning. This may be advantageous from a marketing standpoint. For instance, if low-calorie foods are equally acceptable in terms of taste, convenience, safety, and price, then presumably consumers will have limited resistance to incorporating a new product into their diet. Healthy eating, however, as advocated in the nutrition consensus reports, will necessitate a broader array of food behavior changes to impact on the current food pattern that is high in fat and protein and low in complex carbohydrates and fiber.

Low-calorie foods are predominantly remakes of dairy products (e.g., fluid milk, ice cream, cheese, sour cream), condiments (e.g., salad dressing, mayonnaise), baked products, and beverages. They potentially reduce caloric intake but do not shift food patterns toward increased consumption of non-animal products, namely, fruits, vegetables, breads, and cereal products.

In contrast, some major nutrition issues of yesteryear such as fortification and enrichment required minimal changes in the food pattern. Nutrition surveys indicated that Americans had suboptimal intake of several micronutrients. Consequently, standards were promulgated for adding the specified nutrients to the existing food supply. Foods such as bread products and milk were purposely selected as "carriers" for enrichment and fortification, as they were foods widely consumed by the population and were economically accessible [13].

Essentially no changes were required then in food choices. For example, milk was marketed as a fortified product; it was not widely available with and without fortification necessitating an informed food choice decision. Nutritionists could appropriately assume the role of information disseminators informing the public of the virtues of fortification and enrichment.

Nutrition educators are now encouraged to think in terms of facilitating food behavior changes that will improve eating patterns to achieve the recommendations of the nutrition consensus reports. Nutrition education of the past did not necessarily demand this level of sophistication.

IV. UNDERSTANDING CONSUMER ATTITUDES AND BEHAVIOR

Effective nutrition educators are now beginning to think in terms of conceptual models that explain variables that account for an individual's learning and behavior. Noteworthy among such models is the health belief model (HBM), which suggests that an individual's health behavior reflects readiness to take action plus a sense that the benefits of the health behavior will outweigh the costs [21].

According to the health belief model, people are more likely to follow a health recommendation such as reducing fat intake if they hold certain beliefs. The first belief is *perceived susceptibility*. For example, individuals are more likely to attempt low-fat/low-calorie eating if they perceive that they are susceptible (vulnerable) to negative effects of continuing high-fat/high-calorie eating.

The second belief is *perceived severity*. As the consequences of not following a health recommendation increase in severity, the more likely the individual is to take action. This is often problematic in nutrition/health issues in that disregarding the recommendation for low-fat/low-calorie eating, for instance, may have no immediate consequences. This may indeed explain the discrepancy in food attitudes and food behaviors reported in such consumer surveys as NPD's National Eating Trends Survey. This survey suggests that while food attitudes have changed dramatically over the last decade, the impact on dietary behavior has been less dramatic [22].

The third belief involves *perceived benefits*. That is, to take action on health recommendations such as low-fat/low-calorie eating, the individual must believe that following the recommendations will be effective and that the benefits of following the recommendations outweigh the personal barriers such as economic costs, physical inconvenience, or emotional burden. When the individual does not select foods to meet the dietary goals, for instance, the nutritionist may be effective in facilitating change by focusing on the individual's sense of susceptibility, severity, or perception of barriers.

The Survey of American Eating Habits, a recent survey of dietary attitudes and behaviors co-sponsored by the American Dietetic Association, suggests that Americans cluster into three groups: (1) "Don't bother me", (2) "I know I should, but . . .", and (3) "I'm already doing it" [23]. Most in the first cluster express no interest in changing eating habits, which may be surprising to nutritionists; this group, representing approximately 36% of the population, is in essence neither attitudinally nor behaviorally attuned to healthy eating.

Those in the second group, approximately 38% of the population, indicate that nutrition is important to them but feel they are not doing as much as they could with respect to healthy eating. Thus, they are attitudinally predisposed to healthy eating, but they are lagging behaviorally. The third cluster, 26% of the population, considers diet and nutrition important in their lifestyle, and their attitudes and behaviors reflect healthy eating. Among the "I'm already doing it" group, 76% reported being careful about dietary fat intake compared to 52% in the "I know I should, but . . ." group and 26% in the "Don't bother me" group.

Interpreting these survey results in light of the health belief model offers further insight. For example, the group categorized as "Don't bother me" essentially does not perceive that they are susceptible to poor eating habits or that there are consequences to their current dietary behavior. With no perception of threat, there is no value in changing food behavior, so this group lacks the incentive to substitute, replace, modify, or deliberately exclude food for health reasons.

In terms of the health belief model, the group characterized as "I know I should, but . . ." acknowledges their susceptibility and the severity of consequences to continuing with the status quo. They know that they are vulnerable and that there are potentially negative consequences to their current eating patterns. They value changing their food patterns to be consistent with dietary recommendations of the nutrition consensus reports, but barriers to changing certain food behaviors seem to outweigh the benefits of change. They, therefore, have limited expectation for change. In essence, these individuals are ready to take action, but barriers seemingly impede their implementing the action. Barriers reported in the survey include the belief that a healthy diet would mean forfeiting favorite foods and the thought that healthy eating would require too much time.

The health belief model may be augmented by self-efficacy theories that explain an individual's ability to take action [24]. Self-efficacy is the personal conviction that one can successfully carry out an action such as a dietary recommendation. Individuals may well believe the benefits of a dietary recommendation but find it too difficult. The higher the level of perceived efficacy, the more likely one is to persist in learning a new behavior. Kristal et al.'s food behavior dimension of substitution that encompasses specially manufactured low-fat/calorie foods may be easier to implement as opposed to excluding high-fat/calorie ingredients and preparation techniques, modifying commonly available foods to lower fat/calorie content, or replacing high-fat/calorie foods with lower-fat/calorie alternatives.

As noted earlier, the use of low-calorie foods has limited effect on the food pattern. For example, consuming a no-fat frozen dessert product instead of ice cream indeed results in decreased calorie intake. The use of this "substitute," however, circumvents the idea that calorie intake also could be limited via replacing the ice cream with another food choice, modifying the ice cream selection via portion control, or excluding ice cream from the meal. The no-fat frozen dessert requires no change in the food pattern.

Perhaps this requires less personal conviction, less self-efficacy. Dietary change is thus sought by selecting altered food products rather than by altering the food pattern. For the individual who is predisposed to healthy eating but perceives that barriers to change outweigh the benefits, specially manufactured low-calorie foods may indeed surmount the perceived barriers. Schlicker and Regan note, "Although fat and sugar substitutes will not compensate for poor dietary habits, these ingredients and technologies may be a help to those trying to consume healthful balanced diets" [25].

In the conceptual terms of the health belief model, the survey group characterized as "I'm already doing it" indicated that they perceived a relationship between diet and health, are ready to take action, and perceive that the changes they are making outweigh the costs. The survey revealed that this group, for instance, tends to cook "from scratch," reads nutrition information on packages, actively seeks information about nutrition and healthy eating, purchases low-fat products more often than other groups, and skips meals infrequently.

Similarly, Hudnall [26] concluded,

> Reduced-calorie foods are only *one* weapon in the war against weight. Used alone, they likely will have little impact. . . . Furthermore, attempts to lay the blame for failure at weight management on reduced-calorie foods and ingredients—or on any other single element—perpetuate the myth of a magic cure for weight problems and continue to mislead the public in what can be an extremely destructive search for a lower weight.

This suggests that the cumulative effect of a variety of strategies allows the "I'm already doing it" group to effectively achieve the dietary recommendations. This reflects personal involvement and commitment to change.

V. IMPACT OF LOW-CALORIE FOODS ON NUTRITION EDUCATORS

Product proliferation is, of course, a challenge to nutritionists as well as to consumers. Consumers, as already noted, are confronted with numerous food choices in the marketplace that may unnecessarily compound decision making. Nutritionists are confronted with the challenge of remaining current with a vast and changing array of food products.

Many nutrition educators feel obligated to remain abreast to the marketplace. They, for example, envision that a client may query them about a product and that they may appear uninformed if they have no knowledge of that product. This may, however, be a misdirected focus of nutrition education. In fact, part of the impact of low-calorie foods on nutrition education may be the nutrition community's realization that they are not in command of the marketplace. The dilemma for nutritionists may stretch as far back as their academic preparation. Is the nutrition community preparing professional nutritionists for the complexities of nutrition practice?

Historically, nutritionists have clustered primarily into either nutrition science/research or into dietetics. Both of these groups have tended to be educated in relatively content-laden curricula. The nutrition science professionals have been schooled in nutritional biochemistry as well as research design and laboratory methods in order to further the scientific body of knowledge of nutrition. The dietetic professionals, who traditionally practiced in the hospital setting, have been schooled in the fundamentals of nutrition science as well as the principles of food service as their work focused on optimal feeding of the sick. A third cluster of nutritionists, public health nutritionists, has "ebbed and tided" over the past decades, frequently at the mercy of government funding.

Nutrition scientists generally work at the interface of nutrition and biological sciences with limited experience in nutrition practice or direct service delivery. As skilled clinicians, dietitians traditionally control food choices for the ill via the hospital menu and formulary feedings. Now, however, in considering the impact of low-calorie foods on nutrition education, nutritionists might be working with clients in an ambulatory care clinic, in a managed care facility such as a health maintenance organization, in a worksite wellness program, or in a private practice. In these nontraditional settings the nutritionist has the opportunity to work with clients (particularly clients with chronic diseases such as diabetes, cardiovascular disease, hypertension, or obesity) whose treatment goals frequently include lowering caloric intake. The perplexity in the academic preparation of nutritionists is that few are professionally trained to work with clients to effect changes in food habits.

Thus, when working in the arena of education, nutritionists tend to rely excessively on conveying information to their clients as though lack of knowledge were the primary deficit. Patient education studies indicate, however, that increased knowledge has limited influence on affecting patient behavior (27,28). That is, *telling* a client good sources of low-fat entrees does little to facilitate the client's actual selection of such entrees unless the individual is already motivated to take action.

The focus on information dissemination, however, in the interaction of nutritionists and clients is perhaps a reflection of the content-laden academic preparation of both nutrition researchers and dietitians. Academic preparation of nutritionists has focused almost exclusively on the content of nutrition with limited focus on process skills such as education strategies, counseling skills, or program-planning techniques. While the nutrition community historically has been comfortable with drawing from the biological sciences, nutrition education needs to foster connections with the social sciences to affect behavioral changes, specifically food behavior changes in clients and communities.

VI. CONCLUSIONS

A convergence of stalwart dietary recommendations, technological innovations, and consumer interest in healthy eating accounts for the recent proliferation of low-calorie foods in the marketplace. Although in theory these foods may enable healthful eating [29], their effectiveness in free-living individuals is less certain.

Standardized labeling in the near future may make the labels more intelligible, and consumers may determine that low-calorie foods are a heterogeneous lot. Although too early to assess, consumers may be more receptive to conventional foods in which fat or sugar content has been reduced, whereas low-calorie foods involving fat and sugar substitutes may be dubbed synthetic.

In spite of the vast number of products, the impact on healthful eating is curtailed in two ways. First, low-calorie foods are limited primarily to substitution, one dimension in the repertoire of behaviors that may be invoked to lower fat/calorie intake. Second, substituting low-calorie foods for a conventional counterpart may decrease calorie intake, but substituting one item for another has limited consequence of changing food patterns as suggested by the nutrition consensus reports.

Consumer attitudes toward nutrition and consumer dietary behaviors are not necessarily in concordance. That is, more consumers express an interest in healthy eating than actually attain healthy eating habits. Nutritionists, however, historically focus their efforts on the consumer's knowledge with the hope that increased information will positively influence attitudes and dietary behavior. New knowledge does not invariably result in attitude or behavior change.

Thus, nutritionists are encouraged to augment their professional knowledge base with intervention skills to improve their effectiveness. This will require that nutritionists are more attuned to the expectations and beliefs of those attempting to change dietary behaviors. Exploration of perceived barriers is more conducive to changing behavior than information overload.

Low-calorie foods, despite their vast number, are but one strategy for change. Alone they may have limited impact, but combined with other strategies they may be influential. Changing food habits thus encompasses more than changing food products.

REFERENCES

1. U.S. Department of Agriculture and U.S. Department of Health and Human Services, *Dietary Guidelines for Americans Advisory Committee Report*, USDA/DHHS, Washington, DC (1990).
2. R. R. Butrum, C. K. Clifford, and E. Lanza, NCI dietary guidelines: Rationale, *Am. J. Clin. Nutr.*, *48*(Suppl.): 888 (1988).
3. U.S. Department of Health and Human Services, Public Health Service, *The Surgeon General's Report on Nutrition and Health*, DHHS (PHS) Publication No. 88-50210, Government Printing Office, Washington, DC (1988).
4. National Cholesterol Education Program (NCEP), *Report of the National Cholesterol Education Program Expert Panel on Population Strategies for Blood Cholesterol Reduction*, U.S. Department of Health and Human Services, Public Health Service, National Institutes of Health, National Heart, Lung, and Blood Institute, Washington, DC (February 1990).
5. Committee on Diet, Nutrition, and Cancer, National Research Council, *Diet, Nutrition and Cancer*, National Academy Press, Washington, DC (1982).
6. Committee on Diet and Health, Food and Nutrition Board, Commission on Life Sciences, National Research Council, *Diet and Health: Implications for Reducing Chronic Disease Risk*, National Academy Press, Washington, DC (1989).

7. Subcommittee on the Tenth Edition of the RDAs, Food and Nutrition Board, Commission on Life Sciences, National Research Council, *Recommended Dietary Allowances*, 10th ed., National Academy Press, Washington, DC (1989).
8. American Dietetic Association, The American Dietetic Association's nutrition recommendations for women, *J. Am. Diet. Assoc., 86*: 1663 (1986).
9. American Academy of Pediatrics, Committee on Nutrition, Prudent lifestyle for children: Dietary fat and cholesterol, *Pediatrics, 78*: 521 (1986).
10. American Heart Association, Dietary guidelines for healthy American adults: A statement for physicians and health professionals by the nutrition committee, AHA, *Circulation, 77*: 721A (1988).
11. American Heart Association, American Academy of Pediatrics, American Cancer Society, American Diabetes Association, American Dietetic Association, Centers for Disease Control, National Cancer Institute, National Heart, Lung, and Blood Institute, and U.S. Departments of Agriculture and Health and Human Services, *The Healthy American Diet*, 1990.
12. D. W. Nixon, Nutrition and cancer: American Cancer Society guidelines, programs, and initiatives, *CA Cancer J. Clin., 40* (2): 71 (1990).
13. M. K. Schmidl and T. P. Labuza, The history, current status, and future of nutritional food product development, *Food Product Development: From Concept to the Marketplace* (E. Graf and I. S. Saguy, eds.), Van Nostrand Reinhold, New York, pp. 265–271 (1991).
14. E. Shapiro, New products clog food stores, *New York Times*, May 29, pp. D1, D17 (1990).
15. A. L. Gorman, *Gorman's New Product News*, Gorman Publishing, Chicago, IL (1991).
16. L. Williams, Free choice: When too much is too much, *New York Times*, Feb. 14, pp. C1, C10 (1990).
17. Title 21 (Section 105.66), Label statements relating to usefulness in reducing or maintaining caloric intake or body weight, *Code of Federal Regulations,* pp. 70–72 (April 1, 1992).
18. Regulations for the enforcement of the Nutrition Labeling and Education Act, *Fed. Reg.* (November 27, 1991).
19. A. R. Kristal, A. L. Shattuck, and H. J. Henry, Patterns of dietary behavior associated with selecting diets low in fat: Reliability and validity of a behavioral approach to dietary assessment, *J. Am. Diet. Assoc., 90*: 214 (1990).
20. M. Heasman, Nutrition and technology: The development of the market for "lite" products, *Br. Food J., 92*: 5 (1990).
21. I. M. Rosenstock, Historical origins of the health belief model, *Health Educ. Monogr., 2*: 329 (1974).
22. NPD Group, *National Eating Trends Survey*, NPD Group, Chicago, IL (1989).
23. American Dietetic Association, Kraft General Foods, Good Housekeeping Institute, *Survey of American Dietary Habits*, ADA, Chicago, IL (1991).
24. A. Bandura, Self-efficacy mechanism in human agency, *Am. Psychol., 37*: 122 (1982).
25. S. A. Schlicker and C. Regan, Innovations in reduced-calorie foods: A review of fat and sugar replacement technologies, *Top. Clin. Nutr., 6*: 50 (1990).

26. M. Hudnall, Reduced-calorie foods: Implications for dietary management, *Top. Clin. Nutr., 6*: 61 (1990).

27. E. E. Bartlett, Behavioral diagnosis: A practical approach to patient education, *Patient Couns. Health Educ., 4*: 29 (1982).

28. M. L. Axelson, T. L. Federline, and D. Brinberg, A meta-analysis of food- and nutrition-related research, *J. Nutr. Educ., 17*: 51 (1985).

29. F. X. Pi-Sunyer, Effect of composition of the diet on energy intake, *Nutr. Rev., 48*: 94 (1990).

20

Impact of Low-Calorie Foods on the Development of Low-Calorie and Low-Fat Recipes

Nedra P. Wilson *University of Alabama at Birmingham, Birmingham, Alabama*

Ellen Templeton Carroll Cooking Light, *Birmingham, Alabama*

I. INTRODUCTION

The creation of low-calorie, low-fat foods that fit into meals that reflect current dietary recommendations is a challenge for food manufacturers as well as for people who prepare recipes at home. Food manufacturers have responded by developing foods from appetizers to desserts that contain less fat and sugar and more complex carbohydrates [1]. These are often marketed as low calorie and fit into calorie-controlled eating plans.

American consumers will opt for healthy choices when the taste and quality is good. The proliferation of diet beverages is proof. Consumers state repeatedly that health and nutrition influences their food selections. The Surgeon General stated in his 1988 report that the public would benefit from increased availability of foods low in calories and fat [2]. This should serve as encouragement for food manufacturers to carefully critique product ingredients to include the healthiest options.

The consumer's perception of low-calorie foods is not always positive. Confusion resulting from inconsistent label terminology and limited access to low-calorie products interfere with the incorporation of these foods into meals. As health-conscious young adults assume the responsibility for determining the family food supply, low-calorie foods will be favored. Those foods that are also seen as time-savers will be the most preferred.

Some low-fat, low-calorie food products have been available for decades but have gained greater acceptance as their nutritional virtues are being recognized. Food experimentation has also come to the grass-roots level as educators teach recipe modification to reduce calories, fat, and sugar while retaining the good taste. New low-calorie foods are expected in the near future. The barrier to their availability is deciding which comes first—the product or the desire for the product.

The use of different ingredients and cooking techniques, a willing and adventurous attitude (tempered with common sense toward cooking), and following basic rules for recipe modification can lead to healthier food preparation. There are advantages and limitations to consider. These are discussed within the appropriate food categories that follow.

When low-calorie versions of recipes are sought, the focus should be on fat reduction, as fat is dense in calories. Even though fat has 9 calories per gram and carbohydrate and protein have 4 calories per gram, in past years a reduction in sugar has been the preferred way to decrease calories in foods. Decreasing fat has a greater impact on caloric reduction and on improving the health of Americans.

II. LOW-CALORIE PRODUCTS

A. Meat, Poultry, and Fish

1. Meat

Public concerns about the effect of meat on health has prompted the meat industry to take action. They have responded to the public's concerns and the challenge of the Surgeon General by sponsoring research to produce leaner meat. These products have become the focus of advertising. No longer does advertising depict the "he-man" image of one who eats huge portions of meat at the expense of vegetables. Now, a smaller portion of lean meat is presented alongside vegetables as a part of a healthy meal.

Consumers have recognized their influence over a store's practices. They have learned to reject meat with excess fat. As a result, closely trimmed meats are readily available in the marketplace. Less tender cuts (also moderately priced) are now being marketed in new ways and presented as healthy, lean choices. Some decrease in tenderness can be expected with meats that have less fat. However, with appropriate changes in cooking techniques, a tasty product is possible.

Some cuts require decreased cooking time and temperature to prevent dryness and toughness. Others need increased cooking time and the addition of moisture as in braising or stewing. These methods have the advantage of ease and require less attention by the cook who is seeking time-saving food preparation methods. Marinades are useful to tenderize meat. They work best when they have an acid base such as vinegar. Marinades may be as simple as a bottled, low-calorie Italian dressing. Juices such as pineapple or tomato can also provide an acid base for the marinade, and they can be flavored with other ingredients. Leaner, less tender cuts can also be tenderized by pounding or mechanically cubing.

Deli meat counters are more widely available and healthier options have proliferated. For example, corned beef previously could not have been incorporated into a low-fat diet, but a corned beef cut from the beef round is a healthy option.

2. Poultry

The poultry industry has responded to the public's ready acceptance of their products by providing a greater variety of choices. Chicken is available in a number of forms from cooked, ready-to-eat to premarinated, ready-to-stir-fry slices. Some of the premarinated products may have a high-fat, high-sodium content. Turkey parts and ground turkey are more readily available. Like chicken, some products are nutritionally superior to others. For example, some ground turkey has the skin and fat ground with the lean meat and would not be considered low in saturated fat. Many so-called turkey franks have excess fat—not much lower and sometimes higher in fat than beef and pork franks. It is important to read nutrition labels, so that wise decisions can be made.

Poultry does not require special handling to produce a tender product. It is versatile, and adapts well to a wide variety of cooking methods. Its shorter cooking time (compared to many meats) is seen as a distinct advantage by hurried cooks. It is easily incorporated into favorite recipes as a substitute for other meats.

3. Fish

Fish, naturally low in calories and fat, can be considered an original "fast food." Due to its lack of connective tissue, cooking time is short. However, some ready-to-heat fish products that are prebreaded are high in fat and calories. Plain fish fillets are lower-calorie choices; minimal fat needs to be added to achieve a tasty, finished product.

B. Dairy Products

A multitude of new, low-fat dairy products on the market now makes it easier for individuals to keep this nutritious food group a part of their low-calorie eating plan. Basic items such as low-fat milk, skim milk, low-fat yogurt, and some reduced-fat or fat-free cheeses are standard fare in most supermarkets. However, a wide variety of specialty products is often limited to specific geographic locations and large markets.

1. Milk

The nutrient composition of 2% low-fat, 1% low-fat, and skim milk is virtually the same except for fat content, and thus calorie content. The nutrient profiles are compared in Table 1.

There are few instances where skim milk does not make a suitable replacement for whole milk in recipes. Exceptions include some creamy soups, puddings, and custards. Substituting 1% or 2% low-fat milk or evaporated skim milk in these products usually yields satisfactory results, and the fat and calorie content is still much lower than if whole milk had been used.

Although the name implies a very high-fat product, buttermilk is usually made from skim or 1% low-fat milk. However, in some areas of the country, whole milk buttermilk (150 calories and 8 grams fat per 8 ounces) and nonfat buttermilk (91 calories and 2 grams fat per 8 ounces) are marketed side by side with little to distinguish between the two, so consumers must be careful label readers. Buttermilk can be successfully used in place of higher-fat and higher-calorie dairy products in some soups, beverages, baked goods, salad dressings, and frozen desserts. It is especially useful in some baked goods as a substitute for cream, whole milk, or sour cream. Its natural consistency lends thickness, richness, and texture to soups and sauces. However, it curdles more easily than skim or low-fat milk. Buttermilk's long storage life makes it a convenient item to keep on hand. But its tart taste and high sodium content (compared to some other dairy products) limits its use among some people.

Table 1 Nutrient profile of fluid milk

Item	kcal/8 oz	Fat (g)
Whole milk	138	7.5
2% milk	113	4.3
1% milk	95	2.4
Skim milk	79	0.4

Source: Ref. 4.

Evaporated skim milk (200 calories and 0 grams fat per 8 ounces) is a relatively new product to grocer's shelves. It is a boon to casseroles, soups, and sauces when used in place of heavy cream or half-and-half to lend richness, creaminess, and thickness (when combined with cornstarch or flour) to products. Because it is a shelf-stable item, it is convenient and easy to keep on hand. Drawbacks include the size of the container in which it is sold (it would be helpful to have a small size available as with evaporated whole milk), a metallic taste (as described by some people), and a sweeter flavor due to caramelization of the milk sugars during heat processing. Collectively this flavor is often referred to as a "canned milk flavor," undesirable to some people. Because evaporated skim milk is darker in color than regular fluid milk, it will change the color of some light-colored products.

Instant nonfat dry milk powder (80 calories and less than 1 gram fat per 5 tablespoons) is useful to help add nutritional value to a recipe without adding fat or volume. In its dry form, nonfat dry milk powder helps thicken recipes such as soups and desserts. It also is useful as the basis for a convenient low-fat, low-calorie basic white sauce (to which other ingredients can be added for flavor variety). When whipped with iced water, nonfat dry milk powder increases in volume and makes a good substitute for whipped cream in chilled souffles, or, when other ingredients are added, can add thickness and flavor to a savory sauce.

Instant nonfat dry milk powder is shelf-stable and convenient to use. Although the cost has escalated dramatically in past years, it is still a relatively inexpensive dairy product. Because nonfat dry milk powder is heat-processed, it can be conveniently used in products containing yeast (i.e., yeast breads), unlike fluid milk, which often has to be scalded before use.

Barriers to using nonfat dry milk powder include the fact that when mixed with water, the end product is not well accepted as a beverage (off-flavor being the primary complaint). Thus the dry form of the product is not well accepted as an ingredient in recipes.

2. Yogurt

Yogurt has gained tremendous space in dairy cases in the past 5 years due to better consumer acceptance. Now available as whole milk yogurt, low-fat yogurt, nonfat yogurt, custard-style yogurt, aspartame-sweetened yogurt, and sugar-sweetened, low-fat yogurt, there is a style for everyone regardless of calorie and fat limitations. The nutrient profiles are compared in Table 2.

With more options available, consumers are enjoying yogurt as a snack, a dessert, and a breakfast food. In the preparation of recipes, plain yogurt can be used successfully in place of sour cream as the basis for both sweet

Table 2 Nutrient Profile of Yogurt Products

Item	kcal/8 oz	Fat (g)
Plain whole milk yogurt	138	7.4
Plain low-fat yogurt	143	3.5
Plain nonfat yogurt	127	0.4
Flavored custard-style yogurt	249	4.5
Flavored aspartame sweetened nonfat yogurt	93	0
Flavored sugar-sweetened low-fat yogurt	240	3

Source: Refs. 4, 5.

and savory dips and spreads, salad dressings, and some sauces. It can be stirred into hot dishes such as beef stroganoff and chicken paprikash. As a substitute for sour cream, cream cheese, or whipping cream, it also works well in some desserts.

Yogurt's acidity gives it a distinct flavor that some find disagreeable. This acidity also causes yogurt to react differently in many recipes. While these are not limitations to use, special handling techniques are required when using yogurt in some recipes:

Gently stir yogurt in carton before using.

When processed in an electric blender, yogurt breaks down and gets runny; therefore, it is best to blenderize other ingredients and stir yogurt in at a later point in the recipe.

When heated, yogurt breaks down quicker than sour cream, so it is best to try one of the following techniques: (1) bring yogurt to room temperature before adding it to a hot dish, (2) stir 1 tablespoon flour or cornstarch into each container of yogurt before adding to a hot dish, (3) add yogurt at the end of the cooking period, after the pan or skillet has been removed from the heat.

Nonfat yogurt breaks down and waters out in recipes that are held over a period of time, so low-fat yogurt is usually a better choice for these recipes.

The addition of low-fat or nonfat yogurt to beverages usually causes them to separate upon standing, so it is best to serve them immediately.

When using yogurt in baked goods, compensate for the increased acidity by adding a little more baking soda.

To keep yogurt from watering out upon standing or to give it a thicker, richer, creamier consistency needed for certain recipes, drain it on heavy-duty paper towels for 5 minutes or, for an even thicker product, place it in cheesecloth over a large measuring cup or bowl in the refrigerator overnight. The end product (called yogurt cheese) can be used in a wide variety of applications:

as a binding agent that won't water out in items like potato salad,
piped as a topping that holds its shape on desserts,
as a creamy dessert filling.

Both plain and vanilla low-fat yogurt work well when drained. But yogurt with added stabilizers cannot be drained successfully.
Custard-style yogurt, which has stabilizers added, works especially well for fruit-based or sweet dips. Its creamy texture holds up better than regular low-fat yogurt, which would have to be drained to get a similar product.

3. Sour Cream

With all the knowledge now available about using yogurt in cooking, it will never replace sour cream in the minds of many consumers. As manufacturers have realized this, low-fat and nonfat sour cream alternatives have become more available. The nutrient profiles are compared in Table 3.

In the case of light sour cream alternatives, consumers need to read product labels carefully. While all are somewhat lower in calories and fat, some are much lower than others. From a taste and texture standpoint, the modified products are very acceptable and similar to their original counterpart. However, the newness of the nonfat product at this writing means that little independent testing has been conducted to assess the differences in its physical properties compared to regular sour cream.

4. Cheese

The past 5 years have brought some major breakthroughs in modified cheese products to lower their calorie and fat contents. However, the greatest successes have been with fresh and soft cheeses. There is still work to be done in the area of hard cheese substitutes before tasty ones with similar properties of regular hard cheese are readily available.

Table 3 Nutrient Profiles of sour cream products

Item	kcal/tbsp	Fat (g)
Regular sour cream	26	2.5
Sour half-and-half	20	1.8
Two-thirds-less-fat sour cream	20	1
Nonfat sour cream alternative	20	0

Source: Refs. 4, 5.

Regular, natural hard cheeses get their taste, texture, and physical properties from a high butterfat content, where the largest amount of fat and calories are contained. As researchers have worked to reduce the butterfat content in hard cheese analogs, a decrease in flavor and in melting properties has also occurred. Lack of flavor is sometimes offset by adding herbs, peppers, or smoke flavoring. The melting properties range from good to bad according to brand.

A confusing factor for consumers is that some manufacturers offer modified hard cheeses that really are not different in the amount of calories and fat they contain. Instead, the *type* of fat has been changed—a vegetable oil has been substituted for the butterfat. Often these cheeses carry a "no cholesterol" label, which consumers mistakenly believe to mean low calorie and/or low fat.

When acceptable hard cheese analogs are not available for use in recipes, consumers can decrease the amount of regular hard cheese called for and substitute a stronger-flavored cheese without sacrificing flavor. For example, substitute a smaller amount of extra-sharp cheddar for mild cheddar cheese, and make better use of very pungent cheeses such as blue cheese and Gruyere. Cooks also can increase the perception of cheese flavor by adding a small amount of dry mustard and ground red pepper to many recipes. When carrot purée is added to a reduced-fat cheese soup, it appears to be "cheesier" because of its color. Other problems with cheese analogs include a higher sodium content in processed cheese products.

Some hard cheese is naturally lower in fat and calories than its counterpart, for example, part-skim mozzarella versus whole milk mozzarella. Fortunately for consumers, the part-skim variety has become the market standard.

A confusing issue that consumers have heard for years is that farmer's cheese is a lower-fat cheese. However, farmer's cheese has no standard of identity and can vary from a lower-fat to a high-fat cheese. Consumers need to read the ingredient label to be sure, but generally the softer farmer's cheese is lower in fat and calories than the hard farmer's cheese.

Cottage cheese now comes in 2% low-fat, 1% low-fat, dry curd, and nonfat varieties. Any of the creamed varieties work well as a substitute for 4% butterfat (whole milk) creamed cottage cheese. However, dry curd cottage cheese does not work well as a substitute in most recipes. Substituting the lower-fat varieties means a substantial savings in fat and calories. The nutrient profiles are compared in Table 4.

Cottage cheese can be eaten in its natural form or combined with other ingredients. Processed in an electric blender or food processor, it takes on a smooth thick texture, which makes an ideal substitute for sour cream as a base for dips, salad dressings, and toppings. Thoroughly processed, it has no chalky texture.

Table 4   Nutrient Profile of Cottage Cheese

Item	kcal/4 oz	Fat (g)
Creamed cottage cheese	117	5.1
2% lowfat cottage cheese	101	2.2
1% lowfat cottage cheese	82	1.2
Nonfat cottage cheese	80	0
Dry curd cottage cheese	96	0.5

Source: Refs. 4, 5.

Ricotta cheese comes in a part-skim and a fat-free version as well as regular whole milk ricotta. The nutrient profiles are compared in Table 5. Ricotta can be used in many of the same ways as cottage cheese. It is especially popular as an ingredient in Italian cuisine. In its natural form, ricotta has a finer texture than cottage cheese, but when processed in an electric blender or food processor an undesirable chalky texture is detected. This may make ricotta better suited to cooked dishes. Drawbacks to using cottage cheese and ricotta are that each has a short shelf life and the reduced-fat/calorie versions have a shorter shelf life than the whole milk ones.

Cream cheese comes in four major varieties: regular cream cheese, "light" cream cheese (actually Neufchâtel cheese), light process cream cheese product, and fat-free cream cheese product. The nutrient profiles are compared in Table 6.

Current marketing tactics and labeling terminology confuse consumers as to which type cream cheese they are actually choosing. Light process cream cheese product comes in a tub and is marketed alongside soft regular cream cheese, also in a tub. The "light" cream cheese in a block is marketed alongside regular cream cheese in a block. Also, when light cream cheese is called for in a recipe, consumers do not know whether to choose the block or the tub form, yet the latter is significantly lower in fat and calories.

Table 5   Nutrient Profile of Ricotta Cheese

Item	kcal/oz	Fat (g)
Whole milk ricotta	60	5
Part-skim ricotta	40	3
Fat-free ricotta	20	0

Source: Ref. 5.

Table 6 Nutrient Profile of Cream Cheese

Item	kcal/oz	Fat (g)
Regular cream cheese	99	9.9
"Light" cream cheese		
(Neufchâtel)	74	6.6
Light process cream cheese		
product	60	5.0
Fat-free cream cheese product	30	0

Source: Refs. 4, 5.

Both "light" cream cheese and the light process cream cheese product substitute nicely for regular cream cheese in most recipes. The exception: the light process cream cheese product has a higher (and sometimes more noticeable) sodium content, which may make it less desirable for some desserts and fruit dip recipes. However, combined with other ingredients, it still can be used to produce a lower-fat, lower-calorie cheesecake without undesirable effects. Because the tub-style process product is softer (due to a higher water content) than the "light" cream cheese in the block, it will not set up or lend form to a recipe as well as the "light" cream cheese in the block form. Fat-free cream cheese product is so new to the market little independent testing assessed its attributes and limitations.

Two products with great potential for incorporation into low-calorie recipes have the brand names Fromage Blanc and Quark® . Each of these two soft cheeses has a tart flavor. Fromage Blanc has a silky texture and consistency similar to sour cream. Quark's texture is similar to ricotta cheese. This makes both products desirable substitutes for mayonnaise, sour cream, and even cream cheese in some recipes. (Quark would need to be processed in a food processor for these applications.) However, both are relatively high priced (compared to the products they substitute) and are available only regionally. Quark can be found in the extreme northwestern United States and Fromage Blanc is limited primarily to the northeastern United States.

5. Ice Cream and Frozen Desserts

Ice milk, nonfat frozen desserts, and nonfat and low-fat frozen yogurt have made significant advances into the ice cream market. And when the fat and calorie savings are compared, as shown in Table 7, it's easy to see why.

Each of these modified products is virtually nutritionally equivalent to their regular counterparts, except that sugar has been added and the fat content is lower. From a sensory standpoint, the modified products have an appearance and texture similar to regular ice cream but without the rich taste. These modified products hold up as well as regular ice cream with the exception of nonfat frozen yogurt, which melts quickly.

Table 7 Nutrient Profiles of Ice Cream and Frozen Desserts

Item	kcal/½ cup	Fat (g)
Premium vanilla ice cream (16% fat)	175	11.8
Regular vanilla ice cream (10% fat)	135	7.2
Vanilla ice milk	92	2.8
Vanilla nonfat frozen dessert	90	0
Vanilla low-fat frozen yogurt	74–100	1–3
Vanilla nonfat frozen yogurt	100–110	0
Frozen dairy dessert with fat substitute	134	1

Source: Refs. 4, 5.

A subcategory of these frozen desserts includes those sweetened with aspartame and those containing a fat substitute. Their nutritional advantages over regular ice cream can also be seen in Table 7. These products are becoming more widely available. However, frozen dairy desserts containing a fat substitute have been described by some people as having an undesirably slick rather than creamy texture. Aspartame-sweetened frozen dairy desserts leave an undesirable aftertaste, according to some people.

6. Custards and Puddings

When preparing custards and puddings or other lower-calorie, dairy-based desserts cooked from scratch, special handling techniques are required. Sugar makes a softer custard and helps raise the temperature of coagulation; therefore, a custard or pudding with less sugar will be stiffer and cooking time may be shorter.

Eggs help thicken custards and puddings. When fewer eggs are used to help lower fat and calories in a custard or pudding recipe, more flour, cornstarch, or tapioca will be needed for proper consistency.

C. Fruits and Vegetables

By virtue of their natural composition, fruits and vegetables are low in fat and calories (except coconut and avocado). All fruits and vegetables—even the starchy ones such as potatoes—can be considered low-calorie foods. They contain valuable fiber and have the ability to give a sensation of fullness without contributing significant calories. Fruits in their natural state are guaranteed to be low in fat and calories. Processed and canned fruits present a different picture with varying amounts of added sugar. The nutrient profiles are compared in Table 8.

Table 8   Nutrient Profiles of Raw and Processed Fruit

Item	kcal	Fat (g)
Apple—raw, with skin	81	0.5
Applesauce, sweetened (½ cup)	97	0.2
Applesauce, unsweetened (½ cup)	53	0.1
Peach—raw	37	0.1
Canned peaches—heavy syrup (1 cup)	190	0.3
Canned peaches—light syrup (1 cup)	136	0.1
Canned peaches—juice packed (1 cup)	109	0.1
Canned peaches—water-packed	58	0.1
Dried peaches (10 halves)	311	1.0
Frozen peaches—sweetened (1 cup)	235	0.3

Source: Ref. 6.

Vegetables are especially useful in recipes to extend meat and thereby decrease the percent of calories from fat. Fruits can also serve this purpose, such as apples in tuna salad or grapes in chicken salad. The additional volume, fiber, and flavor are desirable. Vegetable purées made from potatoes or carrots can be used to thicken soups, sauces, or stews in place of a traditional fat-based roux.

Care must be taken in what is added to these low-calorie foods. Potatoes got their reputation as "fattening" because of the high-fat, high-calorie toppings used. Healthier toppings for baked potatoes include:

Reduced-fat cheese
Low-fat yogurt
Part skin mozzarella cheese, grated
Low-fat cottage cheese
Chopped tomatoes with basil or oregano for an Italian flavor
Salsa for a Mexican flavor
Buttermilk (ranch-type) dressing made with skim milk and fat-free mayonnaise

D. Eggs and Egg Products

Eggs are a good source of protein, but people have been limiting their use because they also contain a substantial amount of cholesterol. It is prudent to substitute two egg whites for one egg for half of the eggs called for in most recipes. This will decrease the calories from fat contributed by eggs by one half.

Another option is egg substitute. Made of egg whites, these products are widely available frozen and can be found in a liquid, fresh form in larger grocery stores. These products are convenient and also good for those who find it difficult to discard the yolk from fresh eggs. The frozen type does require time for thawing, and the entire amount may not be needed for one recipe, so there is a potential for waste. This is important because egg substitutes are more expensive than fresh eggs. These products can be useful for most purposes for which fresh eggs are used. However, they do not perform as well as a thickening agent as a whole egg or egg yolk. An omelet or souffle made from egg whites alone will be different from one made from whole eggs. The puffiness is decreased, but the flavor remains tasty, especially with the addition of onions, green pepper, or other distinctively flavored, traditional ingredients.

When using egg substitutes in baking, the leavening agent may need to be increased. Since egg whites are high in protein, cakes may be less tender when made with egg substitutes. A balance may be achieved by using equal amounts of egg substitute and fresh eggs. The fresh eggs can be beaten to incorporate air for additional leavening.

When used in quiches or other egg-based dishes, there may be some watering-out. Again, this might be minimized by the use of equal amounts of egg substitute and whole eggs.

E. Breads, Cereals, and Grains

These foods provide significant contributions to the American diet each day beginning with breakfast, continuing through dinner, and including snacks. Consumers are beginning to see the value of building meals around these foods, which are rich in complex carbohydrates. They fit nicely into fast-paced lifestyles and are particularly attractive to health-conscious consumers because they are naturally low in fat (except quick breads like biscuits) and relatively low in calories. Some breads have fewer calories due to the addition of noncaloric fiber.

1. Grains, Pasta, and Legumes

Cereals are low in fat and calories if they are unadorned. Persons who build breakfast around whole-grain cereals and low-fat milk are making nutritionally sound choices. Cereal labels can give valuable information on fat and sugar content. Some cereals are available with added nonnutritive sweeteners. These have met with limited success partly due to increased cost.

Grains, pasta, and legumes are being touted as good choices for meatless entrees. These foods are applauded by nutritionists and should be promoted more as meat extenders. They provide fiber without fat or excess calories which accompany meat. The toppings for pasta and grains such as high-fat, high-calorie meat sauces can be replaced with fat-free, Italian-seasoned tomato sauce, which is widely available.

2. Baked Goods

a. General. Baked goods have undergone remarkable changes in the past few years. New low-fat cookies have been introduced that utilize fruits such as applesauce or dates to promote tenderness, which is diminished when fat is decreased. Many provide less than 30% of the calories from fat ($\leq$3 g/100 kcal). Several food producers now make cakes, cookies, and coffee cakes with significantly less or no cholesterol or fat and limited sugar, so that the calories do not exceed 100 per serving and have less than 30% of their calories from fat. A corn syrup manufacturer and applesauce producer are providing the public with recipes for fat-free cakes, which are made more tender by the addition of their products. The cake mix manufacturers have responded by introducing light cake and frosting mixes.

At one time crackers were low in fat but specialty crackers were introduced and consumers were attracted because of their buttery flavor, not realizing how much fat they were eating. Saltines, which are low in fat and therefore lower in calories, are receiving renewed interest. Other low-fat specialty crackers have been introduced with added fiber in the form of whole grains and seeds.

The keeping quality and tenderness of baked products are potentially compromised because fat and sugar contribute to these qualities. Consumers may be willing to accept a coarser more crumbly texture, less tenderness, and decreased keeping quality to have products available that are actually healthier. Moderation in serving size remains important because these low-fat products may not be low in calories. Single-serving desserts are available that allow an occasional indulgence without long-term consequence because the temptation of eating several servings has been removed.

b. Cakes. When cakes are made at home with less fat and sugar, creaming of fat and sugar needs to be extended to 5 minutes to help leaven and increase tenderness. (The mixing time after the addition of the flour and liquid should not be increased. This would actually decrease tenderness.)

The following modifications help cut fat and calories:

Instead of greasing pans with shortening and flour, cake pans can be prepared with vegetable cooking spray plus two pieces of waxed paper cut to fit the bottom of the pan to ensure easy removal from pan.

Instead of a buttery icing, dust the baked cake with powdered sugar, perhaps utilizing a paper doily for a stencil design.

Utilize sweet spices such as cinnamon, nutmeg, cloves, and allspice to enhance the perception of sweetness in reduced-sugar baked goods. Sugar can generally be reduced by as much as one third without adversely affecting the final product.

c. Yeast Breads. Yeast breads can be made at home with minimal or no added fat. Most purchased yeast breads are also low in fat and low in calories. Some calories from fat can be avoided by using vegetable cooking spray instead of butter or margarine to coat the surface of loaf breads or rolls. Quick breads are more difficult to modify because they depend on fat and sugar for tenderness. Some alterations that enhance the desirable qualities of quick breads when fat and sugar have been reduced are:

Use cake flour instead of all-purpose flour because it has a lower protein content and will yield a more tender product.

Utilize moist fruits such as applesauce or banana. Even in small amounts that are not detectable when tasted, fruit can provide additional tenderness and moistness.

When a sweet muffin is desired, 1/4 teaspoon of sugar (4 calories) can be sprinkled on top of batter in the muffin pan before baking. The perception of a sweeter product is accomplished by the surface of the muffin coming into direct contact with the taste buds on the front of the tongue.

Two egg whites can be substituted for 1 whole egg.

Yogurt can sometimes be substituted for sour cream in baked goods, but because of its high acidity, recipes may need a little additional baking soda.

Skim milk can be substituted for whole milk.

Using oil instead of shortening does not decrease calories, but a lesser amount can be used for tenderness because the liquid form of fat performs differently.

Extra care must be given to avoid overmixing muffins that have reduced amounts of fat and sugar.

Oatmeal can be utilized as a crunchy topping instead of nuts, which have a higher fat and calorie content.

3. Pastry-Type Crusts

No low-calorie pastry-type crusts are currently available on the market, but a reduced-fat pie crust can be made at home. Pastry must be thoroughly chilled and worked between layers of plastic wrap or waxed paper. If a pie crust is made with less fat, it will be less tender and less flaky—properties contributed by fat. Crumb crusts made from Graham cracker crumbs and a small amount of low-calorie margarine can be an even lower-calorie alternative to a pastry crust.

4. Phyllo Pastry

Phyllo pastry is usually combined with an equal amount of melted butter in traditional rich dessert recipes. To avoid these added calories, each layer can be coated with vegetable cooking spray. Because of problems with shattering of cooked phyllo pastry, it is better to prepare recipes in individual portions versus a large product that has to be cut into servings.

F. Margarines, Spreads, and Dressings

There are more low-calorie products on the market in this food category than others. Still, as with other categories, the availability depends on the market size and location.

1. Margarine and Margarine-Type Products

Margarine, the most popular spread of the 1970s and 1980s, contains about 100 calories and 11.4 grams of fat per tablespoon. It derives 100% of its calories from fat. Pushing their way into the regular margarine market with the possibility of displacing it as the preferred spread of the 1990s and beyond is reduced-calorie margarine (50 calories and 5.6 grams fat per tablespoon), diet imitation margarine (48 calories and 5.4 grams fat per tablespoon), and spreads (70 calories and 7 grams fat per tablespoon) that are all lower in total fat and calories than regular margarine due to incorporation of air and/or water into the product to dilute the fat content.

Reduced-calorie margarine and lower-calorie spreads can be successfully used in a wide variety of recipes. Used in place of regular margarine, they lower the total amount of fat and calories in a recipe. Used in place of butter, they also lower the amount of saturated fat and cholesterol in a recipe.

Reduced-calorie margarine does not have the same physical properties as regular margarine. It doesn't melt as well, and because of the higher water content, it separates when heated or beaten too long. Manufacturers of these products seldom recommend that they be used in baked products. However, it depends on the recipe. Reduced-calorie margarines will work successfully in some baked products, but there is no way to know which ones without testing the specific recipe in question. For example, a reduced-calorie margarine usually works well to hold a Graham cracker crust together, but it causes some cookies to spread too much. For many products, better results can be achieved by simply decreasing the amount of regular margarine by one-third the amount called for in the recipe.

2. Vegetable Cooking Sprays

Vegetable cooking sprays also can make a contribution to reducing fat and calories in recipes when used in place of margarine, butter, or oil to coat cooking utensils (to prevent sticking and for sautéing), to coat phyllo pastry dough sheets, and to promote browning of homemade bread. For example, a recipe might typically call for 1 tablespoon butter, margarine, or oil (about 100 calories and 11.4 grams fat) to coat a 10-inch skillet to prevent sticking. But a 1¼-second spritz of vegetable cooking spray into a nonstick cooking utensil would accomplish similar results for only 7 calories and 1 gram fat.

3. Butter-Flavored Products

Likewise, butter-flavored powders and granules used in place of butter or margarine to "season" or top foods such as vegetables, baked potatoes, and popcorn add as little as 4 calories and 0 grams of fat per ½ teaspoon (butter-flavored powders) to 3 calories and 0 grams of fat for the dry granules. However, their use is limited due to lack of flavor and different physical properties from regular fat; therefore, these products cannot easily be substituted in recipes where fats have a functional property other than flavor.

4. Mayonnaise and Salad Dressing

Mayonnaise provides 100 calories and 11 grams of fat per tablespoon, while spreadable salad dressing provides 70 calories and 7 grams of fat for the same amount. Reduced-calorie mayonnaise contains 50 calories and 5 grams of fat per tablespoon. Thus, regular spreadable salad dressing offers a calorie savings over regular mayonnaise, but reduced-calorie mayonnaise offers even fewer calories per tablespoon. However, the flavor of the two differ, and spreadable salad dressing, which has a slightly sweet flavor, is not as widely accepted as mayonnaise. In early 1991, a fat-free mayonnaise (12 calories and 0 grams of fat per tablespoon) and a fat-free spreadable salad dressing (20 calories and 0 grams of fat per tablespoon) were introduced on the market. These products should be very useful in helping consumers to lower the fat content of many favorite recipes such as potato salad, coleslaw, and meat salads that traditionally use a lot of mayonnaise as a binding agent. The new products have flavor and binding properties similar to the regular mayonnaise and spreadable salad dressings they replace, making them familiar, convenient, and acceptable to consumers.

Reduced-calorie and fat-free mayonnaise and spreadable salad dressing can be used interchangeably as a spread and as a binding agent for foods. However, when used in cooked products such as hot dips or hot salads, the reduced-calorie and fat-free versions may separate.

Regular pourable salad dressings contain 60–70 calories and 6–7 grams of fat per tablespoon. Reduced-calorie salad dressings offer some fat and calorie savings over regular: 16–30 calories and 1–3 grams of fat per tablespoon. But the newer fat-free pourable salad dressings offer the most savings in calories and fat (6–20 calories and less than one-half gram of fat per tablespoon).

Reduced-calorie and fat-free pourable salad dressings have the advantage of similar pourability and "cling" as their regular counterpart. Therefore, the reduced-calorie and fat-free versions can be used in similar application as regular pourable salad dressings. Besides the obvious use on salad greens, they make an excellent base for a wide variety of fat-free marinades. However, when grilling or broiling skinless chicken and lean fish held in a fat-free marinade, there may be a need to add a small amount of oil to the basting marinade to prevent the meat from drying out.

Other limitations include the perception among some people that fat-free pourable salad dressings have an off-flavor or a stronger flavor attributed to garlic, herbs, or vinegar.

G. Sweets: Sugar Substitutes, Jams, Jellies, Pancake Syrups, Fruit-Flavored Gelatin, Etc.

1. Sugar Substitutes

A wide variety of sugar substitutes is now readily available on grocers' shelves, and the specific brands vary from region to region. The nutrient composition of sugar substitutes is virtually calorie-free compared to 16 calories per teaspoon for regular sugar. Sugar substitutes work well in recipes specifically developed for their use. However, there are some limitations. All sugar substitutes cannot be substituted equally for one another. This makes it hard to call for any sugar substitute in a recipe because recipe publishers often are hesitant to mention specific brand names. Other problems include an aftertaste that some consumers find objectionable.

Aspartame-based sugar substitutes cannot be used in cooked products (except some microwave recipes) because they break down upon heating and lose their sweet taste. A major problem with using sugar substitutes in baking goods is that many of them do not provide the bulk of regular sugar.

2. Jams and Jellies

Lower-calorie jams and jellies (fruit spreads) are now widely available. They contain approximately half the calories of regular jams and jellies. Artificially sweetened jams and jellies (imitation jams and jellies) are virtually calorie-free. Both lower-calorie fruit spreads and the imitation products can be used in the same ways as regular jams and jellies with similar results. Lower-calorie fruit spreads are tasty and often have a fruitier flavor than regular jams and jellies. Some people complain that artificially sweetened and imitation products leave an undesirable aftertaste.

The texture of both lower-calorie fruit spreads and imitation jams and jellies are somewhat different from their regular counterparts. The modified versions are more liquid, lose their shape more easily, and tend to water-out upon long storage. The modified products must be kept refrigerated because they do not contain enough sugar to act as a preservative against spoilage.

Consumers easily confuse the lower-calorie fruit spreads with spreadable fruits that contain fruit juice instead of sugar but may not actually be lower in calories. Better labeling regulations and consumer education will help solve this problem.

3. Pancake Syrups

Reduced-calorie pancake syrups contain approximately one third fewer calories than regular pancake syrups. The pourability and flavor is similar to regular pancake syrup so the reduced-calorie product can be substituted in equal amounts for regular pancake syrup.

An advantage to using a reduced-calorie maple-flavored syrup is that it often imparts a stronger maple flavor in cooked products than true maple syrup, so a smaller amount can be used. However, reduced-calorie syrups cannot be used inter changeably with more viscous syrups (such as molasses, corn syrup, or cane syrup) with the same results.

4. Gelatin

Prepared sugar-free gelatin contains 8 calories per ½ cup serving compared to regular sugar-sweetened gelatin at 81 calories for the same amount. Fruit-flavored, sugar-free gelatin is readily available and widely used because consumers are familiar and comfortable with the product, and no special handling is required. It can be used alone as a dessert, in combination with fruit as a dessert or salad, or as an ingredient in punch-type beverages. Its limitation is that it costs more than its regular counterpart and leaves an undesirable aftertaste detectable by some consumers.

H. Frozen Entrees and Dinners

Availability and choices among low-calorie frozen entrees and frozen dinners have increased in recent years due to consumer demand for convenience. Each offering differs in size, calorie, and fat content, but, nutritionally, these items are comparable to their normal counterparts prepared in the same low-calorie, low-fat way.

These entrees and dinners have been readily accepted by consumers who want to keep on hand convenient, quick-to-prepare foods. They also allow variety in the eating plan of a single person or single-dieter household without a lot of food waste.

For consumers who do not own a microwave oven, these foods are not as quick to prepare. Their high sodium content should be a concern for the sodium conscious and those people who make a steady diet of these products. Other drawbacks include the cost. Frozen entrees and dinners are more expensive per serving than traditionally prepared foods. Many of these dinners and entrees begin to taste the same after a while, according to some people who eat them frequently, and people with large appetites may find the portion size skimpy.

When microwaving frozen dinners, it is often hard to get the entree heated thoroughly without overcooking the accompanying vegetables. Consumers need to follow manufacturer's directions closely for the specific wattage of their microwave oven.

Because frozen entrees alone do not constitute an entire meal, the user will need to prepare additional foods, especially from the fruit, vegetable, and dairy groups to ensure a nutritionally balanced meal.

III. DISCUSSION

Low-calorie processed foods are not essential to low-calorie recipes; however, they can add variety and cut shopping and preparation time, an important consideration for today's busy consumer.

Clearly, low-calorie food products have been useful in giving consumers alternative choices. The effectiveness of these low-calorie options depends on how well and how wisely they are used. This explosive market will continue to create a need for nutrition educators to teach the public about a constantly changing food supply. This will be a challenge for the remainder of this century. With most Americans believing that balance, variety, and moderation are the keys to healthy eating but many mistakenly choosing foods based on good food/bad food perceptions, the role of nutrition education is paramount. Misconceptions of consumers such as the notion that a product has been given magical qualities by the addition or deletion of a single ingredient without consideration of the total caloric/fat/sugar/nutrient content will need to be addressed. Nutrition labels on new products will be essential.

Although the number of new, more healthful food products is increasing, many more are needed, especially those listed below:

Ready-to-use, fat-free marinades to encourage use of low-fat cooking methods such as broiling and stir-frying

Fat-free sauces—perhaps fruit juice–based for use on meats and vegetables to enhance the flavors without addition of fat

Fat-free "creamed" condensed soups for use in casseroles and other combination dishes

Canned, reduced-calorie, ready-to-use sauces such as white sauce, "cream" sauce, cheese sauce

Fat-free, ready-to-use whipped topping

Bulking agents to use in baked goods to provide volume, tenderness, and moistness when sugar and fat are reduced

Reduced-fat, ready-to-use pie crusts (regular and crumb-type)

Evaporated skim milk sold as a fresh product much like half-and-half, perhaps in frozen form

Fat-free bread and cracker crumbs and stuffing mixes

Fat-free seasoned coating mixes for meats

Fat-free pasta sauces

Beef, fish, chicken, and vegetable broths that are fat-free, low-cost, and in a convenient liquid form

Low-fat entree mixes, e.g., boxed pasta and chicken casserole mix

Low-calorie peanut butter–type spreads with the similar creaminess and spreading qualities of regular peanut butter

Low-calorie margarine with minimal or no hydrogenation but properties that perform well in baking

These products need to be as close to original counterparts as possible in taste, texture, appearance, and price. These products, when available, must be presented to the public in such a way as to provide nutrition education, familiarity, and trust [3]. This might be accomplished by informative labeling and by using the marketplace for tasting and advice on the use of these products. A word of caution—new products must infringe on the consumer's lifestyle as little as possible. This means they must not require excessive preparation or time (i.e., growing your own fresh herbs).

Whether the increased availability and use of low-calorie foods will reduce the incidence of obesity in our society remains to be seen. Nevertheless, future efforts to develop low-fat/low-calorie foods should be encouraged because of their potential for decreasing the nation's problem with obesity.

REFERENCES

1. A. M. Altschul, Low calorie foods, *Food Technol.*, *43*: 113 (1989).
2. *The Surgeon General's Report on Nutrition and Health*, USDHHS, Public Health Service, DHHS (PHS) Publication No. 88–50210, Washington, DC (1988).
3. A. L. Owen, The impact of future foods on nutrition and health, *J. Am. Diet. Assoc.*, *90*: 1217 (1990).
4. *Composition of Foods, Raw, Processed, Prepared*, USDA Handbook No. 8-1, Washington, DC (1976–1986).
5. Nutritional information obtained from product labels.
6. *Composition of Foods, Raw, Processed, Prepared*, USDA Handbook No. 8-9, Washington, DC (1976–1986).

21

Effect of Diet Composition on Energy Intake

F. Xavier Pi-Sunyer *Columbia University College of Physicians and Surgeons and St. Luke's/Roosevelt Hospital Center, New York, New York*

I. INTRODUCTION

The composition of a diet can be changed by diluting it with noncaloric substances or by varying the macronutrient content (carbohydrate, fat, or protein). In the first instance, the effect is to change the energy density of the diet so that the caloric strength of the total diet is decreased; in the second, to change the nutritional composition, so that the caloric strength of some components is increased and that of others decreased. The challenge to the organism is different in the two instances, so that different physiological responses with respect to energy intake are likely to ensue.

We know very little about what regulates energy intake. The organism may monitor a number of variables, including total energy intake, some function of energy or specific nutrient stores, the rate of energy utilization, or the intake of specific nutrients. While the data are sparse, some are available and will be reviewed in this chapter.

If the energy intake is regulated as a function of the energy expenditure, the expectation would be that if the nutritive density of the diet were altered, an individual would adjust intake appropriately and rapidly. However, this does not seem to occur. There are now numerous instances of populations that have gained weight when they moved from areas where food was of low nutrient density to areas where food was of high nutrient density. Well-known examples are Yemenite Jews who moved to urban Israel from the desert and Australian aborigines who moved from their native areas to the cities. The same phenomenon can be found within countries where the economy has changed rapidly for the better, such as Japan. In these situations, the weight norm tends to increase. Of course, other variables, such as activity patterns, also change, so that not all of the increase in weight can be ascribed to faulty calorie intake regulation, but it is clear that humans do not have a very sensitive monitor of overnutrition that can regulate food intake downwards in the face of excess caloric intake. This may well be a survival vestige of times when food was scarce and hard to find and the usual problem was too little rather than too much food, so that excess food reserves were a benefit [1].

II. DIET DILUTION

A. Diet Dilution with Water

The simplest diluent of a diet is water. The most quoted study of water dilution of a diet was done by Fomon et al. in infants. In their first experiment, 22 normal male infants were studied during their initial 112 days of life [2]. While the control group drank a regular formula with a caloric density of 133 kcal/dl, the experimental group received a diluted formula of 67 kcal/dl. The infants compensated somewhat for the dilution, but not completely. The infants on the diluted formula ate 75–80% of the calories that the control group ate. In a second study, the formula strengths were 100 kcal/dl for the controls and 54 kcal/dl for the study group and again were fed to infants for 112 days [3]. Initially, in the first 41 days, the infants in the experimental group ate about 75% of the control; after 41 days, they ate 85–91% of the intake of the controls. Thus, in both studies, babies given the dilute formula weighed less than those given the more concentrated formula. These studies suggest that, at least in babies, water can be an effective diluent to caloric intake.

In adults, Campbell et al. [4] also used water as a diluent to test the effect on energy intake. Lean and obese subjects were asked to eat exclusively from a formula diet dispensed by machine. The individuals pushed a button and received a certain volume of the formula through a glass straw. The formula was diluted to a strength of 0.75 kcal/ml or 1.5 kcal/ml, and the food intake was measured covertly. Lean volunteers quickly adjusted to the dilution and ate more formula to compensate. Obese individuals did not eat enough of their formula to maintain food intake and did not compensate for dilution. Whether this was due to poor regulatory mechanisms or simply because the obese did not like the formula is unclear. However, Wooley [5] designed a similar experiment in both lean and obese persons and found that both of the groups compensated poorly when the formula was diluted with water. In addition, similar results were obtained by Spiegel [6] in obese subjects. These three studies all suggested a poor ability to match calories to need, particularly in obese persons.

B. Dilution of the Diet with Noncaloric Sweeteners

In our laboratories, Dr. Katherine Porikos undertook a series of studies in which she investigated the effect of diluting the diet with noncaloric sweeteners. She, for the first time in these kinds of experiments, used regular food rather than liquid formula diets. She developed a "platter method" of food presentation by which she was able to achieve what had not been possible with formula diets, that is, to get obese persons while in a metabolic ward or laboratory setting to eat food in quantities adequate to maintain weight. She was aided in her endeavor by having available a noncaloric sweetener, aspartame. With it, she was able to prepare low-calorie desserts, beverages, salad dressings, and other meal items indistinguishable to the subject from those made with sugar.

The "platter method" presents each individual food item on an individual platter and in excess. As a result, the subject can take as much as he or she likes from each of the platters provided. The food can be covertly measured before and after the meal to calculate total caloric intake. In addition, the test subject has available in the room a refrigerator with beverages and snacks that he or she can eat at any time of the day or night. Dr. Porikos had the volunteers live in the metabolic unit for periods of time and fed them by this platter method.

Caloric dilution was accomplished by substitution, without the subjects' knowledge of aspartame for sugar in many meal items: all beverages, all desserts, many gelatin salads and salad dressings, snacks, etc.

Three separate experiments were done [7–9]. These were reviewed in a separate publication [10]. Changing variables in the studies were lengths of time of the trial, gender tested, and whether the volunteers were obese or lean. An initial study [7] was done in men and women at 124–134% of desirable body weight. While the undiluted diet was given on days 1–3 and 10–15, the calorically diluted foods were given on days 4–9. The results are shown in Figure 1.

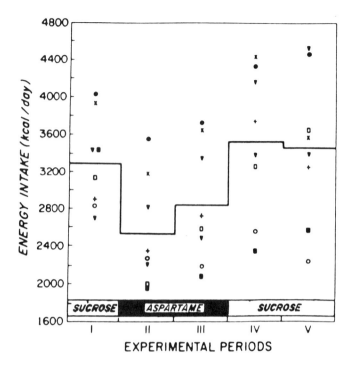

Figure 1 Mean daily energy intake as a function of experimental (sucrose or aspartame) periods for eight obese subjects. Solid line represents daily average intake per 3-day experimental period for all eight subjects. Symbols represent daily average intakes per 3-day period for each individual subject. Reprinted with permission from the American Journal of Clinical Nutrition [ref. 7].

The subjects ate an average of 2667 kcal/day when they were taking the aspartame-diluted diet and 3413 kcal/day when they ate the sucrose-sweetened diet. In the first dilution period they decreased their intake by 23% from baseline. In the second dilution period, they increased their intake by 310 more kcal. When they were returned to the sucrose-sweetened diet, a significant rise in intake occurred to a level even higher than the original baseline. Two conclusions were drawn from this initial study: (1) that obese subjects would voluntarily maintain their weight on such a platter diet; (2) that subjects would accept dilution of food with a noncaloric sweetener for a number of days without accurate compensation.

Because of some indication that the subjects of this first study might have been adapting with an increased food intake during the second dilution period, a second study was done to see if a longer period of dilution would confirm this [8]. As a result, the dilution period was made 24 days long, spanned by an initial and final undiluted period of 6 days each. To remove the variable of excess body weight, all subjects in this second study were lean. The results are shown in Figure 2 and can be seen to be very similar to the results from the first study. The volunteers ate an average of 3632 kcal/day in the undiluted periods and 3010 kcal/day in the diluted periods. They consumed 24% fewer calories in the first dilution period than they had

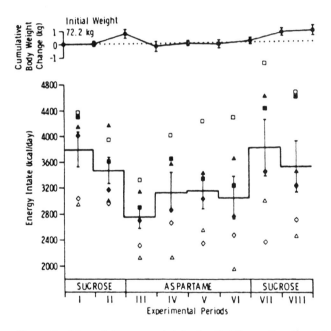

Figure 2   Mean daily energy intake (± SEM) as a function of experimental periods. During periods I, II, VII, and VIII subjects received the sucrose-sweetened diet, and during periods III–VI the aspartame-sweetened diet. The solid line in the lower section of the graph shows the average daily energy intake per 3-day period for the six subjects as a group. The symbols show the same data for each subject individually. The upper section of the graph represents changes in body weight (kg) over the course of the experiment. The dotted line shows the average initial weight of the six subjects (baseline) and the solid line represents the average cumulative change from the baseline at the end of each experimental period. (Reprinted with permission from Physiology and Behavior [ref. 8].

during the baseline period. During the second dilution period, they made some adjustment and increased their intake by 385 kcal/day, but they subsequently made no further changes.

In a third experiment, both lean and obese subjects were studied [9]. The difference in protocol from the second study was that the final baseline was 12 days instead of 6, and the subjects were asked to exercise for 1 hour a day on a treadmill (2.0–2.5 mph, flat grade). The exercise was instituted to try to prevent the slight gain in weight that occurred in the subjects in the undiluted part of the second experiment. The results are shown in Figure 3. On the baseline diet, the obese subjects ate 4131 kcal/day, while on the diluted diet they ate 3464 kcal/day. The lean subjects ate 3419 vs. 2880 kcal/day. This decrease of 21% in the obese and 26% in the lean was very similar and showed that neither group compensated fully for the dilution. Both

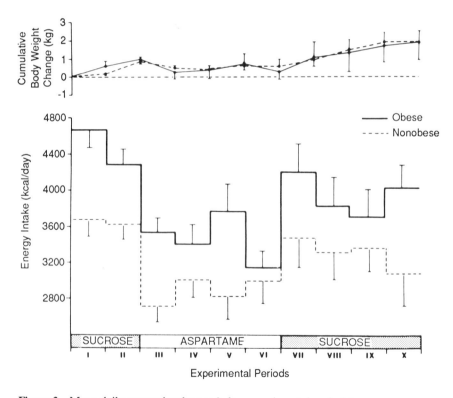

Figure 3   Mean daily energy intake per 3-day experimental period (sucrose or aspartame) and cumulative body weight change (± SE): five obese subjects (---); nonobese subjects (——). (Reprinted with permission from Clinical Endocrinology and Metabolism [ref. 10].

groups gained weight during the initial and final baseline periods, despite the exercise.

In summary, these three studies of noncaloric dilution showed very similar outcomes [10]. With a 25% dilution of calories in the diet, the subjects compensated for only part of this and stabilized at a caloric intake that provided them with about 85% of their baseline intake. Thus, there seemed to be no evident physiological drive to make up all of the calories diluted, even when a 12-day period was allowed to see if this would come about. Clearly, caloric regulation in human beings is not very tight. It is also interesting that the results were remarkably similar in the lean and obese subjects.

Three potential criticisms can be aimed at these studies. One of them is that the subjects did not compensate completely because they had gained some weight in the initial baseline period and were now making up for it. This is unlikely, however, since when the undiluted diet was once again placed before them they quickly increased their intake. Second, it would have been helpful to have a control study where the calorically dense (sugar-sweetened) diet was given throughout. This would have tested whether the sugar diet, which caused high early intake, would have dropped to the level of the diluted diet with time. A third problem with this study is that the subjects were partly coerced in that though they could take as much or as little of the rest of the foods, they had to take a minimum amount of the sweetened foods.

In addition, these studies were done on persons who were not on a diet and whose noncaloric dilution was instituted without their knowledge. It is not easy to extrapolate from these studies what would happen in people who wished to lose weight and who also were aware of the dilution of the diet. Such a study needs to be done.

The short-term effects of the noncaloric sweetener aspartame on food intake have been reviewed by Rolls [11]. Of 17 experiments cited, 15 found no effect on short-term food intake, and two found decreased food intake. Thus, in a one-meal paradigm, it is clear that noncaloric sweeteners do not decrease food intake, that is, they do not replace real calories and have no effect on energy intake. Other well-designed studies of their long-term effects on energy intake are needed.

C. Dilution of the Diet with Noncaloric Fat Substitutes

A number of investigators have studied the effect of diluting the diet with noncaloric fat substitutes, but few of these studies are relatively long term. The longest is that of Glueck et al. [12], who studied the effect of substituting 40 g of a sucrose polyester (SPE) for 40 g of fat in the diet of obese volunteers. After a baseline period to determine caloric intake, two 20-day periods followed randomly, using a placebo and an SPE. The subjects ate 1689 kcal/day during the SPE period vs. 2163 kcal/day during the placebo period. The subjects were obliged to eat a part of their diet (containing the fat or SPE) and then had free access to a number of snacks, which they could eat ad lib. They did not compensate appropriately. While there was a weight loss in both periods, it was greater by 0.42 kg during the SPE period.

D. Dilution of the Diet with Fiber

While fiber has been touted as enhancing weight loss by diluting the calories in the diet, the results are in fact very equivocal. Early rat studies, of which Adolph's [13] are an example, showed rats to compensate well when fiber was added to their diet. This was confirmed by some studies [14,15] but was not shown by Sullivan et al. [16] in obese Zucker rats.

In humans, an interesting study by Porikos and Hagamen [17] evaluated the effect of a 400-kcal preload of either 5.2 g or 0.2 g of crude fiber on a subsequent test meal given 30–45 minutes later. They found that obese subjects ate significantly less after the high-fiber preload. This was suggestive that high fiber might produce a food intake–lowering effect, but it would need to be tested in a longer-term protocol to confirm this.

It has been suggested that dietary fiber may decrease food intake in three ways: (1) it may displace available nutrients; (2) it may decrease the rate of eating by increasing the chewing time; and (3) it may cause a slight reduction in the gut's efficiency of absorption [18]. Whether these statements are in fact correct is unclear. Much more research needs to be done. However, a study by Evans and Miller [19] reports that subjects given 10 g of methylcellulose or 9 g of guar gum with a glass of water 30 minutes before each of two meals a day (lunch and dinner) lost weight. Other trials of fiber and food intake have been reviewed by Blundell and Burley [20], who suggest that fiber does have some effect on short-term food intake. But a recent position statement [21] suggests that the question is open and more long-term trials are in order.

Certainly, if fiber plays a role in regulating the quantity of food intake, the change in the American diet in this century would abet the increased prevalence of obesity. There has been an increase of sugar and fat and a 40% decrease of starch in the diet [22]. The fiber content of the diet has decreased, as shown by the fact that from 1889 to 1961 retail market supplies of carbohydrates decreased by about 28%, while the ratio of complex to simple carbohydrates showed more than a threefold drop [23].

In summary, while there is some evidence that fiber may play a role in modestly decreasing caloric intake in human subjects, the data are sparse and contradictory. More careful, controlled, long-term studies are necessary.

III. Changes in Macronutrient Composition

A. Sucrose

In rats, sucrose can cause obesity if given as a solution [24–30] but is not very effective if it is just added to the diet. An example of the latter is contained in a report by Laube et al. [31] who fed rats 20, 50, and 70% sucrose diets and found that the animals did not manifest any weight differences. Naim et al. [32] fed 25% sucrose diets and found no difference in food intake or body weight in comparison to a control, no-sucrose diet. However, a positive study of the use of a 67% sucrose diet showed a statistically significant increase in food intake and weight gain [33]. It seems that to get an effect in rats, the level of sucrose enrichment necessary to get increase weight is much above what any human group is likely to eat.

It is interesting to note, however, that sucrose in water solution seems to be much more effective in producing obesity than is sucrose added to a dry diet. The mechanism for this phenomenon is unknown. It is possible that the increased sucrose intake raises insulin levels, leading in turn to hypoglycemia and to increased carbohydrate intake in compensation [34]. Such a sequence of events has not been documented, however [30,35,36]. In addition, one can get similar weight gain effects with a high-fructose solution [37], even though insulin levels are only very modestly increased by fructose.

A physiological response to sucrose may be important. For instance, Hill et al. [38] have shown a greater body weight in sucrose-fed than starch- or chow-fed rats, even if all three groups are fed a similar number of calories. This suggests that the body handles the sucrose calories more "efficiently" than the starch or chow ones. Also, studies from our laboratory have shown that if sucrose-fed rats are given acarbose, thereby slowing the digestion of carbohydrates and their rate of absorption, obesity is markedly diminished [39]. While cephalic insulin response may be important in enhancing the obesifying effect of sucrose, this seems negated by studies in which cephalic insulin response is abolished by atropine and yet sucrose intake remains elevated [40,41].

These rat studies have been presented by way of introduction to the problem. However, the range of intake of sucrose in humans is much narrower than the wide range used in animal experiments, where sugar has varied from 4 to 70% of total intake. The average diet in the United States is 18–24% sucrose. Also, it seems precarious to extrapolate from a rat given a single food source of sucrose and humans who may sample a wide variety of foods [42]. For instance, Kratz and Levitsky [43] have shown that if rats are given a wide variety of sucrose and other macronutrient-containing foods, the rats do not gain excess weight and are not hyperphagic. Good long-term studies of the effect of sucrose on food intake and body weight in humans have not been done. It is not possible, therefore, at this time to indict sucrose as the cause of increased overweight in the United States. Also, many other variables have changed as sugar intake has increased. These include an increase in fat, a decrease in fiber, as well as a sedentary lifestyle. Some, all, or none may be involved. We presently do not have a clear enough idea of how individuals compose a diet when they have a wide variety of choices. No clear theory is available and none has been well tested experimentally.

B. Other Sugars

Addition of other sugars to the diet has led to variable effects on food intake. These studies have all been done in rats, not people. Comparative studies of the effect of disaccharides (maltose and sucrose) as compared to monosaccharides (glucose and fructose) suggest that the disaccharides cause more marked weight gain [44,45]. However, two studies that compared glucose vs. sucrose in water solution showed comparable effects of these two sugars [26,46]. Another study comparing fructose, glucose, and sucrose reported similar effects on energy intake and weight gain [47]. No comparable studies have been done in people.

C. Starch

Sclafani has done a series of elegant studies showing that rats have a polysaccharide appetite, which he has reviewed [48]. Given high-starch diets, these animals are hyperphagic and become obese. Like sucrose, the starch is more effective in producing obesity if it is given as a solution than if it is added to the diet. No such data are available for humans. In geographical areas where diets are high in starch, obesity is not common. However, other aspects of lifestyle are generally also different in these societies: lower fat intake, higher fiber intake, lower total caloric intake, and higher activity patterns. Despite these caveats, the epidemiological data does not support an effect of starch in enhancing food intake disproportionately and leading to obesity in humans.

D. Fat

A high-fat diet has been very effective in producing obesity in rats [49] and in other laboratory animals [50,51]. There are at least two known reasons for this: (1) they consume more calories; (2) there is evidence to suggest that the fat calories when eaten in excess are utilized more efficiently than other macronutrients [52]. The principal reason for the increase in body weight with the high-fat diets is that the animals seem to find these diets very palatable and generally increase their caloric intake [53,54]. Part of the increased efficiency is due to the decreased requirement for energy when fat is deposited as reserve than when other macronutrients are converted to fat for deposition [55]. Certainly, the greater efficiency is suggested by studies in which rats on high-fat diets were fed the same number of calories per day as rats fed a low-fat diet yet gained more weight [56]. It is interesting also that the palatability of the fat depends on the kind of fat. For instance, solid fat seems to be more effective than oil. The role of genetics is important, in that the strain of rat makes a difference in terms of the sensitivity to a high-fat diet, but gender seems not to be particularly important [57].

While animal studies are relatively simple to carry out, the same is not true of human experiments. There are, however, a few in the literature. Duncan et al. [58] fed a low-energy diet (LED) and a high-energy diet (HED) to 29 obese and nonobese human subjects. The two diets were tested for their palatability, and the ratings on the two were comparable. While the LED was made up of more fiber, more complex carbohydrate, and little fat and sugar, the HED contained more fat, more sugar, and less fiber. The differing amount of noncaloric bulk is evident in the caloric density of the two diets: the LED was 0.7 kcal/g, while the HED was 1.5 kcal/g. The trial consisted of 5 days on one diet and 5 days on the other, in a counterbalanced design. Each subject could eat freely to satiety at each meal. The subjects ate 1570 kcal on the LED and 3000 kcal on the HED. The satiety ratings were comparable on the two diets. So, even though the subjects ate twice the number of calories on the HED diet than on the LED, the satiety ratings were similar. It is also interesting that these diets were tested in both obese and lean subjects and that both of them responded in a similar fashion. That is, the LED diet was equally successful in both groups in being able to decrease caloric intake very significantly while still preserving satiety intact.

This is a very important study. It was not strictly a high-fat vs. a low-fat trial, since a number of variables were changed. That is, not only fat, but also sugar and fiber were changed. However, the primary change was in the fat content, and the results point out that humans, like rats, respond to a high-fat diet with an increased caloric intake. They seem to be unable to compensate for the higher energy concentration of the diet by decreasing food intake. Since this study was only conducted for 5 days on each diet, it would be interesting to repeat it for a longer period of time to see if the surprisingly large differences in energy intake between the two diets were sustained.

Two other studies have investigated the effect of high-fat vs. low-fat diets on energy intake. Both have been conducted at Cornell University by Levitsky and his collaborators [59,60]. The first studied 24 women for a period of 6 weeks [59]. These women were students who were free-living but came to the metabolic kitchen to eat their meals. For each of two 3-week periods, the women ingested diets consisting of either 15–20, 30–35, or 45–50% fat. The women were intructed to eat as much as they wished at each meal to reach satiety. Intakes on the low-, medium-, and high-fat diets were 2087, 2352, and 2714 kcal per day (Table 1). The dietary fat level seemed to have a major effect on energy intake. As a result, subjects gained weight on the high-fat diet, stayed stable on the moderate-fat diet, and lost weight on the low-fat diet. It is also interesting to note that, as in the Duncan study, the palatability ratings of the three diets were not different. This again suggests that individuals can be satisfied by widely differing caloric contents of diets, depending on the macronutrient composition of these diets.

The above study was carried out for only 5 days on each diet. To explore the phenomenon further, Levitsky and his groups undertook to do a similar but longer study [60]. They fed a high-fat diet and a low-fat diet to volunteers for 16 weeks. The protocol was similar to the previous one, with free-living volunteers coming to the metabolic kitchen to eat their meals. Subjects on the high-fat diet maintained their weight, while subjects on the low-fat diet ate fewer calories and lost weight during the study.

The authors [59] suggest that the compensation seems to be less accurate with diets that have been diluted by removal of fat than with diets that have been diluted with carbohydrate. Their point is that in the Porikos studies [6–10], diets were diluted by replacement of sucrose with noncaloric aspar-

Table 1.   Effects of Fat Level ($n = 24$) on Caloric Intake and Palatability Ratings

	Fat-intake ranges		
	15–20%	30–35%	45–50%
Caloric intake			
(kcal/day)	2087	2352	2714
SEM (56.7)	94	112	105
Palatability ratings	2.63	2.58	2.48
SEM (0.11)	0.12	0.11	0.15
Weighed food intake			
(g/day)	1496	1465	1412
SEM (31.6)	70	72	64
Weight change			
(kg/14 day)	−0.40	−0.03	+0.32
SEM (0.20)	0.16	0.15	0.15

Source: Ref. 59. Reprinted with permission from the *American Journal of Clinical Nutrition*.

tame. Here the compensation was on the order of 37–40%. On the other hand, when diets were diluted with the replacement of fat, the compensation was about 13%, in the study of Glueck where nonabsorbable fat was substituted for absorbable one, the compensation was about 11%, and in the Duncan study, where carbohydrate was substituted for fat, the compensation was about 10%. It is the authors' conclusion that "reducing fat intake may be a more effective strategy for weight loss than consuming artificially sweetened foods and beverages" [59].

IV. SUMMARY

In summing up, one must reflect on why this chapter is written at all. Obesity is increasing to the point where it is a serious liability for the health of the nation. The question is whether the nature of our diet is contributing to this epidemic of obesity. Is the increasing fat content of the diet, the increasing sugar content of the diet, and/or the increasing caloric density of the diet enhancing caloric intake and thus responsible for this fracas? Are human beings unable to regulate food intake when any or all of the above three situations are present? While an inability to regulate may exist, this chapter emphasizes that few studies are available that appropriately document this, and studies that are available have been carried out over very short periods of time. That such an important question has received so little attention is perplexing. Certainly, further and more long-term studies of this phenomenon are in order. The question of how the composition of the diet affects energy intake is a fundamental one in biology and precious little data are available to answer it.

ACKNOWLEDGMENT

This chapter was written under NIH grant NIDDK DK 26687 and R01 DK 40414. Much of this data was previously presented by the author at a symposium in 1989 [61].

REFERENCES

1. J. V. Neel, A thrifty genotype rendered detrimental by "progress", *Am. J. Human Genetics, 14*: 353 (1962).
2. S. J. Fomon, L. J. Filer, Jr., L. N. Thomas, R. R. Rogers, and A. M. Proksch, Relationship between formula concentration and rate of growth of normal infants, *J. Nutr., 98*: 241 (1969).

3. S. J. Fomon, L. J. Filer, Jr., L. N. Thomas, T. A. Anderson, and S. E. Nelson, Influence of formula concentration on caloric intake and growth of normal infants, *Act. Paediatr. Scand.*, *64*: 172 (1975).

4. R. G. Campbell, S. A. Hashim, T. B. Van Itallie, Studies on food intake regulation in man, responses to variations in nutritive density in lean and obese subjects, *New Engl. J. Med.*, *31*: 261 (1971).

5. O. W. Wooley, Long-term food regulation in the obese and nonobese, *Psychosomat. Med.*, *33*: 436 (1971).

6. T. S. Spiegel, Caloric regulation of food intake in man, *J. Comp. Physiol. Psychol.*, *84*: 24 (1973).

7. K. P. Porikos, G. Booth, and T. B. Van Itallie, Effect of covert nutritive dilution on the spontaneous food intake of obese individuals, *Am. J. Clin. Nutr.*, *30*: 1638 (1977).

8. K. P. Porikos, M. F. Hesser, and T. B. Van Itallie, Caloric regulation in normal-weight men maintained on a palatable diet of conventional foods, *Physiol. Behav.*, *29*: 293 (1980).

9. K. P. Porikos and T. B. Van Itallie, Efficacy of low-calorie sweeteners in reducing food intake: Studies with aspartame, *Aspartame: Physiology and Biochemistry* (L. D. Stegink and L. J. Filer, Jr., eds.) Marcel Dekker, New York, 273 (1984).

10. K. P. Porikos and F. X. Pi-Sunyer, Regulation of food intake in human obesity: Studies with caloric dilution and exercise, *Clin. Endocrinol. Metab.*, *13*: 547 (1984).

11. B. J. Rolls, Effects of intense sweeteners on hunger, food intake, and body weight: A review, *Am. J. Clin. Nutr.*, *53*: 872 (1991).

12. C. J. Glueck, M. M. Hastings, C. Allen, E. Hogg, L. Baehler, P. A. Gartside, D. Phillips, M. Jones, E. J. Hollenbach, B. Braun, and J. V. Anastasia, Sucrose polyester and covert caloric dilution, *Am. J. Clin. Nutr.*, *46*: 886 (1987).

13. E. F. Adolph, Urges to eat and drink in rats, *Am. J. Physiol.*, *151*: 110 (1947).

14. G. C. Kennedy, The hypothalamic control of food itnake in rats, *Proc. Roy. Soc.*, *137*: 535 (1950).

15. G. A. Bray and D. A. York, Studies on food intake of genetically obese rats, *Am. J. Physiol.*, *223*: 176 (1972).

16. A. C. Sullivan, J. Triscari, and K. Comai, Caloric compensatory responses to diets containing either nonabsorbable carbohydrate or lipid by obese and lean Zucker rats, *Am. J. Clin. Nutr.*, *31*: 261 (1978).

17. K. Porikos and S. Hagamen, Is fiber satiating? *Appetite*, *7*: 153 (1986).

18. K. W. Heaton, Food fibre as an obstacle to energy intake, *Lancet ii*: 1418 (1973).

19. E. Evans and D. S. Miller, Bulking agents in the treatment of obesity, *Nutr. Metab.*, *18*: 199 (1975).

20. J. E. Blundell and V. J. Burley, Satiation, satiety, and the action of fiber on food intake, *Int. J. Obes.*, *11* (Suppl. 1): 9 (1987).

21. Council on Scientific Affairs: Dietary fiber and health, *JAMA*, *262*: 542 (1989).

22. T. B. Van Itallie, Dietary fiber and obesity, *Am. J. Clin. Nutr.*, *31*: S43 (1978).

23. M. A. Antar, M. A. Ohlson, R. E. Hodges, Changes in retail market food supplies in the United States in the last seventy years in relation to the incidence of coronary artery disease, *Am. J. Clin. Nutr.*, *14*: 169 (1964).

24. R. B. Kanarek and E. Hirsch, Dietary-induced overeating in experimental animals, *Fed. Proc.*, *36*: 154 (1977).
25. R. B. Kanarek and R. Marks-Kaufman, Developmental aspects of sucrose-induced obesity in rats, *Physiol. Behav.*, *23*: 881 (1979).
26. T. W. Castonguay, E. Hirsch, and G. Collier, Palatability of sugar solutions and dietary selections, *Physiol. Behav.*, *27*: 7 (1981).
27. C. A. Maggio, M. Yang, and J. R. Vaselli, Developmental aspects of macronutrient selection in genetically obese and lean rats, *Nutr. Behav.*, *2*: 93 (1984).
28. A. Sclafani and T. H. Kramer, Dietary selection in vagotomized rats, *J. Auton. Nerv. Syst.*, *9*: 247 (1983).
29. A. Sclafani, P. F. Aravich, and M. Landman, Vagotomy blocks hypothalamic hyperphagia in rats on a chow diet and sucrose solution, but not on a palatable mixed diet, *J. Comp. Physiol. Psychol.*, *95*: 720 (1981).
30. J. Vasselli, E. Haraczkiewicz, and F. X. Pi-Sunyer, Effects of Acarbose (Bay g 5421) on body weight, insulin, and oral glucose and sucrose tolerance in sucrose-consuming rats. *Nutr. Behav.*, *1*: 21 (1982).
31. H. Laube, C. Wojcikowski, H. Shatz, and E. F. Pfeiffer, The effect of high maltose and sucrose feeding on glucose tolerance, *Horm. Metab. Res.*, 10: 192 (1978).
32. M. Naim, J. G. Brand, M. R. Kare, and R. G. Carpenter, Energy intake, weight gain and fat deposition in rats fed flavored, nutritionally controlled diets in a multichoice ('cafeteria') design, *J. Nutr.*, *115*: 1447 (1985).
33. A. M. Koh and A. Teitelbaum, Effect of dietary sucrose and starch on oral glucose tolerance and insulin-like activity, *Am. J. Physiol.*, *206*: 105 (1964).
34. P. J. Geiselman and D. Novin, The role of carbohydrates in appetite, hunger, and obesity, *Appetite*, *3*: 203 (1982).
35. K. C. Elwood and O. E. Michaelis, Effect of dietary carbohydrates on blood lipid and glucose levels of lean Zucker rats, *Nutr. Rep. Int.*, *21*: 113 (1980).
36. J. Hallfrish, F. Lazar, C. Jorgensen, and S. Reiser, Insulin and glucose responses in rats fed sucrose or starch, *Am. J. Clin. Nutr.*, *32*: 787 (1979).
37. P. J. Geiselman, Food intake following intraduodenal and hepatic portal infusion of hexoses in the rabbit, *Nutr. Behav.*, *2*: 77 (1984).
38. W. Hill, T. W. Castonguay, and G. H. Collier, Taste or diet balancing? *Physiol. Behav.*, *24*: 765 (1980).
39. J. R. Vaselli, E. Haraczkiewicz, and F. X. Pi-Sunyer, Effects of acarbose (Bay g 5421) on body weight, insulin, and oral glucose and sucrose tolerance in sucrose-consuming rats, *Nutr. Behav.*, *1*: 21 (1982).
40. A. Sclafani and S. Xenakis, Atropine fails to block the overconsumption of sugar solutions by hypothalamic hyperphagic rats, *J. Comp. Physiol. Psychol.*, *95*: 708 (1981).
41. H. P. Weingarten and S. D. Watson, Effects of atropine methyl nitrate on sham feeding in the rat, *Pharmacol. Biochem. Behav.*, *17*: 863 (1982).
42. I. Ramirez, When does sucrose increase appetite and adiposity? *Appetite, 9*: 1 (1987).
43. C. V. Kratz and D. A. Levitsky, Dietary obesity: differential effects with self-selection and composite diet feeding techniques, *Physiol. Behav.*, *22*: 245 (1979).

44. O. E. Michaelis, IV, D. J. Scholfield, C. S. Nance, and S. Reiser, Demonstration of the disaccharide effect in nutritionally stressed rats, *J. Nutr., 108*: 919 (1978).

45. O. E. Michaelis, IV, D. J. Scholfield, L. B. Gardner, and S. Cataland, Metabolic responses of Zucker fatty and lean rats fed carbohydrate diets *ad libitum* or in meals, *J. Nutr., 10*: 1409 (1980).

46. D. L. Trout, N. L. Moy, J. D. Putney, and D. A. Johnson, Dietary regimens for inducing mild hyperphagia, obesity, and hyperinsulinemia in rats, *Nutr. Rep. Int., 18*: 227 (1978).

47. R. B. Kanarek and N. Orthen-Gambill, Differential effects of sucrose, fructose and glucose on carbohydrate-induced obesity in rats, *J. Nutr., 112*: 1546 (1982).

48. A. Sclafani, Carbohydrate taste, appetite, and obesity: An overview, *Neurosci. Biobehav. Rev., 11*: 131 (1987).

49. O. Michelsen, S. Takahashi, and C. Craig, Experimental obesity. I. Production of obesity in rats by feeding high-fat diets, *J. Nutr., 57*: 541 (1955).

50. P. F. Fenton and C. Carr, The nutrition of the mouse: Responses of four strains to diets differing in fat content, *J. Nutr., 45*: 225 (1951).

51. D. R. Romsos, M. J. Hornshuh, and G. A. Leveille, Influence of dietary fat and carbohydrate on food intake, body weight and body fat of adult dogs, *Proc. Soc. Exper. Biol. Med., 157*: 278 (1978).

52. A. Sclafani, Dietary obesity, *Obesity* (A. J. Stunkard, ed.), W. B. Saunders, Philadelphia, p. 166 (1980).

53. H. J. Carlisle and E. Stellar, Caloric regulation and food preference in normal, hyperphagic, and aphagic rats, *J. Comp. Physiol. Psychol., 69*: 107 (1969).

54. C. L. Hamilton, Rat's preference for high fat diets, *J. Comp. Psychol., 58*: 459 (1964).

55. J. P. Flatt, The biochemistry of energy expenditure, *Recent Advances in Obesity Research* (G. Bray, ed.), Newman Publishing Ltd, London, p. 211 (1978).

56. J. D. Wood and J. T. Reid, The influence of dietary fat on fat metabolism and body fat deposition in meal-feeding and nibbling rats, *Br. J. Nutr., 34*: 15 (1975).

57. R. Schemmel, O. Mickelsen, and J. L. Gill, Dietary obesity in rats: Body weight and body fat accretion in seven strains of rats, *J. Nutr., 100*: 1941 (1970).

58. K. H. Duncan, J. A. Bacon, and R. L. Weinsier, The effects of high and low energy density diets on satiety, energy intake, and eating time of obese and nonobese subjects, *Am. J. Clin. Nutr., 37*: 763 (1983).

59. L. Lissner, D. A. Levitsky, B. J. Strupp, H. T. Kalkwart, and D. A. Roe, Dietary fat and the regulation of energy intake in human subjects, *Am. J. Clin. Nutr., 46*: 886 (1987).

60. A. Kendall, D. A. Levitsky, B. J. Strupp, and L. Lissner, Weight loss on a low-fat diet: Consequence of the imprecision of the control of food intake in humans, *Am. J. Clin Nutr., 53*: 1124 (1991).

61. F. X. Pi-Sunyer, Effect of the composition of the diet on energy intake, *Nutr. Rev., 48*(2): 94 (1990).

22

The Impact of Dietary Fat and Carbohydrates on Body Weight Maintenance

J. P. Flatt   *University of Massachusetts Medical School, Worcester, Massachusetts*

I. INTRODUCTION

The regulation of body weight is a complex problem, and many factors are involved in preventing or causing obesity. Some are inherited, others are related to lifestyle and to socioeconomic and dietary variables. Yet, ultimately, the problem of body weight maintenance boils down to two main issues:

1. Why are the cumulative differences between energy intake and expenditure generally so small (less than 1 or 2% when considered over a period of a year) even though substantial short-term deviations from energy balance are frequent and substantial?
2. What factors determine the body weight and shape for which weight stability tends to become established?

The aim of this chapter is to provide a framework to help understand how genetic and circumstantial factors, notably dietary factors, can influence the level at which weight stabilization tends to occur. Such understanding is important in providing a realistic and practical basis for the evaluation of various rationales for weight control and weight reduction.

II. CONTEXT

Let us begin by defining the context in which these two key phenomena operate. In one day, an adult typically might consume 300 g of carbohydrate, 100 g of fat, and 100 g of protein. Carbohydrate and protein provide 4 kcal/g and fat 9 kcal/g, so that this corresponds to an intake of 1200 kcal as carbohydrate, 900 kcal as fat, and 400 kcal as protein. Furthermore, we can note that 15% of the energy consumed is in the form of protein, 45% as carbohydrate, and 40% as fat, which is quite typical for the average American diet. The body of an adult contains about 12 kg of protein and energy reserves comprising 300–400 g of carbohydrate (in the form of glycogen) and 10–20 kg of fat. In obese individuals the amounts of body fat can be much greater, sometimes making up more than half of total body weight. Thus the amount of carbohydrate consumed (and oxidized) in one day is about equal to the body's glycogen stores, whereas the fat consumed in a day corresponds to only 1% or less of the body's fat reserves. If imbalances between intakes and oxidations occur, they will hardly affect the body's fat reserves, but they will alter its glycogen stores noticeably. After a single day without food, glycogen reserves are substantially depleted, while fat and protein contents are hardly affected. It would become urgent to curtail carbohydrate oxidation by switching more and more to the use of fat as a fuel and to seek to replete the carbohydrate stores. The hunger pangs perceived in such situations reveal something about the intensity of the drive to find food before blood glucose levels become too low to meet the brain's need for this essential fuel.

Such considerations illustrate that in order to develop an appropriate set of expectations about the metabolic aspects of body weight maintenance, one has to understand that different principles govern the body's protein, carbohydrate, and fat economies. In particular, it is useful to keep in mind the physical properties of carbohydrates and fats, because these account to a great extent for the differences encountered in the metabolic processing and regulation of these macronutrients. In order to gain a realistic perspective about macronutrients and metabolism, it is important furthermore to understand why energy in the form of protein is of secondary importance in regard to body weight maintenance.

A. Proteins

The intracellular enzymes that catalyze the multiple life-supporting reactions and the muscle fibers that perform physical work are made of proteins.

Other proteins are imbedded in the skeleton and form collagen fibers in the interstitial space between cells; together these make up the body's supporting structures. Because their large size provides for the folding into very specific conformations, proteins can carry out highly specialized functions. But they are therefore also somewhat fragile, being likely to undergo denaturation and proteolysis. Proteins must be constantly replaced, to the tune of about 0.3–0.5 g/kg body weight each day in adults. Accumulation of excess proteins provides little advantage, but adds to the body's maintenance costs and to the bulk which must be moved. The organism has therefore developed mechanisms enabling it to retain as protein only as much of the amino acids absorbed from the intestine as necessary to replace the proteins lost. In childhood, during pregnancy, and during recovery from disease or malnutrition, protein synthesis exceeds protein degradation. This corresponds to periods of *positive nitrogen balance* during which the body's protein content increases due to tissue expansion and growth. The role of dietary protein is thus primarily to replenish the amino acid pools, which permit protein synthesis to proceed at the desirable rate.

Western diets supply far more protein than the minimum needed, often exceeding the Recommended Dietary Allowance (RDA) for protein, which is rather generously set at 0.8 and 1.5 g/kg body weight/day for adults and children, respectively. Amino acids consumed in excess are automatically degraded to intermediates of the metabolic pathways by which carbohydrate and fat are oxidized. They thereby contribute to energy production, but only to a modest extent, since protein makes up only 10–20% of dietary energy. Furthermore, since the body spontaneously maintains a nearly constant protein content (as long as the diet supplies more than enough protein), body weight maintenance is indeed primarily determined by the intake and utilization of carbohydrates and fats.

B. Carbohydrates

Table sugar (also known as sucrose or saccharose) is a highly purified form of carbohydrate that we encounter daily. It is formed by a molecule of fructose linked to a molecule of glucose. Glucose ($C_6H_{12}O_6$) is the main form in which carbohydrate is absorbed, exchanged between tissues, and channeled into metabolic pathways. Some cells depend almost exclusively on glucose to provide energy, notably those of the brain and nervous system, which require about 120 g/day in an adult (i.e., 5 g/hr, or 100 mg/min). The glucose dissolved in the blood must be present at a concentration sufficient to permit it to diffuse into the cells and to support their metabolism. Low blood glucose levels (hypoglycemia) prevail when there is less than 0.6 g of glucose per liter of plasma. The elaborately controlled release of several key hormones (glucagon, epinephrine) regulates the breakdown of glycogen and the rate of glucose release by the liver, so that it is released into the circulation at a rate just appropriate to replace the glucose used and to maintain a circulating concentration of about 1 g per liter of plasma between meals. (At this concentration its sweetness is just about perceivable.)

The most abundant form of edible carbohydrate in plants is starch (in grains, potatoes, etc.). Starches are polymers of glucose in which hundreds of glucose molecules are linked together. They supply the bulk of humans' energy needs, except in affluent Western societies where sucrose now provides almost as many calories as starch. Only simple sugars such as glucose can be absorbed from the intestine. Sucrose and starch must therefore first be hydrolyzed (to monosaccharides) in the gut. The body keeps a reserve of glucose by converting glucose absorbed from the gut into glycogen. Like starch, glycogen is a polymer of glucose, but it has more cross-links between the long strands of connected glucose molecules, making it more suitable for storage in animal tissues. During the complete oxidation of one mole of glucose (180 g), 670 kcal of energy are released, or 3.7 kcal/g. Since one mole of water is removed per mole of glucose polymerized into glycogen or starch, the energy released per gram of glycogen or starch is $3.7 \times 180/162 = 4.18$ kcal/g. People generally consume mixtures of sugars and polysaccharides, so that the energy provided by digestible carbohydrates in foods is usually considered to be 4 kcal/g, as proposed by Atwater. (The Atwater factors for protein and fat are 4 and 9 kcal/g, respectively.)

Meals commonly supply 50–150 g of carbohydrate (e.g., a quarter-pound hamburger with French fries and a milk shake provides about 120 grams). This is much more than the 15–25 grams of free glucose present in the body (5 grams of which are in the blood itself). To avoid hyperglycemia, most of the glucose taken up from the intestine must be rapidly removed from the circulation and stored. This is accomplished primarily by liver and muscle, which take up glucose from the circulation and attach glucose molecules to glucose moieties already part of glycogen. This process is stimulated by insulin, whose secretion increases when blood glucose levels rise.

Glycogen molecules are very large, containing millions of atoms. They are thus effectively trapped in the cells in which they were made, without creating much of an osmotic effect. Two moles of adenosine triphosphate (ATP) are expended to incorporate one mole of glucose into glycogen. Since 36 ATPs are gained during the complete oxidation of a molecule of glucose, 2/36, or about 5% of the energy content of glucose, must be expended to transform it into glycogen. Glycogen in cells is associated with about 3 grams of water per gram. It is therefore a rather bulky form of energy reserve (i.e., only 1 kcal is stored per gram), and its accumulation must be limited to prevent excessive "swelling" of tissues. The glycogen reserves that the body maintains are indeed quite small (some 200–400 g after an overnight fast in an adult). This is not much more than the daily carbohydrate turnover. Glycogen stores are, therefore, readily and markedly affected by daily imbalances between carbohydrate intake and carbohydrate oxidation. This is why fluctuations in the glycogen reserves are likely to affect behavior, for example, in modulating appetite.

C. Fats

In turning our attention to fat, we note the remarkable difference in the interaction of fats and carbohydrates with water. Carbohydrates have a high affinity for water, whereas fats and water do not mix. This is because fats, or lipids, are made up primarily of carbon and hydrogen atoms and contain only very few oxygen atoms, which could interact with water molecules. The roles that lipids play in life are largely predicated by their inability to mix with water, so that they are confined to form a physically separate, non aqueous phase. Thus they can form the cell membranes, which, in spite of their extraordinary thinness, can envelop and separate cells from each other and from the extracellular fluid in which they are bathed. The few oxygen atoms present in plant and animal lipids provide points of attack for chemical reactions, including oxidation as well as linkage to other molecules. The oils and fats found in bulk amounts in plants and animals are made of triglyceride molecules, containing three fatty acid molecules esterified to one molecule of glycerol. Glycerol resembles one half of a glucose molecule and accounts for about 10% of the weight (or 5% of the energy) of fats.

Because of their insolubility in water, triglycerides do not influence the composition and substrate concentrations in the body's aqueous compartments. Thus they remain quite unnoticed, whether present in small or large amounts. Fat can be transported in the blood in the form of tiny droplets; these are surrounded by a surface layer of proteins, which allows them to remain in suspension as an emulsion. Fat droplets (chylomicrons) appear in the blood plasma after fatty meals, making the plasma lactescent (i.e., like milk, whose white appearance is also due to the presence of emulsified fat droplets). Fat is stored without water in adipose tissue, which is made up of cells grossly enlarged by one central fat droplet, much bigger by itself than most of the body's other cells. There is a thin layer of metabolically active cytoplasm around the central fat droplet in these adipocytes and a delicate network of capillary blood vessels between them. But 90% of adipose tissue is fat. Adipocytes can expand or shrink considerably, but once formed, their number cannot be reduced by fasting, only their size. Energy can be stored to the tune of about 8 kcal/g of adipose tissue, which is a much more concentrated form of energy than glycogen (which in its hydrated form holds only 1 kcal/g).

Fat is thus well suited to being accumulated as an energy reserve large enough to allow survival during periods of food deprivation. But one can also appreciate that daily fluctuations in the amount of body fat are unlikely to be perceived, since a gain or loss of even an entire day's portion of fat (50–150 g) is rather trivial compared to a fat reserve of 10–20 kg.

D. Conversion of Carbohydrate into Fat

Conversion of carbohydrate into fat allows animals to build up fat reserves even when their feed contains very little fat. In adult humans such de novo lipogenesis is primarily a hepatic process. Although it has been commonly believed that excess carbohydrate is readily converted into stored body fat, it is now known that even unusually large occasional carbohydrate loads (e.g., 500 g) are handled primarily by expansion of the glycogen stores [1]. The ensuing shift toward a nearly exclusive use of glucose as fuel soon reduces such temporary accumulations of glycogen. To induce rates of lipogenesis exceeding concomitant rates of fat oxidation, the body's total glycogen stores must be considerably raised (i.e., from their usual 4–6 g/kg body weight to more than 8 g of glycogen/kg body weight) [2]. This requires deliberate and sustained overconsumption of large amounts of carbohydrates. Under common conditions of unrestricted access to food, glycogen stores are spontaneously kept well below the range for which conversion of glucose into fat becomes an important pathway for carbohydrate disposal. This observation is important for two reasons: (1) It reveals that there are signals that effectively cause food intake to stop when glycogen levels reach a certain level, and (2) the common belief according to which carbohydrates are readily turned into fat can be dismissed (as well as the frequently made argument that the high metabolic cost of lipogenesis is a cause for greater energy dissipation on high-carbohydrate diets). It should be appreciated, though, that carbohydrate ingestion reduces the need to use fat as a fuel, so that the amounts of carbohydrate ingested remain an important factor in determining how much of the fat consumed will be retained.

Since carbohydrate disposal by lipogenesis appears to be insignificant under habitual dietary conditions [1,3] and since glucose cannot be made from fatty acids, glucose and fat belong to two entirely separate substrate pools. When considered over a few days, changes in the amounts of glycogen stored are so small compared to carbohydrate turnover that glucose oxidation is essentially equal to carbohydrate intake (plus the small amounts of glucose generated by gluconeogenesis from amino acids and triglyceride-glycerol).

III. MAIN FEATURES OF THE BODY'S CARBOHYDRATE AND FAT ECONOMIES

The fact that the body's energy reserves are kept in two distinct forms, in amounts differing by two orders of magnitude, has a number of implications, whose nature can be grasped by consideration of a model shown in Figure 1 [4,5]. The small reservoir is meant to represent the body's limited capacity for storing glycogen, whereas the large reservoir is analogous to the body's ability to store large amounts of fat. The contributions made by the small and by the large reservoirs to the flux through turbine A (upper right panel) are assumed to occur in proportion to the hydrostatic pressures prevailing in the two reservoirs. The small turbine B represents the exclusive use of glucose by the brain under usual conditions. In the two upper and the lower left panels of the figure, 20% of total flux is assumed to occur through turbine B (the same proportion as the brain's energy expenditure in resting humans).

Replenishment occurs from time to time, in portions illustrated by the small containers shown above the reservoirs. The fraction of the total fuel added that falls into the large reservoir is analogous to the fat content of the diet. Given the large cross-sectional area of the large reservoir, the amount of fuel added during one outflow-replenishment cycle will cause only an insignificant change in its level. Changes in its content do not, therefore, provide a favorable site of origin for signals that could be used to trigger fuel replenishment at appropriate intervals. On the other hand, marked changes in the content of the small reservoir occur, which are much more likely to be detectable and, hence, more suitable for triggering replenishment at appropriate intervals. In the model it is thus assumed that fuel addition is elicited whenever the content of the small reservoir has fallen to a particular minimal level (S_1, upper right panel). The model also includes a conduit for the transfer of fuel from the small to the large reservoir (analogous to lipogenesis from carbohydrate). But as is now known to be the case in humans, the fuel content in the small reservoir remains markedly below the level at which this transfer would be induced [2].

The cumulative effect of repeated imbalances between addition and outflow can in time lead to substantial changes in the content of the large reservoir. Ultimately it will come to exert a hydrostatic pressure, which will cause the outflow from the large reservoir to be equal to the amount of fuel added to it in one cycle. Subsequent replenishments, triggered at a frequency appropriate to maintain the content of the small reservoir in its operating range (between S_1 and S_2), will cause no further accumulation or depletion in the large reservoir. A steady state is then reached, which will tend to perpetuate

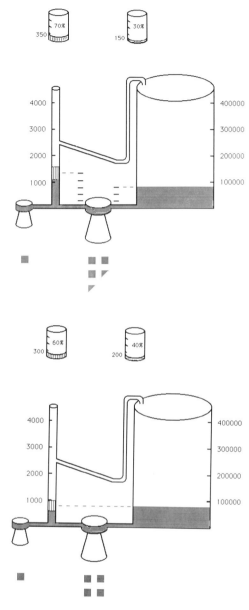

Figure 1 Model used as an analogy for the body's acquisition, storage, and oxidation of carbohydrate (small reservoir) and of fat (large reservoir). Units are chosen to correspond to the amounts of glycogen and triglycerides typically present in the human body, expressed in terms of kcal. Four steady-state situations are illustrated: In the upper left case, 30% of the total influx or 150 kcal are added to the large and 350 to the small reservoir during one outflow-replenishment cycle, replenishment being triggered whenever the content of the small reservoir has declined to a particular level. In the upper right and lower left cases, 40% of the total influx or 200 kcal are added

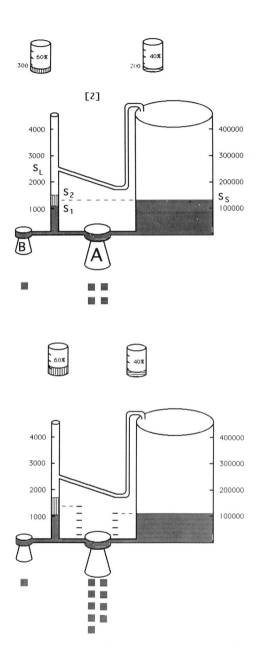

[2]

to the large and 300 to the small reservoir. These influxes are balanced by outflows of 100 kcal through the small turbine and 400 through the large turbine. In the case shown at the lower right, the total outflow is doubled, as 900 kcal are drained through the large turbine in one cycle. This is compensated for by an influx of 400 kcal into the large and 600 kcal into the small reservoir. Note that the outflow through the small turbine is still 100 kcal, but this accounts for only 10% of the total flux, as compared to 20% in the other three situations. (Further explanations are given in the text.) (Ref. 5) itself. It is noteworthy that the steady-state level in the large reservoir establishes itself at some particular height (S_s) without there being a sensor to measure its content, nor any mechanisms that could drive the system to come predetermined set point value.

Changes in the proportion of fuel added to the two reservoirs will cause shifts in the steady-state level reached in the large reservoir. For example, if 40% of the added fuel flows into the large reservoir (upper right panel), the level achieved therein will become stable when the two reservoirs contribute equally to the flux through turbine A, considering that one third of the fuel added to the small reservoir (20% of the total fuel added) escapes through turbine B. The level in the large reservoir thus establishes itself at a height exerting a hydrostatic pressure equal to the average hydrostatic pressure prevailing in the small reservoir. If only 30% of the fuel added falls into the large resevoir, its steady-state level will be lower, corresponding to three fifths of the average level in the small reservoir (upper left panel). The two upper panels in Figure 1 thus illustrate that changes in the fraction of fuel dumped into the large reservoir (i.e., a change in the diet's fat content) causes a shift in its steady-state level when the level that triggers replenishment in the small reservoir remains constant. However, such changes in the content of the large reservoir can be prevented by changing the height for which replenishment is triggered, as shown by comparing the two left side panels, but this requires that the level in the small reservoir be lowered by half.

The model illustrates how changes in the body's glycogen content and in the size of its fat mass contribute to bring about the oxidation of a fuel mix containing glucose and free fatty acids (FFA) in the same relative proportions as provided by carbohydrate and fat in the diet consumed. With regard to the regulation of body weight, these examples illustrate that the fat content of the diet and the range within which glycogen levels are maintained have a very substantial impact in determining the steady-state level in the large reservoir. When these proportions vary, changes in body composition must be expected to occur, until a new body composition is attained for which the relative amounts of glucose and of fat in the fuel mix oxidized are again commensurate with the relative proportions of carbohydrate and fat in the diet.

It is indeed well established that diets with a substantial fat content lead to increases in the adipose tissue mass in most experimental animals, though the extent of this response varies in different strains. This phenomenon is well illustrated in Figure 2, which shows how carcass fat content among ad libitum fed mice varies as a function of the percent of dietary energy provided as fat. The aberration in the dose-response relationship between carcass fat and dietary fat, when the latter is very low, is due to the active rate

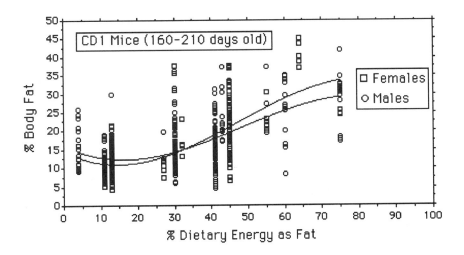

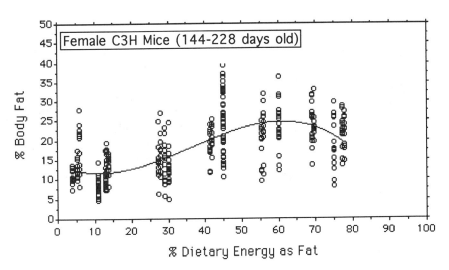

Figure 2 Progressive increase in adiposity elicited by raising the fat content of the diet provided to ad libitum fed male or female CD1 mice (upper panel), and to female C3H mice (lower panel).

of lipogenesis that such diets induce in small animals, providing another source of fatty acids to offset fat oxidation. The considerable variability that is manifest between animals is also noteworthy. It is remarkably high even among mice of a highly inbred strain (C3H).

IV. THE STEADY STATE OF WEIGHT MAINTENANCE

Body composition and hence body weight will only remain stable if the macronutrient mixture consumed is completely oxidized and if this oxidation is sufficient to meet the body's energy needs, so that there is no need to draw additional substrates from the body's substance or from its energy reserves. This means that on average protein oxidation must be equal to protein intake, carbohydrate oxidation to carbohydrate intake, and fat oxidation to fat intake.

A. The RQ/FQ Concept

Information on the composition of the fuel mix oxidized can be obtained by measuring the respiratory quotient (RQ), (i.e., the ratio of the volume of carbon dioxide produced to the volume of oxygen consumed). Proteins are oxidized with an RQ of 0.835 (a more accurate value than that of 0.8 which has been commonly used [6], carbohydrates with an RQ of 1.0, and fats with an RQ of 0.71 (Table 1). As shown in Figure 3, the RQ is not greatly affected by variations in the protein content of the fuel mix oxidized, which rarely provides less than 10% or more than 20% of total energy. RQ measurements thus provide simple means to assess the relative proportions of glucose and fat being oxidized. (One should be aware of the fact that accuracy is more difficult to ensure in obtaining RQ data than in measuring overall energy expenditure [6].) To facilitate the interpretation of data on the adjustment of fuel composition to nutrient intake it is convenient to compare respiratory quotient values to the diet's food quotient (FQ), which describes the ratio of CO_2 produced to O_2 consumed during the biological oxidation of a representative sample of the diet [7]. It is, of course, readily understandable that constant body composition, and hence body weight stability, can only occur when the average RQ is equal to the diet's FQ.

Two equations useful in calculating the FQ are shown in Figure 4. The simpler of the two yields FQ values (FQ ') that are about 1% too high for mixed diets, which means that their actual carbohydrate content is about 3% less than implied by such an FQ value. When such errors are deemed to

Table 1 Respiratory Quotients of Substrate Oxidation

Glucose Oxidation

$$C_6H_{12}O_6 \;+\; 6\;O_2 \xrightarrow{RQ = 1.00} 6\;CO_2 \;+\; 6\;H_2O \;+\; 670\;kcal\,[a]$$

Glucose

Glycogen Oxidation

$$C_6H_{10}O_5 \;+\; 6\;O_2 \xrightarrow{RQ = 1.00} 6\;CO_2 \;+\; 6\;H\;O_2 \;+\; 678\;kcal$$

Glucosyl-

Lipogenesis

$$[b]\;4.5\;C_6H_{12}O_6 \;+\; 4\;O_2 \xrightarrow{RQ = 2.75} 1\;C_{16}H_{32}O_2 \;+\; 11\;CO_2 \;+\; 11\;H_2O \;+\; 630\;kcal$$

Glucose · Palmitate

Palmitate Oxidation

$$C_{16}H_{32}O_2 \;+\; 23\;O_2 \xrightarrow{RQ = .696} 16\;CO_2 \;+\; 16\;H_2O \;+\; 2398\;kcal\,[a]$$

Palmitate

Triglyceride Oxidation

$$C_{57}H_{107}O_6 \;+\; 78\;O_2 \xrightarrow{RQ = .71} 57\;CO_2 \;+\; 52\;H_2O \;+\; 8139\;kcal$$

[c] Triglyceride

Protein Oxidation

Gluconeogenesis and Ketone Body (KB) Production

$$[d]\;\underset{C_{4.6}H_{8.4}O_{1.8}N_{1.25}}{Protein} \;+\; 1.5\;O_2 \;+\; 0.2\;H_2O \xrightarrow{(RQ = .4)} 0.6\;Urea \;+\; 0.6\;CO_2 \;+\; 0.35\;Gluc \;+\; 0.3\;KB$$

Oxidation of Glucose and Ketone Bodies

$$.35\;Gluc \;+\; .3\;KB \;+\; 3.3\;O_2 \xrightarrow{(RQ = 1.0)} 3.3\;CO_2 \;+\; 3.1\;H_2O$$

Complete Oxidation

$$C_{4.6}H_{8.4}O_{1.8}N_{1.25} \;+\; 4.8\;O_2 \xrightarrow{[e]\;RQ = .835} 0.6\;Urea \;+\; 4.0\;CO_2 \;+\; 2.9\;H_2O \;+\; 520\;kcal$$

[d] Protein

[a]*Handbook of Chemistry and Physics*, 57th Ed., CRC Press, Cleveland (1976).
[b]Based on stoichiometry reported for lipogenesis in rat adipose tissue (Flatt, *J. Lip. Res.* 11: 131–143, 1970).
[c]Palmityl-stearyl-oleyl triglyceride, which is representative of the usual fatty acid pattern in human adipose fat.
[d]Approximate composition of a protein mixture chosen to contain 1000 mmoles of amino-acyl residues in 110 g of protein, to have 16% of its weight as N and 50% as C, to be oxidized with an RQ of 0.835 (Livesey and Elia, *Am. J. Clin. Nutr.* 47: 608–628, 1988), and to generate 3.6 g glucose per g of N. ATP stoichiometry is based on McGilvery (*Biochemistry. A Functional Approach*, 2nd Ed., Saunders, Philadelphia, 1979).
[e]Coefficients given by Livesey and Elia (*Am. J. Clin. Nutr.* 47: 608–628, 1988), according to whom protein oxidation yields 4.70 kcal/g and occurs with an RQ of 0.835, which differ from the commonly used values of 4.32 and 0.80, respectively (Lusk, G., *The Elements of the Science of Nutrition*, 4th Ed., p. 68, Johnston Reprint Corp., New York, reprinted 1976).

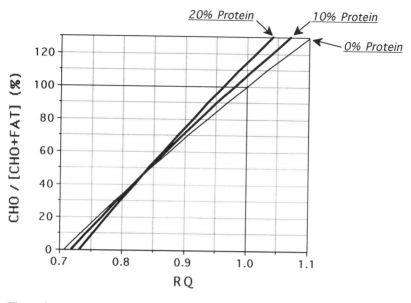

Figure 3 Impact of the protein content in the fuel mix oxidized on the information provided by respiratory quotient (RQ) values on the relative contributions made by carbohydrate and fat to nonprotein substrate oxidation.

excessive, the other equation (FQ″) can be used, with which the deviations from theoretical values are about 10 times less.

B. Nutrient Imbalances and Corrective Responses

A variety of mechanisms are known that operate to limit excessive variations in food intake [8–10]. However, in spite of this diurnal regulation of food intake, daily protein, carbohydrate, fat, and energy balances often deviate substantially from zero [11]. Weight maintenance, therefore, implies that gains or losses of protein, glycogen and fat tend to elicit corrective responses, which tend to restore and sustain steady-state conditions [12]. Three types of corrective responses are possible: changes in energy dissipation, changes in food intake, and/or shifts in the composition of the fuel mix oxidized [13]. The latter are readily and quickly brought about thanks to powerful endocrine and enzymatic regulatory mechanisms. They elicit, for example, the prompt postprandial rise in the RQ that reflects increased carbohydrate

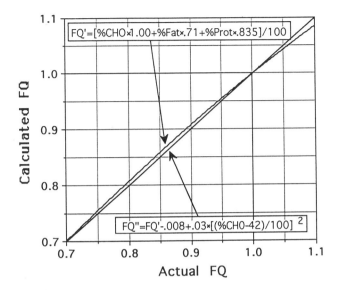

Figure 4 Comparison of food quotients calculated by two abbreviated methods (FQ' and FQ") to the theoretical FQ values computed on the basis of the macronutrient contents of diets containing 10 or 20% of total energy as protein.

oxidation. These responses are dedicated primarily to the goal of minimizing deviations from the carbohydrate balance. Errors in the maintenance of fat balance are consequently much greater than errors in the carbohydrate balance, and gains or losses of fat account for most of the overall errors in the energy balance [14,15]. By themselves, RQ adjustments are ineffective in bringing about corrections for deviations from energy balance. Corrections must be accomplished by altering the rates of energy dissipation and/or by eliciting increases or decreases in food intake. Data obtained under ad libitum feeding conditions in mice show that changes in the energy balance are brought about overwhelmingly by changes in food intake ($R^2 \geq 0.8$), whereas changes in energy expenditure make only a negligible contribution ($R^2 \leq 0.01$) (Fig. 5) [5].

C. Carbohydrate Balance

Since glucose is constantly used, its availability critical, and glycogen reserves small, the carbohydrate economy is particularly important to the well-being of the organism. Not surprisingly, evolution has led to the development of mechanisms giving priority to the maintenance of the carbohydrate

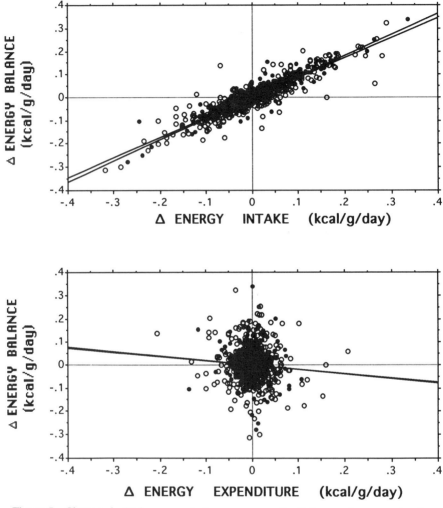

Figure 5 Changes in 24-hr energy balances as a result of changes in energy intake ($R^2 \geq 0.83$; $p \leq 0.0001$) and in energy expenditure in 5 normal weight (O) (body weight = 51.7 ± 3.8g) ($R^2 \leq 0.01$; $p = 0.05$) and 5 overweight (●) (62.3 ± 7.6 g) (N.S.) male CD1 mice maintained ad libitum on diets providing 13, 30, or 41% of dietary energy as fat, 18% as protein, and the balance as starch plus sucrose (1:1). (Reproduced with permission from Flatt, in *Obesity: Dietary Factors and Control* (D. R. Romsos, J. Himms-Hagen, and M. Suzuki, eds.), pp. 239–250, Japan Sci. Soc. Press, Tokyo, and S. Karger, Basel (1991).

balance [16]. They involve hormones to control the storage and mobilization of metabolic fuels, as well as means to set up sensations of hunger or satiety. The endocrine signals serve primarily to adjust carbohydrate oxidation to carbohydrate intake. This works so well that people can readily adapt to various levels of imposed carbohydrate intake and, furthermore, glycogen stores will remain stable, yet not saturated, even when access to food is unrestricted [2].

Since food consumption markedly increases the availability of carbohydrates and stimulates insulin secretion, meals induce an increase in carbohydrate oxidation, as evidenced by the prompt postprandial increase in the RQ (Fig. 6). This rise is related primarily to the amount of carbohydrate consumed, whereas the presence of fat in the meal has little, if any effect on postprandial substrate oxidation [17]. This is imputable in part to the relatively slow rate of fat absorption from the gut. But primarily it is due to the fact that dietary fats appear in the circulation in the form of chylomicrons targeted for deposition in adipose tissue, rather than in the form of free fatty acids, the form in which fat is made available to cells for energy generation.

Fat oxidation is indeed inhibited after meals, even when fat is the major macronutrient in the foods consumed [17]. Thus, *carbohydrate intake promotes carbohydrate oxidation, but fat intake does not promote fat oxidation*! On days with excessive food intake, carbohydrate oxidation increases to prevent excessive glycogen accumulation. Since total substrate oxidation is limited by the rate of ATP expenditure, fat oxidation is curtailed on such days, enhancing fat accumulation [18]. RQs are thus greater than the FQ on such days. On the other hand, RQs are less than the FQ on days with a negative energy balance, when endogenous fat must make a contribution to the fuel mix oxidized (Fig. 7). The upper panel also illustrates that the RQ for which energy balance is achieved varies with the diet's FQ. The relationship between the RQ and the energy balance can be made independent of diet composition and of differences in rates of energy turnover, by relating the ratio of energy intake to energy expenditure to the RQ/FQ ratio (Fig. 7, lower panel).

D. Fat Balance

Fat oxidation is determined by the gap between total energy expenditure and the amounts of energy ingested in the form of carbohydrates and protein [18]. Fat intake, on the other hand, depends on the proportion of energy present as fat in the foods selected and on how much food we are driven to eat to maintain stable glycogen levels or induced to eat by the availability of appetizing foods. Fat oxidation and fat intake are therefore determined in-

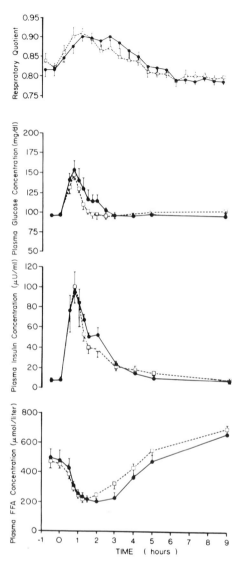

Figure 6 Changes in the nonprotein respiratory quotient, in blood glucose, and in plasma insulin and free fatty acid (FFA) levels observed in seven young men in response to a low-fat breakfast providing white bread, jam, and dried meat (73 g carbohydrate, 6 g fat, and 30 g protein) (●------●) and after consuming the same breakfast on another day with a supplement of 50 g of margarine (41 g of additional fat) (□------□). Means ± SEM. (Reproduced from the *Journal of Clinical Investigation*, 1985, 76:1019–1024, by copyright permission of the American Society for Clinical Investigation)

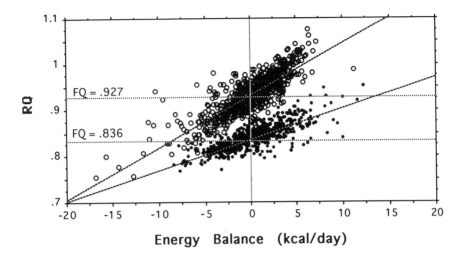

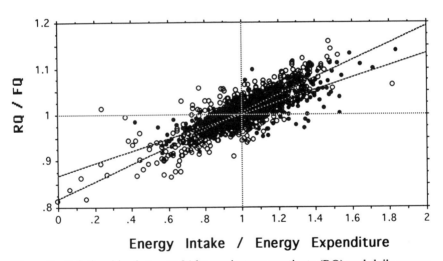

Figure 7 Relationships between 24-hr respiratory quotients (RQ) and daily energy balances in 10 ad libitum fed CD1 mice when maintained on diets providing 13% (○) or 45% (●) of dietary energy as fat, 18% as protein, and the balance as starch plus sucrose (1:1) ($R^2 \geq 0.6$; $p \leq 0.0001$) (upper panel), and energy balances expressed as the ratio of energy intake/energy expenditure in relation to the RQ/FQ ratio ($R^2 \geq 0.6$; $p \leq 0.0001$) (lower panel). (Reproduced with permission from Ref. 18)

dependently. How is it, then, that fat oxidation can nevertheless become adjusted to fat intake, and that people tend to maintain weight even though they eat food mixtures with widely differing fat contents? Some adjustment of fat oxidation to fat intake can be attributed to a lesser postprandial inhibition of fat oxidation when fat-containing meals are consumed, due to the effect of fat in delaying intestinal absorption. Furthermore, to the extent that the presence of fat in the foods consumed results in a lesser intake of carbohydrates [8], glycogen levels will be maintained in a lower range, resulting in lower insulin levels between meals but higher rates of FFA release and oxidation. These indirect effects will not necessarily product an exact compensation, however, and short-term errors in the fat balance are too small to affect the size of the body's fat stores, FFA levels, fat oxidation, or food intake. But substantial accumulation (or depletion) of the adipose tissue fat mass, as may occur over an extended period of time, will in time alter the rate of FFA release from adipose tissue [19] sufficiently to enhance (or reduce) fat oxidation [20] and to bring about the oxidation of a fuel mix whose average RQ matches the diet's FQ. Most individuals will thereby reach a state where fat as well as carbohydrate and protein oxidation rates are commensurate with their particular macronutrient intakes.

E. Regulation of Food Intake and Energy Balance

Data obtained in mice given unrestricted access to food show that changes in the energy balance are achieved by modulation of food intake, rather than by altering rates of energy dissipation [5]. Energy balance is therefore achieved by regulation of food intake. When the fuel mix oxidized has the same average composition as the nutrient distribution in the diet, adjustment of food intake serving to maintain either protein, carbohydrate, or fat balance becomes sufficient, in principle, to achieve overall energy balance as well. This represents a considerable simplification of the problem of energy balance regulation. (In fact, since energy and energy balance are abstract notions, one should not even expect that the energy balance could be the target of biological regulation!) Not surprisingly in view of the importance of maintaining stable glycogen reserves, deviations from the carbohydrate balance appear to be the major factor in eliciting changes in food intake from one day to the next [5]. Thus, regulation of food intake, serving primarily the purpose of maintaining stable glycogen reserves, can be seen to be sufficient to achieve stability of body weights, as proposed many years ago by Mayer and Thomas [16]. This then provides an answer to the first question raised in the introduction. But this allows maintenance of energy balance only when the size of the body's glycogen and fat reserves have drifted toward the particular configuration where they complement the body's metabolic fuel regulatory phenomena in such a manner as to bring about the oxidation of a metabolic fuel mix whose composition matches the nutrient distribution in the diet [12].

V. FACTORS DETERMINING THE WEIGHT MAINTENANCE PLATEAU

The body composition at which different individuals achieve weight stability varies widely, but we now know that it is the one for which the average RQ is equal to the diet's average FQ. The weight maintenance plateau is known to be markedly influenced by genetic factors, by physical activity, by differences in the endocrine state, by age and sex, and by dietary habits (21-23]. The increase in the incidence of obesity in affluent and less affluent societies brought about by changes in food availability and lifestyle, as well as the impact of socioeconomic factors, attest to the influence of such circumstantial (as opposed to inherited) factors as well [24,25]. How can this all be explained in the framework provided by the notion that weight maintenance is brought about by food-intake regulation geared primarily toward the maintenance of carbohydrate balance?

A. Influence of the Adipose Tissue Mass on Energy Expenditure and RQ

Since fat oxidation is not directly determined by fat intake, the contribution made by fat to the fuel mix oxidized is determined indirectly. From the fact that animals and people achieve stable body weights even on high-fat diets, but at a higher degree of adiposity (see Fig. 2), it can be inferred that a change in the size of the fat mass itself plays a role. The increase in body weight due to the enlargement of the adipose tissue mass causes an increase in energy expenditure. If the composition of the fuel mix oxidized were not affected by changes in the size of the adipose mass, this would be offset by increments in food intake and would not lead to the establishment of a new weight maintenance plateau unless total food intake were somehow limited. Expansion of the fat mass, whether due to an increase of the number of fat cells and/or to an enlargement of the adipocytes, causes an increase in FFA release, leading to higher FFA levels [19] with the effect of enhancing fat oxidation relative to glucose oxidation [20] (see Fig. 1). In this regard, it has become evident that the impact of abdominal fat accumulation on FFA levels on intermediary metabolism is greater than that of fat deposition peripherally [26]. By raising FFA levels, enlargement of the fat masses promotes fat oxidation, just as well-filled glycogen stores cause blood glucose and/or insulin levels to be maintained at higher levels after meals, which promotes glucose oxidation. However, whereas food intake elicits prompt responses, which adjust the rate of glucose oxidation to glucose availability, the increase in fat oxidation brought about by expansion of the adipose tissue mass is chronic rather than related to recent fat intake. In cases of extreme obesity, this effect apparently fails to become effective.

B. Regulation of Food Intake

When presented with foods of different macronutrient contents, experimental animals are able to select favorable proportions of nutrients from the choices provided, indicating that the regulation of food intake goes beyond merely influencing the total amount of energy consumed. In humans, who subsist on a variety of foods that provide mixtures of macronutrients, selection of particular items of the diet for physiological or metabolic reasons is not readily demonstrated, and the items consumed appear to be primarily influenced by availability, preferences, cost, and conscious selection and/or avoidance.

The regulation of food intake in humans is especially difficult to elucidate, because numerous circumstantial factors and individual preferences influence food intake. These readily override physiological signals, since substantial short-term deviations from the energy balance are readily tolerated [11,27]. The frequent consumption of meals in portions that are not adjusted to individual needs and the "mirror and scale effect" [28], which induces restraint on food intake in many individuals, further contribute to the difficulty in gaining a realistic perception of the role of physiological factors in controlling food intake in humans [29]. Lack of understanding about the regulation of food intake in humans does not change the fact that this regulation creates powerful, though often undetected, underlying drives. They elicit the indispensible adjustments in food intake necessary to correct for deviations from energy balance, which limit rates of weight gain even in the face of unrestricted food availability and poor dietary habits. Their power is illustrated in children, whose body weights are generally maintained within desirable range in spite of considerable variations in their rates of energy expenditure, and in adults who spontaneously lose weight after a period of deliberate overeating [30]. But these drives also make weight maintenance difficult, as long as body composition differs markedly from that for which the steady state tends to become established spontaneously. This is often the case, in particular, after a period of weight reduction.

C. Impact of the Dietary Carbohydrate-to-Fat Ratio

Nutritionists have long recognized that the high caloric density of fatty foods is a factor favoring the occurrence of positive energy balances [31–34], although some early [8] and delayed [35] compensations for differences in caloric density do occur. At any rate, among mice given free access to one of a series of diets containing different proportions of fat and carbohydrate, the weight maintenance plateau is reached at increasingly higher degrees of adiposity as the proportion of dietary energy provided by fat is raised from 15 to 60% (see Fig. 2). The effect of the dietary fat content on body fat content (as well as on body weight) is progressive and dose-dependent (i.e., the dose being the percentage of dietary energy as fat). This dietary effect is reversible, at least to some extent [13]. It is of interest in this regard that studies on taste preferences in humans show obese individuals to prefer mixtures of cream and sugar that have a higher fat content but a lower sugar content than lean subjects [36]. Positive correlations between dietary fat content and the degree of adiposity have indeed been documented [37–40].

The range of interindividual variations in fatness is much greater on high-fat than on low-fat diets, as even on high-fat diets some animals remain quite lean (see Fig. 2). This pattern seems to reproduce body weight variability in human populations. Since body weights in animals are not influenced by conscious and subconscious motivations as is the case in humans, this diversity suggests that genetic differences could play an important role in determining degrees of obesity. However, remarkably large individual differences are manifest even among highly inbred mice (see Fig. 2). Apparently, even minute individual differences can lead to substantial variability in the size of the adipose tissue mass when food is freely available, particularly when the diets include substantial amounts of fat. This represents an important conclusion in helping to account for the great diversity in body composition encountered in human populations.

D. Impact of Food Palatability and Accessibility

Provision of sucrose solutions or of a selection of highly palatable foods ("supermarket" or "cafeteria" diets) to experimental animals generally causes them to overeat markedly [41], but even under condition of unrestricted access, food intake diminishes spontaneously after some weight gain has occurred [42]. Expansion of the adipose tissue mass, which may be complemented by less obvious changes in glycogen levels, thus appear able to compensate for differences in food palatability, permitting the steady state of weight maintenance to become reestablished, but at a higher degree of adiposity.

Food availability, palatability, and variety can be expected to be even more powerful inducers of obesity in humans than in "cafeteria-fed" animals. To understand this effect in metabolic terms, one should first remember that the range within which glycogen levels are maintained is not fixed, since glycogen levels are maintained far below their level of saturation even under conditions of unrestricted access to food [2]. A varied selection of appealing dishes will enhance meal size, as satiety mechanisms must reach greater intensity to restrict further food intake than in the face of unappealing foods. This and the inducement to eat between meals, a frequent consequence of the ubiquitous availability of foods, have the effect of raising and maintaining high glycogen levels. To compensate for the ensuing curtailment of fat oxidation, a greater expansion of the adipose tissue mass is thus often required to bring about the steady state of weight maintenance where the average RQ matches the FQ.

The diets consumed in affluent societies are commonly referred to as mixed diets because they provide balanced mixtures of carbohydrates, fats, and protein. This endows them with a relatively high fat content, which is without a doubt an important factor in promoting the development of obesity [23,31–40]. But these mixed diets are also remarkable by the wide selection of food items that such a macronutrient distribution makes possible. For the reasons outlined above, these palatability and accessibility characteristics of our food supply need to be taken into consideration as well in trying to recognize measures susceptible to limit the development of obesity.

E. Effects of Exercise on Energy Balance and Body Weight

Having seen that maintenance of stable body weights can be expected in spite of differences in diet composition and food palatability, though the body composition for which this occurs will vary, we are ready to consider the impact of other variables on weight maintenance. The habit of engaging in substantial physical activities, for instance, is generally quite effective in limiting the accumulation of excess weight or in inducing loss of excess adipose tissue [43]. Yet it is generally not well understood why increases in food intake elicited by exercise are sometimes sufficient to assure weight maintenance (i.e., in a physically active individual), but sometimes not (i.e., when someone initiates a physical training program). The data shown in Figure 8 provide some clues. The lower panel describes the increases in energy expenditure and in energy intake elicited by spontaneous running activity in ad libitum fed mice. Running also causes a decrease in the RQ (upper panel), indicating that it promotes the oxidation of fat relative to carbohydrate. The increase in food intake caused by running, being adequate to maintain carbohydrate balance (lower panel), is thus insufficient to compensate for the

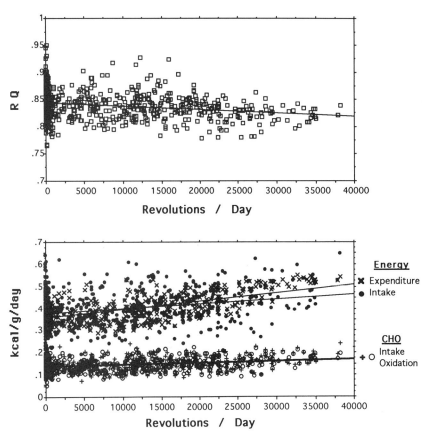

Figure 8 Effects of spontaneous running activity on 24-hr RQ and on daily energy and carbohydrate turnover and balances in 10 ad libitum fed female CD1 mice maintained on a diet providing 45% of dietary energy as fat, 18% as protein and the balance as starch plus sucrose (1:1). The decline in the RQ and the increasingly negative energy balance occur with R^2 values of 0.05 ($p \leq 0.0001$; $N = 769$). (Reproduced with permission from Flatt, in *Obesity: Dietary Factors and Control* (D. R. Romos, J. Himms-Hagen, and M. Suzuki, eds.), pp. 239–250, Japan Sci. Soc. Press, Tokyo, and S. Karger, Basel (1991).

relatively greater increase in fat oxidation. The decrease in the 24-hr RQ elicited by exercise can be attributed to increased substrate oxidation in muscle, which unlike many other tissues uses fatty acids as well as glucose, and/or to the exercise-induced depletion of the glycogen reserves, which leads to a gradual decline in the RQ during the exercise and for some time thereafter. If high-carbohydrate items are selectively consumed following exercise, the amount of food needed to replenish the glycogen reserves will be far less than the energy expended during the exercise period [7].

The fact that the steady state of weight maintenance should be reached with a lesser expansion of the adipose tissue mass when substantial physical activity is part of the daily routine is also predicted by the model (compare the two right panels in Fig. 1). It is noteworthy that the influence of exercise would not be apparent in the model if the small turbine B had not been included, because increases in total flux would then not result in a shift in the relative proportions of fuel drawn from the two reservoirs. It would merely lead to more frequent signals for replenishment, but without affecting the steady-state level in the large reservoir. The fact that flow through turbine B is reduced to 10% of total flux in the case illustrated in the lower right panel is the reason for the decrease in the steady-state level in the large reservoir when flow through A is enhanced. By promoting fat oxidation more than carbohydrate oxidation, exercise decreases the need to expand the adipose tissue mass in order to achieve an RQ as low as the FQ. Thus exercise substitutes for greater adiposity, and greater adiposity substitutes for lack of exercise in bringing about a rate of fat oxidation commensurate with fat intake [44].

Not all kinds of exercise are likely to be equally effective in promoting weight loss. During short periods of physical activity, as well as during strenuous exertion, glycogen is the primary source of fuel, and the fuel mix oxidized has a relatively high carbohydrate content. Heavy exertion (e.g., weight lifting) is thus often associated with a tendency to gain weight. These considerations help in understanding why short bouts of strenuous exertion are less effective for weight control than sustained periods of activities of moderate intensity. The duration and intensity of exercise, the type of muscle fibers involved [45], and its schedule in relation to meals are factors that could influence its impact on fat oxidation and thereby on the regulation of body weight.

F. Impact of Genetic and Endocrine Factors and of Drugs

The genetic influence on body size and shape and on adiposity has been amply demonstrated [21]. In regard to possible metabolic factors promoting obesity, much attention and much work has been devoted to determine whether lower rates of energy expenditure may be an important factor in promoting fat accumulation [46]. But such effects are modest at best [28], and they are clearly outweighed by the increases in resting energy expenditure brought about by expansion of the adipose tissue mass with its supporting component of fat-free mass [47,48]. According to the concept of body weight maintenance discussed here, inherited differences in regulating the relative rates of glucose and fat oxidation can be recognized as individual characteristics susceptible of exerting considerable impact on body weights. Because large variations in the size of the adipose tissue mass are required to exert a noticeable impact on fuel utilization, even minor individual differences can explain wide variability in the degree of adiposity (see Fig. 2). The marked increase in the RQ induced by glucocorticoid administration [49], for instance, provides a simple explanation for the temporary increase in adiposity in patients during treatment with cortisone, which provides a sometimes spectacular illustration of the power of such metabolic changes on body weight regulation.

If individual differences in the adjustment of carbohydrate relative to fat oxidation thus appear to provide an explanation for the expression of genetic influences on body weights, one can for the same reasons come to expect that to be effective in combating obesity, drugs must promote fat oxidation relative to carbohydrate oxidation, rather than merely to increase resting energy expenditure. This may be achieved by a reduction in glycogen levels secondary to inhibition of food intake or by enhancement of fat oxidation, leading to carbohydrate-sparing and to a decrease in the amount of food needed to maintain carbohydrate balance.

VI. STRATEGIES FOR WEIGHT MAINTENANCE AND CONTROL

In metabolic terms, the goal of weight maintenance resides in the achievement of an average RQ equal to the diet's FQ without the need for an undesirable expansion of the adipose tissue mass to satisfy this condition [12,50]. This goal is more readily achieved when a diet with a low fat content is selected, because it is easier to achieve an average RQ lower than the diet's FQ when the FQ is relatively high. Sustained exercise provides additional leverage to keep the average RQ as low as the FQ, because it promotes the oxidation of fat relative to glucose.

Since the body will spontaneously and effectively maintain protein and carbohydrate balances but does not (or cannot) regulate the fat balance nearly as accurately [12–18], it makes sense to direct voluntary efforts at this relatively "soft target." Furthermore, concentrating on the fat balance provides a more specific goal than one based on overall caloric exchanges. Since it is obviously easier to ensure that fat oxidation be at least equal to fat intake when fat intake is kept small, the key measure is therefore to avoid fatty foods and to satisfy one's hunger by eating foods providing most of their energy in the form of carbohydrates [7,33,51].

A word of caution should be included here about sucrose and other rapidly absorbed carbohydrates. It is now known that a slight temporary decline in blood glucose levels is a physiological event often leading to initiation of food intake in rats. In animals consuming a feed of fixed composition, the time elapsed when this event occurs is proportional to the size of the preceding meal [52]. It may well be linked to the end of carbohydrate influx from the gut, when the liver has to shift from a glucose-removing to a glucose-producing state. Rapidly absorbed carbohydrates such as sucrose would be expected to cause this signal to occur not only earlier, but perhaps also more sharply, in view of the high degree of postprandial insulinization and the rapid rates of peripheral glucose utilization that they elicit. One should rather select complex carbohydrates (i.e., carbohydrates in the form of starch still accompanied by natural fiber, vegetables, whole-grain products, etc.), which have a low glycemic index [53] and are, therefore, more likely to exert a prolonged satiating influence.

Awareness of the fact that fatty foods have a particularly high caloric density and that low-fat diets provide more bulk has led dieticians long ago to recommend low-fat diets for weight control [32]. During the last decade, recommendations to reduce fat intake have been increasingly promulgated in dietary guidelines published by government agencies and medical or health-related associations, since limiting fat intake (particularly consumption of the saturated fats predominant in meats, dairy products, chocolate, etc.) appears to be a key measure in lowering blood cholesterol levels and in minimizing the development of atherosclerosis [54]. To these arguments for restricting fat intake we can now add the further consideration that the steady state of weight maintenance can be expected, for metabolic reasons, to be achieved with less adipose tissue on board when the diet's fat content is low [5,12,13].

Selecting foods with a lower fat but higher complex carbohydrate content does not so much entail the discomfort of hunger as it requires avoidance of a whole range of desirable foods. This has the effect of limiting the range of permissible foods and thereby counteracting the impact exerted by the constant availability of appetizing foods [55].

VII. STRATEGIES FOR WEIGHT REDUCTION

New and old methods and regimes for weight reduction are constantly promoted, some based on sound principles, others on unsupported or misleading claims. Some of the major metabolically based rationales are considered below, leaving many other important considerations of a more behavioral and psychological nature to be discussed elsewhere.

A. Avoidance of Dietary Fat

As discussed above and illustrated in Figure 2, a low-fat diet generally allows the steady state of body weight maintenance to become established at a relatively low degree of adiposity. In individuals previously consuming substantial amounts of fat, a sharp reduction in fat intake can therefore be expected to lead to a gradual decline of the adipose tissue mass [35,40]. It is important in this regard to have reasonable expectations about possible rates of weight change after sharply reducing fat intake. For an individual accustomed to a diet providing 45% of total calories as fat, a reduction in fat intake by one third, while protein and carbohydrate consumption remain constant, would create an energy deficit of some 250–450 kcalories per day, depending on body size and energy turnover. This would cause a fat loss of 30–50 grams per day or a weekly reduction of the adipose tissue mass by ½ to 1 pound. This is not likely to sustain much enthusiasm in an obese individual who needs to shed much weight. These numbers also serve to illustrate that the admonition to eat carbohydrate freely while cutting fat intake, though perhaps reasonable for individuals aiming to maintain weight, is counterproductive for overweight subjects, as it will attenuate the impact of a reduction in fat intake on the energy balance. To be effective as a measure for weight correction, a reduction in fat intake should be complemented by efforts to limit (or at least to not increase) carbohydrate intake. This should be implemented primarily by restricting sugar intake, while selecting preferentially complex carbohydrates with a low glycemic index [53]. Finally, as mentioned earlier, avoidance of foods with a substantial fat and sugar content has the advantage of restricting food choices, reducing the obesity-promoting influence of the wide food variety provided by mixed diets.

B. Balanced Weight Reduction

Many weight-reduction diets prescribe intakes of 1000–1500 kcal/day without stressing major shifts in the relative proportions of carbohydrates, fats, and proteins. In order to ensure an adequate protein intake, selection of foods with a relatively high protein content is important, even in such balanced weight-reduction diets. Given that weight loss is less rapid, the likelihood of staying on course long enough is generally far less than with the more severely restricted PSMF and VLCD regimes (discussed below) on which discomfort due to hunger is generally rated to be less [56]. However, balanced weight-reduction diets have the considerable advantage of emphasizing reasonable food selection and control of portion size and developing knowledge about foods and control of eating behavior, which are essential for long-term success in weight control.

C. Acute Weight Reduction

Since fat oxidation is limited to the gap between total energy expenditure and carbohydrate plus protein intake [18], a considerable reduction in carbohydrate intake is essential to induce rapid fat oxidation. Near total avoidance of carbohydrate forces the body to cover most of its energy needs by burning fat. Depending on body size and activity, this may induce the oxidation of 150–250 grams of fat per day. Thus many weight-reducing diets emphasize strict avoidance of carbohydrates. But this will be beneficial only to the extent that enhanced fat oxidation is not compensated by high fat intakes. Total starvation creates the greatest energy deficit and a spectacularly rapid initial weight loss, due to the natriuresis of fasting, which leads to a decrease in the extracellular volume during the first days of carbohydrate deprivation. Prolonged starvation can be tolerated for many weeks, as the liver will produce ketone bodies to replace glucose as a fuel for the brain [57]. Quite remarkably, hunger is substantially attenuated after a few days. But the great disadvantage of total starvation is that it causes major losses of body protein. Such losses can fortunately be effectively minimized by consuming protein. Protein-sparing modified fasting (PSMF) [58] and very low calorie diets (VLCD) [59] have been developed, which take advantage of the relative suppression of hunger associated with total starvation, while preventing significant losses of lean body mass.

To maintain or approach nitrogen balance during periods of severely negative energy balance, it is necessary to maintain a rather high protein intake [60]. This fact has sometimes been obscured by comparing the average dose of protein needed to achieve nitrogen balance on restricted diets with the normal RDA for protein, which is set at two standard deviations above the average protein intake needed for nitrogen balance when energy needs are met. In PSMF regimes, 1.2–1.5 g protein/kg ideal body weight/day are usually prescribed, in the form of lean meat and fish [58], whereas somewhat lower doses of 70 g protein/day are considered to be sufficient with the VLCD formulas, since they also provide 30–45 g of glucose/day [59]. (In less obese subjects, in obese adolescents, and in adults engaging in substantial physical activity, slightly more carbohydrate or glucogenic precursors appear to be necessary for maintenance of nitrogen balance.) Due to the appreciable intake of glucogenic precursors with PSMF or to the small dose of glucose allowed with VLCD, ketogenesis proceeds at lower rates and ketone body levels are less than half than those prevailing during total starvation. The hyperuricemia induced by total starvation (due to inhibition of renal uric acid excretion by ketone bodies) is thereby substantially attenuated as well.

When proteins of high biological value are provided, complemented with adequate supplements of minerals, vitamins, potassium, and salt, the PSMF and VLCD regimens provide efficient and safe programs for rapid weight loss [59]. They are most appropriate for markedly obese subjects, who appear to be best able to reduce their need for glucogenic precursors and for whom there is a special incentive to lose weight as rapidly as possible. Losing fat at a rate of ⅓ to ½ pound per day still requires several months to achieve the substantial reduction in the adipose tissue that obese individuals may wish to achieve, but at least it offers some hope and motivation. It stands to reason that long periods of severe nutritional restriction may present some dangers to health and that they should only be undertaken under medical supervision to ensure adequate intakes of all the nutrients needed to maintain health (protein, minerals, electrolytes, notably potasssium, which is a prescription item, and vitamins) as well as safe management of drug dosages and sound advice about individual problems [59,61].

D. Weight Regain: Pitfalls

While weight reduction depends on defeating the natural tendency to regulate food intake, weight maintenance is a situation in which one should be able to rely to some extent on spontaneous control of food intake (or at least to minimize the struggle against it). It is, therefore, important to recognize that the logic for nutrient selection during weight maintenance and weight reduction is not the same! This is not commonly appreciated, in part no doubt because such notions are not germane to considerations based merely on the overall energy balance. Failure to appreciate the differences pertaining to weight maintenance and to weight reduction can be conducive to rapid regain of weight lost. Avoidance of carbohydrate in trying to achieve acute weight reduction drastically reduces food choices and compels the organism to operate with low glycogen reserves to enhance fat oxidation; it allows rapid adaptation to the starvation state where hunger is less intense [56], but only as long as carbohydrate intake is kept very low [58]. After such a bout of weight reduction, when carbohydrate intake is no longer as severely curtailed and weight tends to be regained, one will remember how rapid weight reduction was achieved by avoiding carbohydrates while relying on meat and fish. Thus reinforced in the common belief that carbohydrates are major culprits in causing weight gain, one may again be enticed to more liberally consume foods known for their low carbohydrate, but high protein content (i.e., chiefly meats, cheese, and nuts). But now that carbohydrate intake is not severely restricted, this bias is counterproductive, because these foods are high in fat, thereby thwarting the central strategy for weight maintenance, which is to prevent a positive fat balance by limiting fat intake.

VIII. CONCLUSIONS

In summary, we have seen that variations in the size of the adipose tissue mass are well tolerated and that this can be ultimately traced to the fact that fats are insoluble in water. Fat stores can therefore become very large. Errors in the fat balance have consequently deserved a much lower priority in biological evolution than the need to maintain appropriate glycogen stores and a suitable lean body mass. In view of the priority accorded by the body's regulatory mechanisms to the adjustment of carbohydrate and protein balances, the steady state of weight maintenance becomes established when food intake, in amounts appropriate to maintain carbohydrate balance, also brings in fat in amounts commensurate with the average rate of fat oxidation. To avoid fat accumulation, it is sufficient to burn as much fat as one eats, though this is made difficult when the consumption of a diet with substantial amounts of fat is combined with a sedentary lifestyle [44]. If one fails to limit fat intake, or to maintain glycogen levels low enough to facilitate fat oxidation, or to exercise enough to increase fat oxidation in muscle, the increase in fat oxidation required to make fat oxidation commensurate with fat intake is ultimately brought about by expansion of the adipose tissue mass. The degree of adiposity for which this occurs is determined by the particular set of inherited traits and circumstantial conditions—lifestyle and eating pattern —characteristic for each individual. As long as circumstantial factors remain unchanged, this configuration tends to be restored had it been temporarily disturbed. It thus appears as if the organism preferred to operate at a particular body weight and was able to regulate the energy balance. This has led to the concept of defense of body weight around a predetermined setpoint [62] and to speculations about the possible existence of a ponderostat [63], according to which individuals would be destined to have a particular body weight. These concepts do not readily allow one to take into account the influence of circumstantial factors, however [64]. When one understands that weight maintenance becomes established whenever the particular body composition allows the RQ to be equal to the FQ [12,13] these concepts are in fact not needed to explain why body weights are generally quite stable. Obesity thus appears to be caused not so much by a defect in the ability to regulate the energy balance as by a tendency to maintain energy balance, but only in the presence of an unacceptably high amount of adipose tissue. The constant availability of highly appetizing foods, by stimulating food consumption and by reducing the intervals between meals and snacks, has the effect of keeping glycogen reserves high, thereby curtailing fat oxidation. A high incidence of obesity in affluent societies is thus to be expected.

The arguments presented here suggest that a reduction in fat intake, if substantial, may represent a long-term measure capable of significantly reducing the need for an expanded adipose tissue mass in achieving the steady state of spontaneous weight maintenance. Instead of the usual principle based on counting calories ingested and expended, this provides an alternative strategy for weight maintenance, founded on measures that favor the occurrence of periods where metabolism operates at a relatively low RQ compared to the diet's FQ. This is obviously facilitated by consuming a diet with a high FQ (i.e., a diet with a high carbohydrate-to-fat ratio). Additional leverage can be obtained by physical activities likely to induce a decline in the RQ (i.e., sustained exercise of moderate intensity). Seriously limiting fat intake also appears to be a crucial dietary measure helping to limit or delay weight regain after periods of dieting, inasmuch as fat accumulation in individuals consuming mixed diets occurs by storage of dietary fatty acids, rather than by conversion of carbohydrate into fatty acids. Such regain must of course be expected to occur, unless at least one of the parameters involved in determining the weight maintenance plateau has been permanently and significantly altered.

There is insufficient information as of now to judge to what level the percentage of total energy intake consumed in the form of fat must be reduced to prevent obesity, and this limit is in fact likely to vary for different individuals. It seems likely that the 30% target proposed by current guidelines [65] will not by itself be sufficient to prevent excess weight among individuals prone to develop obesity. However, even if limiting fat intake to 30% does not guarantee or restore ideal body weights, such a dietary measure can be expected to have a significant impact, particularly because a cap on fat intake could substantially alter the dietary habits of obese subjects, who often have a predilection for fatty foods [36]. In this regard, it is worth mentioning that a recent study indicates that energy consumed in the form of alcohol should be included with that provided by fat, since ethanol intake selectively reduces fat, but not carbohydrate oxidation [66].

It is certainly feasible to reduce fat to 25% or even 20% of total caloric intake, but this requires a sustained commitment to an increasingly exclusive selection of food items, differing substantially from the assortment of foods preferred in Western societies. In addition to the metabolic leverage thereby achieved and to the reduction in caloric density of the allowed foods, this has the probably very significant advantage of facilitating weight control by reducing the diversity of the food mix provided by mixed diets.

ACKNOWLEDGMENTS

This work was supported by NIH grant DK 33214. The collaboration of K. E. G. Sargent and D. Demers is gratefully acknowledged.

REFERENCES

1. K. Acheson, Y. Schütz, T. Bessard, E. Ravussin, E. Jéquier, and J. Flatt, Nutritional influences on lipogenesis and thermogenesis after a carbohydrate meal, *Am. J. Physiol., 246*: E62 (1984).
2. K. Acheson, Y. Schütz, T. Bessard, K. Anatharama, J. Flatt, and E. Jéquier, Glycogen storage capacity and de novo lipogenesis during massive carbohydrate overfeeding in man, *Am. J. Clin. Nutr., 48*: 240 (1988).
3. M. K. Hellerstein, M. Christiansen, S. Kaempfer, C. Kletke, K. Wu, J. S. Reid, K. Mulligan, N. S. Hellerstein, and C. H. L. Shackleton, Measurement of de novo hepatic lipogenesis in humans using stable isotopes, *J. Clin. Invest., 87*: 1841 (1991).
4. J. P. Flatt, The difference in the storage capacity for carbohydrate and for fat, and its implications in the regulation of body weight, *Ann. N.Y. Acad. Sci., 499*: 104 (1987).
5. J. P. Flatt, Differences in the regulation of carbohydrate and fat metabolism and their implication for body weight maintenance, *Hormones, Thermogenesis and Obesity* (H. Lardy and F. Stratman, eds.), Elsevier, New York, pp. 3–17 (1989).
6. G. Livesay and M. Elia, Estimation of energy expenditure, net carbohydrate utilization, and net fat oxidation and synthesis by indirect calorimetry: Evaluation of errors with special reference to the detailed composition of fuels, *Am. J. Clin. Nutr., 47*: 608 (1988).
7. J. P. Flatt, The biochemistry of energy expenditure, *Rec. Adv. Obesity Res., 11*: 211 (1978).
8. R. Foltin, M. Fischman, T. Moran, B. Rolls, and T. Kelly, Caloric compensation for lunches varying in fat and carbohydrate content by humans in a residential laboratory, *Am. J. Clin. Nutr. 52*: 969 (1990).
9. H. Koopmans, Satiety signals from the gastrointestinal tract, *Am. J. Clin. Nutr., 42*: 1044 (1985).
10. R. Mattes, C. Pierce, and M. Friedman, Daily caloric intake of normal-weight adults: Response to changes in dietary energy density of a luncheon meal, *Am. J. Clin. Nutr., 48*: 214 (1988).

11. O. Edholm, J. Adam, M. Healey, H. Wolff, and R. B. Goldsmith, Food intake and energy expenditure of army recruits, *Br. J. Nutr., 24*: 1091 (1970).
12. J. P. Flatt, Importance of nutrient balances in body weight regulation, *Diabetes/ Metabolism Reviews, 4*: 571 (1988).
13. J. Flatt, Dietary fat, carbohydrate balance and weight maintenance: Effects of exercise, *Am. J. Clin. Nutr., 45*: 296 (1987).
14. W. Abbott, B. Howard, L. Christin, D. Freymond, S. Lillioja, V. Boyce, T. E. Anderson, C. Bogardus, and E. Ravussin, Short-term energy balance: Relationship with protein, carbohydrate, and fat balances, *Am. J. Physiol., 255*: E332 (1988).
15. Y. Schütz, J. Flatt, and E. Jéquier, Failure of dietary fat intake to promote fat oxidation: A factor favoring the development of obesity, *Am. J. Clin. Nutr., 50*: 307 (1989).
16. J. Mayer and D. Thomas, Regulation of food intake and obesity, *Science, 156*: 328 (1967).
17. J. Flatt, E. Ravussin, K. Acheson, and E. Jéquier, Effects of dietary fat on postprandial substrate oxidation and on carbohydrate and fat balances, *J. Clin. Invest., 76*: 1019 (1986).
18. J. Flatt, Opposite effects of variations in food intake on carbohydrate and fat oxidation in ad libitum fed mice, *J. Nutr. Biochem., 2*: 186 (1991).
19. P. Björntorp, H. Bergman, E. Varnauskas, and B. Lindholm, Lipid mobilization in relation to body composition in man, *Metabolism, 18*: 841 (1969).
20. L. Groop, R. Bonadonna, M. Shank, A. Petrides, and R. DeFronzo, Role of free fatty acids and insulin in determining free fatty acid and lipid oxidation in man, *J. Clin. Invest., 87*: 83 (1991).
21. C. Bouchard, L. Pérusse, C. LeBlanc, A. Tremblay, and G. Thériault, Inheritance of the amount and distribution of human body fat, *Int. J. Obes., 12*: 205 (1988).
22. G. Pitts and L. Bull, Exercise, dietary obesity, and growth in the rat, *Am. J. Physiol., 232*: R38 (1977).
23. E. J. Danforth, Diet and obesity, *Am. J. Clin. Nutr., 41*: 1132 (1985).
24. G. Bray, *Obesity in America*, NIH Publication No. 79-359, Bethesda, MD (1979).
25. J. Sobal and A. Stunkard, Solcioeconomic status and obesity: A review of the literature, *Psychol. Bull., 105*: 260 (1989).
26. P. Björntorp, The associations between obesity, adipose tissue distribution and disease, *Acta Med. Scand., 723*: 121 (1988).
27. H. Kissileff and T. Van Itallie, Physiology of the control of food intake, *Ann. Rev. Nutr., 2*: 371 (1982).
28. J. S. Garrow, Energy balance in man—an overview, *Am. J. Clin. Nutr., 45*: 114 (1987).
29. G. Bray, Obesity, a disorder of nutrient partitioning: the MONA LISA hypothesis, *J. Nutr., 121*: 1146 (1991).
30. S. B. Roberts, V. R. Young, P. Fuss, M. A. Fiatarone, B. Richard, H. Rasmussen, S. Wagner, J. Lyndon, E. Holehouse, and W. Evans, Energy expenditure and subsequent nutrient intakes in overfed young men, *Am. J. Physiol., 259*: R461 (1990).

31. L. Lissner, D. Levitsly, B. Strupp, H. Kalkwarf, and D. Roe, Dietary fat and the regulation of energy intake in human subjects, *Am. J. Clin. Nutr., 46*: 886 (1987).
32. K. H. Duncan, J. A. Bacon, and R. L. Weinsier, The effects of high and low energy density diets on satiety, energy intake, and eating time of obese and non-obese subjects, *Am. J. Clin. Nutr. 37*: 763 (1983).
33. A. Tremblay, G. Plourde, J. Després, and C. Bouchard, Impact of dietary fat content and fat oxidation on energy intake in humans, *Am. J. Clin. Nutr., 49*: 799 (1989).
34. J. Hill, J. Peters, G. Reed, D. Schlundt, T. Sharp, and H. Greene, Nutrient balance in humans: effects of diet composition, *Am. J. Clin. Nutr., 54*: 10 (1991).
35. A. Kendall, D. Levitsky, B. Strupp, and L. Lissner, Weight loss on a low-fat diet: Consequence of the imprecision of the control of food intake in humans, *Am. J. Clin. Nutr., 53*: 1124 (1991).
36. A. Drewnowski, J. Brunzell, K. Samde, and P. Iverius, Sweet tooth reconsidered: Taste responsiveness in human obesity, *Physiol. Behav., 35*: 617 (1985).
37. I. Romieu, W. Willett, M. Stampfer, G. Colditz, L. Sampson, B. Rosner, C. H. Hennekens, and F. E. Speizer, Energy intake and other determinants of relative, *Am. J. Clin. Nutr., 47*: 406 (1988).
38. D. Dreon, B. Frey-Hewitt, N. Ellsworth, P. William, R. Terry, and P. Woud, Dietary fat: carbohydrate ratio and obesity in middle-aged men, *Am. J. Clin. Nutr., 47*: 995 (1988).
39. V. George, A. Tremblay, J. Després, C. Leblanc, and C. Bouchard, Effect of dietary fat content on total and regional adiposity in men and women, *Int. J. Obes., 14*: 1085 (1990).
40. T. Prewitt, D. Schmeisser, P. Bowen, P. Aye, T. Dolecek, P. Langenberg, T. Cole, and L. Brace, Changes in body weight, body composition, and energy intake in women fed high- and low-fat diets, *Am. J. Clin. Nutr., 54*: 304 (1991).
41. A. Sclafani and D. Springer, Dietary obesity in rats: Similarities to hypothalmic and human obesity syndromes, *Physiol. Behav., 17*: 461 (1976).
42. P. Rogers, Returning "cafeteria-fed" rats to a chow diet: negative contrast and effects of obesity on feeding behavior, *Physiol. Behav., 35*: 493 (1985).
43. B. Andersson, X. Xu, M. Rebuffé-Scrive, K. Terning, M. Krotkiewski, and P. Björntorp, The effects of exercise training on body composition and metabolism in men and women, *Int. J. Obes., 15*: 75 (1991).
44. J. Stern, Is obesity a disease of inactivity?, *Eating and Its Disorders* (A. J. Stunkard and E. Stellar, eds.), Raven, New York, pp. 131–139 (1984).
45. A. J. Wade, M. M. Marbut, and J. M. Round, Muscle fiber type and aetiology of obesity, *Lancet, 335*: 805 (1990).
46. E. Jéquier, Does a thermogenic defect play a role in the pathogenesis of human obesity? *Clin. Physiol., 3*: 1 (1983).
47. P. Avons and P. T. James, Energy expenditure of young men from obese and nonobese families, *Human Nutr. Clin. Nutr., 40*C: 259 (1985).
48. J. C. Waterlow, Metabolic adaptation to low intakes of energy and protein, *Annu. Rev. Nutr., 6*: 495 (1986).

49. J. P. Flatt, Effects of corticosterone on RQ food intake and energy balance, *Int. J. Obes., 13*: 552 (1989).
50. F. Zurlo, S. Lillioja, A. Esposito-Del Puente, B. L. Nyomba, I. Raz, M. F. Saad, B. A. Swinburn, W. C. Knowler, C. Bogardus, and E. Ravussin, Low ratio of fat to carbohydrate oxidation as predictor of weight gain: study of 24-h RQ, *Am. J. Physiol., 259*: E650 (1990).
51. W. C. Miller, A. K. Lindeman, J. Wallace, and M. Niederpruem, Diet composition, energy intake, and exercise in relation to body fat in men and women, *Am. J. Clin. Nutr., 52*: 426 (1990).
52. J. LeMagnen, The metabolic basis of dual periodicity of feeding in rats, *Behav. Brain Sci., 4*: 561 (1981).
53. D. Jenkins, T. Wolever, and A. Jenkins, Starchy foods and glycemic index, *Diabetes Care, 11*: 149 (1988).
54. Report of the National Cholesterol Education Program Expert Panel on detection, evaluation, and treatment of high blood cholesterol in adults, *Arch. Intern. Med., 148*: 36 (1988).
55. E. Sims, Energy balance in human beings: The problem of plentitude, *Vit. Horm., 43*: 1 (1986).
56. T. A. Wadden, A. J. Stunkard, S. C. Day, R. A. Gould, and C. J. Rubin. Less food, less hunger: Reports of appetite and symptoms in a controlled study of a protein-sparing modified fast, *Int. J. Obes., 11*: 239 (1987).
57. G. F. J. Cahill, Starvation in man, *N. Engl. J. Med., 282*: 668 (1970).
58. P. G. Lindner, and G. L. Blackburn, Multidisciplinary approach to obesity utilizing fasting modified by protein-sparing therapy, *Obesity/Bariatric Med., 5*: 198 (1976).
59. T. A. Wadden, A. J. Stunkard, and K. D. Brownell, Very low calorie diets: Their efficacy, safety, and future, *Ann. Int. Med., 99*: 675 (1983).
60. L. J. Hoffer, B. R. Bistrian, V. R. Young, G. L. Blackburn, and D. E. Matthews, Metabolic effects of very low calorie weight reducing diets, *J. Clin. Invest., 73*: 750 (1984).
61. B. R. Bistrian, Clinical use of a protein-sparing modified fast, *J.A.M.A., 240*: 2299 (1978).
62. R. Keesey, A set-point analysis of the regulation of body weight, *Obesity* (A. J. Stunkard, ed.) WB Saunders, Philadelphia, pp. 144–165 (1980).
63. M. Cabanac, Role of set-point theory in body weight regulation, *FASEB J., 5*: 2105 (1991).
64. R. B. S. Harris, Role of set-point theory in regulation of body weight, *FASEB J., 4*: 3310 (1990).
65. P. R. Thomas, *Improving America's Diet and Health. From Recommendations to Action,* National Academy Press, Washington, D.C. (1991).
66. P. M. Suter, Y. Schutz, and E. Jaquier, The effect of ethanol on fat storage in healthy subjects, *N. Engl. J. Med., 326*: 983 (1992).

23
Effect of Lowering Dietary Fat on Health Status

Mary M. Flynn   *The Miriam Hospital at Brown University, Providence, Rhode Island*

Peter N. Herbert   *Yale University School of Medicine and Hospital of Saint Raphael, New Haven, Connecticut*

I. ROLE OF FAT IN THE DIET

The average person consumes more dietary fat than is physiologically necessary. Humans require 1–2% of their calories as fat [1]. The fat requirement is necessary to supply linoleic acid, a polyunsaturated fatty acid. Humans lack the capacity to synthesize this polyunsaturated fat and must obtain linoleic acid in their diet. They can synthesize both saturated and monounsaturated fatty acids from the metabolic end products of any excess calories [2].

The average American ingests approximately 36–37% of his or her calories as fat [3]. This value was as high as 40–42% 40 years ago [4]. Consumption of saturated fat has been decreasing, with a concomitant rise in polyunsaturated fat [3]. Americans have also been decreasing their total caloric intake since the 1940s [4].

Despite a steady decline in fat consumption over several decades, many health professionals recommend further reductions in fat intake. Levels approximating 30% of total calories are recommended [3]. Some guidelines further stipulate that a maximum of 10% of these calories come from saturated fat and 10% from polyunsaturated fats.

How are these dietary recommendations translated into food choices? Is there a minimum level of dietary fat intake, below which optimum health may be jeopardized? Does the dietary fat requirement change throughout the life cycle? What type of diet results when fat calories are reduced? These questions are addressed in the following sections.

II. TYPES OF LOW-FAT DIETS

Low-fat diets have been developed by both health professionals and nutrition charlatans. Diets low in fat are recommended to reduce the risk of cancer [5] or heart disease [6] and to promote weight loss. Excess body fat, moreover, may be a risk factor for several diseases.

Fat is the most concentrated source of energy in the diet. Caloric intake can be shown to be less precisely regulated when fat calories are surreptitiously altered in a conventional diet [7]. A caloric deficit that leads to weight loss can occur when subjects are unaware that they are consuming a low-fat diet [7].

There are a variety of ways to select and combine foods in a low-fat diet. Some examples follow.

1. Very low-calorie diets (VLCD): Very low-calorie diets [8] represent the extreme in low-fat diets. VLCD allow a maximum of 800 calories a day and are often composed solely of a very low-fat liquid formula drink. Some VLCDs allow one or two low-fat/low-calorie meals. The use of a liquid diet reduces food planning and decision making and therefore limits the opportunities to cheat. Examples of VLCDs include Optifast, Slimfast, and Herbalife.
2. Novelty or fad diets: These [8] are composed of a limited number of food items and often have rules for how foods can be combined and when they can be eaten. A rationale for these diets, having little basis in fact, is usually described. Novelty diets are low in fat and total calories due to a reduction in total food consumption. Examples include Fit for Life, The Beverly Hills Diet, and the Rotation Diet.
3. Vegetarian diets: Vegetarian diets [9] excluding animal products tend to be low in fat and especially low in saturated fat. A range of fat content can be found in vegetarian diets, depending on the amount and types of both dairy products and vegetable fat sources, such as nuts and oils. The following types of diets are included under the rubric of vegetarian:

a. Vegan or total vegetarian—exclude all animal products.
b. Lacto-vegetarian—permit dairy products, but no other animal products.
c. Lacto-ovo-vegetarian—consumption of dairy products and eggs is permitted.
d. Semi- or partial vegetarians—animal products are avoided only in part. Red meat is often not eaten, but poultry and seafood may be included.

It should be stressed that any strict or semivegetarian diet may be low in fat, but use of large quantities of vegetable fat is theoretically and practically possible.

4. Fat-restricted diets: Fat calories may be either severely or moderately restricted by reducing the intake of high-fat, calorie-dense foods [8]. Fat calories are partially replaced with carbohydrate calories. Diets severely restricted in fat calories recommend an elimination of all dietary fat sources. The result is a diet such as the Pritikin Diet, which has less than 10% of calories as fat. The Rice Report Diet and The Macrobiotic Diet are other examples. Fat calories are moderately restricted when fat comprises no more than 30% of total calories. Moderately fat-restricted diets often emphasize a severe reduction in saturated fat with the balance of fat calories from unsaturated fats. Examples include the diets for lowering blood lipids recommended by the American Heart Association [10] and the National Cholesterol Education Program [11] and that recommended by the American Cancer Society [5]. It must be appreciated that wholesale substitution of vegetable products for animal products may result in a reduction in the quantity and quality of dietary protein [12]. The long-term implications of such a change are not yet understood.

The rest of this chapter will examine the wisdom and consequences of following a low-fat diet throughout the human life cycle.

III. LOW-FAT DIETS DURING PREGNANCY

Low-fat diets that do not provide adequate energy may have an adverse effect on pregnancy outcome. The maternal requirement for energy, protein, and several vitamins and minerals increases during pregnancy to provide for the growing fetus [13]. The requirement for energy is the most important to fulfill as the levels set for the other nutrients are based upon adequate energy intake [14].

Inadequate energy intake during pregnancy, as reflected by poor maternal weight gain, is associated with a high incidence of low-birthweight infants (<2.5 kg) [15–17]. Caloric supplementation of women initially at risk for inadequate energy intake will produce infants with higher birthweights relative to the birthweights of infants born to similar women not receiving caloric supplementation [18,19]. The growing fetus normally deposits a large quantity of fat during the second half of gestation [20]. Body fat content at birth is the determining factor for birthweight [21]. The incidence of low-birthweight infants is therefore particularly striking when maternal undernutrition occurs during the final trimester of gestation [22,23].

Low birthweight is associated with increased infant mortality and morbidity and a range of development delays [24,25]. There is evidence to suggest that the mental delays continue throughout childhood [26]. Low-birthweight infants that ranked low on tests of mental development at 6–7 years of age were shown to have similar mental impairment when retested at 8–10 years of age [26].

Fetal body composition seems to be unrelated to the maternal dietary intake during the first two trimesters of gestation [27,28]. Maternal undernutrition during the final trimester results in a decrease in (1) fetal fat content [27,29], (2) infant size [28,29], and (3) organ weights, especially for the liver and the adrenal glands [28,29].

Vegetarians constitute the most common population of women consuming low-fat diets during pregnancy. Careful dietary planning is necessary to ensure that all the nutrient demands of pregnancy are met by the vegetarian diet [30]. Particular care is needed to meet the energy requirement, as vegetarian diets are inherently low in caloric density [31]. Vegetarians tend to gain less weight during pregnancy compared with omnivores [32]. However, women following vegan diets who continued these diets throughout pregnancy have been shown to produce infants equal in birthweight to omnivore controls without clinically adverse effects on themselves [33].

Requirements for most vitamins and minerals increase with pregnancy [13,14]. The dietary intake of several of these vitamins and minerals may be decreased on a low-fat diet. Low-fat diets that eliminate animal products may be low in iron, zinc, folate, and vitamin B_{12}. But if legumes are substituted for meat, iron and folate intakes may be higher than those consumed by pregnant omnivores [34]. Elimination of milk and dairy products greatly reduces the chances of meeting the increased demands for calcium. However, compared to a high-fat diet, a diet moderately low in fat may provide greater amounts of most vitamins and minerals [35].

IV. LOW-FAT DIETS DURING LACTATION

A low-fat diet during lactation has the potential to influence human milk fatty acid composition and the total volume of milk produced. The type and amount of dietary fat consumed and the energy available from the diet strongly influence human milk. Human milk can provide the total nutrient needs of the infant. It contains adequate water, lipids, protein, carbohydrate, vitamins, and minerals [36]. Only the vitamin and lipid composition of human milk are reflective of the mothers' dietary intake [37], with the lipids being the most variable component [36].

Human milk contains 3-4.5% fat on average [38-40]. However, a large variation can be seen between women [38,41] depending in part on the method of analysis utilized [42]. The fats present in human milk originate from mammary gland synthesis, subcutaneous fat mobilization, and maternal dietary intake [43-45]. The mammary gland can synthesize capric, lauric, and myristic acids. The mammary gland can also synthesize palmitic acid, but at one-half the rate it synthesizes capric, lauric, and myristic [45]. Palmitic acid in human milk is derived primarily from the immediate maternal diet [46,47], but also from mobilized maternal fat stores [47]. The rest of the fatty acids in human milk are derived from the maternal plasma triglycerides [46], which reflect the dietary intake and the fat mobilized from adipose stores. The mammary gland can potentially modify dietary and depot fat as it can insert double bonds in both saturated and monounsaturated fatty acids [39,43]. The linoleic acid content of human milk is from the maternal diet [46].

The total lipid content of human milk does not seem to vary greatly with changes in maternal diet composition [38,43,48], including large variations in fat intake [44,49-52]. Only the severe general malnutrition found in developing countries seems to yield a reduction in human milk fat content [53, 54]. However, maternal intakes of energy, fat, and/or carbohydrate exert significant influence on the fatty acid pattern of human milk (Table 1). The carbohydrate content of the maternal diet is thought to be primarily responsible for the changes in fatty acid composition seen with maternal dietary manipulation [47,54,55].

The linoleic acid content of human milk correlates with the amount of linoleic acid in the maternal diet [48,51,58,59]. The degree of correlation varies greatly among women [43]. Levels of linoleic acid between 1 and 43% have been found in human milk [38], with most samples being close to 10% [60]. The proportion of linoleate-rich vegetable fat in the American diet rose between 1947 and 1972 from 15 to 39% of total dietary fat [39]. This dietary change was reflected in an almost doubling in the linoleic acid content of breast milk [39].

Linoleic acid contents greater than 10% in human milk are thought to result in an increased requirement for vitamin E to prevent potential peroxidation of cell membranes [38]. Fortunately, breast-fed infants receive large quantities of vitamin E from colostrum during their first week of life [61]. Likewise, the vitamin E content of human milk is closely related to both the total lipid and the linoleic content [42,61].

Table 1 Influence of Maternal Diet on Human Milk Fat Composition

Maternal diet variable	Human milk fat	Ref.
Energy: inadequate for weight maintenance	Reflects maternal subcutaneous fat stores	49, 54
Energy: weight maintenance Fat: unrestricted	Reflects fatty acid pattern of maternal diet	48,49,54
Energy: weight maintenance Fat: low Carbohydrate: high	Increase in capric, lauric, myristic	44,47,49,55–57

The volume of human milk produced is fairly constant over a wide range of maternal energy intakes [62]. However, energy intake below approximately 1500 kcal/day will reduce the volume of milk produced [62,63]. Adequate energy intake during pregnancy may be at least as important to successful lactation. Failure to gain sufficient weight during pregnancy, which allows for maternal subcutaneous fat deposition, is associated with a decreased ability to produce milk [64]. The mobilization of these fat stores may be limited, however [65,66]. Women who successfully breast-feed consume more calories than women who are unsuccessful in lactation, yet weight loss is present in both groups [64,65].

The vitamin content of human milk, especially the water-soluble vitamins, can vary with dietary intake [14]. Fat-soluble vitamins are less reflective of the immediate diet due to the storage of considerable amounts of all the fat-soluble vitamins. Insufficient information is available regarding the relationship between dietary intake of minerals and human milk mineral content [14]. Low-fat diets have the potential to contain higher amounts of many of the vitamins and minerals compared to traditional Western diets, which may result in increased amounts in human milk [35]. However, this is based on diets that replace fat-containing foods with complex carbohydrates, fruits, vegetables, and nonfat or low-fat protein sources [35].

V. LOW-FAT DIETS DURING INFANCY

Energy requirements per pound of body weight are greatest during infancy [67]. Total energy needs vary not only with body size, but with rate of growth and activity level. An average requirement is 90–120 kcal/kg [68]. There is no defined absolute total fat requirement during infancy, and the optimal amount has not been determined [69]. Dietary recommendations for infants suggest a minimum of 30% and a maximum of 54% of calories from fat [70].

Recommendations for feeding infants up to 5–6 months of age are for human milk or commercially prepared formulas that have been designed to meet the known nutrient needs of the infant [71]. Bottle-fed infants tend to be heavier and longer than breast-fed infants by 3 months of age [72], but studies have repeatedly shown that the type of infant feeding will not determine the infant's body fatness [69].

Fat supplies 40–50% of the calories of both human milk and commercial formulas [67,68]. The high percentage of fat is advantageous to the rapidly growing infant. The volume of liquid that an infant can consume is limited, and fat provides a maximum number of calories per given volume of food [67]. Despite the apparent large fat intake, the actual fat available to the infant is less. Infants have a decreased ability to absorb fat until about 6–9 months old [67], with the fat in human milk more readily absorbed by the infant than the fat in formulas [73].

Infants, like adults, have a small requirement for linoleic acid [67,68]. This requirement is estimated to be 2–4% of total calories [68]. This level has a margin of safety since infants maintained on natural diets containing less than 1% of calories as linoleic acid do not manifest essential fatty acid deficiency [74]. Linoleic acid deficiency in humans has only been demonstrated after prolonged use of fat-free parenteral nutrition [74]. Linoleic acid deficiency in infants manifests as skin lesions and a reduction in somatic growth [75].

Recent evidence suggests that linolenic acid, or its longer-chain derivative docosahexaenoic acid (DHA), may also be essential to humans, particularly during early life [76]. DHA and arachidonic acid, a derivative of linoleic acid, have been shown to be rapidly deposited in the cerebral membranes in the last trimester of pregnancy and in the first 3 months of life [77,78]. High levels of DHA are found in cell membranes of the developed human brain and retina [76]. Evidence for the essentiality of linolenic acid and its derivatives derives from the specific cerebral cortex and retinal changes seen in animals maintained on diets deficient in these fats [76].

Human milk contains DHA, while most commercially prepared infant formulas do not [76,79]. Infants fed human milk have significantly higher amounts of DHA in their red blood cells than do infants fed formulas [79, 80]. Some infant formulas contain linolenic, the precursor of DHA [79]. However, linolenic acid conversion to DHA seems to be limited [79–81]. Infants fed formulas containing large amounts of linolenic acid have significantly less DHA in their red blood cells compared to infants fed human milk [79]. Continued research is needed to establish whether linolenic acid and/or its derivatives are essential for optimum human development.

The total amount of fat provided by human milk and commercial formulas is comparable, but the constituent fatty acids are quite different. The fat in commercially prepared formulas is from vegetable oils and the fatty acids will reflect the oil used [68]. The fatty acid profile of human milk reflects the maternal diet. The total calories, percentage of calories from carbohydrate, and the amount of linoleic acid in the maternal diet can each exert an influence on the human milk fatty acid profile and result in a predictable fatty acid profile in the breast milk produced.

The plasma lipids of infants will respond to the fatty acids in their diet [82,83]. It can be shown that the fat in an infant's diet will influence the contemporary lipid values, but will not affect the lipid values of childhood unless the diet remains the same [84,85]. The long-term benefits or consequences of infants consuming dramatically different fatty acid patterns has not been defined. Children maintained on a low saturated fat diet from infancy until 3 years of age were compared to a control group of children eating an unrestricted diet [86]. There was no difference in any physical or developmental parameter measured. The only difference between the two groups was a lower serum cholesterol in the group eating the low-saturated fat diet.

Low-fat diets during infancy can result if the infant is fed products other than human milk or formula. Reduced-fat milk is not recommended for infants [71]. Infants are occasionally fed reduced-fat milk in an effort to avoid obesity or atherosclerosis [87]. Fomon et al. [87] compared infants from 112 days of age fed either commercial infant formula or skim milk. Both groups were allowed commercially prepared strained foods. After 56 days, infants fed skim milk gained significantly less weight, yet consumed a larger volume of both milk and food. Total energy consumed for the skim milk group was lower and skinfold thickness measurements decreased by 24%, indicating fat mobilization.

Human growth will proceed satisfactorily for the first 3 months of life almost regardless of the calories available [88]. Infants that are undernourished after 4 months of age are more likely to suffer from delays in both physical growth and mental development in later childhood [89]. The growth retardation correlates positively with the length of time the inadequate nutrition occurs during the first year of life [89].

Infants weaned to low-fat diets may not maintain normal growth rates. Infants aged 7–22 months that were fed low-fat diets developed a "failure-to-thrive" syndrome [90]. The parents had consciously instituted a low-fat diet in an effort to avoid obesity and atherosclerosis [90]. Normal growth patterns were restored when the dietary restrictions were eliminated.

Infants weaned to vegetarian diets seem to be at a particularly high risk for inadequate growth velocities [89,91]. Vegetarian diets for children tend to be too low in calories and nutrient density due to their low fat content [92–94]. A low-fat diet is not considered appropriate for an infant because of their limited stomach capacity and high energy needs [92]. Vegetarian infants have more variability in their growth velocities than omnivore children because of the heterogeneity of vegetarian diets [95]. Infants weaned to very strict vegetarian diets of limited variety and quantity are more likely to experience multiple nutritional deficiencies [96].

VI. LOW-FAT DIETS FOR CHILDREN AND ADOLESCENTS

Low-fat diets that do not provide sufficient energy may interfere with the normal growth and development of children and adolescents. Caloric intake is thought to be a principal variable in determining the rate at which a child will grow [97]. After infancy the rate of growth decreases, but normal growth is associated with a steady increase in height and weight throughout childhood [98]. Children eating low-fat diets that do not provide sufficient energy tend to be shorter and weigh less than children eating unrestricted diets [97, 99]. The rate of growth increases again as a child enters adolescence [98]. The energy needs of adolescence vary, but inadequate energy intake during this time may delay or stunt the adolescent growth spurt [100].

Vegetarian diets low in fat, energy density, and digestibility may not meet the energy needs of growth [101]. There is a heterogeneity of growth patterns in vegetarian children due to the range of food intakes that are encompassed by "vegetarian diets" [99,101]. Normal growth is difficult to achieve in children on vegan or macrobiotic diets [97,99,101,102]. Children being raised on a vegetarian diet that includes some animal products, however, are more likely to achieve normal growth rates [101–103]. A group of growth-delayed vegan children that began to eat a vegetarian diet that included dairy products experienced an increase in growth with the change to less restrictive diet [104].

The velocity of growth in vegetarian children over 2 years of age approximates that found in children eating unrestricted diets [95]. However, children raised from infancy on vegetarian diets experience significantly lower mean weight and length velocities than norms before the age of 2 years [95]. This results in vegetarian infants beginning their childhood at a smaller size [95]. A continuation of a diet that does not allow sufficient energy for "catch-up" growth results in a smaller child [88,95].

The issue of recommending low-fat diets for all children over 2 years of age to reduce the risk of hyperlipidemia is controversial. The American Academy of Pediatrics questions whether cholesterol-lowering diets will support growth and development in children and adolescents and if diet will decrease their serum lipids [105,106]. The American Heart Association (AHA) contends that, although some potential hazards may exist, there have not as yet been any adverse experiences with children eating diets to lower their blood cholesterol [107]. The AHA therefore advises that dietary modifications not only appear to be safe for all children, but they may be beneficial [107].

Fat-modified diets will lower blood lipids in both normal and hyperlipidemic children and adolescents [108,109]. There may, however, be a minimum level of dietary fat below which normal growth and development is compromised. Diets that contain a minimum of 30% fat continue to support growth and development in children and adolescents [109,110], while diets with less than 30% fat have been associated with growth retardation [108,110]. Diets that contain less than 30% fat also contain less energy relative to diets with at least 30% fat [108,110]. Diets that are lower in fat but contain adequate calories, protein, vitamins, and minerals to support growth and development are feasible, but they require careful planning [111,112].

The use of hypocaloric–low-fat diets for weight loss in the first two decades of life may interfere with normal increases in height. The timing of caloric restriction relative to growth periods seems to determine the subsequent effects on height velocity. Both a very low-caloric diet (350 kcal/day) [113] and a moderately hypocaloric diet (66% of usual intake) [114] can result in pronounced growth retardation when used in obese children and young adolescents. Changes in height velocity in older adolescents are not as frequently associated with hypocaloric diets [115,116].

VII. LOW-FAT DIETS FOR ADULTS

Low-fat diets are recommended to lower blood lipids in adults. These lipid-lowering diets have 25–50% less total and saturated fat than diets eaten by most Americans [10,11]. The carbohydrate content of these diets is increased to compensate for the caloric deficit created by the decrease in dietary fat. These diets can be shown to lower total cholesterol, low-density lipoprotein cholesterol (LDL-c), and high-density cholesterol (HDL-c) in both hyperlipidemic [117] and normolipidemic [118–120] subjects. However, the increase in carbohydrate content of these diets often results in an increase in triglycerides [119,121]. The combination of elevated triglycerides and lowered HDL-c resulting from these diets could be detrimental to a hyperlipidemic patient.

Very recent studies by the authors indicate that the calorie content of low-fat diets is critical in determining the clinical response. Diets rich in carbohydrate and low in fat, but containing enough calories to prevent any weight loss, have potential to produce distinctly undesirable lipid profiles [122]. Conversely, qualitatively similar diets with fewer calories produce much more desirable changes in blood lipids [123].

REFERENCES

1. Lipids, *Recommended Dietary Allowances,* 10th ed., National Academy Press, Washington, DC, p. 44 (1989).
2. W. G. Linscheer and A. J. Vergroesen, Lipids, *Modern Nutrition in Health and Disease* (M. E. Shils and V. R. Young, eds.), Lea & Febiger, Philadelphia, p. 72 (1988).
3. Data sources, key nutrients, and selection of targets for change, *Designing Foods. Animal Product Options in the Marketplace*, National Academy Press, Washington, DC, p. 9 (1988).
4. A. M. Stephen and N. J. Wald, Trends in individual consumption of dietary fat in the United States, 1920-1984, *Am. J. Clin. Nutr., 52*: 457 (1990).
5. American Cancer Society, Nutrition and cancer: Cause and prevention. An American Cancer Society Special Report, *CA, 34*: 121 (1984).
6. American Heart Association, Dietary guidelines for healthy adult Americans, *Circulation, 74*: 1465a (1986).
7. L. Lissner, D. A. Levitsky, B. J. Strupp, H. J. Kalkwart, and D. A. Roe, Dietary fat and the regulation of energy intake in human subjects, *Am. J. Clin. Nutr., 46*: 886 (1987).
8. C. L. Rock and A. M. Coulston, Weight-control approaches: A review by the California Dietetic Association, *J. Am. Diet. Ass., 88*: 44 (1988).
9. N. A. Raper and M. M. Hill, Vegetarian diets, *Nutr. Rev.,* Suppl, (July): 29 (1974).
10. S. M. Grundy, D. Bilheimer, H. Blackman, V. Brown, P. O. Kwiterovich, F. Mattson, G. Schonfeld, and W. H. Weidman, Rationale of the diet heart statement of the American Heart Association, *Circulation, 65*: 839A (1982).
11. Expert Panel Report of the National Cholesterol Education Program, Expert Panel on detection, evaluation, and treatment of high blood cholesterol in adults, *Arch. Intern. Med., 148*: 36 (1988).
12. A. E. Harper, Dietary goals—a skeptical view, *Am. J. Clin. Nutr., 31*: 310 (1978).
13. R. M. Pitkin, Nutritional influences during pregnancy, *Med. Clin. North Am., 61*: 3 (1977).
14. A. G. Whitehead, Pregnancy and lactation, *Modern Nutrition in Health and Disease* (M. E. Shils and V. R. Young, eds.), Lea & Febiger, Philadelphia, p. 931 (1988).
15. H. C. Miller and K. Hassanein, Fetal malnutrition in white newborn infants: Maternal factors, *Pediatrics, 53*: 504 (1973).
16. A. S. Ademowore, N. G. Courey, and J. S. Kime, Relationships of maternal nutrition and weight gain to newborn birth weight, *Obstet. Gynecol., 39*: 460 (1972).
17. D. M. Campbell and I. MacGillivray, The effect of a low calorie diet or a thiazide diuretic on the incidence of pre-eclampsia and on birth weight, *Br. J. Obstet. Gynecol., 82*: 572 (1975).
18. A. Lechtig, H. Delgado, R. Lasky, C. Yarbrough, R. E. Klein, J. P. Habicht, and M. Béhart, Maternal nutrition and fetal growth in developing countries, *Am. J. Dis. Child., 129*: 553 (1975).

19. A. Lechtig, J. P. Habicht, H. Delgado, R. E. Klein, C. Yarbrough, and R. Martorell, Effect of food supplementation during pregnancy on birth weight, *Pediatrics, 56*: 508 (1975).
20. F. M. Widdowson, Body composition and energy metabolism before and after birth, *The Body Weight Regulatory System: Normal and Disturbed Mechanism* (L. A. Cioffi, W. P. T. James, and T. B. VanItallie, eds.), Raven Press, New York, p. 223 (1981).
21. G. Enzi, V. Zanardo, F. Caretta, E. M. Inelmen, and F. Rubaltelli, Intrauterine growth and adipose tissue development, *Am. J. Clin. Nutr., 34*: 1785 (1981).
22. C. A. Smith, Effects of maternal undernutrition upon the newborn infant in Holland (1944-1945), *J. Pediatr., 30*: 229 (1947).
23. A. N. Antonov, Children born during the siege of Leningrad in 1942, *J. Pediatr., 30*: 250 (1947).
24. L. Bergner and M. W. Susser, Low birth weight and prenatal nutrition: An interpretative review, *Pediatrics, 46*: 946 (1970).
25. V. Eisner, J. V. Brazie, M. W. Pratt, and A. C. Hexter, The risk of low birth weight, *Am. J. Public Health, 69*: 887 (1979).
26. G. Wiener, R. V. Rider, W. C. Oppel, and P. A. Harper, Correlates of low birth weight. Psychological status at eight to ten years of age, *Pediatr. Res., 2*: 110 (1968).
27. Fetal growth and maternal nutrition, *Nutr. Rev., 30*: 226 (1972).
28. R. L. Naeye, W. Blanc, and C. Paul, Effects of maternal nutrition on the human fetus, *Pediatrics, 52*: 494 z)1973).
29. R. L. Naeye, M. M. Diener, and W. S. Dellinger, Urban poverty: Effects on prenatal nutrition, *Science, 166*: 1026 (1969).
30. J. Dwyer, Health implications of vegetarian diets, *Compr. Therapy, 9*: 23 (1988).
31. P. K. Johnston, Counseling the pregnant vegetarian, *Am. J. Clin. Nutr., 48*: 901 (1988).
32. J. Dwyer, Vegetarian diets in pregnancy, *Alternative Dietary Practices in Pregnancy*, Proceedings of a workshop, National Academy Press, Washington, DC, pp. 61–83 (1982).
33. J. Thomas and F. R. Ellis, The health of vegans during pregnancy, *Nutr. Soc. Proc., 36*: 46A (1977).
34. Position paper on the vegetarian approach to eating, *J. Am. Diet. Assoc., 77*: 61 (1980).
35. R. M. Dougherty, A. K. H. Fong, and J. M. Iacono, Nutrient content of the diet when the fat is reduced, *Am. J. Clin. Nutr., 48*: 470 (1988).
36. American Academy of Pediatrics, Committee on Nutrition: Nutrition and lactation, *Pediatrics, 68*: 435 (1981).
37. B. S. Worthington-Roberts, Lactation and human milk: Nutritional considerations, *Nutrition in Pregnancy and Lactation* (B. S. Worthington-Roberts, J. Vermeersch, and S. R. Williams, eds.), The C.V. Mosby Company, St. Louis, p. 155 (1981).
38. R. G. Jensen, M. M. Hagerty, and K. E. McMahon, Lipids of human milk and infant formulas: a review, *Am. J. Clin. Nutr., 31*: 990 (1978).

39. H. A. Guthrie, M. F. Picciano, and D. Sheehe, Fatty acid patterns of human milk, *J. Pediatr., 90*: 39 (1977).
40. J. N. Udall and K. A. Kilbourne, Selected aspects of infant feeding, *Nutrition, 4*: 409 (1988).
41. B. Hall, Uniformity of human milk, *Am. J. Clin. Nutr., 32*: 304 (1979).
42. S. E. Collins, M. B. Jackson, C. J. Lammi-Keefe, and R. G. Jensen, The simultaneous separation and quantification of human milk lipids, *Lipids, 24*: 746 (1989).
43. E. Vuori, K. Kiuru, S. M. Makinen, P. Vayrynen, R. Kara, and P. Kiutunen, Maternal diet and fatty acid pattern of breast milk, *Acta Paediatr. Scand., 71*: 959 (1982).
44. G. H. Silber, D. L. Hachey, R. J. Schanler, and C. Garza, Manipulation of maternal diet to alter fatty acid composition of human milk intended for premature infants, *Am. J. Clin. Nutr., 47*: 810 (1988).
45. B. J. Thompson and S. Smith, Biosynthesis of fatty acids by lactating human breast epithelial cells: An evaluation of the contributions to the overall composition of human milk fat, *Pediatr. Res., 19*: 139 (1985).
46. D. L. Hachey, M. R. Thomas, E. A. Emken, C. Garza, L. Brown-Booth, R. O. Adlolf, and P. D. Klein, Human lactation: Maternal transfer of dietary triglycerides labeled with stable isotopes, *J. Lipid. Res., 28*: 1185 (1987).
47. W. W. C. Read, P. G. Lutz, and A. Tashjian, Human milk lipids III. Short-term effects of dietary carbohydrate and fat, *Am. J. Clin. Nutr., 17*: 184 (1965).
48. J. M. Potter and P. J. Nestel, The effects of dietary fatty acids and cholesterol on the milk lipids of lactating women and the plasma cholesterol of breast-fed infants, *Am. J. Clin. Nutr., 29*: 54 (1976).
49. W. Insull, J. Hirsch, T. James, and E. H. Ahrens, The fatty acids of human milk II. Alterations produced by manipulation of calorie balance and exchange of dietary fats. *J. Clin. Invest., 38*: 443 (1959).
50. A. R. P. Walker, B. F. Walker, D. Bhamjee, and Y. Ntola, Serum lipids in long-lactating African mothers habituated to a low-fat intake, *Atherosclerosis, 44*: 175 (1982).
51. D. A. Finley, B. Lonnerdal, K. G. Dewey, and L. E. Grivetti, Breast milk composition: Fat content and fatty acid composition in vegetarians and non-vegetarians, *Am. J. Clin. Nutr., 41*: 787 (1985).
52. L. A. Nommsen, C. A. Lovelady, M. J. Heining, B. Lonnerdal, and K. G. Dewey, Determinants of energy, protein, lipid, and lactose concentrations in human milk during the first 12 months of lactation: The DARLING Study, *Am. J. Clin. Nutr., 53*: 457 (1991).
53. M. A. Crawford and P. Stevens, Lipid composition of human milk: Comparative studies on African and European mothers, *Nutr. Soc. Proc., 33*: 50A (1974).
54. D. B. Jelliffe and E. F. P. Jelliffe, The volume and composition of human milk in poorly nourished communities. A review, *Am. J. Clin. Nutr., 31*: 492 (1978).
55. W. W. C. Read, P. G. Lutz, and A. Tashjian, Human milk lipids II. The influence of dietary carbohydrates and fat on the fatty acids of mature milk. A study in four ethnic groups, *Am. J. Clin. Nutr., 17*: 180 (1965).

56. M. W. Borschel, R. G. Elkin, A. Kirksey, J. A. Story, O. Galal, G. G. Harrison, and N. W. Jerome, Fatty acid composition of mature human milk of Egyptian and American women, *Am. J. Clin. Nutr., 44*: 330 (1986).

57. G. Silber, J. Hopkinson, D. Hachey, and C. Garza, Modification of fatty acid composition in human milk, *Am. J. Clin. Nutr., 40*: 688 (1986).

58. T. A. B. Sanders, F. R. Ellis, and J. W. T. Dickerson, Studies of vegans: The fatty acid composition of plasma choline phosphoglycerides, erythrocytes, adipose tissue, and breast milk, and some indicators of susceptibility to ischemic heart disease in vegans and omnivore controls, *Am. J. Clin. Nutr., 31*: 805 (1978).

59. M. J. Mellies, T. T. Ishikawa, P. S. Gartside, K. Burton, J. MacGee, K. Allen, P. M. Steiner, D. Brady, and L. J. Glueck, Effects of varying maternal dietary fatty acids in lactating women and their infants, *Am. J. Clin. Nutr., 32*: 299 (1979).

60. M. A. Crawford, A. G. Hassam, and J. P. W. Ruers, Essential fatty acid requirements in infancy, *Am. J. Clin. Nutr., 31*: 2181 (1978).

61. L. Jansson, B. Akesson, and L. Holmberg, Vitamin E and fatty acid composition of human milk, *Am. J. Clin. Nutr., 34*: 8 (1981).

62. W. A. Coward, A. A. Paul, and A. M. Prentice, The impact of malnutrition on human lactation: Observations from community studies, *Fed. Proc., 43*: 2432 (1984).

63. M. A. Strode, K. G. Dewey, and B. Lonnerdal, Effects of short-term caloric restriction on lactational performance of well-nourished women, *Acta Paediatr. Scand., 75*: 222 (1986).

64. D. J. Naismith and C. D. Ritchie, The effect of breast-feeding and artificial feeding on body-weights, skinfolds measurements and food intakes of forty-two primiparous women, *Nutr. Soc. Proc., 34*: 116A (1975).

65. M. J. Whichelow, Success and failure of breast-feeding in relation to energy intake, *Nutr. Soc. Proc., 35*: 62A (1976).

66. M. M. Brewer, M. R. Bates, and L. P. Vannoy, Postpartum changes in maternal weight and body fat depots in lactating vs. non-lactating women, *Am. J. Clin. Nutr., 49*: 259 (1989).

67. P. L. Pipes, Energy and energy producing nutrients: Proteins, fats and carbohydrates, *Nutrition in Infancy and Childhood*, The C.V. Mosby Company, St. Louis, p. 25 (1981).

68. W. C. Heird and A. Cooper, Nutrition in infants and children, *Modern Nutrition in Health and Disease* (M. E. Shils and V. R. Young, eds.), Lea & Febiger, Philadelphia, p. 944 (1988).

69. J. N. Udall and K. A. Kilbourne, Selected aspects of infant feeding, *Nutrition, 4*: 409 (1988).

70. C. W. Woodruff, The science of infant nutrition and the art of infant feeding, *JAMA, 240*: 657 (1978).

71. S. J. Fomon, L. J. Filer, T. A. Anderson, and E. E. Ziegler, Recommendations for feeding normal infants, *Pediatrics, 63*: 52 (1979).

72. C. D. Ritchie and D. J. Naismith, A comparison of growth in wholly breast-fed infants and artificially fed infants, *Nutr. Soc. Proc., 34*: 118A (1975).

73. A. L. Jarvenpaa, Feeding the low-birth-weight infant IV. Fat absorption as a function of diet and duodenal bile acids, *Pediatrics, 72*: 684 (1983).
74. W. F. J. Cuthbertson, Essential fatty acid requirements in infancy, *Am. J. Clin. Nutr., 29*: 559 (1976).
75. Z. Friedman, Essential fatty acids revisited, *Am. J. Dis. Child., 134*: 397 (1980).
76. M. Neuringer, N-3 Fatty acids in the brain and retina: Evidence for their essentiality, *Nutr. Rev., 44*: 285 (1986).
77. M. T. Clandinin, J. E. Chappell, S. Leong, T. Helm, P. R. Swyer, and G. W. Chance, Intrauterine fatty acid accretion rates in human brain: Implications for fatty acid requirements, *Early Hum. Develop., 4*: 121 (1980).
78. M. T. Clandinin, J. E. Chappell, S. Leong, T. Heun, P. R. Swyer, and G. W. Chance, Extrauterine fatty acid accretion in infant brain: Implications for fatty acid requirements, *Early Hum. Develop., 4*: 131 (1980).
79. J. C. Putnam, S. E. Carlson, P. W. DeVoe, and L. A. Barness, The effect of variations in dietary fatty acids on the fatty acid composition of erythrocyte phosphatidylcholine and phosphatidylethanolamine in human infants, *Am. J. Clin. Nutr., 36*: 106 (1982).
80. S. E. Carlson, P. G. Rhodes, and M. G. Ferguson, Docosahexaenoic acid status of preterm infants at birth and following feeding with human milk or formula, *Am. J. Clin. Nutr., 44*: 798 (1986).
81. M. A. Crawford, A. G. Hassam, and G. Williams, Essential fatty acids and fetal brain growth, *Lancet, 1*: 452 (1976).
82. J. P. Van Biervliet, N. Vinaumont, H. Caster, R. Vercaemst, and M. Roseneu, Plasma apoprotein and lipid patterns in newborns: Influence of nutritional factors, *Acta Paediatr. Scand., 70*: 851 (1981).
83. M. J. Sweeney, J. N. Etteldorf, W. T. Dobbins, B. Sommervill, R. Fischer, and C. Ferrell, Dietary fat and concentrations of lipids in the serum during the first six to eight weeks of life, *Pediatrics, 50*: 765 (1961).
84. J. K. Huttunen, U. M. Saarinen, E. Kostiainan, and M. A. Siimes, Fat composition of the infant diet does not influence subsequent serum lipid levels in man, *Atherosclerosis, 46*: 87 (1983).
85. R. P. Farris, M. S. Hyg, G. C. Frank, L. S. Webber, S. R. Srinivasan, and G. S. Berenson, Influence of milk source on serum lipids and lipoproteins during the first year of life, Bogalusa Heart Study, *Am. J. Clin. Nutr., 35*: 42 (1982).
86. G. Friedman and S. J. Goldberg, An evaluation of safety of a low-saturated fat, low-cholesterol diet beginning in infancy, *Pediatrics, 58*: 655 (1976).
87. S. J. Fomon, L. J. Filer, E. E. Ziegler, K. E. Bergmann, and R. L. Bergmann, Skim milk in infant feeding, *Acta Paediatr. Scand., 66*: 17 (1977).
88. A. M. Thompson, The evaluation of human growth patterns, *Am. J. Dis. Child., 120*: 398 (1970).
89. H. P. Chase and H. P. Martin, Undernutrition and child development, *N. Engl. J. Med., 282*: 933 (1970).
90. M. T. Pugliese, M. Weyman-Dawn, N. Moses, and F. Lifshitz, Parental health beliefs as a cause of non organic failure to thrive, *Pediatrics, 80*: 175 (1987).

91. J. T. Dwyer, R. Palumbo, H. Thorne, I. Valadian, and R. B. Reed, Preschoolers on alternate life-style diets, *J. Am. Diet. Assoc., 72*: 264 (1978).
92. C. Jacobs and J. R. Dwyer, Vegetarian children: Appropriate and inappropriate diets, *Am. J. Clin. Nutr., 48*: 811 (1988).
93. D. D. Truesdall and P. B. Acosta, Feeding the vegan infant and child, *J. Am. Diet. Assoc., 85*: 837 (1985).
94. American Academy of Pediatrics, Committee on Nutrition: Nutritional aspects of vegetarianism, health foods, and fad diets, *Pediatrics, 59*: 460 (1977).
95. M. W. Shull, R. B. Reed, I. Valadian, R. Palumbo, H. Thorne, and J. T. Dwyer, Velocities of growth in vegetarian preschool children, *Pediatrics, 60*: 410 (1977).
96. E. Zmora, R. Gorodischer, and J. Bar-Zin, Multiple nutritional deficiencies in infants from a strict vegetarian community, *Am. J. Dis. Child., 133*: 141 (1979).
97. T. A. B. Sanders, Growth and development of British vegan children, *Am. J. Clin. Nutr., 48*: 822 (1988).
98. P. L. Pipes, Nutrition: Growth and development, *Nutrition in Infancy and Childhood*, The C.V. Mosby Company, St. Louis, p. 1 (1981).
99. J. T. Dwyer, E. M. Andrew, C. Berkey, I. Valadian, and R. B. Reed, Growth in new vegetarian preschool children using the Jenss-Bayley curve filling technique, *Am. J. Clin. Nutr., 37*: 815 (1983).
100. J. Dwyer, Nutritional requirements of adolescence, *Nutr. Rev., 39*: 56 (1981).
101. W. C. Maclean and G. C. Graham, Vegetarianism in children, *Am. J. Dis. Child., 134*: 513 (1980).
102. W. A. van Staveren and P. C. Dagnelie, Food consumption, growth, and development of Dutch children fed on alternative diets, *Am. J. Clin. Nutr., 48*: 819 (1989).
103. M. Tayter and K. L. Stanek, Anthropometric and dietary assessment of omnivore and lacto-ovo-vegetarian children, *J. Am. Diet. Assoc., 89*: 1661 (1989).
104. C. M. Trahms, Catch up growth in children previously deprived of animal protein, *Fed. Proc., 36*: 1181 (1977).
105. American Academy of Pediatrics, Committee on Nutrition: Prudent lifestyle for children: Dietary fat and cholesterol, *Pediatrics, 78*: 521 (1986).
106. Committee on Nutrition: Toward a prudent diet for children, *Pediatrics, 71*: 78 (1983).
107. C. J. Glueck, H. C. McGill, R. E. Shank, and R. M. Lauer. Value and safety of diet modification to control hyperlipidemia in childhood and adolescence, *Circulation, 58*: 381A (1978).
108. E. Vartiainen, P. Puska, P. Pietinen, A. Nissinen, U. Leuno, and U. Uusitalo, Effects of dietary fat modifications on serum lipids and blood pressure in children, *Acta Paediatr. Scand., 75*: 396 (1986).
109. E. A. Stein, J. Shapero, C. McNerney, C. J. Glueck, T. Tracy, and P. Gartside, Changes in plasma lipid and lipoprotein fractions after alteration in dietary cholesterol, polyunsaturated, saturated, and total fat in free-living normal and hypercholesterolemic children, *Am. J. Clin. Nutr., 35*: 1375 (1982).

110. P. Lifshitz and N. Moses, Growth failure: A complication of dietary treatment of hypercholesterolemia, *Am. J. Dis. Child., 143*: 537 (1989).

111. P. O. Kwiterovich, Biochemical, clinical, epidemiologic, genetic, and pathologic data in the pediatric age group relevant to the cholesterol hypothesis, *Pediatrics, 78*: 349 (1986).

112. J. Dwyer, Diets for children and adolescents that meet the dietary goals, *Am. J. Dis. Child., 134*: 1073 (1980).

113. C. G. D. Brook and J. K. Lloyd, Rapid weight loss in children, *Br. Med. J., 2*: 44 (1974).

114. W. H. Dietz and R. Hartung, Changes in height velocity of obese preadolescents during weight loss, *Am. J. Dis. Child., 139*: 705 (1985).

115. E. H. Archibald, J. E. Harrison, and P. B. Pencharz, Effect of a weight-reducing high-protein diet on the body composition of obese adolescents, *Am. J. Dis. Child., 137*: 658 (1983).

116. M. R. Brown, W. J. Klish, J. Hollander, M. A. Campbell, and G. B. Forbes, A high protein, low calorie liquid diet in the treatment of very obese adolescents: long-term effect on lean body mass, *Am. J. Clin. Nutr., 38*: 20 (1983).

117. C. Ehnholm, J. K. Huttunen, P. Pietinen, U. Leino, M. Mutanen, E. Kostiainen, J. Pikkarainen, R. Dougherty, J. Iacono, and P. Puska, Effect of diet on serum lipoproteins in a population with a high risk of coronary heart disease, *N. Engl. J. Med., 307*: 850 (1982).

118. S. M. Grundy, D. Nix, M. Whelan, and L. Franklin. Comparison of diets of different fat content and composition on plasma lipids and lipoproteins, *Circulation, 72*: III-452 (1985).

119. J. H. Brussard, G. Dallinga-Thie, P. H. E. Groot, and M. B. Katan, Effects of amount and type of dietary fat on serum lipids, lipoproteins and apolipoproteins in man, *Atherosclerosis, 36*: 515 (1980).

120. S. M. Grundy, D. Nix, M. F. Whelan, and L. Franklin, Comparison of three cholesterol-lowering diets in normolipidemic men, *JAMA, 256*: 2351 (1986).

121. H. Ginsberg, J. M. Olefsky, G. Kimmerling, P. Crapo, and G. M. Reaven, Induction of hypertriglyceridemia by a low-fat diet, *J. Clin. Endocrinol. Metab., 42*: 729 (1976).

122. P. N. Herbert, M. M. Flynn, A. M. Nugent, S. E. Peloquin, M. J. Pucci, C. B. Chenevert, P. D. Thompson, and S. P. Sady. Efficacy of the American Heart Association diets in men with coronary heart disease, *Circulation, 76*: IV-292 (1987).

123. M. M. Flynn, S. P. Sady, and P. N. Herbert, Modest caloric restriction augments blood lipid response to a fat modified diet, *Clin. Res., 39*: 146A (1991).

24
Lessons Learned from Attempts to Implement Long-Term Low-Fat Diet Regimens

Maureen M. Henderson, Elizabeth R. Burrows, and Holly Henry
Fred Hutchinson Cancer Research Center, Seattle, Washington

I. INTRODUCTION

Numerous studies and programs have been undertaken to reduce the fat and calories that people eat, and most of them have had limited success. Many of the programs have been focused on the reduction of cardiovascular disease, while others have been part of weight-loss programs. Most of the dietary goals in these programs have been aimed at reducing fat intake to approximately 30% of energy. Success rates in these trials have varied; initial reductions of 10–25% of baseline fat consumption are reported to be common. However, long-term maintenance, even in well-motivated, high–clinical risk populations, has not been good [1].

Currently, it is widely recommended that we reduce our consumption of dietary fat. These recommendations come from both national [2,3] and local organizations, as well as private physicians. There have also been intensive educational efforts by local offices of the American Heart Association and Cancer Society to help the public implement the suggested recommendations. Some dietary changes have been reported in response to community education programs [4]. However, success has been limited and little is known about how to help free-living individuals initiate and maintain lower-fat eating habits.

The Women's Health Trial (WHT) was successful in dramatically reducing the fat intake of women [5]. The purpose of this chapter is to share some insights learned from the behavior of women in that study about techniques that help to lower dietary fat intake. First we will describe the WHT and its participants. Then we will share information about the basic changes they made in their food intake, including the variety of ways in which they manipulated their use of food groups and specific foods to achieve these changes. Finally, we will discuss maintenance of dietary changes—which changes were easiest to maintain and which were more difficult.

II. THE WOMEN'S HEALTH TRIAL

The Women's Health Trial was designed in 1985 as a multicentered randomized trial to evaluate the effectiveness of a low-fat diet on reducing the incidence of breast cancer. The study was to be a long-term dietary intervention in free-living women, but it was aborted in 1988. A total of 2064 intervention women 45–69 years of age were enrolled in the study. They had been in the intervention process for varying lengths of time when the study ended. One group (feasibility study) had completed approximately 36 months of intervention, while a second group (full-scale study) had participated for an average of 10 months. The information shared in this chapter is based on the 3-year experience of the initial group of 303 women.

The participants in this study were typical, healthy, middle-class women. They were all at average or above-average risk of breast cancer. However, as a group, their risk of breast cancer was lower than the heart disease risk of the men included in earlier randomized dietary intervention trials [7]. None of the women who volunteered and were accepted into this trial had a history of cancer, coronary heart disease, or diabetes, and none was on physician-prescribed or self-imposed low-fat or low-calorie diets. All were less than 150% above ideal body weight, and all had agreed to commit the time needed each week to follow the study protocol for up to 10 years.

They lived in three large, widely separated U.S. cities with substantial differences in local food habits and preferences. All were sufficiently well motivated to fulfill the relatively demanding admission requirements. The majority were white, married (78%), postmenopausal (80%), and had some college education (65%). Approximately two out of five were employed outside their homes [5,6].

The goal for the entire intervention group of women was to lower daily fat consumption from an average of 39% to an average of 20% of baseline daily calories. Each woman was given her own working goal, which was the number of grams of fat from all sources equal to 20% of the calories estimated from her baseline, 4-day food record. For most, the fat intake goal was approximately half of the baseline intake. The women in this particular trial were advised to cut in half the fat eaten from all sources and not to try to change the existing balance of fatty acids from predominantly animal or vegetable sources.

The instruction for dietary intervention followed an established protocol. It consisted of a detailed nutritional and behavioral program delivered to small permanent groups of 8–12 women. Each group had eight weekly classes, six biweekly sessions, and six monthly sessions and was supervised by the same intervention counselor throughout.

The dietary intervention provided the knowledge and skills necessary to make food selections needed to achieve the low level of 20% of calories from fat. Reductions of the major fat-containing food groups—fats and oils, red meats, dairy foods, and high-fat grain products—were emphasized. The women were encouraged to use complex carbohydrates such as grains and legumes and fruits and vegetables to replace fat calories. The distinction between this and many other dietary intervention programs was the absence of any menu plans or rigid diets. Change was planned to be gradual. Participants were encouraged to set their own goals, their own rates of change, and to monitor their own progress. They were also taught how to monitor their daily use and consumption of fat, how to determine the sources of fat in their own diets, and how to identify the food groups and foods where they could most easily make reductions in the amount of fat they were currently eating.

III. CHANGING FROM A HIGH- TO A LOW-FAT DIET

A 4-day food record and a semi-quantitative food-frequency questionnaire were used to collect dietary data at baseline and at 6, 12, and 24 months into the intervention. All the food record dietary information was coded by trained nutritional personnel and analyzed using the University of Massachusetts Nutrient Data Base [8].

A. Long-Term Changes

As a group the 184 women who followed the dietary intervention made successful long-term changes in their fat consumption. Detailed descriptions of their eating patterns during the first 24 months of intervention have been published [5,6,9]. The maintenance of those changes up to 36 months was described in the final report of the WHT [10]. This final report also described similar but necessarily short-term (average 10 months) changes in the 699 intervention participants recruited into the truncated full-scale trial.

An independent follow-up study was completed approximately 4 years after the first group of women and 1½ years after the second group of women began their intervention. It confirmed the maintenance of the intervention women's lowered fat intake [11].

Eighty percent of the women were successful in reaching their goal by 6 months, and 67% were maintaining that level 2 years later. Education and income did not appear to have much influence on the rate of success. Those women with the lowest incomes and the least education were able to make and maintain virtually the same dietary changes as the women who had more extensive personal resources (Table 1). It is important to remember that these volunteers had already decided that they were ready to change if randomized into the intervention group.

No nutritional inadequacies were reported by the women who were following a low-fat pattern. The overall quality of their diet compared well with that of the control group of women in terms of vitamins and minerals (Table 2). The relatively severe changes in fat consumption did not appear to compromise the overall nutrient quality of diet, and the women had no excess symptoms or morbidity of any kind.

Table 1 Fat[a] Eaten by Intervention Subjects by Socioeconomic Status Characteristics

		Months of intervention			
	n	0	6	12	24
Completed years of education					
High school	68	72.7	29.3	28.5	33.4
College	85	77.5	31.3	31.9	33.8
Graduate	26	79.7	31.8	35.1	36.3
Income (in thousands)					
Less than 30	64	74.1	30.5	29.9	34.3
30–50	64	77.9	30.2	32.1	34.3
over 50	43	76.5	30.6	29.6	31.9
Working outside the home	96	77.3	30.2	31.6	34.2
Not working outside the home	83	74.9	31.0	30.7	33.8

[a]Amount of fat (g/day) averaged according to 4-day food records. *n* = number of women.

Table 2 Mean Daily Intake of Calories and Micronutrients
Reported by Intervention and Control Subjects[a]

		Months in Group					
		Intervention			Control		
		0	12	24	0	12	24
Nutrient[b]	n	184	173	158	119	114	101
Calories (kcal)		1728	1300	1355	1702	1576	1613
Vitamin A (IU)		6470	7336	7966	6559	7028	7536
Vitamin C (mg)		132.9	147.0	144.0	127.9	135.5	134.7
Calcium (mg)		717.0	750.3	720.6	704.9	703.7	738.7
Iron (mg)		13.1	12.0	13.0	12.9	12.7	12.9
Alcohol (kcal)[c]		50.8	33.0	29.1	50.0	40.6	38.2
Riboflavin (mg)		1.7	1.6	1.6	1.6	1.6	1.6
Niacin (mg)		34.5	31.6	32.3	32.7	32.5	32.8
Thiamin (mg)		1.4	1.2	1.3	1.2	1.2	1.3
Vitamin B_6 (mg)		1.2	1.3	1.4	1.1	1.3	1.3
Vitamin B_{12} (μg)		3.5	3.3	3.5	3.1	4.0	3.6

[a]Four-day food record.
[b]Without reported supplements.
[c]Includes calories from mixers and other nonalcoholic ingredients.

Weight loss was not a focus of the intervention; it was neither encouraged nor discouraged. During the first 6 months, the women reduced their average consumption of food energy from 1731 to 1295 kcal/day and fat from 76 to 31 grams with proportionate cuts in saturated, polyunsaturated, and monounsaturated fatty acids (Table 3). Between 12 and 24 months, their consumption of fat and calories remained at approximately the same average levels. The women lost an average of 3.0 kg in weight during the first year, gradually gained some of it back during the second, and eventually stabilized at a lower-than-average baseline weight.

The gradual increase in average weight without a reported increase in total calorie consumption has been criticized and proposed as evidence of inaccurate recording. However, a recent analysis of the detailed information on the women's weight changes suggested that the changes were complex. The weight changes observed were much more closely linked to changes in fat intake than to changes in total calories. The changes in weight were also confounded by use of therapeutic drugs and by the decision of a very small number of women to use short-term, severe calorie restriction for weight management [12].

Table 3 Mean Weights and Daily Intake of
Calories and Fat in the Intervention Group[a]

	Months in Group			
	0	6	12	24
Weight (kg)	68.8	65.7	65.9	67.4
Kilocalories	1731	1295	1295	1349
Fat (g)				
Total	76	31	31	34
Saturated	27	10	10	11
Monounsaturated	27	10	11	12
Polyunsatured	13	5	5	6
Cholesterol (mg)	318	162	146	159

[a]n = 179; 4-day food record.

B. Sources of Fat

The majority of the dietary fat came from four food groups: fats and oils, red meats, dairy foods, and grain products. These groups provided 80% of the women's daily fat intake. No one or even two food groups were sufficiently predominant that they could absorb all the necessary fat reduction. All four food groups had to be cut to some extent. So the real choice was the relative extent of the cuts from each of the four.

Table 4 shows the average grams of fat eaten from each food group after 6, 12, and 24 months of intervention. Similar reductions were made in fats from fats and oils, red meats, and dairy products, with slightly smaller changes occurring in grain products and "other" groups.

In general, the women did not replace fat calories with calories from other sources. If they added back any calories over the years, they were fat calories. The extensive use of non- or low-fat dairy products made a sizeable increase in carbohydrate calories from this source and there was some small increase in the use of fruit. There were no significant increases in the use of sugars or alcohol. In fact, the average calories from alcohol and sweets decreased from 239 to 158 between baseline and 24 months, a drop of approximately 80 kcals.

The limited number of carbohydrate calories added to the diet on average spoke to the difficulty in, or resistance to, replacing some fat with nonfat calories. This is an important issue if healthy diets are to be absolutely, as well as relatively, higher in fruits, vegetables, and grains and the macro- and micronutrients they provide.

Table 4 Mean Daily Grams of Fat from
Food Groups

	Months in intervention			
Food groups	0	6	12	24
Fats and oils	19	6	7	8
Red meat	16	5	6	6
Dairy foods	13	5	5	6
Grain products	13	7	7	7
Other	15	8	6	7
TOTAL	76	31	31	34

IV. PATTERNS OF CHANGE

Although the women were successful overall, they fell naturally into three more or less successful subgroups. These three groups had separated themselves out by 6 months and maintained their positions based on fat intake relative to each thereafter. The most successful women (Group 1) reached their goal of lowered fat intake by 6 months and maintained those levels over the course of the trial. At 24 months, they were consuming an average of 19% of their calories from fat. Most of the group of slightly less successful women (Group 2) had reached their goal at 6 months but met that goal at only one of the other two follow-up visits. This group consumed approximately 20% of their calories from fat for the first and most of the second year, but by 24 months they reported eating an average of 25% of their calories as fat. The third group of women never achieved the level of 20% of calories from fat (Group 3), but they did manage to reduce their fat consumption to approximately 30% of daily calories and maintained this level up to 24 months. There was a close link between changes in fat consumption and changes in body weight in these three subgroups of intervention women (Table 5).

The most successful women reduced their average calorie consumption by 548 kcal and lost an average of 3.6 kg. Furthermore, they continued to eat fewer calories and their weight loss persisted. Over the course of 12 months, their mean weight loss was 4.1 kg. By 24 months, their weights had risen slightly but were still an average of 3.0 kg lower than baseline levels.

The second group of women lost weight during the first 6 months (average 2.5 kg) but then slowly drifted back toward baseline levels. By 24 months their mean weights were only about 1 kg lower than baseline values.

Table 5   Average Body Weight (kg)
in Intervention Groups

Group	Months in group			
	0	6	12	24
All Intervention (n = 179)	68.8	65.7	65.9	67.4
Subgroup 1[a] (n = 91)	68.6	65.0	64.5	65.6
Subgroup 2[b] (n = 47)	69.1	66.6	67.2	68.4
Subgroup 3[c] (n = 41)	69.1	66.3	67.6	69.0

[a]Reached goal of reduced fat intake at three follow-up visits.
[b]Reached goal of reduced fat intake at two follow-up visits.
[c]Never reached goal.

The least successful intervention subjects also lost some weight during the first 6 months (average 2.8 kg) when their reported caloric intake was lowest. However, over the next 18 months both their average caloric intake and body weight gradually increased back to starting levels.

Whether they ranked at the top or bottom in terms of overall success in lowering fat and maintaining low fat consumption, virtually all the women made the same proportionate cuts in fats from the four food groups. The only real differences between women who were successful and those who were unsuccessful were in the extent of cuts made in the fat coming from each of the food groups. None of the groups made incremental reductions over time. The extent of the initial cut was the best single predictor of long-term success.

The most successful group of women (Group 1) made the most substantial fat reductions in all four food groups and maintained these original reductions extremely well. They lowered their fat from fats and oils, red meats, and dairy foods more than 70%. Fats from grain products, which include desserts and snacks, were reduced 60% (Table 6).

Although there was some opportunity to make individual decisions about the food groups and foods in which to make fat reductions, the overall impact of the intervention was to reduce the amount of variability in fat consumption from foods in all four groups. There was still, however, some personal variation even among these successful women. The grams of fat eaten from fats and oils at 6 months ranged from zero to 17; from red meats, dairy

Table 6 Percent Reduction from Baseline in the Average Grams of Fat Eaten from Each Food Group According to Long-Term Success

	All Intervention	Subgroups		
		1	2	3
	(n)	(91)	(47)	(41)
		Percent		
Fats and Oils				
6 months	68	75	69	49
24 months	58	72	48	27
Red Meat				
6 months	69	76	66	42
24 months	63	70	61	34
Dairy Foods				
6 months	62	70	55	53
24 months	54	68	47	42
Grain Products				
6 months	46	61	44	22
24 months	46	59	45	24
Other				
6 months	47	52	40	49
24 months	50	61	45	40

Subgroup 1 = Reached goal of reduced fat intake at three followup visits.

2 = Reached goal of reduced fat intake at two followup visits.

3 = Never reached goal.

products, and grain products, it ranged from zero to 16. At 24 months those figures were, respectively, 0–19 and 0–16; 0–16 and 0–27. As many as one-fourth of the women ate no red meat while they were keeping their food records, and more than half of them ate at the most only one small serving of very lean meat. On the other hand, 25% were able to eat as much as one serving of lean red meat a day such as trimmed beef or pork tenderloin.

Fifty percent added no fats or oils or only one serving of a low-calorie fat or oil product to their food. Only 10% allowed themselves as much as an average tablespoon of fat a day. Fifty percent ate less than 4 g of fat a day from dairy products including cheese. In other words, 50% were using low-fat dairy products and eating neither cheese nor ice cream. Only 5% were eating enough fat from dairy products (average 11 g) to be allowing themselves any servings of either cheese or ice cream.

The least successful women (Group 3) took a longer time to make changes, and the reductions they made were more limited. Fats and oils, red meats, and dairy products were only cut in half, and grain products, which include desserts and sweets, were reduced by less than a quarter.

Although conceptually they could have made slow, incremental improvements as their instruction progressed, they made no stepwise advances. On the contrary, they began to slowly increase their average fat consumption again beginning at 6 months.

V. CHANGES IN SPECIFIC FOODS

These three subgroups of women provided as broad as possible a picture of eating pattern changes. Their food frequency questionnaires (FFQs) were used to identify specific foods that were easier or more difficult to change. Since different FFQs were used at different points in time, comparisons were limited to foods that were described in exactly the same manner on all forms. Because women tended to maintain their initial level of fat reduction throughout the intervention, comparisons of a group of 50 women reaching an average 17% and a group of 30 women reaching an average of 28% of their baseline calories from fat at 3 months were examined in more detail. Figures 1 through 4 portray the changes in servings of specific foods over the course of the intervention.

As far as fats and oils were concerned, the women used less regular salad dressing and less spread products. Looking at the servings, it appears that all the women initially reduced their use of salad dressings and then added them back to their diet. The most successful women maintained a reduced intake of fat even when they added back salad dressings primarily by substituting diet products for regular products. The least successful women used diet salad dressings, but they also continued to use regular dressings about half of the time (Fig. 1) In addition, the most successful women restricted their use of butter and margarine on bread and as a seasoning on vegetables. At 24 months, they reported only three servings per week, whereas the least successful group reported six servings a week.

In the dairy group of foods there were major changes in the consumption of whole milk, cheese, and ice cream. All the women reduced their consumption of whole milk. Almost all of the women in the most successful group switched to nonfat milk. In the least successful group, about half of the women were drinking 2% milk and half nonfat milk.

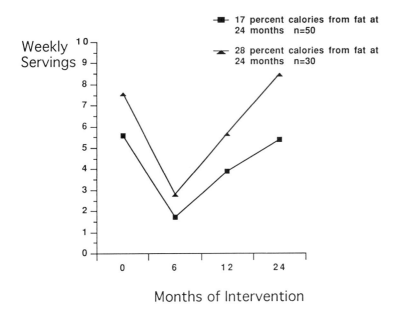

Figure 1 Number of servings per week of salad dressing associated with relative levels of long-term success.

At baseline, cheese was the major source of fat from the dairy products group. The women were eating four to five servings of regular cheese a week, which provided about 30 g of fat. The best performers chose to use regular cheese only once a week, whereas the poor performers cut back initially to two but eventually relapsed to three servings a week (Fig. 2). All of the women used low-fat cheese to replace some of the high-fat cheeses. They reported an average of two servings of low-fat cheese a week.

Ice cream was the second major source of fat from dairy products (Fig. 3). The women reduced their consumption of ice cream and increased their consumption of sherbet.

Most fat from red meats came from beef and pork. The baseline average was four servings a week. By 6 months, two to three servings per week were being eaten. At 2 years, the most successful intervention women reported one serving per week and the least successful reported one and a half servings (Fig. 4). Both groups changed their intake of beef and pork more slowly than their intake of other foods. Hamburger was only eaten about once a week at baseline. The best performers reduced their consumption of hamburger by 70%. The poor performers seemed to find this change difficult and continued to eat hamburger almost once a week.

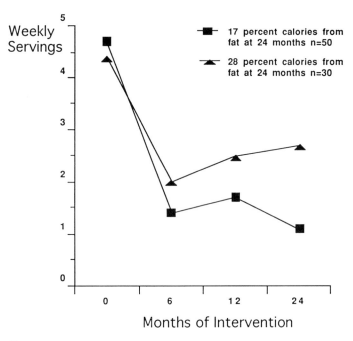

Figure 2 Number of servings per week of cheese associated with relative levels of long-term success.

In spite of the limited number of foods that could be compared across different instruments, the FFQ comparisons provide interesting insights into differences in consumption of specific foods over time. Very few of the most successful women showed any backsliding. The reductions they made in fat consumption achieved during the first 6 months were well maintained, and for some food groups were increased up to 24 months. For example, they consumed less fat from dressings and red meat at 24 months than they did at 6 months.

On the other hand, recidivism was observed among the group of women who were least successful. Even in this group, however, although participants slipped, they did not return to their original fat intake for any food item. The patterns of recidivism give some illustration of the particular difficulties the women had to deal with in maintaining a very low-fat diet.

Originally more fat calories were cut from fats and oils than any other food group. Those cuts were harder for the least successful women to maintain. They had more trouble with salad dressings and seemed to be unable to substitute diet products to the same extent as the more successful women.

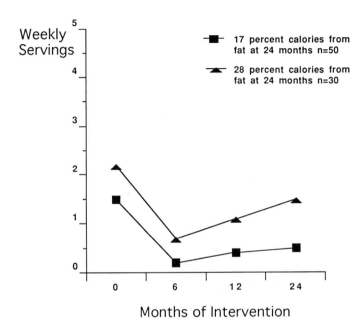

Figure 3 Number of servings per week of ice cream associated with relative levels of long-term success.

Changes in cheese and ice cream were the most difficult dairy food changes to maintain. All three subgroups increased their intake of ice cream between 6 and 24 months. The best group increased their use of ice cream from less than once a month to an average of twice a month and the least successful intervention women from less than once a week to approximately six times a month (see Fig. 3). Difficulties in maintaining infrequent use of cheese have already been mentioned.

It seemed to be much easier to maintain changes in red meats. Consumption of beef and pork continued to decline throughout the duration of the trial (see Fig. 4). There was some slippage in the use of hamburger, bacon, and hot dogs by the least successful group of women; however, these foods were still eaten infrequently (less than once a week on average).

VI. SUMMARY AND CONCLUSIONS

These patterns of dietary behavior have given some insight into both the way women make major dietary changes and into the changes that are easier and

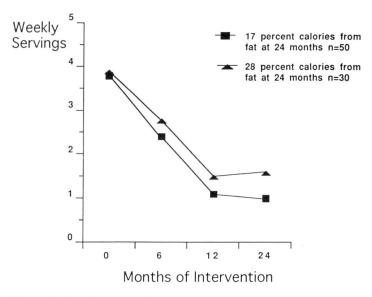

Figure 4 Number of servings per week of beef and pork associated with relative levels of long-term success.

harder to make and maintain. For example, under the circumstances of this intervention, it seemed to be easier to make a one-time reduction in fat consumption and maintain it than to make several incremental changes. As far as specific foods are concerned, some changes in fat consumption that are most successful in the short term are least successful in the long term.

A few other summary observations can be made:

Women find it easiest to change their use of easily identified fat. They often find it hard to maintain these changes. Those who are successful learn to use substitutes.

It may take longer to complete the reductions in fat eaten from foods that do not obviously provide a lot of fat, but these changes may be more persistent once they are made. They often involve modification and substitution from the beginning (e.g., cheese, red meats, and grain products). The changes may be slower because they depend upon changes in cuisine.

Cutting down fat eaten from desserts and snacks is one of the most difficult changes to make. The use of sweets as a reward and family tastes may account for some of this difficulty.

Although not studied specifically, the maintenance of dietary change appeared to be enhanced by the availability of acceptable lower-fat substitutes.

REFERENCES

1. K. Glanz, Nutrition education for risk factor reduction and patient education: A review, *Prev. Med.*, *9*: 787 (1985).
2. National Cancer Institute, Division of Cancer Prevention and Control, *Cancer Control Objectives for the Nation: 1985–2000* (P. Greenwald and E. J. Sondik, eds.), NIH Publication No. 86–2880, Number 2 (1986).
3. National Research Council Committee on Diet and Health, *Diet and Health: Implications for Reducing Chronic Disease Risk*, National Academy Press, Washington, DC (1989).
4. L. Rastam, R. V. Luepker, and P. L. Pirie, Effect of screening and referral on follow-up and treatment of high blood cholesterol levels, *Am. J. Prev. Med.*, *4*: 244 (1988).
5. W. Insull, M. M. Henderson, R. L. Prentice, D. J. Thompson, C. Clifford, S. Goldman, S. Gorbach, M. Moskowitz, R. Thompson, and M. Woods, Results of a randomized feasibility study of a low-fat diet, *Arch. Intern. Med.*, *150*: 421 (1990).
6. M. M. Henderson, L. H. Kushi, D. J. Thompson, S. L. Gorbach, C. K. Clifford, W. Insull, M. Moskowitz, and R. S. Thompson, Feasibility of a randomized trial of low-fat diet for the prevention of breast cancer: Dietary compliance in the Women's Health Trial Vanguard Study, *Prev. Med.*, *19*: 115 (1990).
7. Multiple Risk Factor Intervention Trial Group, Statistical design considerations in the NHLI Multiple Risk Factor Intervention Trial (MRFIT), *J. Chronic Dis.*, *30*: 261 (1977).
8. University of Massachusetts Nutrient Data Base, Release 5, University of Massachusetts, Amherst, MA (1985).
9. S. L. Gorbach, A. Morrill-LaBrode, M. N. Woods, J. T. Dwyer, W. D. Selles, M. Henderson, W. Insull, S. Goldman, D. Thompson, C. Clifford, and L. Sheppard, Changes in food patterns during a low-fat dietary intervention in women, *J. Am. Diet. Assoc.*, *90*: 802 (1990).
10. Women's Health Trial final report for National Cancer Institute. National Institutes of Health, June 1988 (unpublished).
11. E. White, A. L. Shattuck, A. R. Kristal, N. Urban, R. L. Prentice, M. M. Henderson, W. Insull, M. Moskowitz, S. Goldman, and N. Woods, Maintenance of a low-fat diet: Follow-up of the Women's Health Trial, *Cancer Epidemiology, Biomarkers and Prevention, 1*: 315 (1992).
12. L. Sheppard, A. R. Kristal, and L. H. Kushi, Weight loss in women participating in a randomized trial of low fat diets, *Am. J. Clin. Nutr., 54*: 821 (1991).

25
Low-Calorie Foods and the Prevalence of Obesity

Adam Drewnowski *University of Michigan, Ann Arbor, Michigan*

I. INTRODUCTION

The typical American diet derives almost 60% of its calories from two ingredients, simple sugars and fat [1–3]. Fat accounts for 37% of total daily calories, while sugars, both natural and added, contribute a further 20%. Diets that are high in fat but low in complex carbohydrates and fiber have been associated with a high prevalence of obesity and with increased risk of coronary heart disease and some forms of cancer [4,5]. The standard dietary advice is to moderate sugar consumption and to restrict fat intake to 30% of daily calories or less.

Excessive fat consumption is thought to be the number one problem in the American diet [4]. However, the present health focus on fats is relatively new. Two decades ago, starchy foods were regarded as extremely fattening, while sugar, in particular, was viewed as the main source of empty calories. Accordingly, popular weight-loss diets of the time typically allowed the consumption of both protein and fat, but completely eliminated all sweets and starchy foods [6]. Dietary recommendations were largely concerned with reducing sugar intake, and desirable low-calorie foods were mostly those that were sugar-free.

Fat rather than sugar is currently reputed to play a major role in the development of human obesity [4]. New dietary guidelines, neutral with respect to sugar, have actively promoted the consumption of complex carbohydrates at the expense of foods rich in fat [4,5]. In 1988, the *Surgeon General's Report on Nutrition and Health* [4] recommended replacing foods high in fat, saturated fat, and cholesterol with vegetables, fruits, and whole grain foods. In 1989, the *Diet and Health* report of the National Academy of Sciences [5] recommended increasing intake of carbohydrates to 55% of total daily calories by doubling the intake of vegetables and fruits. Most recently, the United States Department of Agriculture (USDA) recommended consuming two to four servings of fruit and three to five servings of vegetables per day [7]. The nutritional rehabilitation of starchy foods has been accompanied by a shift in health emphasis from dietary sugars to fat.

However, reducing the fat content of the American diet has proved to be a difficult task. Many people enjoy the taste of sweet or fat-rich foods and are reluctant to give them up [8–10]. Fats endow foods with their characteristic texture and flavor, and they play a major role in determining the palatability of the diet [9]. In contrast, diets composed of natural low-calorie foods, largely vegetables and grains, tend to be viewed as bland, monotonous, and unsatisfying. According to conventional wisdom, healthy foods always taste bad, while good-tasting foods are bound to be unhealthy.

Poor compliance with dietary guidelines is partly due to ingrained taste preferences and dietary habits [8]. Foods rich in sugar and fat are an integral component of the American diet. Fats and oils, meat, and dairy products are an ever-growing segment of the U.S. food supply [3]. In contrast, the consumption of vegetables and fruits is no higher now than it was 50 years ago. Indeed, USDA survey data indicate that the consumption of vegetables and fruits by women 19–50 years old actually declined between 1977 and 1985 [11].

Advances in food technology have made possible the development of reduced-calorie equivalents of the popular sweet and fat-rich foods [12]. Most low-calorie foods developed by the food industry can be divided into those that are low in sugar and those that are low in fat. While sugar substitutes have been available for decades [13], industry emphasis on fat replacements is relatively new. The public's realization that fat rather than sugar provides the bulk of excess calories in the American diet has led to an industrywide search for acceptable fat replacement products. Since fat is calorically more dense than sugar (9 kcal/g vs. 4 kcal/g), replacing fat in foods offers greater caloric savings to the consumer.

The question arises whether the wide availability of sugar and fat replacements has effectively diminished the prevalence of obesity in the United
States and had a measurable impact on public health. In order to assess the
impact of low-calorie foods on weight control, we need to examine nutrient
content of the typical American diet and the role of dietary factors, particularly sugar and fat, in the development and maintenance of human obesity.
Although it is generally assumed that there is a direct connection between
overeating and overweight, the evidence from clinical and survey studies has
not always been clear. While there is little evidence to link sugar consumption with obesity [14], there seems to be a developing consensus that the habitual diet of obese men and women tends to be rich in fat [15,16].

II. THE AMERICAN DIET

A. Historical Trends

According to food disappearance data collected by the USDA, complex carbohydrates in the U.S. food supply have been gradually replaced by simple
sugars and fat [17]. Carbohydrate use declined more than 20% between 1910
and 1982. However, a 50% drop in complex carbohydrates (primarily potatoes and grain products) has been partly offset by a greatly increased use of
sugars. The estimated consumption of sugars was only 65 lb per capita in
1910, but reached a high of 142.5 lb in 1984. More than half of this amount
was fructose, largely consumed in the form of carbonated soft drinks. Recent USDA statistics indicate that natural and added sugars contribute approximately 20% of total calories to the U.S. diet [18].

The use of fats has also risen. Fats contribute 37% of calories to the U.S.
diet, with fat consumption estimated at 64 g/day for women and 98 g/day
for men [1]. Three food groups—fats and oils; meat, poultry, and fish; and
dairy products—still provide approximately 90% of all fats in the food supply [19]. However, there has been a major shift from animal to vegetable
fats. While the use of butter declined from 18 lb per capita to 4 lb between
1910 and 1982, the use of margarine rose from 1 to 11 lb, and the use of oils,
chiefly salad and cooking oils, rose from 2 to 23 lb. Increased use of cooking
oils largely accounts for the observed net increase in fat consumption. In
the meat group, a major reduction in beef fat has been more than offset by
a threefold increase in fat from poultry. Similarly, decreased use of whole
milk, butter, and cream has been offset by increased use of low-fat milks,
cheeses, and frozen desserts [20].

B. Nutrient Sources of Sugar and Fat

What foods contribute the most calories, sugar, and fat to the current American diet? Some answers can be found in a remarkable analysis of data from

the National Health and Nutrition Examination Survey, 1976–80 (NHANES II), compiled and published by Block et al. [21]. That study quantified the contributions of 147 food categories representing foods most frequently eaten by 11,658 adult respondents, according to the number of people consuming them. The calculation of each food's contribution to the percent intake of calories, carbohydrate, or fat was based on its nutrient content as well as on the estimated frequency of consumption.

The top 10 nutrient sources of calories in the U.S. diet are listed in Table 1. White bread, rolls, and crackers provided 9.6% of total calories. This food group was followed by the category of doughnuts, cookies, and cake (5.7%); and by alcoholic beverages (5.6%), whole milk (4.7%), and beef products, including hamburgers (4.4%) and steaks (4.1%). Regular soft drinks accounted for 3.6% of dietary calories, provided mostly in the form of simple sugars. These 10 food categories accounted for a cumulative 46% of calories in the population diet.

The top 10 nutrient sources of carbohydrate are shown in Table 2. White bread, rolls, and crackers accounted for 15.0% of all carbohydrate calories. This category was followed by regular soft drinks (8.6%); doughnuts, cookies, and cake (7.5%); and table sugar (3.5%). Although the NHANES II database does not distinguish between complex carbohydrates and simple sugars, it can be seen that regular soft drinks, doughnuts, and table sugar contributed almost 20% of the carbohydrate calories to the U.S. diet. Since sugar is a major component of sweets and soft drinks, the use of artificial sweeteners in these product categories is likely to have a significant impact on caloric intake.

Table 1 Chief Nutrient Sources of Calories in the U.S. Diet

Food type	Caloric intake (%)	Cumulative caloric intake (%)
1. White bread, rolls	9.6	9.6
2. Doughnuts, cookies, cake	5.7	15.3
3. Alcoholic beverages	5.6	20.9
4. Whole milk	4.7	25.6
5. Hamburger, cheeseburger	4.4	30.0
6. Beef steaks, roasts	4.1	34.1
7. Regular soft drinks	3.6	37.7
8. Hot dogs, ham, lunch meats	3.2	40.9
9. Eggs	2.5	43.5
10. French fries	2.5	46.0

Source: NHANES II survey, 1976–1980 (Ref. 21).

Table 2   Chief Nutrient Sources of Carbohydrate in the U.S. Diet

Food type	Carbohydrate intake (%)	Cumulative carbohydrate intake (%)
1. White bread, rolls	15.0	15.0
2. Regular soft drinks	8.6	23.6
3. Doughnuts, cookies, cake	7.5	31.1
4. Sugar	3.5	34.6
5. Whole milk	3.5	38.1
6. French fries, fried potatoes	3.3	41.4
7. Alcoholic beverages	3.3	44.7
8. Whole wheat, dark breads	3.1	47.8
9. Orange juice	3.0	50.8
10. Potatoes, excl. fried	2.3	53.1

Source: NHANES II survey, 1976–1980 (Ref. 21).

The top 10 nutrient sources of fat are summarized in Table 3. Hamburgers and cheeseburgers were the chief sources of dietary fat (7.0%); followed by hot dogs, ham, and lunch meats (6.4%); whole milk (6.0%); and doughnuts, cookies, and cake (6.0%). Taken together, all beef items contributed 15% of total fat to the diet. Cheeses, margarine, mayonnaise, and other spreads contributed a total of 13.3% of fat calories.

Lowering the sugar and fat contents of selected foods can have a major impact on the population diet. Of course, the impact will be greatest for those food categories that are important sources of calories, sugar, or fat. Thus, a more dramatic lowering of dietary calories can be achieved by re-

Table 3   Chief Nutrient Sources of Fat in the U.S. Diet

Food type	Fat intake (%)	Cumulative fat intake (%)
1. Hamburger, cheeseburger	7.0	7.0
2. Hot dog, ham, lunch meat	6.4	13.4
3. Whole milk	6.0	19.4
4. Doughnuts, cookies, cake	6.0	25.4
5. Beef steaks, roasts	5.4	30.8
6. White bread, rolls	4.9	35.7
7. Eggs	4.6	40.3
8. Cheeses, excl. cottage cheese	4.5	44.8
9. Margarine	4.5	49.3
10. Mayonnaise, salad dressing	4.3	53.6

Source: NHANES II survey, 1976–1980 (Ref. 21).

placing sugar in soft drinks (3.6% of diet calories) than by replacing sugar in jellies or jams (0.5% of diet calories). Similarly, limiting or replacing fat in hamburgers, processed meats, deep-fried doughnuts, or table spreads is likely to have greater impact on the population fat intake than replacing cocoa butter in chocolate. Chocolate candy contributes only 1.0% of fat calories to the typical American diet.

C. Changing Dietary Habits, 1976–1985

The current dietary recommendations are to replace meats and full-fat dairy products with grain products, vegetables, and fruits. How effective are such guidelines in influencing food choices? We are often told that American consumers are increasingly receptive to low-calorie food products as they become more concerned with issues of nutrition and health. Systematic USDA surveys of changing food habits are helpful in assessing the effectiveness of dietary guidelines as a function of sex, ethnic status, education, and income [22].

Dietary recommendations of a decade ago identified sugars and starches as the chief sources of unwanted calories. As might be expected, consumers modified their behaviors accordingly. Data from a 1976 USDA survey [23] showed that 64% of 1353 respondents modified dietary intakes over the preceding 3 years for reasons of health and nutrition. The chief reason given for such changes was weight control. Among dietary changes listed, 30% of respondents reported reducing the intake of sugar and sweet foods, 14% reported using low-sugar cereals, while 14% used low-calorie soft drinks. Restricting fat consumption was given secondary priority. Reducing meat consumption was listed by only 15% of respondents, while 10% reduced the use of whole milk, butter, and other fats and oils [23].

The current advice is to reduce the consumption of fats, especially saturated fats contained in meat and full-fat dairy products. Dietary changes made by women between 1977 and 1985 have been summarized in a USDA report [11]. That study compared intake data from the 1977 Nationwide Food Consumption Survey (NFCS) with the 1985 Continuing Survey of Food Intakes of Individuals (CSFII).

As part of CSFII, 1503 women aged 19–50 years reported what they ate at home and away from home for 6 days during 1985. The first day's intake data were compared with a day's data for 2228 women of comparable age interviewed in the 1977 NCFS. Dietary intake assessment was based on the same epidemiological technique of 24-hour recall [11].

In 1985, the women ate less meat and fewer full-fat dairy products than in 1977. The consumption of meat (beef, pork, lamb, veal, sausages, and luncheon meats) dropped by a third, as did the consumption of whole milk and eggs. However, the consumption of meat-containing mixtures, mostly sandwiches and stews, increased by 35%, while the consumption of skim and low-fat milk increased by 60%. The consumption of cheese and frozen desserts also increased substantially [11].

The women also appeared to eat more grains, including bread and cereals. However, the greatest increase in the grains category was observed for such fat-containing foods as pizza and pasta with sauce. In contrast, there was an overall decrease in the consumption of fruits and vegetables, with the greatest drop (21%) reported by low-income women.

The consumption of carbonated soft drinks showed a sharp increase. Low-calorie soft drinks, in particular, increased 123% between 1977 and 1985. The greatest increase was seen among upper-income women: by 1985 47% of their soft drinks were low-calorie drinks, compared to only 17% among low-income women [11]. Industry sources indicate that noncaloric soft drinks now represent 23.1% of the soft drinks market, up from 10% in 1975 [18]. The typical American lunch of a decade ago may have been a hamburger and a glass of milk. It appears to have been replaced by a pizza and a diet Coke.

Education and income are often correlated with greater health awareness and better compliance with healthy diets. According to the USDA surveys, the greatest decline in meat consumption since 1977 was observed among high-income women. However, while high-income women consumed less meat, eggs, and whole milk, they ate more cheese, cream and milk desserts, baked goods, table fats, and salad dressings. Total fat intake (37% of total calories) was essentially independent of both education and income [22].

These findings suggest that many consumers have simply learned to trade sources of dietary fat and to replace one fat source with another [22]. While sugar intake has been reduced by the widespread use of intense sweeteners, excessive fat consumption remains a major problem in the U.S. diet.

III. OBESITY IN THE UNITED STATES

A. Prevalence Rates

A large proportion of American adults are obese [4,5]. The 1971–74 National Health and Nutrition Examination Survey (NHANES I) found that 23.7% of men and 26.0% of women aged 20–74 were obese. Obesity was defined as body weight exceeding the 85th percentile of body mass index (BMI = kg/m^2) of men and women in the third decade of life [4].

Subsequent health surveys pointed to an increase in the prevalence of obesity [24,25]. The 1976–80 Health and Nutrition Examination Survey (NHANES II) found that 24.4% of men and 26.7% of women were obese

[26]. According to recent reports, obesity is also becoming more prevalent among children, teenagers, minorities, and newly immigrant ethnic groups [27].

The chief features of the obese population have been described elsewhere (see Chapter 2). Briefly, more people become obese as they get older. While obesity among men peaked between 35 and 64 years of age, the prevalence of obesity among women increased with each age decade [4]. Obesity in women (but not men) has also been linked to ethnicity and socioeconomic status. The NHANES II survey showed that obesity was almost twice as common among black women (45.1% prevalence rate) as among white women (24.6% prevalence rate). Peak prevalence rate of 61.2% was observed among black women aged 45–54. In the same age range, 54.1% of poor women were obese, as compared to 32.5% in the total female population [4].

Weight management has become a multibillion dollar industry. The typical dieter likely to use low-calorie foods is an overweight woman in her late thirties or early forties. However, despite major advances in obesity research, the status of obesity treatment is much the same as it was decades ago. With some modifications, obese patients are still advised to eat less and to exercise more. Since most obese people are dieting at some point in their lives, the effectiveness of low-calorie foods in helping weight control is a topic of great clinical and public health interest.

B. Obesity and Energy Intake

Experts agree that genetic, biological, psychological, and sociocultural factors all contribute in different ways to the development and maintenance of the obese state [28–30]. Although the precise role of dietary factors is far from clear, excessive caloric intake is likely to be among the key contributing factors.

However, dietary intake assessments have often failed to link obesity with excess calories. In clinical studies, obese patients often ate no more than lean controls. Survey studies, including NHANES I data, actually pointed to an inverse relationship between overeating and overweight [31]. According to the NHANES I dataset, admittedly based on a single 24-hour food recall, obese women actually ate fewer calories per day than did lean women [31]. However, the standard 24-hour food recall is probably unsuitable for use with an obese population, where binge days may alternate with periods of dieting and caloric restriction. Other investigators have suggested that food intake records of obese individuals tend to be characterized by underreporting and bias [32].

Studies using doubly labeled water technique to measure energy expenditure have recently shown that obese people have elevated resting energy expenditure (REE) values and probably consume more calories than do lean controls [33]. Both clinical and epidemiological studies have also linked obesity with overconsumption of dietary fat [15,16]. In some studies, percent body fat was linked to percentage of fat calories in the habitual diet [15] and with sensory preferences for elevated levels of fat in foods [34]. In other studies, obesity was linked to elevated proportion of fat in the diet and lower carbohydrate-to-fat ratios [15,16].

A series of studies with humans and rats has now shown that a diet that is rich in fat may promote obesity and the deposition of body fat [35,37]. While excess carbohydrate calories tend to be dissipated as heat, excess fat calories are more likely to be stored in adipose tissue [35]. Fat-rich diets characterized by a low carbohydrate-to-fat ratio may thus be more fattening than equicaloric diets that are low in fat [36,37]. Some investigators have also noted that repeated cycles of weight loss and weight regain may lead to increased metabolic efficiency and enhanced fat storage [38,39].

In contrast, no study has successfully linked obesity with sugar intake. On the contrary, a nationwide survey of almost 1000 adolescents (5–18 years old) found no significant link between body fatness and self-reported intake of sweet snacks [40]. Neither the frequency of snack consumption nor the amount of sugar consumed were linked to the status of body weight [41]. Data from the Ten State Nutrition Survey found no relationship between triceps skinfold of teenagers and reported intakes of sugar-containing foods, including jams, honey, candies, and soft drinks [14].

C. Human Obesities: Genetic or Diet-induced?

Studies of human obesities increasingly suggest that not all obese people are alike. Some obesities clearly represent a familial trait. Obesity in the child is to some extent predicted by whether first-degree relatives (parents and siblings) are also obese [30]. More compelling data for a genetic component in obesity have been provided by studies of monozygotic and dizygotic twins [28] and by adoption studies correlating body build of children with those of natural and adoptive parents [30].

The current view is that obesity may result from an interaction between genetic predisposition and exposure to environmental stimuli, including diet. Human obesities may therefore range from those that are familial or genetic to those more likely to be diet-induced [42]. In some cases of familial obesity, reduced metabolic rate rather than overeating may be the key factor. Reduced rates of energy expenditure observed among obese adults and among infants of obese mothers may be, in some cases, the chief cause of body weight gain [43].

The contribution of dietary factors may also depend on genetic predisposition to the obese state. For example, depending on genetic predisposition, some obese people may be more susceptible than others to the effects of dietary challenge. One type of challenge may involve exposure to foods rich in fat, sugar, or both. Consequently, the role of diet in the expression of obesity may vary from one obese individual to another. By the same token, the effectiveness of low-calorie foods in weight control may vary among different groups of susceptible obese individuals. Caloric restriction through the use of foods reduced in sugar and fat content may prove beneficial to some obese persons but not to others.

Repeated dieting and weight loss may also lead to significant metabolic changes, notably increased metabolic efficiency and enhanced energy storage [39]. These changes may make subsequent loss more difficult, while facilitating weight regain [44]. Weight fluctuations in humans have also been linked to elevated sensory preferences for calorie-dense mixtures of sugar and fat [45]. Preferences and cravings for calorie-dense foods may be one behavioral mechanism by which obese people gain and regain body weight.

D. Weight-Loss Strategies

Women diet more often than men [46]. Women are more concerned with body image and body weight than are men [47]. Survey studies have shown that one in three adult women is dieting to lose weight, while a majority have attempted to diet at least once during the past year. In weight reduction programs, women typically outnumber men 4 to 1 [48].

While clinical reports have suggested that 95% of patients will fail at long-term weight loss, limited data from the general population are less gloomy. It is actually possible to lose weight and maintain weight loss over a substantial period of time. Jeffery et al. [46] found that one third of overweight people had successfully reduced over a 5-year span. However, an almost equal number of people became overweight during that time. One reason why clinic studies report uniformly low success rates may be that many clinic patients are preselected for diet failure [49]. Clinic populations usually overrepresent massively obese middle-aged women who have previously tried and failed to lose weight. There are at present no data as to whether clinic populations oversample the predominantly genetic form of human obesity.

The concern with weight and body image among young women usually begins after puberty. Fear of fatness has been named as one reason for increasing attention to weight control and the subsequent increase in the prevalence of eating disorders, such as anorexia nervosa and bulimia. However, while in the past, psychiatrists blamed sugar avoidance and "carbohydrate phobia" for the refusal to accept sufficient calories, current studies indicate that anorectic women reject not starches but fats [50]. Fat avoidance and not carbohydrate phobia is the characteristic dietary behavior in anorexia nervosa [50,51].

Increasing concern with dietary fats has also been reflected in the popular strategies for weight reduction. Two decades ago, the conventional belief was that starches and sugars were highly fattening. Most weight-loss diets of the period were high-protein, high-fat formulations, and patients were advised to eliminate carbohydrates, especially sugars, from their diet [52]. This advice was also followed by the general public. In 1980, approximately one half of college men and three quarters of college women reported using saccharin at least once a week [53]. However, following the popularization of high-carbohydrate diets by athletes, most weight-loss diets became low in fat. The current strategy for weight loss is to consume more carbohydrates, moderate protein intake, and restrict the amount of calories from fat. The typical weight-reducing diet now contains 60% of calories from carbohydrate, 20% from protein, and 20% from fat. Given the shift of emphasis from sugar to fat, it is not surprising that the industry search for sugar substitutes has given way to the search for fat replacements.

IV. SENSORY ROLE OF SUGAR AND FAT

Consumers like the taste of sweet and high-fat foods and are reluctant to give them up [54,55]. The study of taste and sensory preferences for dietary fats has thus acquired new importance in obesity research. Preliminary data indicate that taste responsiveness profiles to sugar/fat mixtures may help distinguish between different subgroups of obese individuals. Such subgroups may be characterized by familial risk of obesity, early age of onset, or by past attempts at weight reduction. There is also evidence from studies in humans and rats [45,56] that taste and food preferences may be modified by a history of weight cycling or "yo-yo" dieting. Although human data are scarce, there is new evidence that obese weight cyclers show elevated sensory response to sweet, fat-rich foods [45].

A. Sweet Tooth Versus Fat Tooth

While past studies on obesity and taste preferences were largely restricted to sugar solutions in water, more recent studies have focused on the role of fat in determining food acceptance. Instead of sweet solutions, these studies used more realistic stimuli such as milkshakes, cream cheese, cake frostings, or ice cream [44,51,54,55]. Such foods are reported as highly preferred by overweight women and are often mentioned in the context of food cravings and eating binges [57–59]. Anecdotal reports suggest that cravings for sweet, fat-rich desserts are especially common among women dieters.

Studies on sensory acceptability of sugar/fat mixtures [45,54,55] showed that preferences for sugar versus fat may help discriminate between clinical populations of women patients at extremes of body weight. A series of sensory evaluations using 20 different mixtures of milk, cream, and sugar conducted with groups of obese and anorectic patients showed that obese women preferred stimuli that were rich in fat, but were relatively low in sugar [55]. In contrast, anorectic women liked sweet taste, but showed reduced preferences for the oral sensation of dietary fat [51].

B. Food Preferences

What foods do overweight people say they like to eat? In a large study of U.S. Army personnel, Meiselman et al. [60] showed that overweight people selected red meat dishes rather than desserts. A study of several hundred obese patients confirmed that self-reported food preferences of obese males typically include steaks and roasts, hamburgers, french fries, pizza, and ice cream. In contrast, obese women tended to list bread, cake, cookies, ice cream, chocolate, pies, and other desserts. In other words, obese men tended to prefer protein/fat mixtures (i.e., meats), while obese women listed carbohydrate/fat mixtures, notably those that were sweet. Although food preferences of obese women have been characterized as "carbohydrate cravings" [7,58], preferences for fat, sugar, or both often seem closer to the mark.

Some past studies have suggested that food cravings were independent of the sensory qualities of food. For example, obese people were said to crave a specific macronutrient, carbohydrate, because of a deficiency in central serotonin metabolism [57,58]. Selective consumption of carbohydrate-rich foods in the absence of protein was said to redress serotonin imbalance and improve mood in susceptible obese individuals. Overconsumption of carbohydrate calories was in turn regarded as a major contributing factor in the development of obesity.

However, both clinical and survey studies have failed to link excess carbohydrate consumption with overweight. To the contrary, clinical observations suggest that the most common targets of food cravings are sweet desserts such as chocolate candy, cakes, and ice cream. In other studies, obese men and women were said to crave chocolate candy (Snickers bars and M&M's), chocolate cupcakes, chocolate chip cookies, cakes, frozen pastries, and other desserts [57-59]. These foods are composed largely of two ingredients, sugar and fat, and are usually sweet. Clearly, sensory response to sugar and fat is an important variable in determining food preferences.

V. REPLACING SUGAR AND FAT

A. New Technologies

The food industry's search for sugar substitutes has given way to a new emphasis on low-fat foods. However, technological problems in replacing fat in foods are perhaps even more complex. A successful fat-replacement product must mimic the texture, mouthfeel, and flavor of the original fat [12]. In the past, this has been accomplished using mixtures of starch, protein, and water. Fat substitutes used in such products as margarine, salad dressings, cake frostings, and frozen desserts were typically based on modified starches and gums. The products are partially or fully digestible and provide between 1 and 4 kcal/g. For example, polydextrose, a bland, partially absorbable starch polymer (Pfizer), supplies creamy mouthfeel qualities normally provided by sugar and fat [12]. It has been used as a partial fat substitute in frozen desserts, puddings, and cake frostings.

Mixtures of protein and water can also serve as fat replacements. The microparticulated protein product Simplesse (NutraSweet) consists of small round particles of milk casein and egg albumin that resemble emulsified dairy fat in size and shape. Since food particles less than $3\mu m$ in diameter are not individually perceived by the oral cavity, the substance feels creamy and smooth. Simplesse can replace fat in products that are not cooked (e.g., ice cream, creamy salad dressings, or margarine). Because their globular structure traps water, products like Simplesse contain only 1–2 kcal/g [12].

Additional fat-replacement products based on modified fats are under development. These products contain fatty acids and have the mouthfeel and texture of fats. Olestra (Procter & Gamble) is the name for a set of esters of sucrose that combine a sucrose molecule with six to eight fatty acids derived from edible soils: soybean, corn, and cottonseed. The resulting molecule is too bulky to be digested by lipases, is not absorbed or metabolized, and contributes no calories to the diet. The proposed use for olestra is in such foods as deep-fried snacks (potato chips) and fried foods, including fried chicken and doughnuts. Another new fat-replacement product, caprenin, is a triglyceride composed of caprylic, capric, and behenic fatty acids. Since behenic acid is only partly absorbed by the body, the product contains 5 kcal/g. Its proposed use is as a replacement for cocoa butter in confectionery use. The development of further heat-stable fat replacements for use in baking and frying is currently under way.

B. New Products

The development of new fat-reduced products has become a public health issue. A recent report from the Secretary of Health, Education and Welfare

[61] stated the following objective: "Increase to at least 5,000 brand items the availability of processed food products that are reduced in fat and saturated fat". A specific aim of the proposal is that such food items should be made available to schools and low-income families (objective 2.15).

Consumers appear to want low-calorie, low-fat foods. A Gallup survey of 1035 people 18 and over conducted for the Calorie Control Council pointed to increasing consumption and acceptance of "light" food products [62]. Between 1987 and 1989, the number of new light foods increased by 47%. In 1989 alone, 130 new dairy foods described as low in fat, low in cholesterol, and light/lite were introduced. In addition to diet beverages, light items included cheese, yogurt, ice cream and frozen desserts, cakes and other baked goods, snack foods, and dinner entrees. Most recently, the category of low-fat food products was extended to hamburgers.

The potential size of the market for low-fat foods is a topic of major interest. According to USDA figures [63], the annual production of butter, ice cream, yogurt, and natural and processed cheeses totaled 12.1 billion pounds in 1987. Since dairy products vary in fat content from 3% for yogurt to 81% for butter, the potential use of fat replacements in dairy products has been estimated at 2.8 billion pounds per year [63]. Other targets for fat replacement include baking and frying fats, salad and cooking oils, and margarine. This category accounted for almost 14 billion pounds in 1987 [63].

Fat-replacement products may be used differently by men and women. As noted above, overweight men and women tend to prefer different foods. While obese men list hamburgers, steaks, and french fries among their favorite foods, obese women are more partial to sweets and desserts. Consequently, sugar substitutes (Aspartame) and dairy fat replacements (Simplesse) would be expected to have greatest impact on the diets of overweight women. In contrast, replacing fat in meat products and fried foods might be more useful in dietary management of obesity in men.

C. Regulation of Intake

The question arises whether replacing dietary sugar and fat with low-calorie substitutes leads to caloric compensation, or even rebound eating. It has been suggested [64] that the consumption of noncaloric sweeteners actually promotes hunger and enhanced food intake. Other studies have claimed that low-calorie soft drinks are ineffective in the management of body weight. There is no evidence for either contention [65]. Most investigators have found the use of aspartame-sweetened soft drinks associated with decreased or unchanged hunger ratings [66]. While hunger ratings are a poor predictor of food intake, other studies showed that the use of low-calorie sweeteners was associated with reduced or unchanged food consumption. In an early clinical study [67], sucrose was covertly replaced with aspartame to achieve a 26% calorie reduction. The subjects reduced their intakes by 15% and remained at that level for 20 days [67]. Analysis of 1985 CSFII data [68] showed that the use of intense sweeteners reduced caloric intakes from 1670 kcal/day to 1505 kcal/day. In another study, the use of aspartame-sweetened soda for 3 weeks significantly reduced caloric intakes of both females and males relative to when no soda was given [69].

Intense sweeteners have never been found to cause weight gain in humans. The use of aspartame-sweetened sodas for 3 weeks helped decrease body weights of males but not of females [69]. In another study [70], aspartame-sweetened foods used as adjuncts to a balanced weight-loss diet improved compliance with the clinical regimen.

One epidemiological study [71] is often cited as evidence that the use of low-calorie sweeteners is ineffective in the management of body weight. However, the analysis of sweetener use in relation to weight loss was peripheral to the main purpose of the study, which was designed to examine cancer incidence in a large female population. The study, which specifically excluded women who had made major changes in their diet, found that casual use of intense sweeteners in the absence of other lifestyle changes did not lead to a clinically significant weight loss. Needless to say, low-calorie diet products can only serve as adjuncts in weight reduction, and major dietary changes are a prerequisite for weight loss [65,72].

The data on the short-term effectiveness of fat replacements are even more limited [73]. Current data on replacing dietary fat with olestra suggest that caloric compensation eventually does occur—not at the next meal, but following a longer time interval. However, there is no evidence that this compensation is nutrient-specific [73]. In other words, the use of fat replacements is not followed by a specific craving for fats. As a result, one of the consequences of fat replacement is a net decrease in the proportion of fat calories in the habitual diet and increased carbohydrate-to-fat ratio.

VI. IMPACT ON PUBLIC HEALTH

Has the use of low-calorie foods diminished the prevalence of obesity and had a measurable impact on public health? We have seen that fat and sugar together account for almost 60% of daily calories in the typical American diet [2,3]. While obesity has never been convincingly linked with excess sugar consumption, there are indications that the habitual diet of obese men and women may be rich in fat [15,16]. The use of low-calorie foods containing sugar substitutes and fat replacements offers major caloric savings to the consumer [75].

Reducing the amount of sugar and fat in the diet is an effective way to reduce calories and so promote weight loss. Studies with low-fat diets have shown that maintaining dietary fats below 30% of daily calories led to a spontaneous reduction in body weight. In one study [74], subjects were offered only low-fat food options and did not supplement their diets with fat from other sources. Other studies have suggested that the habitual use of low-calorie soft drinks was associated with lower calorie intakes [68]. Eliminating sugars and fats from the diet has long been the key weight-loss strategy, as outlined in several popular diet books.

However, the success of any calorie-restricted diet largely depends on consumer compliance. High-carbohydrate diets devoid of sugars and fat are often regarded as bland and unsatisfying, and adherence rates are low. Poor dietary compliance is a recognized clinical problem in the dietary management of dyslipidemias, using diets that are very low in fat. Obese dieters oftem report cravings for sweet, fat-rich desserts, and eating binges are blamed for diet failure and subsequent weight regain.

Clinical studies have reported that the use of aspartame-sweetened soft drinks increased compliance with a dietary regime and so promoted weight loss [70]. The impact of noncaloric soft drinks on the diet of the general population is more difficult to assess, since there is no information as to how many people might become overweight if noncaloric sweeteners were not available. Noncaloric soft drinks are widely used by dieters, not all of them overweight, and are viewed as a valuable tool in the management of body weight. USDA statistics further suggest that consumers have not replaced the sugar in soft drinks with sugar from other sources. In other words, the provision of noncaloric sweet taste may prevent increased consumption of other sweets.

The available data on fat consumption are more problematic. USDA surveys indicate that women who reduced the consumption of milk and meat increased the consumption of fat from other sources, notably mixed foods, cheeses, and desserts [22]. The overall level of fat consumption remained much the same. However, obvious sources of fat (butter, cream) were sometimes replaced with foods where the presence of fat was more difficult to detect. While the sweet taste of sugar makes it readily identifiable as a source of calories, oral assessment of fat content is far more complex, especially in solids foods. As a result, low- and high-calorie food choices often coexist. The same person who orders fat-laden cheesecake may sweeten her coffee with aspartame.

Sugar substitutes and fat replacements provide the sensory qualities of sweet and fat-rich foods without providing excess calories. Their major role in weight management may be to promote dietary compliance. Far from being the major cause of weight loss, the use of low-calorie food products should be regarded as an adjunct to a comprehensive weight-reduction regime.

The current guidelines for implementing dietary recommendations [76] have identified three types of strategy. The first involves altering the food supply, primarily by reducing the fat content of the diet. The second strategy is to increase the number of food choices for a healthy diet. Increasing the availability of low-calorie foods should reduce the amount of available fats and provide a wider range of options for selecting healthful diets. The third strategy involves improved nutritional education. The common assumption has been that greater nutritional awareness aids the acceptance of healthful eating patterns. For example, USDA survey data indicate that the consumption of low-calorie food products (both low-calorie softs drinks and low-fat items) is greatest among highly educated and high-income women. Other studies have also shown that group to be most concerned with dieting and body weight. High-income women also show the lowest prevalence of obesity. However, such cross-sectional correlative data do not allow us to postulate direct cause and effect, especially since many other factors (health status, income, access to health care) are also likely to be involved.

In the past, dieters had few palatable food options, and the most common weight-loss strategy was to eliminate all good-tasting foods from the habitual diet. Providing a broader range of palatable low-calorie food options to the consumer seems to be the most promising weight-loss strategy. What we need is more low-calorie foods available to all income levels and a coherent strategy for implementing existing dietary recommendations among the general public.

REFERENCES

1. M. D. Carroll, S. Abraham, and C. M. Dresser, Dietary intake source data: United States 1976-80, National Center for Health Statistics, *Vital and Health Statistics Series 11-No 231,* DHHS Pub. No. (PHS) 83-1681, U S Government Printing Office, Washington DC (1983).
2. W. H. Glinsman, H. Irausquin, and Y. K. Park, Evaluation of health aspects of sugars contained in carbohydrate sweeteners, *J. Nutr., 116*(11S): 1-216 (1986).
3. U.S. Department of Health and Human Services and U.S. Department of Agriculture, *Nutrition Monitoring in the United States,* DHHS Pub. No (PHS) 89-1225, Public Health Service, Washington DC (1989).
4. U.S. Department of Health and Human Services, *The Surgeon General's Report on Nutrition and Health,* DHHS (PHS) Pub. No. 88-50210, U.S. Government Printing Office, Washington, DC (1988).

5. National Academy of Sciences, Committee on Diet and Health, Food and Nutrition Board, *Diet and Health*, National Academy Press, Washington DC (1989).
6. A. Drewnowski, Diet and health: A commentary on current dietary recommendations and their use in public health, *Diet and Health* (P. Leathwood and P. Horisberger, eds.) (in press).
7. Human Nutrition Information Service, USDA, *Dietary Guidelines and Your Diet*, Pub. HG 232-1-7, U.S. Government Printing Office, Washington, DC (1990).
8. A. Drewnowski, Body weight and sensory preferences for sugar and fat, *J. Can. Inst. Food Sci. Technol., 20*: 327 (1987).
9. A. Drewnowski, Fats and food texture: Sensory and hedonic evaluations, *Food Texture* (H. R. Moskowitz, ed.), Marcel Dekker, New York, pp. 217–250 (1987).
10. A. Drewnowski, Sensory preferences for fat and sugar in adolescence and adult life, *Nutrition and the Chemical Senses in Aging* (C. Murphy, W. S. Cain, and D. M. Hegsted, eds.), *Ann. N.Y. Acad. Sci., 561*: 243 (1989).
11. B. B. Peterkin and R. L. Rizek, Diets of American women: Looking back nearly a decade, *Natl. Food Rev.* (Summer): 12 (1986).
12. A. Drewnowski, The new fat replacements: A strategy for reducing fat consumption, *Postgrad. Med., 87*: 111 (1990).
13. M. B. McCann, M. F. Trulson, and S. C. Stulb, Non-caloric sweeteners and weight reduction, *J. Am. Diet. Assoc., 32*: 327 (1956).
14. S. M. Garn, M. A. Solomon, and P. E. Cole, Sugar-food intake of obese and lean adolescents, *Ecology Food Nutr., 9*: 219 (1980).
15. D. M. Dreon, B. Frey-Hewitt, N. Ellsworth, P. T. Williams, R. B. Terry, and P. D. Wood, Dietary carbohydrate-to-fat ratio and obesity in middle-aged men, *Am. J. Clin. Nutr., 47:* 995 (1988).
16. L. Lissner, D. A. Levitsky, B. J. Strupp, H. J. Kalkwarf, and D. A. Roe, Dietary fat intake and regulation of energy intake in human subjects, *Am. J. Clin. Nutr., 46*: 886 (1987).
17. R. M. Marston and N. R. Raper, The nutrient content of the food supply, *Natl. Food Rev., 29*: 5 (1985).
18. Drewnowski, Sweet foods and sweeteners in the U.S. diet, *Diet and Obesity*, (G. A. Bray, J. LeBlanc, S. Inoue, and M. Suzuki, eds), Japan Scientific Societies Press, Tokyo, pp. 153–161 (1988).
19. B. Schneeman, Fats in the diet: Why and where?, *Food Technol., 40* (10): 115 (1986).
20. J. J. Putnam, Food consumption, *Natl. Food Rev.,* (July-Sept.): 1 (1990).
21. G. Block, C. M. Dresser, A. M. Hartman, and M. D. Carroll, Nutrient sources in the American diet: Quantitative data from the NHANES II survey, *Am. J. Epidemiol., 122*: 27 (1985).
22. D. Putler and E. Frazao, Diet/Health concerns about fat intake, *Natl. Food Rev., 1*: 16 (1991).
23. J. L. Jones and J. Weimer, Health related food choices, *Fam. Econ. Rev., 2*: 16 (1981).

24. W. R. Harlan, J. R. Landis, K. M. Flegal, C. S. Davis, and M. E. Miller, Trends in body mass in the United States, 1960-1980, *Am. J. Epidemiol., 128*: 1065 (1988).
25. K. M. Flegal, W. R. Harlan, and J. R. Landis, Trends in body mass index and skinfold thickness with socioeconomic factors in young adult women, *Am. J. Clin. Nutr., 48*: 535 (1988).
26. M. F. Najjar and M. Rowland, Anthropometric reference data and the prevalence of overweight, United States 1976-80, National Center for Health Statistics, *Vital and Health Statistics, 11*(238):1-73, DHHS Pub. No. (PHS) 87-1688, U.S. Government Printing Office, Washington, DC (1987).
27. S. L. Gortmaker, W. H. Dietz, A. M. Sobol, and C. A. Wehler, Increasing pediatric obesity in the United States, *Am. J. Dis. Child., 141*: 535 (1987).
28. C. Bouchard, Inheritance of human fat distribution, *Fat Distribution During Growth and Later Health Outcomes* (C. Bouchard and F. E. Johnston, eds.), Alan R. Liss, New York, pp. 103-125 (1988).
29. J. Rodin, Psychological factors in obesity, *Recent Advances in Obesity Research III* (P. Bjorntorp, M. Cairella, and A. N. Howard, eds.), J. Libbey, London, pp. 106-123 (1981).
30. A. J. Stunkard, T. I. A. Sorensen, C. Hanis, T. W. Teasdale, R. Chakraborty, W. J. Schull, and F. Schulsinger, An adoption study of human obesity, *N. Engl. J. Med., 314*: 193 (1986).
31. L. E. Braitman, E. V. Adlin, and J. L. Stanton, Obesity and caloric intake: The National Health and Nutrition Examination Survey of 1971-1975 (HANES I), *J. Chron. Disease. 38*: 727 (1985).
32. D. Lansky and K. D. Brownell, Estimates of food quantity and calories: Errors in self-report among obese patients. *Am. J. Clin. Nutr., 35*: 727 (1984).
33. A. M. Prentice, A. E. Black, W. A. Coward, H. L. Davies, G. R. Goldberg, P. R. Murgatroyd, J. Ashford, M. Sawyer, and R. G. Whitehead. High levels of energy expenditure in obese women, *Br. Med. J., 292*: 983 (1986).
34. D. J. Mela and D. A. Sacchetti, Sensory preferences for fats: Relationships with diet and body composition. *Am. J. Clin. Nutr. 53*: 908 (1991).
35. J. P. Flatt, Efficiency of carbohydrate and fat utilization for oxidation and storage, *Diet and Obesity* (G. A. Bray, J. LeBlanc, S. Inoue, and M. Suzuki, ed), Japan Scientific Societies Press, Tokyo, pp. 87-100 (1988).
36. R. S. Schwartz, E. Ravussin, M. Massari, M. O'Connell, and D. C. Robbins, The thermic effect of carbohydrate versus fat feeding in man, *Metabolism, 34*: 285 (1985).
37. A. Tremblay, G. Plourde, J. P. Despres, and C. Bouchard, Impact of dietary fat content and fat oxidation on energy intake in humans, *Am. J. Clin. Nutr., 49*: 799 (1989).
38. T. J. Yost and R. H. Eckel, Fat calories may be preferentially stored in reduced-obese women: A permissive pathway for resumption of the obese state, *J. Clin. Endocrinol. Metab., 76*: 259 (1988).
39. S. N. Steen, R. A. Opplinger, and K. D. Brownell, Metabolic efects of repeated weight loss and regain in adolescent wrestlers, *JAMA, 260*: 47 (1988).

40. K. J. Morgan and M. E. Zabik, Amount and food sources of total sugar intake by children aged 5 to 12 years, *Am. J. Clin. Nutr., 34*: 404 (1981).
41. K. J. Morgan, S. R. Johnson, and G. L. Stampley, Children's frequency of eating, total sugar intake and weight/height stature, *Nutr. Res., 3*: 635 (1983).
42. A. Sclafani, Animal models of obesity, *Dietary Treatment and Prevention of Obesity* (R. T. Frankle, J. Dwyer, L. Moragne, and A. Owen eds.), John Libbey, London, pp. 105–123 (1985).
43. S. B. Roberts, J. Savage, W. A. Coward, B. Chew, and A. Lucas, Energy expenditure and intake in infants born to lean and overweight mothers, *N. Engl. J. Med., 318*: 461 (1988).
44. G. L. Blackburn, G. T. Wilson, B. S. Kanders, L. J. Stein, P. T. Lavin, J. Adler, and K. D. Brownell, Weight cycling: The experience of human dieters, *Am. J. Clin. Nutr., 49*: 1105 (1989).
45. A. Drewnowski, C. L. Kurth, and J. E. Rahaim, Taste preferences in human obesity: Environmental and familial factors, *Am. J. Clin. Nutr., 54*: 635 (1991).
46. R. W. Jeffery, A. R. Folsom, R. V. Luepker, D. R. Jacobs, R. F. Gillum, H. L. Taylor, and H. Blackburn, Prevalence of overweight and weight loss behavior in a metropolitan adult population: The Minnesota Heart Survey experience, *Am. J. Publ. Health, 74*: 349 (1984).
47. A. Drewnowski and D. Yee, Men and body image: Are males satisfied with their body weight? *Psychosom. Med., 49*: 626 (1987).
48. A. R. Price, A. J. Stunkard, R. Ness, T. Wadden, S. Heshka, B. Kanders, and A. Cormillot, Childhood-onset (age <10) obesity has high familial risk, *Int. J. Obesity, 8*: 491 (1990).
49. S. Schachter, Recidivism and self-cure of smoking and obesity, *American Psychologist, 37*: 436 (1982).
50. A. Drewnowski, B. Pierce, and K. A. Halmi, Fat aversion in eating disorders. *Appetite 10*: 119 (1988).
51. A. Drewnowski, K. A. Halmi, B. Pierce, J. Gibbs, and G. P. Smith, Taste and eating disorders, *Am. J. Clin. Nutr., 46*: 442 (1987).
52. R. C. Atkins, *Dr. Atkins' Diet Revolution*, Bantam Books, New York (1972).
53. E. S. Parham and A. R. Parham, Saccharin use and sugar intake by college students, *J. Am. Diet. Assoc., 76*: 560 (1980).
54. A. Drewnowski and M. R. C. Greenwood, Cream and sugar: Human preferences for high-fat foods, *Physiol. Behav., 30*: 629 (1983).
55. A. Drewnowski, J. D. Brunzell, K. Sande, P. H. Iverius, and M. R. C. Greenwood, Sweet tooth reconsidered: Taste preferences in human obesity, *Physiol. Behav. 35*: 617 (1985).
56. D. R. Reed, R. J. Contreras, C. Maggio, M. R. C. Greenwood, and J. Rodin, Weight cycling in female rats increases dietary fat selection and adiposity, *Physiol. Behav. 42*: 389 (1989).
57. J. J. Wurtman, The involvement of brain serotonin in excessive carbohydrate snacking by obese carbohydrate cravers, *J. Am. Diet. Assoc., 84*: 1004 (1984).
58. J. J. Wurtman, R. J. Wurtman, J. H. Growdon, P. Henry, A. Lipscomb, and S. H. Zeisel, Carbohydrate craving in obese people: Suppression by treatments affecting serotoninergic transmission, *Int. J. Eating Disorders, 1*: 2 (1981).

59. E. S. Paykel, P. S. Mueller, and P. M. de la Vergne, Amitryptiline, weight gain and carbohydrate craving: a side effect, *Br. J. Psychiat., 125*: 501 (1973).
60. H. L. Meiselman, D. Waterman, and L. E. Symington, Armed Forces Food Preferences, *Technical Report 75-63-FSL*, U.S. Army Natick Development Center, Natick, MA (1974).
61. U.S. Department of Health and Human Services, *Healthy People 2,000*, U.S. Government Printing Office, Washington, DC (1991).
62. Americans to make "lighter" choices in the 90's, *Calorie Control Commentary 12*: 1 (1990).
63. R. M. Morrison, The market for fat substitutes, *Natl. Food Rev., 4*: 24 (1990).
64. J. E. Blundell and A. J. Hill, Paradoxical effects of an intense sweetener (aspartame) on appetite, *Lancet, 1*: 1092 (1986).
65. B. J. Rolls, Effects of intense sweeteners on hunger, food intake, and body weight: A review, *Am. J. Clin. Nutr., 53*: 872 (1991).
66. D. J. Canty and M. B. Chan, Effects of consumption of caloric vs noncaloric sweet drinks on indices of hunger and food consumption in normal adults, *Am. J. Clin. Nutr. 53*: 1159 (1991).
67. K. P. Porikos, M. F. Hesser, and T. B. Van Itallie, Caloric regulation in normal-weight men maintained on a palatable diet of conventional foods, *Physiol. Behav., 28*: 293 (1982).
68. J. L. Smith and J. P. Heyback, Evidence for the lower intake of calories and carbohydrates by 19-50 year old female aspartame users from the continuing survey of food intakes by individuals (CSFII85), *FASEB J., 2* (5): A1197 (1988).
69. M. G. Tordoff and A. M. Alleva, Effect of drinking soda sweetened with aspartame or high-fructose corn syrup on food intake and body weight, *Am. J. Clin. Nutr., 51*: 963 (1990).
70. B. S. Kanders, P. T. Lavin, M. B. Kowalchuk, I. Greenberg, and G. L. Blackburn, An evaluation of the effect of aspartame on weight loss, *Appetite, 11* (Suppl.1): 73 (1988).
71. S. D. Stellman and L. Garfinkel, Artificial sweetener uses and one-year weight change among women, *Prev. Med., 15*: 195 (1986).
72. B. J. Rolls, L. S. Jacobs, and M. Heatherington, Sweeteners and energy regulation, *Appetite, 7*: 291 (1986).
73. R. W. Foltin, M. W. Fischman, T. H. Moran, B. J. Rolls, and T. H. Kelly, Caloric compensation for lunches varying in fat and carbohydrate content by humans in a residential laboratory, *Am. J. Clin. Nutr., 52*: 969 (1990).
74. A. Kendall, D. A. Levitsky, B. J. Strupp, and L. Lissner, Weight loss on a low-fat diet: Consequence of the imprecision of the control of food intake in humans, *Am. J. Clin Nutr. 53*: 1125 (1991).
75. A. M. Altschul, Low-calorie foods, *Food Technol., 4*: 113 (1989).
76. Institute of Medicine, Committee on Dietary Guidelines Implementation, *Improving America's Diet and Health: From Recommendations to Action* (P. R. Thomas, ed.), National Academy Press, Washington, DC (1991).

26
Psychological Aspects of the Use of Low-Calorie Foods: Changing Beliefs and Preferences

Paul Rozin   *University of Pennsylvania, Philadelphia, Pennsylvania*

I. INTRODUCTION

Low-calorie foods are seen by many health professionals as desirable alternatives to many common foods in the American diet. The problem this creates is how to increase acceptance and intake of low-calorie foods. This chapter will address that issue from the psychological perspective.

Promoting a diet composed of low-calorie foods is actually appropriate for only a minority of all human beings—basically, people who live in modern, industrialized cultures. These people constitute approximately 16% of all living human beings (calculated as all the people in Europe including the former Soviet Union, plus Canadians, Americans, and Japanese, divided by the total number of people in the world). These nutritionally privileged people face a surplus of foods and are more threatened by overconsumption of food than underconsumption of food. For this substantial minority of human beings, hereafter called "prosperous people," what are the threats presented by the current diet that low-calorie foods can address?

First, the promotion of low-calorie foods would affect the physical health of prosperous people. Promoting low-calorie foods may decrease the prevalence of obesity and decrease morbidity due to obesity. Because Americans consider obesity ugly, obesity *also* affects their mental health. American women probably use low-calorie foods more for the effects on their appearance rather than on health. For American women, appearance seems to be more important in controlling food intake than health. However, as it happens, attempts (made in moderation) to improve appearance may encourage the weight loss that is valuable in improving health. In addition to the fact that controlling appearance is a better motivator than improving health in making dietary changes, the rewards of making these changes are more apparent in the area of appearance. The effects of calorie reduction on appearance occur much more rapidly than the effects on health. Second, promoting low-fat foods may reduce morbidity resulting from cardiovascular (and some other) diseases.

The reduction of obesity and the risk of cardiovascular disease (the two are obviously related) by increased employment of low-calorie foods offer very different prospects for success from the point of view of public health. Replacement of animal fats by fat substitutes would be very likely to decrease cardiovascular risk. However, replacement of high-calorie foods with lower-calorie foods would not necessarily affect obesity, since, to the extent that people regulate their energy intake, they will compensate for an increase in low-calorie foods by eating more food (see Chapter 25). As a result, the most encouraging prospect for low-calorie foods may be the use of fat substitutes as a means of changing the nutrient content of the diet, rather than necessarily reducing obesity (see also Chapters 21 and 22).

II. CHANGING FOOD HABITS

From the psychological perspective, eating is an extraordinarily personal activity. Eating threatens the self because it involves incorporation of material from the outside world into the self. It is not surprising that people have very strong feelings about what goes in their mouths. Biologically, these reactions reflect both the vital importance of the ingestion of nutrients and the opposing real risks of consuming natural toxins or nutritionally inadequate diets. Humans, as omnivorous animals, eat a very wide range of foods. Fortunately, cultural transmission makes it unnecessary for them to individually discover what potential foods are safe, edible in only small quantities, or toxic.

Biologically, food is a source of energy and nutrients. Psychologically, it serves many other functions. Food is one of the great sources of pleasure to human beings, a pleasure that no doubt evolved to motivate ingestion. Furthermore, for most humans (less so in the United States), food assumes a variety of social and moral functions [1,2]. These multiple motivations for consuming or avoiding particular foods make the manipulation of food choices particularly difficult.

The actual intake of specific foods by people is largely determined by two nonpsychological factors: cost and availability. Psychological factors become more important as availability ceases to be a constraint (as in the American supermarket) and as financial constraints decrease. Under such circumstances, one repeatedly finds in consumer surveys that the prime determinant of food selection by humans is sensory properties. Generally, people choose foods that taste good to them. The predominance of taste (at least in an affluent society) produces the major deterrent to changing diets in order to improve health.

Two robust sensory promoters of food ingestion in humans are sweet tastes and fatty textures. There is abundant evidence that a desire for sweets is an innate feature of human food choice [3-5]. We are not certain whether the desire for fatty textures is innate, but it is certainly a powerful influence on choice for adults and children around the world. The bias to ingest sweet tastes and fatty textures is quite understandable biologically. Both are indicators of the presence of energy in nature. This useful and adaptive bias becomes problematic in a society facing overabundance. The fat/sugar preference presents a double-barreled problem: foods containing both fat and sugar are particularly palatable [6]. Therefore, one problem with calorie control is that we naturally seek sensory properties that are, in nature, associated with calories. The development of substitutes for fat and sugar that share many sensory properties with fat or sugar is one way of addressing this problem.

Concern about health also motivates people's choice of food. However, the continued ingestion of high animal-fat diets and excessive calories attests to the fact that health concerns are generally secondary to pleasure. The extraordinary measures that have had to be taken in order to reduce smoking in the United States also testify to the inadequacy of health risk *alone* in producing a major modification in intake. The problem is that people like both the sensory aspects and the physiological effects of smoking.

People tend to eat what they like, and what they like is not always optimal for health. However, the problem is not simply a mismatch between what people think is good for them and what they like. People also do not know what is good for their health. Americans have a poor understanding of the major costs and benefits of particular dietary patterns. They are not educated, in the school system or at home, about either the fundamentals of nutrition and risk or about the balancing of costs and benefits. The normal human urge to simplify complex situations causes people to think of foods as either good or bad for health. The biological and psychological importance of food makes the stakes much higher and encourages strong advocacy of a wide variety of positions: the superiority of natural foods, the toxicity of sugar, and, more generally, the emerging idea among many Americans that food is a toxin. The desire for a simplified set of nutritional guidelines is accompanied by the constant barrage from laboratories and the media suggesting that intake of X is either harmful to health or prevents disease. In some cases, claims that X is harmful to health are later countered with claims that X is actually beneficial to health. Risks that are extremely difficult to comprehend, such as an increase in mortality of one in one million, are either ignored or treated as if they are among the major risks in life.

The desire to classify everything as good or bad, plus a basic belief that objects transfer properties to other objects by physical contact [7], induces great overreactions to substances of questionable or minimal toxicity [8,9]. Many people treat sugar and salt as potent toxins. Their presence in even tiny amounts in the diet is perceived as having negative effects on health, as if, for example, contact with a tiny amount of sugar transmits "sugarness" and all its purported evil properties into a food [10]. Substances with "empty calories" are thought of as poisons. There is a commonly held view that if something may be harmful to a person in large amounts, then it is necessarily harmful in small amounts [10]. Sugar and fat are lumped together as risk factors for cardiovascular disease and health in general, where there is in fact no convincing evidence that sugar in moderate levels is harmful to health. "Natural" foods are thought to be necessarily more healthful than processed foods, and natural toxins are considered less dangerous than toxins that are part of food processing [8].

Finally, food is a social and moral instrument, even in America. Certain foods, such as animal products, have taken on negative moral characteristics, as has smoking cigarettes. In general, people seem surprisingly poor at distinguishing health from moral concerns. This appears clearly in attitudes to a trim body, to AIDS [11], and in explanations of illness: cross-culturally, moral transgression is the most common explanation for illness [12]. Consumption of certain foods and avoidance of others has social significance, because it aligns people with groups that they respect or abhor.

Amid this chaotic mixture of true and false nutritional information, large and small risks, social/moral concerns about foods and body appearance, somewhat irrational attitudes about foods, and poor education about nutrition and risk management, it is not surprising that individuals have trouble centering on a few dietary changes that might make a big difference in their lives. It might be easier to get people to make *important* health-related changes in their lives, like stopping smoking, wearing seat belts, driving less, and cutting down on animal fats, if they would also stop worrying about issues that pose only minimal risks to health, such as exposure to pesticides.

In summary, Americans face two problems: focusing on a very few significant changes in diet and then implementing these changes.

III. SOLUTIONS TO THE SENSORY PROBLEM

Since desire for good tastes is the prime motivator of food choice, duplication of the desired tastes in healthier foods should go a long way in improving health. Artificial sweeteners have been available for some time, and fat substitutes are now becoming available. Such products may indeed contribute to the control of obesity and cardiovascular disease. However, there are some factors that limit the effect of the currently available substitutes. First, sugars do not seem to be major contributors to either obesity or cardiovascular disease. Unfortunately, the best substitutes we have are for sugar and not for fats. Second, the substitutes are far from perfect sensory mimics. Aspartame is perhaps the most successful substitute, but all fat and sugar substitutes have some sensory effects that differentiate them from their target substances. For artificial sweeteners, these include bitter and unusually long aftertastes. Current research indicates that there are a number of different sugar receptors [13]. This allows for the possibility that some artificial sweeteners may initiate a sweet sensation that differs from those produced by sugars.

Third, and most significantly, there is abundant evidence that humans regulate their food intake and weight. The relative stability of the weight of most people over a period of years speaks most directly to this point. Insofar as an underlying regulatory mechanism modulates hunger, and hence the tendency to eat, the removal of calories from a diet will simply increase intake of available, lower-calorie foods. Hence, it is at least possible that even perfect sugar and fat substitutes will have no long-term effect on obesity. There is a growing literature on this subject, which is reviewed in Chapters 21 and 25. The current evaluation offered in that review is that there seems to be some net calorie reduction in at least some studies that have monitored the food intake of humans using fat or sugar substitutes.

The future of fat substitutes in producing a reduction in fat (or animal fat) intake is much more promising. As far as we know, there is not a specific fat-intake regulatory mechanism. Fat substitutes might satisfy the desire for fatty textures and facilitate consumption of a diet in which carbohydrates replace many fats.

IV. CHANGING TASTES

Many foods available have desirable nutritional profiles and are relatively low in calories. Unfortunately, these foods as a group are less popular in the United States and many other countries than desserts, meats, and dairy products. One way to improve the makeup of the American diet, if not to control obesity, would be to shift intake away from high-fat (especially animal fat) foods. For example, if people came to dislike animal foods and came to like vegetables more, their diet would naturally become healthier. I have already pointed out that reducing health risks has rarely been a sufficient motivation for changing people's food choices. A much more powerful way is to develop likings for the tastes of foods that are healthy and dislikes for foods that are unhealthy. This section will discuss what is known about how people come to like or dislike foods. First it will present a psychological taxonomy of foods, and then discuss how foods come to move from one of these categories to another.

A. The Adult Classification of Edibles and Inedibles

Every adult in every culture has a set of attitudes toward objects in the world as to these objects' appropriateness and desirability as food. The acquisition of this categorization, and the assignment of objects to appropriate categories, may be a major feature of food enculturation. Fallon and Rozin [14–16] have explored these attitudes in American adults using a combination of questionnaires and interviews. The results indicate that there are three reasons for accepting or rejecting potential foods. Each of these (Table 1), in one form, motivates acceptance, and, in the opposite form, motivates rejection.

1. Sensory-Affective Factors

Some items are accepted or rejected because of a liking or disliking for their sensory properties: taste, smell, and, to a lesser extent, appearance. Items accepted primarily on such grounds are "good tastes," while those rejected on such grounds are "distastes." Most commonly, when we say we like or dislike a food, we are referring to sensory-affective factors. Individual differences in liking for particular sensory-affective factors probably account for most within-culture variance in food preferences (e.g., liking for hot pepper, lima beans, beer, yogurt) [17].

2. Anticipated Consequences

Some items are accepted or rejected primarily because of beliefs about the consequences of ingesting them. These may be rapid effects, such as satiation,

Table 1 Psychological Categories of Acceptance and Rejection

Dimensions	Rejections				Acceptances			
	Distaste	Danger	Inappropriate	Disgust	Good taste	Beneficial	Appropriate	Transvalued
Sensory-affective	−			−	+			+
Anticipated consequences		−				+		
Ideational		?				?	+	+
Examples	Beer, chili, spinach	Allergy foods, carcinogens	Grass, sand	Feces, insects	Saccharine	Medicines	Ritual food	Leavings of heroes or deities

Source: Ref. 14.

nausea, or increased social status. Or they may be more delayed effects, such as gaining weight or increased risk of developing cancer. Items accepted because of positive anticipated consequences are called beneficial, while those rejected because of negative anticipated consequences are called dangerous (see Table 1).

3. Ideational Factors

Some substances are rejected or accepted primarily because of our knowledge of what they are, their origins, or their symbolic meanings. Ideational factors probably play a modest role in food acceptance, but they play a major role in food rejection. There are two distinct categories of ideational rejection.

a. Inappropriate. Inappropriate items are considered inedible, and hence are refused. They account for most items in the world: bark, sand, paper, grass, etc. These items may or may not be viewed as bad-tasting or dangerous. They are inoffensive. The primary reason for rejection is that they are not considered to be food. Most culturewide rejections seem to fall into this category.

b. Disgusting. Disgusting items are also rejected on ideational grounds, but they are considered offensive. They have a strong negative sensory-affective loading and are likely to elicit nausea. They are so offensive that they are contaminants. In other words, if they touch an edible food, they tend to render it inedible. Disgusting items (see Table 1), unlike other categories of items, are heavily loaded on two dimensions in our taxonomy: negative ideation and negative taste. Almost all substances that elicit disgust are animals or animal products, with feces as the apparently universal disgust substance [18,19].

This taxonomy represents an oversimplification. Most rejections and acceptances are motivated by reasons that fall into more than one category. Thus, milk is good-tasting and beneficial; cockroaches are disgusting, but may also be dangerous. Nonetheless, many items fall within a single category. That is, there is a primary reason for accepting or rejecting them.

B. Intrinsic Value and Food: Getting to Like and Dislike Foods

The issue of intrinsic value, or internalization, is fundamental in understanding preferences. The critical distinction is between consuming a food because of costs or consequences of ingestion and consuming food for its own sake, that is, because it tastes good [15,20]. As indicated in the discussion above of classification of foods by adults, accepted foods fall into two categories: those that are "beneficial" (e.g., medicines) and those that are "good tastes." The parallel distinction on the negative side generates foods that are avoided but not disliked (dangerous entities) and those that are disliked (distastes). For example, people with shellfish allergies (shellfish in the dangerous category) usually like shellfish and would return to eating them if assured that they would no longer show an allergic reaction. On the other hand, people who got food-poisoning with associated nausea and vomiting from shellfish typically dislike the taste of shellfish, even though they know that shellfish would not normally make them sick [21]. A critical variable that causes a change in intrinsic value in the aversion situation is nausea [21]. This seems to be a form of Pavlovian conditioning, in which the food (a conditioned stimulus) is paired with nausea (an unconditioned stimulus). In general, Pavlovian conditioning in humans, in which the value or liking for an object has been changed, is called evaluative conditioning [22,23]. This seems to be a potentially potent mechanism for the changing of likes and dislikes.

The phenomenon of acquired taste aversions (taste-nausea pairings) in animals and humans is extremely robust [24]. Nausea is like a "magic bullet" for creating dislikes (distastes). Bad consequences of ingesting a food, other than nausea, tend to cause that food to be thought of as dangerous, rather than distasteful [21].

There does not seem to be a "magic bullet' for creating good tastes. Although people often come to like particular foods, it is usually more gradual than acquired distastes of food, and the forces at work are less clear [20, 25–27].

Under a wide variety of circumstances, exposure to (ingestion of) a food or other event leads to enhanced liking [28,29]. This has been described as the "mere exposure" effect. This effect is not presently understood. That is, we are not sure whether exposure per se is a sufficient cause for liking. It may simply provide the opportunity for Pavlovian conditioning or other processes to operate. In any event, a good way to get people to like a food is to induce them to try it on a few occasions.

Pavlovian (evaluative) conditioning has been implicated in a number of ways in the acquisition of food likes by humans [23,27,30]. Under some conditions, postingestional events such as satiety (an unconditioned stimulus) can enhance the liking of foods that precede them [30]. Alternatively, when a flavor is paired with an already positive (sweet) taste, the flavor may become enhanced in taste [31]. Preparation of a new food with already familiar and palatable accompaniments may be a powerful way of establishing positive evaluative conditioning.

Social factors seem to be the predominant forces in producing likes [32, 33]. These may work, in part through Pavlovian processes, such as exposure to a food in the presence of positive facial expressions of other people.

Empirical work, largely by Birch [32], indicates that a child's perception that a respected other likes a food seems to foster liking. Parents report particular efficacy in inducing preferences for new foods by involving the child in the preparation of the food [34]. This may be a major arena for the communication of positive social messages.

Birch's findings fit well with the research of Lepper [35] and Deci and Ryan [36], which emphasize the destructive effect of coercion or apparent compliance on intrinsic value. Forcing a child to perform a previously liked activity seems to reduce the intrinsic value of that activity. This is sometimes called the overjustification effect. Birch and colleagues [37] have shown the operation of the overjustification effect in the area of food preferences. Rewarding a child for consuming a food tends to *reduce* the child's liking for the food below baseline after the rewards cease. One explanation for this effect is that when a child consumes a food, she looks for accounts of why she has done so. If she has been coerced or bribed, this is a sufficient account. If the child cannot identify an external cause of the ingestion, she is likely to explain her own action as a liking for the food in question. In at least some contexts, liking for a food can be enhanced by using it as a reward rather than by rewarding its ingestion [38]. Although American parents seem aware of the inefficacy of rewarding ingestion of a specific food in order to increase preference for that food, they are unaware of the virtue of using a target food as a reward in order to enhance liking [34].

The predominance of social factors and the overjustification effect fit well with the natural history of acquisition for liking for chili pepper by children in Mexico [39]. The critical factor seems to be participation by preschoolers in a family meal context in which the older members clearly enjoy the chili pepper. Specific rewards for consuming piguant foods are not provided.

We presume that some of these same social factors are at work with adults. If they are, they presage trouble for inducing liking for "healthy" foods. If people believe they are eating a food because it is healthy, they might be less likely to come to like it. Indeed, one study reports that people rarely come to like the tastes of oral medicines, and accounts for this on the grounds that the salience of medicinal effects blocks (by overjustification) the acquisition of a liking [40].

C. Preference Transmission Across Generations: The Family Paradox

All models of preference acquisition, from mere exposure through social influence, point to the parents as the main vehicle of transmission of both culturewide preferences and individual differences in preferences. Parents dictate the foods offered, create the context in which the foods are consumed, and are the main source of social exchange at meal time. The particularities of a family's preferences should be communicated in the same way as the culturewide preferences. However, a series of studies have reported low (0.0 to approximately 0.3) correlations between the food preferences of parents and their children [41–44]. This surprisingly weak relationship appears whether the offspring subjects are young children or young adults, and whether preferences are determined by ratings of offered foods or by verbal reports. This is the "family paradox" [44]. In other words, the family appears to be a powerful force for instilling culturewide preferences, but a very weak one for instilling family-specific preferences.

One explanation for the family paradox is that the child receives a totally consistent message about culturewide food preferences from both parents and all others. On the other hand, although there is some concordance on preferences varying within culture between parents [43,45], parents will often be discordant on particular preferences. Hence, the low parent-child correlations might result from the child receiving mixed messages. However, when only parents who are concordant for the preference in question are considered, the parent-child correlation goes up only slightly [44]. Hence, parental discordance is not a sufficient explanation of the low family correlations.

The paradox is deeper yet. The mother has a special role in the food socialization of her children. The nursing process provides a powerful mother-child linkage. Furthermore, even in most modern cultures, the mother handles most of the food preparation and child feeding. Hence, one would reasonably predict that the mother's food preferences should correlate more highly than the father's with the preferences of their children. This obvious prediction is not consistently supported by the data. Three studies report no difference between mother-child and father-child food preference correlations [42,46,47], and only two find a slight effect favoring the mother [41,43]. There is a possible explanation for this anomaly. Mothers may be more influenced by the father's food preferences than by their own preferences in making food purchases [46,48]. Insofar as parents induce preferences by providing exposure to particular foods, the father might have a greater influence. However, insofar as emotional displays while consuming foods are critical, one would still expect a dominant role for the mother. These results imply that changing parents' preferences is not a very effective way of inducing corresponding changes in their children's preferences.

D. Moralization: Turning Preferences into Values

Although preferences (for foods and other things, like music) run only weakly in families, values show much more substantial parent-child correlations

[44,49]. (We will define values as attitudes that can be described as right or wrong as opposed to defining them as matters of individual taste.) Choices are strongly affected by values, and values may be powerful forces in inducing likes and dislikes. For example, dislikes or strong intrinsic negative reactions are manifested to certain potential foods in terms of the emotion and food class of disgust [19].

There is a relationship between disgust and moral offense. Two recent examples relevant to food and health come to mind. One is the recent change in attitudes to cigarette smoking. Smoking has become less of a preference and more of a (negative) value. In line with this, more and more people report a strong disgust response to cigarette smoke and ashes. A second example involves the rise of vegetarianism. Beginning vegetarians often find renouncing meat difficult, because they still find it palatable. Many vegetarians who have maintained a no-meat regime for some time come to actually dislike or be disgusted by meat [50]. The disgust response to meat is more likely to occur in people who are "moral" vegetarians (those who reject meat because it involves killing animals, etc.) than those who are "health" vegetarians (those who reject meat because it is bad for health) [51]. Endowing a food with disgust properties is a powerful way to eliminate it from one's diet and to eliminate any temptation to eat it. However, this does not always work. Centuries of "moralization" of negative properties of sugar have not succeeded very much in reducing intake [52,53].

On the positive side, it is also possible that moralization can produce likes for foods through emphasizing the values associated with the food (e.g., its environment-sparing quality). This may happen to some vegetarians with respect to some of the vegetable foods they consume. In many cases, such vegetables become much more attractive with time.

V. CHANGING BELIEFS AND COGNITIONS

The second aspect of promoting low-calorie foods is to focus the goals of individuals on a few particularly important dietary changes. This involves changing beliefs and cognitions. Changing beliefs and cognitions about health and nutrition presents less of a challenge on the theoretical level to psychology than does changing likes. The problem is primarily in education, public relations, and the media. We have to think about educating people about risks, weighing costs and benefits in decision making, and the basics of nutrition. People must learn about the importance of dose levels, the interchangeability of many nutrients, the inevitability of certain low risks, and making compromises between health and pleasure [54]. At the same time, we must discourage the press and scientists from publicizing preliminary findings suggesting that common foods and substances have possible harmful effects on health. Incorporating basic nutritional wisdom in convenient forms and promoting basic guidelines such as variety and moderation at the expense of short-lived dietary scares and fads would also be highly desirable. At a minimum, a better educated public would be more likely to focus on big problems and control them.

VI. CONCLUSION

Increased consumption of low-calorie foods at the expense of high-calorie foods can be promoted by letting people focus on such foods as a principal health/nutrition goal, and by encouraging associations that would promote a liking for low-calorie foods and a disliking of high-calorie foods. It is odd that although it is easier to create dislikes than likes, almost all efforts are directed towards creating likes for the healthier foods. It is also important to change people's beliefs so that they don't think of food as a toxin. People must come to realize that they should create a compromise between pleasure and health, and that they can continue to eat their favorite foods, but simply in smaller amounts [54]. With this relatively palatable diet, it may be possible to insert new low-calorie foods into the diet, in appetizing settings, with palatable preparations. Under these circumstances, exposure, associations, and habit may conspire to produce an enduring liking for low-calorie foods.

ACKNOWLEDGMENTS

This paper was prepared with the assistance of funding from the John D. and Catherine T. MacArthur Foundation Research Program on Determinants and Consequences of Health-Promoting and Health-Damaging Behavior. Thanks to Deidre Byrnes for comments on the manuscript.

REFERENCES

1. A. Appadurai, Gastropolitics in Hindu South Asia, *Am. Ethnol., 8*: 494 (1981).
2. P. Rozin, Social and moral aspects of eating, *The Legacy of Solomon Asch*: *Essays in Cognition and Social Psychology* (I. Rock, ed.), Lawrence Erlbaum, Potomac, Maryland, pp. 97–110 (1990).
3. C. Davis, Self-selection of diets by newly weaned infants: An experimental study, *Am. J. Diseas. Child., 36*: 651 (1928).

4. J. Steiner, Human facial expressions in response to taste and smell stimulation, *Advances in Child Development and Behavior*, Vol. 13 (H. W. Reese and L. P. Lipsitt, eds.), Academic Press, New York, pp. 297–328 (1990).

5. P. Rozin, The selection of foods by rats, humans, and other animals, *Advances in the Study of Behavior*, Vol. 6 (J. Rosenblatt, R. A. Hinde, C. Beer, and E. Shaw, eds.), Academic Press, New York, pp. 21–76 (1976).

6. A. Drewnowski and M. R. C. Greenwood, Cream and sugar: Human preferences for high-fat foods, *Physiol. Behav., 30*: 629 (1983).

7. P. Rozin and C. J. Nemeroff, The laws of sympathetic magic: A psychological analysis of similarity and contagion, *Cultural Psychology: the Chicago Symposium* (J. Stigler, G. Herdt, and R. A. Shweder, eds.), Cambridge University Press, Cambridge, England (1989).

8. B. M. Ames, R. Magaw, and L. S. Gold, Ranking possible carcinogenic hazards, *Science, 236*: 271 (1987).

9. A. Wildavsky, *Searching for Safety*, Transaction Publishers, New Brunswick, NJ (1988).

10. P. Rozin and M. Markwith. The monotonic mind: Contagion and psychological dose insensitivity in response to risks (submitted).

11. P. Rozin, M. Markwith, and C. R. McCauley, Aversion to indirect contact with AIDS: A composite of aversion to strangers, infection, moral taint, and misfortune (submitted).

12. G. P. Murdock, *Theories of Illness: A World Survey*, University of Pittsburgh Press, Pittsburgh (1980).

13. L. M. Bartoshuk, Is sweetness unitary? An evaluation of the evidence for multiple sweets, *Sweetness* (J. Dobbing, ed.), Springer-Verlag, London, pp. 33–46 (1988).

14. A. E. Fallon and P. Rozin, The psychological bases of food rejections by humans, *Ecol. Food Nutr., 13*: 15 (1983).

15. P. Rozin and A. E. Fallon, Psychological categorization of foods and nonfoods: A preliminary taxonomy of food rejections, *Appetite, 1*: 193 (1980).

16. P. Rozin and A. E. Fallon, The acquisition of likes and dislikes for foods, *Criteria of Food Acceptance: How Man Chooses What He Eats. A Symposium* (J. Solms and R. L. Hall, eds.), Forster, Zurich, pp. 35–48 (1981).

17. H. G. Schutz and D. S. Judge, Consumer perceptions of food quality, *Research in Food Science and Nutrition: Food Science and Human Welfare*, Vol. 4 (J. V. McLoughlin and B. M. McKenna, eds.), Boole, Dublin, pp. 249–242 (1984).

18. A. Angyal, Disgust and related aversions, *J. Abnorm. Soc. Psychol., 36*: 393 (1941).

19. P. Rozin and A. E. Fallon, A perspective on digust, *Psychol. Rev., 94*: 23 (1987).

20. P. Rozin, The acquisition of food habits and preferences, *Behavioral Health: A Handbook of Health Enhancement and Disease Prevention* (J. D. Matarazzo, S. M. Weiss, J. A. Herd, N. E. Miller, and S. M. Weiss, eds.), John Wiley, New York, pp. 590–607 (1984).

21. M. L. Pelchat and P. Rozin, The special role of nausea in the acquisition of food dislikes by humans, *Appetite, 3*: 341 (1982).

22. I. Martin and A. B. Levey, Evaluative Conditioning, *Adv. Behav. Res. Ther., 1*: 57 (1978).

23. P. Rozin and D. A. Zellner, The role of Pavlovian conditioning in the acquisition of food likes and dislikes, *Ann. N.Y. Acad. Sci., 443*: 189 (1985).
24. J. Garcia, W. G. Hankins, and K. W. Rusiniak, Behavioral regulation of the milieu interne in man and rat, *Science, 185*: 824 (1974).
25. D. A. Booth, Learned ingestive motivation and the pleasures of the palate, *The Hedonics of Taste* (R. C. Bolles, ed.), Lawrence Erlbaum, Hillsdale, NJ (1991).
26. P. Rozin and J. Shulkin, Food selection, *Handbook of Behavioral Neurobiology*, Vol. 10, *Food and Water Intake* (E. M. Stricker, ed.), Plenum, New York, pp. 297-328 (1990).
27. D. A. Zellner, How foods get to be liked: Some general mechanisms and some special cases, *The Hedonics of Taste* (R. C. Bolles, ed.), Lawrence Erlbaum, Hillsdale, NJ, pp. 199-217 (1991).
28. R. B. Zajonc, Attitudinal effects of mere exposure, *J. Pers. Soc. Psychol., 9*(II): 1 (1968).
29. P. Pliner, The effects of mere exposure on liking for edible substances, *Appetite, 3*: 283 (1982).
30. D. A. Booth, M. Lee, and C. McAleavey, Acquired sensory control of satiation in man, *Br. J. Psychol., 67*: 137 (1976).
31. D. A. Zellner, P. Rozin, M. Aron, and C. Kulish, Conditioned enhancement of human's liking for flavors by pairing with sweetness, *Learn. Motiv., 14*: 338 (1983).
32. L. L. Birch, Children's food preferences: Developmental patterns and environmental influences, *Ann. of Child. Dev.*, Vol. 4 (G. Whitehurst and R. Vasta, eds.), JAI Press, Greenwich, CT (1987).
33. P. Rozin, Social learning about foods by humans, *Social Learning: A Comparative Approach* (T. Zentall and B. G. Galef, Jr., eds.), Erlbaum, Hillsdale, NJ, pp. 165-187 (1988).
34. R. Casey and P. Rozin, Changing children's food preferences: Parent opinions, *Appetite, 12*: 171 (1989).
35. M. R. Lepper, Social control processes and the internalization of social values: An attributional perspective, *Social Cognition and Social Development* (E. T. Higgins, D. N. Ruble, and W. W. Hartup, eds.), Cambridge University Press, New York, pp. 294-330 (1983).
36. E. L. Deci and R. M. Ryan, *Intrinsic Motivation and Self-Determination in Human Behavior*, Plenum, New York (1985).
37. L. L. Birch, D. Birch, D. W. Marlin, and L. Kramer, Effects of instrumental eating on children's food preferences, *Appetite, 3*: 125 (1982).
38. L. L. Birch, S. I. Zimmerman, and H. Hind, The influence of social-affective context on the formation of childrens' food preferences, *Child. Dev., 51*: 856 (1980).
39. P. Rozin and D. Schiller, The nature and acquisition of a preference for chili pepper by humans, *Motiv. Emot., 4*: 77 (1980).
40. P. Pliner, P. Rozin, M. Cooper, and G. Woody, Role of specific postingestional effects and medicinal context in the acquisition of liking for tastes, *Appetite, 6*: 243 (1985).
41. L. L. Birch, The relationship between children's food preferences and those of their parents, *J. Nutr. Ed., 12*: 14 (1980).

42. P. Pliner, Family resemblance in food preferences, *J. Nutr. Ed., 15*: 137 (1983).
43. P. Rozin, A. E. Fallon, and R. Mandell, Family resemblance in attitudes to food, *Devel. Psychol., 20*: 309 (1984).
44. P. Rozin, Family Resemblences in food and other domains: The family paradox and the role of parental congruence, *Appetite, 16*: 93 (1991).
45. R. A. Price and S. G. Vandenberg, Spouse similarity in American and Swedish couples, *Behav. Gen., 10*: 59 (1980).
46. J. V. Burt and A. A. Hertzler, Parental influence on the child's food preference, *J. Nutr. Ed., 10*: 127 (1978).
47. P. Pliner and M. L. Pelchat, Similarities in food preferences between children and their siblings and parents, *Appetite, 7*: 333 (1986).
48. G. Weidner, S. Archer, B. Healy, and J. D. Matarazzo, Family consumption of low fat foods: Stated preference versus actual consumption, *J. Appl. Soc. Psychol., 15*: 773 (1985).
49. L. L. Cavalli-Sforza, M. W. Feldman, K. H. Chen, and S. M. Dornbusch, Theory and observation in cultural transmission, *Science, 218*: 19 (1982).
50. P. R. Amato and S. A. Partridge, *The New Vegetarians: Promoting Health and Protecting Life*, Plenum Press, New York (1989).
51. P. Rozin, M. Markwith, and C. Stoess, Becoming a vegetarian: Development of the vegetarian ideology, attitudes, and preferences. (1991). Unpublished manuscript.
52. C. Fischler, Attitudes toward sugar and sweetness in historical and social perspective, *Sweetness* (J. Dobbing, ed.), Springer-Verlag, London, pp. 83–98 (1988).
53. P. Rozin, Sweetness, sensuality, sin, safety, and socialization: Some speculations, *Sweetness* (J. Dobbing, ed.), Springer-Verlag, London, pp. 99–110 (1988).
54. P. Rozin, Disorders of food selection: The compromise of pleasure, *Ann. N.Y. Acad. Sci., 575*: 376 (1989).

27
Reflections on the Role of Low-Calorie Foods

Aaron M. Altschul *Georgetown University School of Medicine, Washington, D.C.*

I. INTRODUCTION

Although the title of this book is *Low-Calorie Foods Handbook*, this book attempts to be more. It is really about the low-calorie foods phenomenon. As such it provides a description of low-calorie foods and deals with their impact on public eating behavior.

The problem with the description of the foods themselves is that this is a dynamic area. New products are introduced at a rapid and accelerating pace. New ways of using these food products are presented daily in the food sections of newspapers and magazines. We can only provide an idea of the status of low-calorie foods in a cross section of time, the time that it took to prepare this volume. It is even too early to try to imagine what the situation might be when the field stabilizes. Nevertheless, the reader gets an idea of what is happening and the trends. And short-term projections are reasonable.

Ramifications are more difficult to deal with. Has the existence of low-calorie food choices had an impact on obesity? Is there less obesity now than

10 years ago? Is there even any way of knowing whether the prevalence of obesity and the presence of low-calorie foods are in any way related? Yet this is what the whole idea is about: to manage the available food choices so that dietary control is easier for those who want it.

Many talented and knowledgeable individuals contributed chapters to this volume. The purpose of this chapter is to try to tie it all together, if possible, if not as a coherent explanation of the low-calorie foods phenomenon, at least to provide an approach to understanding this phenomenon and dealing with it.

II. AN ENIGMA

There is no question that the number and types of low-calorie foods is increasing rapidly, even dramatically. Any number of ways of measuring the market situation support this conclusion. More types available, more shelf space in the food market, more per capita consumption, more individuals admitting that they used a low-calorie food within the past week or month, more dollar sales, more research and development resources devoted to improving and increasing the choices: all these attest to low-calorie foods as an important and growing part of the food industry.

In some instances, the low-calorie version has replaced or is on the verge of replacing the original food as the norm for that type. Sales of low-fat fluid milk now exceed those of whole milk; artificially sweetened soft drinks are 30% of all soft drink sales; low-calorie sweetener sales are 14% of all sweeteners sales; low-fat and non-fat pourable dressings approach 50% of that market.

Low-calorie foods are now "regular" foods. They are no longer in the diet category. They take their place on the shelf alongside the "classical" foods. They are "mainstream" products. The greatest growth among new products is in the low-calorie lines.

The demand by consumers for low-calorie items is affecting menu planning in restaurants and recipe planning. Over 60% of retailers said that menu planning was influenced by consumers' nutrition concerns. This is one fact. The other is that obesity has not diminished in the United States and may still be increasing [1]. It is increasing among children. The prevalence of severe obesity is increasing; the obese are becoming more obese.

So here we have it: an exciting change in the food industry, providing and aggressively marketing low-calorie food choices designed to attract and assist those who wish to control weight; a positive response by the consumer who is buying the idea and the products; but no apparent effect on the public health problem it purports to solve.

Perhaps this is an unfair question. Causal relationships are difficult to prove. Most chronic diseases, including obesity, are multifactorial. Under such circumstances, it becomes difficult to tease out the particular effect of a single intervention in the complex of environmental and individual conditions.

But billions of dollars are involved: billions of dollars worth of new food products and billions of dollars in added health-care costs resulting from obesity and its consequences. The coexistence of low-calorie foods and obesity is worth pursuing further.

III. POSSIBLE EXPLANATIONS

Several possible explanations for the coexistence of a healthy and growing low-calorie foods industry and a stable pattern of obesity emerge from the preceding chapters. Any of the following or combinations of several of them could be operative.

1. It may be that the pattern of obesity is not stable, that it is decreasing among certain groups but the trend is hidden in overall averages. Obesity among high-income women is lower than for any other group and may be decreasing. These women are also using more artificially sweetened soft drinks and low-fat items. But obesity is higher and increasing in other groups, especially those with lower general education and socioeconomic status.

Another way of expressing it is that the prevalence of obesity may be decreasing among health-conscious individuals who are patronizing health-oriented foods. It is also possible that obesity might have become more prevalent had less low-calorie foods been available and choices more limited. But this is a matter that cannot easily be verified.

2. It could be that sedentary living is the greater determinant of energy balance so that changes in food intake are less likely to influence weight if work and exercise pattern are not changed concomitantly. Some call obesity an exercise-deficiency syndrome [2].

Some would argue that it is all in the genetic predisposition toward obesity. Hence, the food system should not make any difference: those preordained by their inheritance to become obese will do so no matter what. This view is not generally held. As Drewnowski put it, "The current view is that obesity may result from an interaction between genetic predisposition and exposure to environmental stimuli."

3. Despite the availability of more low-calorie choices, or, perhaps because of it, the consumer is confused. While manufacturers are increasing the number of low-calorie and low-fat options, the information that they

present in marketing these new products is often confusing and sometimes misleading. The government has the responsibility to devise and enforce labeling regulations. But the consumer ultimately must take the responsibility for knowing what is needed and making the best choice. He or she, if not careful, is apt to trade one source of calories for another or one source of fat for another so that the caloric and fat intake are the same but the sources differ (e.g., pizza instead of hamburger). And the consumer may neglect to consider the value of traditional low-calorie foods such as fruits and vegetables and whole grain cereals.

4.   The early emphasis on low-calorie foods was to replace sugar and other caloric sweeteners with artificial sweeteners. Now, the emphasis is on low-fat foods. This is a more useful concept, and it is only just beginning to take effect. Only very recently, for example, has consumption of skim milk increased significantly above a long-standing plateau.

Trends in fat consumption might be considered to anticipate trends in obesity. Thus far the changes are modest, as described in Chapters 4 and 25. The level of fat in the diet is lower than the maximum in this century of 43% of calories as fat to around 37%. Those who are more compliant with dietary and health guidelines take in closer to 30% of the calories as fat; the others are closer to 40%.

The patterns of change are complex. People are eating less red meat and more poultry and fish, but are eating more cheese, and they are eating more away from home, meals that are generally higher in energy, fat, saturated fat, and sodium.

Once many more choices to reduce dietary fat become available, the pattern of obesity may change. The changes will probably first be observed among the higher socioeconomic classes and among the better educated who have lower opportunity costs in adopting change.

5.   There are problems with taste and acceptance of the present versions of low-fat foods. Nutrition sells, and this is a major change in food marketing. But the food must taste good to sell. Present technology may not be sufficient to meet the needs of the marketplace. New fat substitutes and mimetics may be needed, and new flavor combinations developed to provide the consumer with the kinds of food that he or she can accept regularly.

6.   The idea of low-calorie foods is to "fool" the physiological signal-producers so that they signal for satiety even when the amount of calories "expected" from the sight, smell, and taste of food are not provided. Evidence from relatively short-term experiments with covert substitution of low-calorie foods for their regular counterparts show that compensation by eating more of other foods is incomplete. This is encouraging.

Does the same hold true for overt substitution of low-calorie foods? This is the paradigm of the low-calorie foods phenomenon: incomplete compensation is essential. Yet so little is known. As Pi-Sunyer states, "That so important a question as the nature of the diet and obesity has received so little attention is perplexing."

Of the most successful women in the experiment reported in Chapter 24 few showed any backsliding of their reduction in fat intake. They consumed less fat from salad dressings and red meat at 24 months than they did at 6 months. Processed low-calorie foods, in this instance, were relatively unimportant as a way of reducing fat intake.

So far, there has been no decrease (actually an increase) in total caloric sugar consumption despite the huge gains in consumption of artificially sweetened foods and beverages [3]. What will happen to fat consumption once more low-fat foods become available?

7. It may turn out that nothing automatic can be expected from the proliferation of low-calorie foods as long as our society provides an abundance of calories and promotes obesity. Change must start with the decision by the individual to eat more healthfully, to make *qualitative* as well as *quantitative* dietary changes, to restrain the amount of less-desirable foods eaten, and to reduce the level of sedentary living. Then the available low-calorie foods, natural and commercially produced, can help compliance with a decision to eat more healthfully.

If normal weight and a lifestyle that reduces risk to major chronic diseases are considered socially desirable, then society must help each individual, rich or poor, to undertake a way of living that promotes that goal. This means education about the relationship between eating and behavior to health, improving the clarity of description of the foods to minimize confusion, and specific advice on what to do and how to use all available food choices. Much of this is being done but, obviously, not enough, especially to reach and help the poor who suffer most from obesity and the other diseases and who have difficulty giving dietary change a high enough priority above problems of jobs, housing, and education. As stated by Rozin in Chapter 26, "People eat what they like and what they like is not always optimal for health. . . . People also do not know what is good for their health."

Chapter 3 mentions how children receive mixed signals in this regard when they are exposed on Saturday morning TV to six eating episodes within an hour showing thin models who show no effect of overeating. The same is true for adults who on a Sunday afternoon are exposed, as they watch an athletic event, to six episodes per hour of drinking and eating by types who show no effects of such behavior.

We are living in an energy-abundant environment. At this time, it is also an environment that promotes obesity in many of the signals that it emits. The objective of public health measures should be to change it into an environment that does not promote but rather discourages behaviors that lead to greater risk of obesity and other chronic diseases.

IV. SUGAR VERSUS FAT

A calorie is a calorie is a calorie. So it shouldn't make any difference how the calories are removed from the diet, whether as sugar or as fat. Caloric intake can be reduced when calories provided by caloric sweeteners are eliminated by substituting with artificial sweeteners or sugar substitutes. And many new sugar substitutes are becoming available, thereby making it easier for the food manufacturer and the consumer to find the best combination. One should not forget that the original rationale for artificially sweetened foods was to help diabetics comply with their dietary restrictions. In real life, many fatty foods are also sweet. Hence reduction in sugar content could be beneficial, although according to Pi-Sunyer "It is not possible at this time to indict sugar as the cause of increased overweight in the United States."

But several authors point out the advantages of removing the calories primarily as fat. There is no evidence that replacement is nutrient-specific. Fat removed from the diet may not necessarily be replaced with fat; it just as well could be carbohydrate, hence providing a net loss in calories even if the food removed is replaced weight for weight with other food.

Moreover, there seems to be less physiological control over excess consumption of fat compared with carbohydrate. If more carbohydrate is eaten one day, the chances are that less will be eaten the next day. That is not true for fat. Hence, there would be special advantage to reducing dietary fat as compared with general reduction in caloric intake.

Counting calories is difficult. Counting fat may be equally difficult, although that is exactly what the women in the experiment reported by Henderson et al. (Chapter 24) did. But it is easy to categorize foods as high, low, or medium in fat content as defined by percentage of calories contributed by fat. This information is often on the label or can be easily calculated. A strategy for losing weight or of maintaining a normal weight would be to eat fewer high-fat foods and more low-fat foods so that the percentage of calories as fat would be less than 30%. It may be that if the fat intake is controlled, so will be the caloric intake without further particular effort [4].

White bread, rolls, and crackers provide almost 10% of the calories consumed. High-fiber, reduced-calorie (mostly reduced-fat) bakery products have been marketed since the mid-1970s, and the number is increasing.

The dairy industry, a major contributor of dietary fat, has made great strides in providing low-fat alternatives. Considerable research effort is underway to find ways to reduce fat further in products such as cheese and frozen desserts.

The meat industry is also a major contributor of dietary fat. It seeks to retain its markets by reducing the fat content of its products. Gains have been made in this regard, and considerable effort is underway to lower fat content further. The gains already made make it possible to include some meat and poultry products in health-oriented diets.

Food scientists are showing considerable talent in developing ways of "fooling the tongue." Ways are being developed to provide fat mimics to replace fat so that foods with less or no fat will be accepted equally or almost as equally as the original fatty foods. And fatlike materials are being synthesized that have the physical and organoleptic properties of natural lipids, yet are not digested.

These activities portend a revolution in the kinds of foods that will be eaten in the twenty-first century. It puts a burden on regulators and health professionals to ensure that the departure from the "norm" does not bring with it unexpected dietary imbalances and new health problems.

Low-fat diets are not recommended for all, particularly children and pregnant and nursing women. There is a danger of insufficient dietary energy to support the synthesis of new tissue and the additional requirements of nursing. There is also the danger that visible fat will be reduced preferentially, thereby reducing the level of dietary polyunsaturated fatty acids.

V. CONSIDERATIONS FOR THE FUTURE

First, there is no quick technological fix to the problem of obesity. Obesity is a chronic disease and can only be contained when treated as such. In an environment of overabundance of food, despite the availability of many choices, natural or commercially produced, for lowering fat and caloric intake, the action is with the individual. The individual must decide to exercise restraint. The individual must decide to increase energy output. The individual must decide on a strategy. As Rozin (Chapter 26) puts it: "to focus on a very few significant changes in the diet; to create a compromise between pleasure and health; and to implement these changes." Then the availability of low-calorie options helps compliance with the strategy.

From the public health viewpoint, the idea is to increase the proportion of the population that is health-conscious and to make it easier to select health-oriented foods. This means, in part, that health professionals should be prepared not only to provide information but also to help the public take advantage of the information.

The second most important point is the need for more emphasis on fat intake. This is happening, albeit slowly. With more education and with the increased availability of attractive low-fat foods, this can happen faster. The fact that lower dietary fat (especially lower saturated fat) is considered important for lowering risk to heart disease provides an added incentive to reduce total fat intake. And Americans have learned to reduce risk factors for this disease, in part by changing their diet [5].

The third point is to give special emphasis to reaching the poor [6]. Health education for the poor is far less effective than for the middle class and the rich. Many of the new foods are not available in inner city stores. Many of the new foods are more expensive than the old. And strategies on how to take best advantage of available choices, natural and processed, are not clearly spelled out. Instead, there is confusion about goals of dieting and about the role of foods.

VI. SCIENCE AS AN ENGINE FOR CHANGE

Science is an engine for change. Low-calorie and low-fat foods are products of food science and technology. We can try to assess the public health effects of the present state of the development, as we did in this volume. But aside from that, we must recognize that we are describing a revolution in food science and technology generated by the public's desire for more healthful foods that look and taste much like the foods to which they have been accustomed. This takes on the properties of a self-propelling phenomenon. These technical achievements have the broad potential to change eating habits much as the invention of bread and pasta did in their time. Who can tell where this will end and how food science as an engine for change will itself influence the food culture that created it.

But this burst of technological activity exposes the grim paradox of two worlds coexisting on this planet. In one, technology is utilized to remove excess calories and fat for the sake of better health, yet to provide pleasant eating; in the other, despite available technology, food supply is insufficient; famine, hunger, and malnutrition secondary to nutrient deficiency are commonplace. This is taking place on a planet constantly shrinking in its ability to provide for its inhabitants, and on a cozier planet, made so by advances in communication technology, so that anyone from one world can look into the kitchen of the other.

REFERENCES

1. M. Shah, P. J. Hannan, and R. W. Jeffery, Secular trend in body mass index in the adult population of three communities from the upper-midwestern part of the USA: the Minnesota Heart Health Program, *Int. J. Obesity, 15*: 499 (1991).
2. W. Willett and F. M. Sacks, Chewing the fat: How much and what kind, *N. Engl. J. Med., 324*: 121 (1991).
3. J. J. Putnam, Food consumption, prices, and expenditures, 1967-1988, *Statistical Bulletin No. 804*, U.S. Department of Agriculture, Economic Research Service, Washington, DC (1990).

4. L. Sheppard, A. R. Kristal, and L. H. Kushi, Weight loss in women participating in a randomized trial of low-fat diets, *Am. J. Clin. Nutr., 54*: 821 (1991).
5. A. Leaf and T. J. Ryan, Prevention of coronary heart disease: A medical imperative, *N. Engl. J. Med., 323*: 1416 (1990).
6. R. W. Jeffery, Population perspectives in the prevention and treatment of obesity in minority populations, *Am. J. Clin. Nutr., 53*: 1621S (1991).

Index